MGH Cardiology Board Review

MGH Cardiology
Board Review

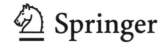 Springer

Editors

Hanna K. Gaggin
Cardiology Division
Department of Medicine Massachusetts
General Hospital
Boston
Massachusetts
USA

James L. Januzzi, Jr.
Cardiology Division
Department of Medicine
Massachusetts General Hospital
Boston
Massachusetts
USA

ISBN 978-1-4471-4482-3   ISBN 978-1-4471-4483-0   (eBook)
DOI 10.1007/978-1-4471-4483-0
Springer London Heidelberg New York Dordrecht

Library of Congress Control Number: 2013939842

Printed on acid-free paper

Springer is part of Springer Science+Business Media (www.springer.com)

Foreword

When I was asked to write a foreword for this remarkable cardiology board review book, I could not help but hark back to the time when I finished my cardiology training half a century ago. Our knowledge base and our ability to treat patients with cardiovascular diseases were so limited then. Our board exams consisted of a written part with only multiple choice questions and a clinical exam in which we worked up and—with considerable trepidation—presented patients to some of the most distinguished clinicians in American cardiology. Computers and high tech were still years away. The avalanche of amazing advances in the diagnosis and treatment of heart disease was just beginning.

Fast forward to today. Current cardiology board examinations are administered using a computer terminal with complex multiple choice questions, often accompanied by high resolution images of not only electrocardiograms and x-rays that were the mainstays of diagnosis 50 years ago, but also dynamic images of coronary arteriograms, echocardiograms and other techniques currently used in the diagnosis of cardiovascular diseases. Therapy has also become ever more complex—from pharmacology to interventions to medical devices to guidelines.

The increased emphasis on board examinations for initial certification coupled with the need for periodic recertification poses a big challenge for the test-taker, given the incredible breadth of knowledge that is now required to pass the board examinations. Compounding the problem is the further subspecialization within the specialty of cardiovascular diseases itself. Indeed, while in the course of a busy day, a cardiologist may encounter a broad range of important problems represented on the examination, there are many topics in cardiology which he or she may not frequently face. As examples, the general cardiologist may not easily decipher the intracardiac electrograms that are second nature to the electrophysiologist. Pediatric cardiologists adept in complex congenital heart disease (a topic that instills fear in the hearts of many board-takers) may not have much experience in the management of acute coronary syndromes. Yet wherever one finds his or her niche in cardiology there is a level of knowledge encompassing the whole breadth of cardiovascular diseases that one is expected to possess. That is what the board examinations are all about.

Getting ready for the board examinations requires the diligent use of available board preparation resources. It is in this context that I am so enthusiastic about the publication of the Massachusetts General Hospital (MGH) Cardiology Board Review Book by Drs. Gaggin and Januzzi, Jr. of our Division of Cardiology. Representing contributions by a broad array of the best and brightest from our Division, this comprehensive review book has a concise, easy-to-read, visually appealing layout that will assist both those who are taking the boards initially as well as those seeking recertification after many years of practice. The authors and editors are careful not to overwhelm the reader with irrelevant information so commonly found in board review books, some of which are as long as a standard cardiology textbook. Indeed the contents of this book are designed to contain the most important, most pertinent and most often tested topics in each subject—essentially, what the authors and editors believe the reader needs to know in order to pass the board examinations. Furthermore, the inclusion of a multi-media format—easily accessed from the publisher's website—that displays video loops of coronary arteriograms, ventriculograms and echocardiograms corresponding to still images in the textbook simulate the actual experience of taking the boards, and adds an extra dimension that is lacking from most board review books. And importantly, the added value of multiple choice questions designed by people who recently sat for the exams further enhances the value of this book for board takers.

It gives me great pride to see the name of the MGH Cardiac Division on this book. Since the Division was founded by Dr. Paul Dudley White in 1917, the MGH has enjoyed a rich tradition of excellence in the practice and the teaching of clinical cardiology. Dr. White's single-authored textbook—*Heart Disease*—first published in 1931 was the definitive reference text in cardiology for many years. Subsequently the MGH Cardiac Division published a highly acclaimed textbook—*The Practice of Cardiology*. Numerous members of the MGH Cardiac Division have either published or contributed to textbooks in cardiovascular diseases. This Board Review Book edited by Drs. Gaggin and Januzzi, Jr. is an important new educational resource, and adds further luster to the long tradition of the MGH for excellence in clinical teaching.

Roman W. DeSanctis, M.D.
James and Evelyn Jenks,
Professor of Medicine, Harvard Medical School
Physician and Director of Clinical Cardiology Emeritus,
Massachusetts General Hospital,
Boston, MA, USA

Preface

It has been quite a journey—from the inception of this book's concept while a fellow at the University of Pittsburgh Medical Center 5 years ago to working with the fearless authors at Mass General who took on this challenge, and now the submission of the completed book.

All I can think of are the people who made this possible. Dr. James Januzzi, Jr. my super mentor and co-editor, and Dr. G. William Dec, for bringing me into Mass General and supporting my ambitious concept with all their resources. All the authors of this book who worked tirelessly, sometimes edits after edits, to make it of quality and of substance. It was my pleasure to have gotten to know them and their dedication to education through this book. Drs. Doug Drachman, Eric Isselbacher, Randy Zusman, Igor Palacios, Ik-Kyung Jang, Quynh Truong, Rory Weiner and Aaron Baggish for their advice and for being the first brave ones to sign up for the book.

I can't thank enough Drs. Barry London and Mike Mathier from UPMC who entrusted me with the Board Review Conference. Dr. John Gorcsan for opening my eyes to the art of research and presentation whose teachings on organization of material for learning I have used again and again. Drs. Fred Crock, Mark Schmidhofer, Prem Soman, Jenifer Lee, Bill Katz and the great late Jim Shaver for always being available. Too numerous to name, all the fellows and faculty members at the University of Pittsburgh Medical Center who contributed to the Board Review Conference.

Everything I learned, I learned from Drs. Robert Vorona and J. Catesby Ware at the Eastern Virginia Medical School. I always strive to emulate their work ethic, character and compassion.

On a personal note, I have to credit my mom, Hee Jung Kim, for making sure that I pursue what I love and for being the wisest, strongest woman I know. My sisters, Han Holmberg and Dr. Amy Pollak for always giving me the brutal truth. My very special angels, Ruth and Jim Clark—their sense of curiosity, adventure and philanthropy are inspirational. My best friends, Drs. Ranjith Shetty and Mattie Campbell for making sure that I appreciate life outside of work.

But above all, I would like to thank my ultimate partner-in-crime and love, Robert T. Gaggin. I didn't know such a wonderful, amazing person existed. I will work hard to make you proud.

Boston, MA, USA   Hanna K. Gaggin, MD, MPH

It is a marvelous thing to teach. An effective teacher leaves an indelible mark on the student, and can result in a profound effect on a person's career. I remember exact lessons taught to me by my first mentor and physician/teacher—my father—even before I went to medical school, while some of the most powerful bedside physical diagnosis lessons taught to me by Dr. Jack Chadbourne in medical school, Dr. Eugene Braunwald in residency, or Drs. Roman DeSanctis and Dolph Hutter during fellowship similarly remain with me years later. These powerful forces inspired me to teach—something that remains a major focus for my career. In parallel, I have also realized the importance of preparing for assessment exams such as the Cardiology Boards, thus it is in this context that I am so very proud to have worked with my colleague Dr. Hanna Gaggin together with members from the MGH Division of Cardiology to write this important textbook.

I am grateful to all my colleagues that supported this effort—there is nothing more satisfying than coming to work every day surrounded by a group of peers that inspire me to work harder, learn more, and help patients on a daily basis. I would also like to recognize my Chief of Cardiology, Dr. G. William Dec, who enthusiastically supported this textbook. In addition, it goes without saying that I would like to thank my mentor, Dr. Roman W. DeSanctis, from whom I learned more clinical cardiology than most textbooks could ever teach.

Finally, to my daughters Caterina and Julianne, and especially my wife Roberta: thank you for endlessly supporting my dreams and my efforts—without you and your love and support, I would never be able to do what I do.

Boston, MA, USA   James L. Januzzi, Jr., MD, FACC, FESC

How to Ace the Boards

The cardiovascular board exam is expensive, often stressful and time-consuming. A well thought out preparation is especially important as you want to pass it the first time you take it! This is also a great opportunity to consolidate your experience and knowledge, brush up on rare disorders, while familiarizing yourself with the latest clinical practice guidelines. In this book, we have pooled the talents, expertise and teaching experience of the best and brightest at Mass General to help you do all of the above.

This book is not meant to be all-inclusive—there are several excellent text books for that—but rather, it is meant to be a primer for the highlights of the cardiology topics (including board-style questions, electrocardiograms [ECG] and imaging studies) covered in the Cardiovascular Disease Board exam for the busy clinicians and fellows. The inspiration for this book came from the board review course run by Dr. Gaggin while at the University of Pittsburgh Medical Center and the feedback from the fellows and faculty members who recently took the exam. Dr. Januzzi, Jr. is a frequent faculty member of board review courses and multiple clinical practice guideline committees, and has won many teaching awards for his role in the education of fellows and residents at Mass General. Importantly, Dr. Gaggin herself recently sat for the initial board exam in cardiology, while Dr. Januzzi, Jr. recently re-certified. Here are our thoughts on how to ace the boards.

1. Basic exam information
2. What's new in 2012–2013
3. Exam tips
4. The Plan when you have a year before your certification
5. The Plan when you have a month before your certification
6. When you are re-certifying—the basics.
7. The Plan for your maintenance of certification.

BASIC EXAMINATION INFORMATION

■ You **MUST** visit the official American Board of Internal Medicine (ABIM) website first and **obtain exact dates and requirements as they often change**: (*http://www.abim.org*), *get information by specialty, Cardiovascular Disease*

■ Key dates, *initial certification*

- Register early—as soon as registration opens up (typically March 1)—in order to get your first choice in testing center.

  ■ Registration deadline: typically May 1.

- The examination is at the end of October/early November after completing clinical cardiology fellowship.
- If you must cancel, make sure to do it within the designated time (typically September 1).

■ **Key dates**, *re-certification*

- Beginning in the sixth year of your certification you can schedule a seat for the exam.
- Importantly, you must be enrolled in the Maintenance of Certification (MOC) at least 2 weeks prior to the seat scheduling deadline.
- Exams are offered twice a year, typically in the Spring and Fall.
- Exams are offered at Pearson VUE Test Centers; you must register online in order to reserve a spot for the test.
- If you must cancel, you typically have until 11:59 PM EST 3 days prior to the exam.

NEW IN 2012–2013

■ The exam format and content has been changed in the multiple choice, ECG and Imaging Studies section.

- The multiple choice questions section now contains audio-based questions with heart sounds.
- The Imaging Studies section now only contains echocardiograms and angiograms.
- Ventriculograms and aortograms are covered under the multiple choice questions section.
- The answer options list has been updated and will look different also.

EXAM TIPS

A. **The test**
   ■ **Initial certification format**: typically 50 questions per one 2-h session (there are four 2-h sessions total). 2.4 min/question. Time yourself. In addition, you must pass both the ECG/Imaging section and the multiple choice question sections in order to pass the board exam.
   ■ **Maintenance of certification format**: similar to the initial certification format, but there is no separate ECG or imaging section—these are included in the flow of the exam.
   ■ In the multiple choice questions section, you don't get penalized for guessing, so do not leave any questions unanswered!
   ■ A recent test composition was as follows:

MEDICAL CONTENT CATEGORY	%
Arrhythmias	13.0
Coronary artery disease	12.5
Acute coronary syndrome	12.0
Valvular heart disease	12.0
Congenital heart disease	5.0
Pericardial disease	4.0
Aortic/peripheral arterial diseases	9.0
Hypertension/pulmonary diseases	7.0
Pharmacology	5.0
Heart failure	13.0
Physiology/biochemistry	6.0
Miscellaneous	1.5

- Know where your weaknesses are, and expect there will be questions in that area. There is nothing more satisfying than getting lots of questions in a prior area of weakness that you prepared well in!

- While there are no guarantees, there are certain things you can well-expect on the examination:

  - You must know the latest American College of Cardiology (ACC)/American Heart Association (AHA) Clinical Practice Guideline recommendations.

    - There is <u>heavy</u> emphasis on Class I recommendations (what to do) and Class III recommendations (what not to do). If there is controversy about a topic, it will not be tested.

  - Good, old fashioned clinical evaluation is emphasized on the exam: know your history and physical (see Chap. 1 of this text), and know how the findings on history and physical tie in to management.

- Don't be discouraged by questions that seem out of nowhere. About 10 % of the questions are new questions that are being explored for use and do not count toward your score.

B. **Some thoughts about multiple choice questions:**
  - Get used to board-style exam questions, they are long-winded, and often have an extended "stem" that can mis-lead you from the real reason for the question.

    - More than 75 % of questions are based on patient presentations, with the majority requiring integrating numerous aspects of the data presented—but not all of it!

      - Our advice is to read the question and the answers list first, then circle back to read the long description of the situation.

C. **ECG section (for those taking the initial exam)**
  - We cannot emphasize how important it is to **KNOW THE ANSWER OPTIONS LIST BY HEART** that the ABIM provides on its website.

    - Download the *Tutorial* and the *Answer Key*. **PAY SPECIAL ATTENTION TO THE *ANSWERS* AND THE *SCORING OF SAMPLE CASES*** as they provide priceless insight into the way ABIM will score your ECG's.
    - **Know the answer options list by heart** (how many times can we say this?), so you can rapidly find the diagnoses you seek

  - **Format**: typically 37 ECG's in one 2-h session. 3.2 min/ECG. Time yourself.
  - Most people fail the board exam because they failed the ECG section. **The most frequent comment was that they ran out of time, usually because they wasted too much time looking for the location of the answer in the answer options list.**
  - **You DO get penalized for overcoding** or guessing in this section, so code only what you need.

D. **Imaging studies section**
  - Similar to the ECG section. Know the Answer options list.
  - **Format**: typically 39 cases in one 2 h and 15 min session. 3.5 min/case. Time yourself.
  - **You DO get penalized for overcoding** or guessing in this section, so code only what you need.

E. **Audio-based heart sounds**
  - Practice, practice, practice.
  - **Know your maneuvers** to differentiate between heart murmurs (see Chap. 1 of this text)

WHAT TO STUDY WHEN YOU HAVE A YEAR: A CHECK LIST FOR INITIAL TEST-TAKERS

■ Study materials

- *MGH Cardiology Board Review book*
- *ACCSAP* (comprehensive but lengthy. Great if you have the time.)
- Braunwald's Heart Disease, a textbook of cardiovascular medicine (A great text book, pay special attention to the sections on ACC/AHA guidelines)
- Michael J. Barrett's Heart Songs audio (Basic, Intermediate and Complex) available through Cardiosource

■ Multiple choice questions: we are big believers in the importance of getting into the swing of test taking, so practice tests are crucially important.

- *Questions and Answers sections from the MGH Cardiology Board Review book*
- *ACCSAP* (Essential for the well-written, accurate practice exam questions. Very similar to the actual ABIM question format)

■ ECG

- Chapter 36 of the *MGH Cardiology Board Review Book*
- *The Complete Guide to ECG's* by James O'Keefe, et al (basic foundation)
- *ECGSAP* (its scoring system gives you an insight to the way ABIM will score, especially for penalties for overcoding, but the system is a little different from ABIM)
- ABIM Answer Options List
- *Podrid's Real World ECGs* by Philip Podrid et al

■ Imaging Studies section

- Multimedia website and Chap. 35 of the *MGH Cardiology Board Review Book* that includes almost all the diagnosis from the ABIM Answer Options list.
- Still images from the *Mayo Clinic Cardiology: Concise Textbook* (The book itself is great, but it is NOT concise: the 3rd edition is 1584 pages long)
- ABIM Answer Options List

■ Consider attending the Mayo Cardiovascular Review Course

- A week-long intensive course in late September/early October, Rochester, MN (expensive and time-consuming, but it's worth it. Extremely well organized and taught)

WHAT TO STUDY WHEN YOU HAVE A MONTH: A CHECK LIST FOR INITIAL TEST TAKERS

■ *MGH Cardiology Board Review book and its multimedia website for the moving images for the imaging section as well as practice questions*
■ *The Complete Guide to ECG's* by James O'Keefe
■ *ACCSAP* practice examination questions and answers
■ Consider Mayo Cardiovascular Review Course
■ Michael J. Barrett's Heart Songs audio (Basic, Intermediate and Complex) available through Cardiosource

WHEN YOU ARE RE-CERTIFYING

■ Subspecialists certified in 1990 or later must complete the Maintenance of Certification (MOC) program, which includes 100 MOC points of self-evaluation plus the examination.

■ The enrollment fee includes one secure examination and access to an unlimited number of self-evaluation products.

THE PLAN FOR YOUR MOC

■ Begin your MOC early. You must complete the 100 points by the time you sit for the exam. You acquire these points by completing self-evaluations from two categories:

- Self-Evaluation of Medical Knowledge: open-book modules that test clinical practical knowledge.
- Self-Evaluation of Practice Performance: modules that focus on practice improvement, which may include the American Board of Internal Medicine Practice Improvement Modules.
- You **must** start your MOC early! These modules take time, so do not wait until the last minute to start the modules—in the midst of a busy career, you do not want to have to cram the MOC modules plus prepare for the examination!

■ Study materials

- *MGH Cardiology Board Review Book and its multimedia website for moving images and practice questions*
  ACCSAP
- Consider the Mayo Cardiovascular Review Course

■ As above, multiple choice questions are crucially important to get into the swing of things!

> That's it—happy studying, and we wish you all the best!

Boston, MA, USA   Hanna K. Gaggin, MD, MPH
Boston, MA, USA   James L. Januzzi, Jr., MD

Contents

Contributors

FARHAD ABTAHIAN, MD
Clinical and Research Fellow, Harvard Medical School
Cardiology Division, Department of Medicine, Massachusetts General Hospital,
Boston, MA, USA

IMAD AHMADO, MD
Clinical and Research Fellow, Harvard Medical School
Cardiology Division, Department of Medicine, Massachusetts General Hospital,
Boston, MA, USA

KARIM M. AWAD, MD
Clinical and Research Fellow, Harvard Medical School
Department of Medicine, Brigham and Women's Hospital, Boston, MA, USA

AARON L. BAGGISH, MD
Assistant Professor of Medicine, Harvard Medical School
Associate Director, Cardiovascular Performance Program, Cardiology Division,
Department of Medicine, Massachusetts General Hospital, Boston, MA, USA

CONOR D. BARRETT, MB BCh
Instructor in Medicine, Harvard Medical School
Cardiac Arrhythmia Service, Cardiology Division, Department of Medicine,
Massachusetts General Hospital, Boston, MA, USA

AMI B. BHATT, MD
Instructor in Medicine and Pediatrics, Harvard Medical School
Director, Adult Congenital Heart Disease Program, Cardiology Division,
Department of Medicine, Massachusetts General Hospital, Boston, MA, USA

RON BLANKSTEIN, MD
Assistant Professor of Medicine and Radiology, Harvard Medical School
Cardiovascular Medicine, Department of Medicine and Radiology,
Brigham and Women's Hospital, Boston, MA, USA

ANNE M. BORDEN, RN MPH
Cardiology Division, Department of Medicine, Massachusetts General Hospital,
Boston, MA, USA

JONATHAN CLARKE, MD
Clinical and Research Fellow, Harvard Medical School
Cardiology Division, Department of Medicine, Massachusetts General Hospital,
Boston, MA, USA

STEPHAN B. DANIK, MD
Instructor in Medicine, Harvard Medical School
Director, Experimental Electrophysiology Laboratory, Cardiac Arrhythmia Service,
Cardiology Division, Department of Medicine, Massachusetts General Hospital,
Boston, MA, USA

DOUGLAS E. DRACHMAN, MD
Assistant Professor of Medicine, Harvard Medical School
Director, Cardiology Fellowship Program, Associate Director, Interventional Cardiology
Fellowship Program, Cardiology Division, Department of Medicine,
Massachusetts General Hospital, Boston, MA, USA

DAVID M. DUDZINSKI, MD, JD
Clinical and Research Fellow, Harvard Medical School
Cardiology Division, Department of Medicine, Massachusetts General Hospital,
Boston, MA, USA

BRIAN L. EDLOW, MD
Clinical and Research Fellow, Harvard Medical School
Department of Neurology, Massachusetts General Hospital, Boston, MA, USA

SAMMY ELMARIAH, MD, MPH
Instructor in Medicine, Harvard Medical School
Interventional Cardiology, Cardiology Division, Department of Medicine,
Massachusetts General Hospital, Boston, MA, USA

AIDAN W. FLYNN, MD, PhD
Clinical and Research Fellow, Harvard Medical School
Cardiology Division, Department of Medicine, Massachusetts General Hospital,
Boston, MA, USA

HANNA K. GAGGIN, MD, MPH
Instructor in Medicine, Harvard Medical School
Cardiology Division, Department of Medicine, Massachusetts General Hospital,
Boston, MA, USA

RAJESH TIM GANDHI, MD
Associate Professor of Medicine, Harvard Medical School
Division of Infectious Diseases, Department of Medicine,
Massachusetts General Hospital, Boston, MA, USA

Ragon Institute of MGH, MIT and Harvard, Cambridge, MA, USA

JOSEPH M. GARASIC, MD
Assistant Professor of Medicine, Harvard Medical School
Director, Peripheral Vascular Intervention, Cardiology Division,
Department of Medicine, Massachusetts General Hospital, Boston, MA, USA

HENRY GEWIRTZ, MD
Associate Professor of Medicine, Harvard Medical School
Director, Nuclear Cardiology, Cardiology Division, Department of Medicine,
Massachusetts General Hospital, Boston, MA, USA

LAUREN G. GILSTRAP, MD
Resident in Medicine, Harvard Medical School
Department of Medicine, Massachusetts General Hospital, Boston, MA, USA

JAY S. GIRI, MD, MPH
Assistant Professor of Medicine, Perelman School of Medicine at the
University of Pennsylvania
Director, Peripheral Intervention, Cardiology Division, Hospital of the University of
Pennsylvania, Philadelphia, PA, USA

SHAWN A. GREGORY, MD
Assistant Professor of Medicine, Harvard Medical School
Cardiology Division, Department of Medicine, Massachusetts General Hospital,
Boston, MA, USA

DAVID M. GREER, MD, MA
Zimmerman and Spinelli Professor of Neurology and Neurosurgery,
Yale University School of Medicine
Vice Chairman, Department of Neurology, Director,
Neurology Residency Program, Director Neurosciences Intensive Care Unit,
Department of Neurology, Yale-New Haven Hospital,
New Haven, CT, USA

BRIAN C. HEALY, PhD
Assistant Professor of Neurology, Harvard Medical School
Instructor in Biostatistics, Harvard School of Public Health
Biostatistics Center, Department of Neurology, Massachusetts General Hospital,
Boston, MA, USA

JASON HOMSY, MD, PhD
Clinical and Research Fellow, Harvard Medical School
Cardiology Division, Department of Medicine, Massachusetts General Hospital,
Boston, MA, USA

PAUL L. HUANG, MD, PhD
Professor of Medicine, Harvard Medical School
Director, MGH Cardiology Metabolic Syndrome Program, Cardiology Division,
Department of Medicine, Massachusetts General Hospital,
Boston, MA, USA

JUDY W. HUNG, MD
Associate Professor of Medicine, Harvard Medical School
Associate Director, Echocardiography, Cardiology Division,
Department of Medicine, Massachusetts General Hospital,
Boston, MA, USA

ROCIO M. HURTADO, MD DTM&H
Instructor in Medicine, Harvard Medical School
Division of Infectious Diseases, Department of Medicine,
Massachusetts General Hospital, Boston, MA, USA

EMILY P. HYLE, MD
Instructor in Medicine, Harvard Medical School
Division of Infectious Diseases, Department of Medicine,
Massachusetts General Hospital, Boston, MA, USA

ERIC M. ISSELBACHER, MD
Associate Professor of Medicine, Harvard Medical School
Associate Director, MGH Heart Center
Co-Director, MGH Thoracic Aortic Center
Cardiology Division, Department of Medicine,
Massachusetts General Hospital, Boston, MA, USA

FAROUC A. JAFFER, MD, PhD
Associate Professor of Medicine, Harvard Medical School
Interventional Cardiology, Cardiology Division, Department of Medicine,
Massachusetts General Hospital, Boston, MA, USA

IK-KYUNG JANG, MD, PhD
Professor of Medicine, Harvard Medical School
Director, Cardiology Laboratory for Integrative Physiology and Imaging:
CLIPI, Interventional Cardiology, Cardiology Division,
Department of Medicine, Massachusetts General Hospital,
Boston, MA, USA

JAMES L. JANUZZI, JR., MD
Associated Professor, Harvard Medical School
Roman W. Desanctis Endowed Distinguished Clinical Scholar, Director,
Cardiac Intensive Care Unit, Cardiology Division, Department of Medicine,
Massachusetts General Hospital, Boston, MA, USA

WILLIAM J. KOSTIS, PhD, MD
Clinical and Research Fellow, Harvard Medical School
Cardiology Division, Department of Medicine, Massachusetts General Hospital,
Boston, MA, USA

RODRIGO M. LAGO, MD
Clinical and Research Fellow, Harvard Medical School
Cardiology Division, Department of Medicine, Massachusetts General Hospital,
Boston, MA, USA

THOMAS A. LAMATTINA, MD
Clinical Instructor in Medicine, Harvard Medical School
Interventional Cardiology, Cardiology Division, Department of Medicine,
Massachusetts General Hospital, Boston, MA, USA

GREGORY D. LEWIS, MD
Assistant Professor of Medicine, Harvard Medical School
Director, Mass General Cardiopulmonary Exercise Laboratory,
Cardiology Division, Department of Medicine,
Massachusetts General Hospital, Boston, MA, USA

RICHARD R. LIBERTHSON, MD
Associate Professor in Pediatrics, Harvard Medical School
Director, Adult Congenital Heart Disease Program, Cardiology Division,
Department of Medicine and Pediatrics, Massachusetts General Hospital,
Boston, MA, USA

STEVEN A. LUBITZ, MD, MPH
Instructor in Medicine, Harvard Medical School
Cardiac Arrhythmia Service, Cardiology Division, Department of Medicine,
Massachusetts General Hospital, Boston, MA, USA

ANDREAS C. MAUER, MD
Clinical and Research Fellow, Harvard Medical School
Cardiology Division, Department of Medicine, Massachusetts General Hospital,
Boston, MA, USA

PRAVEEN MEHROTRA, MD
Clinical and Research Fellow, Harvard Medical School
Cardiology Division, Department of Medicine, Massachusetts General Hospital,
Boston, MA, USA

ELI M. MILOSLAVSKY, MD
Clinical and Research Fellow, Harvard Medical School
Division of Rheumatology, Department of Medicine,
Massachusetts General Hospital, Boston, MA, USA

SHRIRAM NALLAMSHETTY, MD
Clinical Instructor, Harvard Medical School
Cardiology Division, Department of Medicine, Massachusetts General Hospital,
Boston, MA, USA

PRADEEP NATARAJAN, MD
Clinical and Research Fellow, Harvard Medical School
Cardiology Division, Department of Medicine, Massachusetts General Hospital,
Boston, MA, USA

OYERE K. ONUMA, MD
Clinical and Research Fellow, Harvard Medical School
Cardiology Division, Department of Medicine, Massachusetts General Hospital,
Boston, MA, USA

IGOR F. PALACIOS, MD
Associate Professor of Medicine, Harvard Medical School
Director, Knight Catheterization Laboratory, Director, Interventional Cardiology,
Cardiology Division, Department of Medicine, Massachusetts General Hospital,
Boston, MA, USA

J. CARL PALLAIS, MD, MPH
Assistant Professor of Medicine, Harvard Medical School
Division of Endocrinology, Department of Medicine, Massachusetts General Hospital,
Boston, MA, USA

MARCELLO PANAGIA, MD, D.PHIL
Clinical and Research Fellow, Harvard Medical School
Cardiology Division, Department of Medicine, Massachusetts General Hospital,
Boston, MA, USA

KIMBERLY A. PARKS, DO
Instructor in Medicine, Harvard Medical School
Advanced Heart Failure and Cardiac Transplantation, Cardiology Division,
Department of Medicine, Massachusetts General Hospital, Boston, MA, USA

JORGE PLUTZKY, MD
Associate Professor of Medicine, Harvard Medical School
Director, Vascular Disease Prevention Program, Cardiovascular Medicine,
Department of Medicine, Brigham and Women's Hospital, Boston, MA, USA

PHILIP J. PODRID, MD
Professor of Medicine and Professor of Pharmacology and Experimental
Therapeutics, Boston University School of Medicine
Lecturer in Medicine, Harvard Medical School, Boston, MA, USA

Associate Chief of Cardiology, Department of Medicine,
VA Boston Healthcare System, West Roxbury Division, West Roxbury,
MA, USA

JEREMY N. RUSKIN, MD
Associate Professor of Medicine, Harvard Medical School
Director, Cardiac Arrhythmia Service, Cardiology Division, Department of Medicine,
Massachusetts General Hospital, Boston, MA, USA

MARC S. SABATINE, MD, MPH
Associate Professor of Medicine, Harvard Medical School
Chairman, TIMI Study Group, Cardiology Division, Departments of Medicine,
Massachusetts General Hospital and Brigham & Women's Hospital, Boston, MA, USA

GABRIEL SAYER, MD
Clinical and Research Fellow, Harvard Medical School
Cardiology Division, Department of Medicine, Massachusetts General Hospital,
Boston, MA, USA

MARC J. SEMIGRAN, MD
Associate Professor of Medicine, Harvard Medical School
Medical Director of the Heart Failure and Cardiac Transplant Program,
Cardiology Division, Department of Medicine, Massachusetts General Hospital,
Boston, MA, USA

RAVI V. SHAH, MD
Clinical and Research Fellow, Harvard Medical School
Cardiology Division, Department of Medicine, Massachusetts General Hospital,
Boston, MA, USA

EMILY J. KARWACKI SHEFF, MS, RN, CMSRN, FNP, BC
School of Nursing, Massachusetts General Hospital Institute of Health Professions,
Boston, MA, USA

JAGMEET P. SINGH, MD, DPHIL
Associate Professor, Harvard Medical School
Cardiac Arrhythmia Service, Cardiology Division, Department of Medicine,
Massachusetts General Hospital, Boston, MA, USA

JOHN H. STONE, MD, MPH
Professor of Medicine, Harvard Medical School
Director, Clinical Rheumatology, Division of Rheumatology,
Allergy and Immunology, Department of Medicine,
Massachusetts General Hospital, Boston, MA, USA

JACKIE SZYMONIFKA, MA
Department of Biostatistics, Massachusetts General Hospital, Boston, MA, USA

TIMOTHY C. TAN, MBBS, PhD
Clinical and Research Fellow, Harvard Medical School
Cardiology Division, Department of Medicine, Massachusetts General Hospital,
Boston, MA, USA

WAI-EE THAI, MD
Research Fellow, Harvard Medical School
Cardiac MR PET CT Program, Department of Radiology,
Massachusetts General Hospital, Boston, MA, USA

QUYNH A. TRUONG, MD, MPH
Assistant Professor of Medicine, Harvard Medical School
Cardiology Division, Department of Medicine and Cardiac MR PET CT Program,
Department of Radiology, Massachusetts General Hospital, Boston, MA, USA

GAURAV A. UPADHYAY, MD
Clinical and Research Fellow, Harvard Medical School
Cardiology Division, Department of Medicine, Massachusetts General Hospital,
Boston, MA, USA

BRYAN WAI, MD
Research Fellow, Harvard Medical School
Cardiac MR PET CT Program, Department of Radiology,
Massachusetts General Hospital, Boston, MA, USA

NANCY J. WEI, MD, MMSc
Instructor in Medicine, Harvard Medical School
Division of Endocrinology, Department of Medicine,
Massachusetts General Hospital, Boston, MA, USA

RORY B. WEINER, MD
Assistant Professor of Medicine, Harvard Medical School
Cardiovascular Performance Program, Cardiology Division,
Department of Medicine, Massachusetts General Hospital, Boston, MA, USA

M. BRANDON WESTOVER, MD, PhD
Instructor in Neurology, Harvard Medical School
Department of Neurology, Massachusetts General Hospital, Boston, MA, USA

MALISSA J. WOOD, MD
Assistant Professor, Harvard Medical School
Co-director MGH Heart Center Corrigan Women's Heart Health Program,
Cardiology Division, Department of Medicine, Massachusetts General Hospital,
Boston, MA, USA

DOREEN DeFARIA YEH, MD
Instructor in Medicine, Harvard Medical School
Adult Congenital Heart Disease Program, Cardiology Division,
Department of Medicine, Massachusetts General Hospital, Boston, MA, USA

JODI L. ZILINSKI, MD
Clinical and Research Fellow, Harvard Medical School
Cardiology Division, Department of Medicine, Massachusetts General Hospital,
Boston, MA, USA

RANDALL M. ZUSMAN, MD
Associate Professor, Harvard Medical School
Director, Hypertension, Cardiology Division, Department of Medicine,
Massachusetts General Hospital, Boston, MA, USA

CHAPTER 1

Hanna K. Gaggin and Douglas E. Drachman

History and Physical Examination

CHAPTER OUTLINE

ABBREVIATIONS

ABI	Ankle/brachial index
ACS	Acute coronary syndrome
AR	Aortic regurgitation
AS	Aortic stenosis
ASD	Atrial septal defect
AV	Aortic valve
BB	Beta blocker
BNP	B-type natriuretic peptide
BP	Blood pressure
CAD	Coronary artery disease
CI	Confidence interval
CMP	Cardiomyopathy
CP	Chest pain
CXR	Chest x-ray
DCM	Dilated cardiomyopathy
DM	Diabetes mellitus
ECG	Electrocardiogram
EP	Electrophysiology
HCM	Hypertrophic cardiomyopathy
HF	Heart failure
HR	Heart rate
HTN	Hypertension
JVD	Jugular venous distension
JVP	Jugular venous pressure
LA	Left atrium
LBBB	Left bundle branch block
LLSB	Left lower sternal border
LR	Likelihood ratio
LV	Left ventricle
LVEDP	Left ventricular end diastolic pressure
LVEF	Left ventricular ejection fraction
LVH	Left ventricular hypertrophy
MI	Myocardial infarction
MR	Mitral regurgitation
MS	Mitral stenosis
MV	Mitral valve
MVP	Mitral valve prolapse
OS	Opening snap
PCWP	Pulmonary capillary wedge pressure

PDA	Patent ductus arteriosus
PH	Pulmonary hypertension
PMI	Point of maximal impulse
PND	Paroxysmal nocturnal dyspnea
PR	Pulmonic regurgitation
PS	Pulmonic stenosis
PV	Pulmonic valve
PVD	Peripheral vascular disease
RA	Right atrium
RBBB	Right bundle branch block
RV	Right ventricle
RVH	Right ventricular hypertrophy
SOB	Shortness of breath
TR	Tricuspid regurgitation
TS	Tricuspid stenosis
TV	Tricuspid valve
VSD	Ventricular septal defect

INTRODUCTION

With technological advances in laboratory testing, imaging studies, and invasive procedures in cardiology, it is easy to discount the relevance of the history and physical examination. It is precisely the astute performance of the focused history and physical examination, however, that informs appropriate and efficient diagnostic testing. In the current climate emphasizing cost-effective practice, the strategic and parsimonious use of diagnostic testing is of paramount importance. Moreover, the determination of pretest probability—based on history and physical examination findings—may enhance the accuracy and clinical interpretation of subsequent diagnostic findings. In this manner, the classic teachings of the history and physical examination, coupled with the advanced capabilities of contemporary diagnostic technology, may provide optimal insight into the care of the patient.

HISTORY

General History

General history is comprised of the following (from the patient or the family).
Chief complaint
- Common presenting symptoms for patients with suspected or known cardiovascular disease: chest pain (CP) or discomfort, shortness of breath (SOB) or dyspnea, edema, palpitations, dizziness, syncope, and fatigue or weakness.
- Asymptomatic patients with incidental findings on physical examination, electrocardiogram (ECG), chest x-ray (CXR) or other imaging modalities
- Asymptomatic patients who require pre-operative evaluation.
- Sudden cardiac death.
- Similar symptoms may stem from different underlying cardiovascular disorders and paying attention to history and examination findings will reveal clues to diagnosis.

History of the presenting illness
- Description, location, onset, radiation, precipitating factors, associated symptoms, duration, alleviating factors.
- Semi-quantitative assessment of symptom severity may enable serial evaluations for a change in clinical status.
- Recent health status, events.

Past medical history
- Known cardiac disorders
- Known vascular disorders such as peripheral vascular disease (PVD) or stroke
- Relevant risk factors for cardiovascular disease such as hypertension (HTN), hypercholesterolemia, metabolic syndrome, diabetes mellitus (DM), smoking status, obesity, exercise
- Others: sleep apnea, chest surgery or radiation, mental stress.
- Baseline functional capacity assessment is very important; a sedentary patient may never experience exertion-associated symptoms. Exercise capacity also has important prognostic implications [1]. Despite limitations, frequently used classification systems include the New York Heart Association classification, Canadian Cardiovascular Society classification and Specific Activity Scale [2].

Previous cardiovascular test results
- ECG, echocardiogram, CXR, noninvasive imaging, stress test, catheterization, electrophysiologic (EP) evaluation.

Medications
- Cardiac medications and compliance
- Relevant non-cardiac medications with implications for diagnosis and management of the cardiovascular disease, such as: phosphodiesterase inhibitors taken for erectile dysfunction; anticoagulation for venous thromboembolism; metformin in patients exposed to iodinated contrast from cardiac catheterization

Allergies
- Drug and contrast allergies and reaction should be documented.

Family history
- Premature coronary artery disease (CAD), history of hypertrophic cardiomyopathy (HCM), dilated cardiomyopathy (DCM) or sudden cardiac death.

Social history
- Cocaine and alcohol intake, smoking status, job, family or home situation.

Review of systems
- Neurologic, pulmonary, gastrointestinal, urinary, infectious, hematologic, immunologic, musculoskeletal, endocrine and psychiatric systems should be reviewed (Table 1-1).

Common Chief Complaints

Chest discomfort or pain (Table 1-2)
- **Classic angina** [3]: exertional or stress-related, substernal discomfort, resolves with rest or nitroglycerin; response to nitroglycerin in the emergency department is not predictive of cardiac etiology [4] (Table 1-3).

  - **CP equivalents**: Presenting symptoms in a retrospective study of 721 patients with acute myocardial infarction presenting to the emergency department [5]

TABLE 1-1

MAJOR CAUSES OF CHEST PAIN

Cardiac: ACS, aortic dissection, valvular heart disease, HF, myocarditis, pericarditis, variant angina, syndrome X, cocaine abuse, stress-induced cardiomyopathy

Pulmonary: PE, pleuritis/serositis, pneumonia, pneumothorax, reactive air way disease, PH and cor pulmonale, lung malignancy, sarcoidosis, pleural effusion

Gastrointestinal: GERD, esophageal spasm, esophageal tear or rupture, mediastinitis, esophagitis, peptic ulcer disease, cholecystitis, biliary colic, pancreatitis, kidney stones

Musculoskeletal: Costochondritis, spinal disease, fracture, muscle strain, herpes zoster

Psychogenic: anxiety, panic disorder, depression, hypochondriasis

ACS acute coronary syndrome, *GERD* gastroesophageal reflux disease, *HF* heart failure, *PE* pulmonary embolism, *PH* pulmonary hypertension

TABLE 1-2	CARDIAC	NON-CARDIAC
LIFE-THREATENING CAUSES OF CHEST PAIN	**Acute coronary syndrome** substernal, radiating to arm, dyspnea on exertion, diaphoresis, worse with exertion	**Acute pulmonary embolism** sudden onset, pleuritic, dyspnea, tachycardia, tachypnea, hypoxia, evidence of lower extremity deep venous thrombosis
	Aortic dissection sudden onset, severe, tearing, radiating to the back (associated with neurologic deficits, AR), unequal arm BP >20 mmHg, wide mediastinum	**Tension pneumothorax** sudden onset, sharp, pleuritic, decreased breath sounds and chest excursion, hyperresonant percussion, hypoxia
	Acute pericarditis & tamponade sudden onset, pleuritic, better with sitting forward, radiating to the back, pericardial rub, ± tamponade (distant heart sounds, hypotension, JVD)	**Esophageal rupture/perforation** severe, increase with swallowing, fever, abdominal pain, history of endoscopy, foreign body ingestion, trauma, vomiting

AR aortic regurgitation, *BP* blood pressure, *JVD* jugular venous distension

TABLE 1-3	INCREASE THE LIKELIHOOD	LR (95 % CI)	DECREASE THE LIKELIHOOD	LR (95 % CI)
CHEST PAIN CHARACTERISTIC AND LIKELIHOOD RATIO FOR ACUTE CORONARY SYNDROME [10]	Radiates to the right arm or shoulder	4.7 (1.9–12)	Pleuritic	0.2 (0.1–0.3)
	Radiates to both arms or shoulders	4.1 (2.5–6.5)	Sharp	0.3 (0.2–0.5)
	Precipitated by exertion	2.4 (1.5–3.8)	Positional	0.3 (0.2–0.5)
	Radiates to the left arm	2.3 (1.7–3.1)	Reproducible with palpation	0.3 (0.2–0.4)
	Associated with diaphoresis	2.0 (1.9–2.2)		

ACS acute coronary syndrome, *CI* confidence interval, *CP* chest pain, *LR* likelihood ratio

- Chest, left arm, jaw, or neck complaint (53 %), SOB (17 %), cardiac arrest (7 %), dizziness/weakness/syncope (4 %), abdominal complaints (2 %), miscellaneous (trauma, gastrointestinal bleeding, altered mental status, nausea/vomiting, palpitations, and other) (17 %)
- Atypical presentation is associated with an increased risk of adverse outcomes and common in women, elderly and patients with diabetes mellitus [6, 7]

- **Pericarditis:** abrupt onset, sharp, pleuritic and positional (better with sitting forward and worse with lying down), radiating to the back, recent fever or viral illness

  - Look for evidence of associated pericardial effusion (muffled or distant heart sounds) and **tamponade** (distant heart sounds, hypotension, jugular venous distension (JVD), dyspnea, tachycardia, pulsus paradoxus) [8]

    - Think constrictive pericarditis if a history of chest radiation, cardiac or mediastinal surgery, chronic tuberculosis or malignancy and right-sided heart failure (HF) symptoms/signs.
- **Aortic dissection:** Having (1) sudden, severe, tearing CP (or equivalent), maximal at onset with radiation to the back, (2) Unequal arm blood pressure (BP) >20 mmHg and (3) Wide mediastinum on CXR had a positive likelihood ratio of 66.0 (CI 4.1–1062.0) [9]

  - Look for neurologic deficits, aortic regurgitation (AR), history of HTN, bicuspid aortic valve (AV), coarctation of the aorta, Marfan's syndrome, Ehlers-Danlos syndrome, Turner syndrome, giant cell arteritis, third-trimester pregnancy, cocaine abuse, trauma, intra-aortic catheterization, history of cardiac surgery

Palpitations [11]
- Often described as flutters, heart skipping, pounding sensation
- A history of cardiac disease increases the likelihood for cardiac arrhythmia (Likelihood ratio [LR] 2.0, 95 % confidence interval [CI] [1.3–3.1])
- Palpitation associated with a regular, rapid-pounding sensation in the neck was strongly predictive in one study of atrioventricular nodal re-entry tachycardia with a LR of 177, 95 % CI (25–1,251)

Dyspnea
- Differential diagnosis includes cardiac, pulmonary, neuromuscular, obesity, deconditioning, anemia and psychiatric.
- Cardiac causes can be divided into the following

  - **Heart failure (may be due to a variety of causes including valvular disease, arrhythmia, etc.):**

    - Lack of adequate forward flow (fatigue, weakness, exercise intolerance)
    - Increased systemic venous or pulmonary pressures or congestion (dyspnea, orthopnea, paroxysmal nocturnal dyspnea [PND], abdominal discomfort from hepatic congestion or ascites, edema).
    - Acute HF tends to present with dyspnea while chronic HF tends to present with edema, fatigue, anorexia.

  - **Myocardial ischemia:** typically presents as dyspnea on exertion. Caused by acute coronary syndrome (ACS) or demand supply mismatch (left ventricular hypertrophy [LVH], HCM, valvular disease, bradycardia or tachycardia)
  - **Pericardial disease:** mainly due to increased pulmonary pressures

Claudication [12, 13]
- **Types of claudication:**

  - Classic: exertional calf pain that resolves with 10 min of rest causes the patient to stop walking.
  - Atypical: non-calf pain, does not resolve with rest, does not keep the patient from walking, rest as well as exertional leg pain (concurrent DM, neuropathy, spinal stenosis)

- **Differential diagnosis of arm or leg pain**

  PVD: claudication associated with edema and skin discoloration
  - Other arterial disease: aneurysm, dissection, injury, trauma, radiation therapy, vasculitis, ergot use, artery entrapment/kinking (cyclists)
  - Deep vein thrombosis: associated with unilateral edema, pain worse with dependency
  - Musculoskeletal disorders: arthritis
  - Peripheral neuropathy: radiation of pain, sharp pain, back pain
  - Spinal stenosis: muscular weakness, worse after standing for a long time, back pain

- In PVD, the location of the pain depends on the level of arterial narrowing (Table 1-4)
- In new outpatients patients diagnosed with PVD 47 % did not have claudication, 47 % had atypical claudication and only 6 % had classic claudication [13].
- Functional and exercise capacity determination is paramount as a patient may not have any symptoms if sedentary.

TABLE 1-4

LOCATION OF THE ARTERIAL STENOSIS AND THE PAIN

PAIN	BUTTOCK OR HIP	THIGH	UPPER 2/3 OF THE CALF	LOWER 1/3 OF THE CALF	FOOT
Location	Aortoiliac	Aortoiliac or common femoral	Superficial femoral	Popliteal	Tibial or peroneal

PHYSICAL EXAMINATION

General Examination

Vital signs

■ Any abnormality in BP, heart rate (HR), respiratory rate and oxygenation should be explored.

■ Blood pressure

– Significant difference in pulses and BP in arms: >20 mmHg in BP is associated with aortic coarctation or dissection, subclavian artery disease, supravalvular (right>left in BP) and aortic stenosis (AS)

– Significant difference in the pressure in legs compared with arms: >20 mmHg higher than arms is associated with the Hill sign in severe AR or extensive and calcified lower extremity peripheral arterial disease. A delay in pulse from radial to femoral in a patient with HTN is associated with aortic coarctation

– **Pulse pressure** is defined as systolic pressure – diastolic pressure

   ■ Wide pulse pressure is associated with AR, older age, atherosclerosis

   ■ Narrow pulse pressure is associated with HF (a pulse pressure of <25 % of the systolic pressure is associated with a cardiac index of <2.2 L/min/m^2) [14], HCM

■ **Orthostatic blood pressures:** measure BP and HR after standing for 1–3 min.

   – Orthostatic hypotension: a drop in systolic BP >20 mmHg, a drop in diastolic BP >10 mmHg or HR rise >10 bpm.

■ **Valsalva response**

   – Normal Valsalva sinusoidal response (Fig. 1-1)

   – Abnormal response pattern (in patients not taking a beta blocker [BB])

      ■ Absent overshoot response: no Phase 4 rise in systolic BP, associated with moderately decreased left ventricular ejection fraction (LVEF)

      ■ Square wave response: presence of Korotkoff sounds during the entire straining phase and no Phase 4 rise in systolic BP, associated with severely decreased LVEF

FIGURE 1-1

Normal valsalva sinusoidal response. *BP* blood pressure (Courtesy of Dr. Hanna Gaggin)

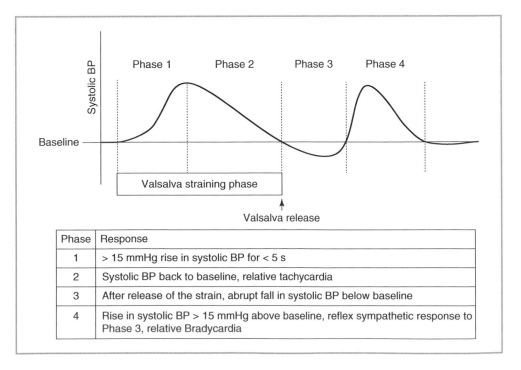

Phase	Response
1	> 15 mmHg rise in systolic BP for < 5 s
2	Systolic BP back to baseline, relative tachycardia
3	After release of the strain, abrupt fall in systolic BP below baseline
4	Rise in systolic BP > 15 mmHg above baseline, reflex sympathetic response to Phase 3, relative Bradycardia

■ **Pulsus paradoxus**

- Fall in systolic BP >12 mmHg with inspiration has a sensitivity of 98 % and specificity of 83 % for the diagnosis of pericardial tamponade [8]
- Can also be positive in hypovolemia, anything that results in right-sided failure (pulmonary embolism, chronic lung disease), constriction, HF

General appearance

■ The first assessment before any history or physical examination should be the global overview. Is the patient acutely ill? Diaphoresis, tachypnea, cyanosis, decreased mental status all signify serious conditions. The result of this assessment will determine how focused and timely the history and examination should be.

The skin

■ Identify evidence of poor perfusion such as cold and clammy skin (cardiogenic shock, HF or PVD), cyanosis (congenital heart disease or shunts), bronzing of the skin (iron overload or hemochromatosis), ecchymoses (antiplatelet or anticoagulation medication), xanthomas (hypercholesterolemia), lupus pernio, erythema nodosum or granuloma annulare (sarcoidosis).

■ Look for dialysis fistulas (end stage renal disease and in acutely ill patients, likely metabolic disarray).

■ Skin findings that increase the likelihood of PVD [15]

- Cool to touch LR 5.9 (95 % CI 4.1–8.6)
- Wounds or sores LR 5.9 (95 % CI 2.6–13.4)
- Skin discolorations LR 2.8 (95 % CI 2.4–3.3)

Head and neck

■ Elevated jugular venous pressure (HF), high arched palate (Marfan's), large protruding tongue (amyoloidosis), ptosis and ophthalmoplegia (muscular dystrophies), hypertelorism, low-set ears, micrognathia, webbed neck (Noonan, Turner and Down syndromes), proptosis, lid lag and stare (Grave's hyperthyroidism).

■ **Jugular venous pressure** (Table 1-5)

- Calculation of jugular venous pressure (JVP) in mmHg
  1. Determine vertical distance above the sternal angle to the top of the venous pulsation (in cm water)
  2. Add to above, 5 cm if incline is at 0–45° or 10 cm if incline is at 45 + ° [16]
  3. Divide by 1.36

- Normal RA pressure is <8 mmHg
- Clinical assessment of the presence of an elevated JVP (rather than exact JVP) is fairly accurate in predicting elevated right atrial (RA) pressure and the pulmonary capillary wedge pressure (PCWP)

  ■ JVP <11 cm in predicting invasively measured RA pressure <8 mmHg: negative predictive value =82 % [17]
  ■ Presence of elevated JVP at rest or hepatojugular reflux in predicting PCWP >18 mmHg: sensitivity =81 %, specificity =80 %, predictive accuracy =81 % (in the absence of cirrhosis, volume overload in renal diseases and right-sided cardiac disease) [18]

- When three or more signs (JVD, S3, tachycardia, low pulse pressure, rales, abdomino-jugular reflux), >90 % likelihood of increased filling pressures if severe left ventricular (LV) dysfunction was not known. 1 or 0 symptoms or signs <10 % likelihood of increased filling pressures [19]. In chronic HF, rales, edema, JVD and pulmonary edema on CXR can be often absent.

Chest

■ Look for venous collaterals (venous obstruction), pectus carinaturm or excavatum (connective tissue disorders), barrel chest (emphysema), kyphosis (ankylosing spondylitis)

TABLE 1-5	FINDING AND RA TRACING	EXAMPLES
JUGULAR VENOUS WAVEFORMS	Normal 	

	Prominent a wave
	
		Obstruction to RA emptying
		  TV abnormalities: TS, RA myxoma, carcinoid heart disease, lupus endocarditis, RA thrombus, tricuspid atresia
		  Distal to tricuspid valve: decreased RV compliance such as in RVH, RV outflow obstruction such as in PS
		  PH
		  Uncommon in conditions with VSD or ASD

	Cannon a wave
	
		RA contraction against a closed TV
		  A-V dissociation
		  Premature atrial, junctional or ventricular beats
		  1st degree AVB

	Flutter a wave	Atrial flutter

	Absent a wave
	
		No effective atrial contraction
		  Atrial fibrillation
		  Ebstein's anomaly

	Equal a wave and v wave 	ASD TR
	Prominent v wave 	ASD without PH
	Prominent x descent 	ASD Early cardiac tamponade
	Blunted or absent y descent 	Late pericardial tamponade TS Severe RVH
	Steep y descent 	Constrictive pericarditis (classic M or W contour with prominent x and y descents) Restrictive cardiomyopathy Severe right side HF TR

ASD atrial septal defect, *AVB* atrioventricular block, *PH* pulmonary hypertension, *PS* pulmonic stenosis, *RA* right atrial, *RV* right ventricle, *RVH* right ventricular hypertrophy, *TR* tricuspid regurgitation, *TS* tricuspid stenosis, *TV* tricuspid valve, *VSD* ventricular septal defect

Abdomen

- Hepatomegaly and ascites (right-sided HF, constrictive pericarditis), enlarged abdominal aorta (the positive predictive value for abdominal aortic aneurysm is only 43 % [20])
- Abdominal bruit: systolic-diastolic bruit that lateralizes to one side is suggestive of renovascular disease in hypertensive patients (39 % sensitivity and 99 % specificity) [20], diffuse bruit is more likely due to aneurysm.

Extremities

- Symmetric edema (HF), asymmetric edema (venous thrombosis or lymphatic obstruction), nontender Janeway lesions and painful Osler's nodes (endocarditis), "fingerized" thumb (Holt-Oram syndrome), arachnodactyly (Marfan syndrome).

Vascular examination

- **Arterial bruits**

  - Caused by turbulent flow through narrowed arteries, arteriovenous fistulas or high flow through normal arteries
  - Weak correlation between the presence of bruit and the presence of significant arterial narrowing
  - **Carotid bruits**: sensitivity of carotid auscultation for a 70–99 % stenosis of the common or internal carotid artery was 56 % and specificity was 91 %. Positive predictive value of a bruit was 27 % and the negative predictive value of a normal carotid auscultation was 97 % [21].
  - **Femoral bruits**: in asymptomatic patients, the presence of a femoral bruits increases the likelihood of PVD (LR 4.8, 95 % CI 2.4–9.5) [15].

- **Pulses**

  - Bilateral carotid, radial, brachial, femoral, popliteal, posterior tibial and dorsalis pedis pulses should be examined
  - Carotid pulse most closely represents central aortic pulse (Table 1-6)
  - The ability to determine the presence or absence of a dorsalis pedis and the tibialis posterior arterial pulses (best with a cutoff point of ankle/brachial index [ABI]=0.76) is better than the ability to reliably determine a diminished pulse.
  - **Differential diagnosis of unequal or delayed pulses**: PVD, aortic disease (dissection, aneurysm, coarctation), Takayasu disease, supravalvular aortic stenosis (right>left upper extremity pulses)
  - **Pulsus paradoxus**: >10–12 mmHg fall in systolic BP with inspiration associated with cardiac tamponade, pericardial or severe pulmonary disease, hypovolemic shock, constrictive pericarditis, restrictive cardiomyopathy
  - **Pulsus alternans**: associated with cardiac tamponade, severe LV systolic HF, severe AR, HTN and hypovolemic state, ectopy

		TABLE 1-6
Bounding	AR, arteriovenous fistula, hyperkinetic states such as fever, anemia, thyrotoxicosis	CAROTID ARTERY PULSE
Bifid	Pulsus bisferiens (both peaks during systole)	
	Significant AR, HCM, arteriovenous fistula, large PDA	
	Dicrotic pulse (one peak in systole and one peak in diastole)	
	Severe HF, cardiac tamponade, intra-aortic balloon counterpulsation, immediate post operative aortic valve replacement, hypovolemic shock, hyperkinetic states	
Weak and delayed	Severe AS	
Abrupt carotid upstroke with a rapid fall-off	Severe AR (waterhammer or Corrigan pulse), PDA, large arteriovenous fistulas, hyperkinetic states, older patients with HTN and wide pulse pressures	
Bruit	Arterial stenosis, arteriovenous fistulas, hyperkinetic state	

AR aortic regurgitation, *HCM* hypertrophic cardiomyopathy, *HF* heart failure, *AS* aortic stenosis, *PDA* patent ductus arteriosus

Cardiac Examination

Inspection
- Look for visible pulsations, sternotomy scars and implanted devices such as pacemakers or defibrillators

Palpation
- **Normal Point of Maximal Impulse (PMI)**

    - Adults: LV apex (midclavicular line at the fifth intercostals space), <2 cm in diameter, quick
    - Children and adults with thin chest: Left parasternal at the fifth intercostals space

- **Abnormal PMI** (Table 1-7)

    - Double impulse: severe dilated CMP, HCM
    - Prominent a wave: due to elevated left ventricular end diastolic pressure (LVEDP) and decreased compliance (LVH, AS, HTN, HCM, CMP, ischemic CMP, LV aneurysm)
    - Paradoxical (inward with systole and outward with diastole): constrictive pericarditis

Auscultation (Table 1-8)
- **Distant heart sounds:** pericardial effusion, pneumothorax, mechanical ventilation, obstructive lung disease, obesity, large breasts

Pericardial rub is pathognomonic for the diagnosis of pericarditis
- A waxing and waning pericardial rub (not very sensitive, but almost 100 % specific)

    - A leathery, scratchy sound
    - Up to three components (atrial systole, ventricular systole and rapid-filling phase of the ventricle)
    - Can be localized or widespread

Heart Sounds (Fig. 1-2)
Normal S1
- Best heard over the apex and left lower sternal border with S1 > S2 in intensity
- The intensity of S1 increases as the distance and the speed over which the leaflets of the mitral valve (MV)-to a lesser extent, tricuspid valve (TV), must travel in systole

Accentuated S1
- Early stages of rheumatic mitral stenosis (MS), tricuspid stenosis (TS), atrial myxoma, or RA mass
- Hyperkinetic states: patent ductus arteriosus (PDA), ventricular septal defect (VSD), atrial septal defect (ASD), high output states
- Short P-R intervals: pre-excitation syndrome and tachycardia

Soft S1
- Late stages of rheumatic MS and rheumatic mitral regurgitation (MR)
- Presystolic semiclosure of the AV: severe acute AR, significant AS, dilated CMP, Long P-R intervals
- BB, left bundle branch block (LBBB)

Wide splitting of S1: right bundle branch block (RBBB), LV pacing, pre-excitation syndrome, Ebstein's anomaly, TS, ASD
Reverse splitting of S1: premature right ventricular (RV) ectopy, severe MS and left atrial (LA) myxoma

Normal S2
- Best heard over the left and right upper sternal border with S2 > S1 in intensity
- **Normal (physiologic) S2 splitting**: A2 and P2 are coincident during expiration; during inspiration, P2 is relatively delayed, resulting in physiologic splitting.

TABLE 1-7

ABNORMAL POINT OF MAXIMAL IMPULSE

LEFT SECOND INTERSPACE	LEFT PARASTERNAL		APEX		DISPLACED LATERALLY	RIGHT PARASTERNAL
	Hyperdynamic	Sustained	Hyperdynamic	Sustained		
Dilated PA	RV volume is increased	Significant RVH				RV dilation
Severe PH	ASD	PH	Severe MR	LVOT obstruction	**Dilated heart**	Ebstein's anomaly
Severe ASD	TR	Right-sided tension pneumothorax	Severe AR	HTN	Pulmonary fibrosis	Large ASD
		Massive pleural effusion	Large PDA	Dilated CMP	Right sided tension pneumothorax	Severe MS
		Absent left pericardium	Large VSD	Ischemic heart disease	Massive pleural effusion	
		MS	Hypermetabolic state	AR with decreased LVEF	Thoracic deformity	
			Thyrotoxicosis			
			Anemia			
			Normal after rigorous exercise			

AR aortic regurgitation, ASD atrial septal defect, CMP cardiomyopathy, HTN hypertension, LVEF left ventricular ejection fraction, LVOT left ventricular outflow track, MR mitral regurgitation, MS mitral stenosis, PA pulmonary artery, PDA patent ductus arteriosus, PH pulmonary hypertension, RV right ventricle, RVH right ventricular hypertrophy, TR tricuspid regurgitation, VSD ventricular septal defect

TABLE 1-8

DIFFERENTIAL DIAGNOSIS OF HEART
SOUNDS AND MURMURS

SYSTOLIC		DIASTOLIC		CONTINUOUS
Murmurs	Sounds	Murmurs	Sounds	Murmurs
Early	■ MVP click	**Early**	■ Opening snap	■ PDA
■ Acute severe or mild chronic MR/TR	■ Ejection click from bicuspid aortic or pulmonary valve disease	■ AR/PR	■ Pericardial knock	■ Ruptured sinus of Valsalva aneurysm
■ VSD	■ Ejection click from aortic or pulmonic root dilation	**Mid-to late diastolic**	■ Atrial myxoma	■ Arteriovenous fistulas
Midsystolic		■ MS/TS	■ Other tumor plops	■ Benign
■ AS/PS		■ Atrial myxoma		– Cervical venous hum
■ Supra and subvalvular stenosis		■ Complete heart block		– Mammary souffle of pregnancy
■ HCM		■ Acute rheumatic mitral valvulitis		
Midsystolic ejection murmur				
■ Benign flow murmur				
■ Aortic sclerosis				
■ Healthy children and adolescents				
■ High flow across valve				
– Pregnancy				
– Hyperthyroidism				
– Anemia				
– AR				
– ASD				
Late systolic murmur				
■ MVP				
Holosystolic				
■ VSD				
■ MR/TR				

AS aortic stenosis, *AR* aortic regurgitation, *ASD* atrial septal defect, *HCM* hypertrophic cardiomyopathy, *MR* mitral regurgitation, *MS* mitral stenosis, *MVP* mitral valve prolapse, *PDA* patent ductus arteriosus, *PR* pulmonic regurgitation, *PS* pulmonic stenosis, *TR* tricuspid regurgitation, *TS* tricuspid stenosis, *VSD* ventricular septal defect

FIGURE 1-2

Heart sounds. *M* mitral,
T tricuspid, *A* aortic, *P* pulmonary,
C click, *E* ejection sound, *OS*
opening snap, *K* pericardial
knock (Courtesy of Dr. Hanna
Gaggin)

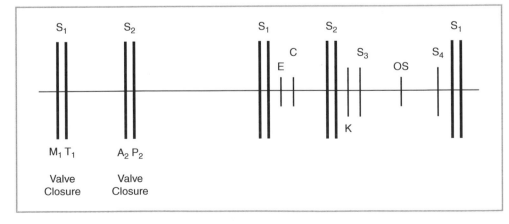

Accentuated P2: P2 > A2 at the left upper sternal border or P2 can be heard at the apex
- Pulmonary hypertension (PH), ASD (not necessarily with PH), Soft A2 (relative intensity)

Wide but preserved respiratory variation on S2 splitting
- Delayed activation of RV: RBBB, ectopy/arrhythmia originating from LV such as Wolff-Parkinson White syndrome
- PH with RV failure, RV outflow obstruction (pulmonic stenosis [PS], pulmonary embolism)
- Severe MR (due to premature AV closure), VSD, constrictive pericarditis

Wide and Fixed splitting of S2
- Ostium secundum ASD
- Severe RV failure

Reversed or paradoxical, splitting of S2 due to a pathologic delay in AV closure
- Delay in LV activation: complete LBBB and ectopy/arrhythmia from RV, RV pacing
- Delayed LV ejection: severe AS, HCM, AR, PDA, myocardial ischemia

Single S2: AV or pulmonic valve (PV) abnormalities or fused A2 and P2 (Eisenmenger's VSD, common ventricle)

S3
- Normal in healthy people <40 years of age or in high output states (pregnancy, thyrotoxicosis)
- A low-pitched sound best heard over the LV apex/PMI in the left lateral decubitus position with the bell; a right-sided S₃ is best heard at the lower left sternal border (LLSB) or subxiphoid position with the patient supine, and may become louder with inspiration
- Associated with HF: elevated LVEDP, reduced LVEF, or elevated B-type natriuretic peptide (BNP) – sensitivity 32–52 %, specificity 87–92 % [22]
- Associated with MR, not necessarily indicative of HF

S4
- Low-pitched sound best heard over the LV apex in the left lateral decubitus position with the bell
- Common in patients with accentuated atrial contribution to ventricular filling such as LVH
- Associated with abnormal LV compliance: hypertensive heart disease, AS, HCM, acute myocardial infarction (MI), MR, AR

Aortic ejection sound
- A high-pitched early to mid systolic sound widely transmitted, best heard at the LLSB > base of the heart
- Congenital bicuspid AV (including in the absence of stenosis) or aortic root dilation with a normal AV
- Absent in subvalvular and supravalvular AS

Pulmonary ejection sound
- Similar in quality to the aortic ejection sound, but best heard at the left upper and lower sternal border and decreases with inspiration
- Congenital bicuspid PV or pulmonic root dilation with a normal PV

Nonejection click
- A systolic click heard after the upstroke of the carotid pulse

Midsystolic click
- A systolic click best heard over right or left upper sternal border from mitral valve prolapse (MVP)

Opening snap (OS)
- A high-pitched diastolic opening snap of MV in MS, best heard over left upper and lower sternal border

TABLE 1-9

2006 ACC/AHA GUIDELINE
RECOMMENDATIONS FOR
INDICATIONS FOR
ECHOCARDIOGRAPHY IN PATIENTS
WITH CARDIAC MURMURS [23]

Class I recommendations (definitely perform echocardiography)

Patients with cardiac symptoms

Asymptomatic patients with the following murmurs

  Diastolic murmurs

  Continuous murmurs

  Holosystolic murmurs

  Late systolic murmurs

  Murmurs associated with ejection clicks

  Murmurs that radiate to the neck or back

  Grade 3 or louder mid-peaking systolic murmurs

Class IIa recommendations

Murmurs associated with abnormal physical findings, ECG or CXR

Patients with likely noncardiac findings, but cardiac disease cannot be excluded by standard evaluation

Class III recommendations (do not perform echocardiography)

Grade 2 or softer midsystolic murmurs considered innocent or functional by an experienced observer

ECG electrocardiogram, *CXR* chest x-ray

Pericardial knock
- A high-pitched early diastolic sound (between S2 and S3) best heard at the lower right sternal border
- Results from abrupt cessation of ventricular expansion after atrioventricular valve opening in constrictive pericarditis-prominent y descent seen in JVP waveform

Tumor plop
- A low-pitched diastolic sound caused by prolapse of tumor (usually atrial myxoma) across the MV

VALVULAR DISEASES AND MURMURS

Systolic murmurs (Tables 1-8 and 1-10)

Benign systolic murmur
- An isolated grade 1 or 2 midsystolic crescendo-decrescendo (also known as ejection) murmur **in the absence of symptoms or other signs of heart disease**

Aortic stenosis
- **Classic**: a crescendo-decrescendo, harsh or musical midsystolic murmur best heard over the right upper sternal border with radiation to the neck and both carotids
- A soft and single S2
- **Severe AS:**

  - A late-peaking murmur, a soft or paradoxically split S2, a soft or absent A2
  - Pulsus tardus (slowly rising carotid upstroke) and pulsus parvus (decreased carotid pulse amplitude)
  - Commonly associated with mild AR
  - A single finding is not very sensitive, but specific (sensitivity 25–32 %, specificity 86–99 %) [24]

- **Gallavardin phenomenon**: a loud, harsh, blowing murmur at the apex associated with AS (easily confused with MR or HCM often and can be differentiated by maneuvers)
- **Maneuver:**

  - Increase in murmur intensity: handgrip, standing or sitting up, Valsalva (phase 2), amyl nitrate
  - Decrease in murmur intensity: squatting and first beat after a premature beat or after a long cycle length in atrial fibrillation
  - Stronger the carotid pulse, the louder the murmur of AS and vice versa.

Bicuspid aortic valve

- A midsystolic murmur best heard over the right upper sternal border
- Preceded by an aortic systolic ejection sound, a short early diastolic murmur, normal carotid pulse upstroke and S2 (very specific for the diagnosis of bicuspid AV)
- Does not require outflow obstruction for the findings above

Supravalvular aortic stenosis

- A midsystolic murmur best heard above the right upper sternal border
- Radiation is louder in the right carotid than left carotid

Subvalvular aortic stenosis

- A midsystolic murmur best heard over left lower sternal border or over the apex with minimal radiation to the neck

Hypertrophic cardiomyopathy

- A midsystolic crescendo-decrescendo murmur best heard over the apex and LLSB
- Unlike fixed aortic outflow obstruction such as AS, the initial upstroke of the carotid pulse is usually sharp and the amplitude is normal
- **Maneuvers:**

  Increase in murmur intensity: standing (best discriminator vs. AS); sitting up; long beat-to-beat cycle length in atrial fibrillation or post-extrasystolic beat, resulting in **Brockenbrough sign** (postextrasystolic potentiation due to increased LV outflow gradient and decreased or unchanged pulse pressure); Valsalva (phase 2); or amyl nitrate (early)

  - Decrease in murmur intensity: handgrip, squatting
  - Unlike fixed aortic outflow obstruction: Carotid pulse decreases or remains unchanged with Valsalva (phase 2) and amyl nitrate (early) while the murmur intensity increases

Pulmonic stenosis

- **Classic**: a harsh midsystolic murmur best heard over the left upper sternal border with radiation to the left carotid, increases in intensity with inspiration
- Associated with a widely split S2 with preserved respiratory variation, decreased intensity of P2 and a pulmonic ejection sound at the onset of the murmur
- **Severe PS:** a late-peaking murmur and evidence of right ventricular hypertrophy (RVH) and/or RV failure

Dilation of the aortic root or pulmonary artery without PH

- A midsystolic murmur with an ejection sound

Mitral regurgitation

- **Classic**: a high-pitched, blowing, holosystolic murmur best heard over the cardiac apex

  - Radiates anteriorly and to the base (prolapsed or flail posterior mitral leaflet) or posteriorly and to the axilla (anterior leaflet involvement)

- Variable onset, duration, quality and radiation depending on the mechanism and severity

  - Early systolic in timing (chronic mild, due to dilated CMP or mitral annular calcification)
  - Blowing (due to chronic annular dilatation)
  - Harsh or musical, late-peaking (ruptured chordae tendinae or from a floppy mitral valve)
  - Associated with one or more clicks in MVP

- **Acute severe:**

  - Murmur often soft or absent, but when present, may be decrescendo, early in systole, and best heard at the LLSB or the axilla rather than the apex
  - Look for other associated signs of left and right-sided failure, although may be absent

■ **Chronic severe**

  – Evidence of chronic remodeling: enlarged, displaced, dynamic PMI, apical systolic thrill
  – Mid-diastolic filling complex (an S3 and a short low-pitched murmur)
  – Wide but physiologic splitting of S2 due to early aortic valve closure
  – Loud P2 or RV lift

Tricuspid regurgitation (TR)
■ **Classic**: holosystolic murmur over LLSB, right lower sternal border or along the left sternal border, may radiate to the epigastrium, increases with inspiration (Carvallo's sign), associated with a prominent v wave in the jugular venous pulse
■ **Severe TR**: associated with a mid-diastolic flow murmur simulating TS (from increased flow across TV) and RV S3 but the typical murmur may be absent or early systolic if severe RV failure exists
■ **Primary TR**: Early decrescendo, systolic murmur with normal RV pressures
■ **Secondary TR**: evidence of PH

Evidence of PH
■ Prominent left parasternal impulse
■ Narrowly split S2
■ Accentuated P2
■ Pulmonary ejection sound and pulmonary regurgitation (PR) murmur due to dilated pulmonary artery
■ TR murmur

Mitral valve prolapse
■ **Classic:** one or more midsystolic non-ejection click followed by a mid to late systolic murmur (due to MR) at the apex; findings may be intermittent and subtle
■ Most common cause of a late systolic murmur
■ **The click and murmur onset and duration are highly sensitive to LV volume status**

  – Decreased LV volume: standing, sitting, Valsalva (phase 2), amyl nitrite

    ■ Earlier onset of prolapse, resulting in earlier onset of the click and murmur with a longer duration of the systolic murmur, decreased intensity of the murmur

  – Increased LV volume: squatting, passive leg raise, hand grip

    ■ Delayed onset of prolapse, resulting in later onset of the click and murmur with shorter duration of the systolic murmur, increased intensity of the murmur

■ Associated with skeletal deformities including straight back, pseudohypertrophic muscular dystrophy, longer arm span than height and relatively tall R waves in V1 or V2.

Ventricular septal defect
■ **Classic**: loud, holosystolic murmur with a thrill at the left upper sternal border (exact location depends on the level of the VSD), usually due to a small VSD (no evidence of PH and a normal S2)
■ The intensity and quality of the murmur depend on the VSD size and hemodynamic:

  – **Large VSD**: an early systolic and early peaking murmur, associated with evidence of PH and RVH
  – **Eisenmenger complex**: a single S2, no murmur as ventricular pressures are equal, but possibly with a midsystolic murmur due to dilated pulmonary trunk

Diastolic murmurs (Tables 1-8 and 1-12)
Aortic regurgitation
■ **Classic**: high-pitched, decrescendo, blowing, early to mid-diastolic murmur at the upper left (primary valvular) or right (root dilation and secondary) sternal border
■ **Technique**: leaning forward, after a full exhalation with a diaphragm
■ Variable radiation and duration, sometimes associated with a systolic ejection sound
■ Associated with a soft midsystolic murmur from the increased flow across AV, resulting in a "to-and-fro" murmur at the cardiac base in moderate or severe AR, bisferiens pulse

MANEUVER	THEORY	AS	HCM	MR
Inspiration		↓	↓	↓
Handgrip or exercise (can be variable and best for AS vs MR)	↑Afterload	↓	↓	↑
Squatting or passive leg raising	↑Preload ↑Afterload	↑	↓	↑
Standing	↓Preload ↓Afterload	↓	↑	↓
Valsalva (Phase 2, the straining phase)	↓Preload ↓Afterload	↓ ↓Carotid pulse	↑ ↓ or ↔ Carotid pulse	↓
First beat after a premature beat or after a long cycle length in atrial fibrillation	↑Preload ↑Contractility	↑	↑	↔ or ↓
Amyl nitrite (Early)	↓Afterload, hypotension	↑ ↑Carotid pulse	↑ ↓ or ↔ Carotid pulse	↓ or ↔
Amyl nitrite (Late)	↑HR ↑Preload			

TABLE 1-10

MANEUVERS TO DIFFERENTIATE SYSTOLIC MURMURS

AS aortic stenosis, *HCM* hypertrophic cardiomyopathy, *MR* mitral regurgitation

- A musical diastolic 'whoop': thought to be due to a flail everted aortic cusp
- **Austin-Flint murmur:** low-pitched mid- to late diastolic rumble with a presystolic accentuation at the apex associated with a severe AR, responds to maneuvers similarly to AR
- **Acute severe:**
  - **Presentation**: evidence of acute HF, pulmonary edema and cardiogenic shock: S3, accentuated P2, hypotension
  - **Murmur**: short, low-pitched, early, decrescendo, blowing diastolic murmur, but the murmur may be absent
  - Absence of evidence of chronic compensation: a normal PMI and no peripheral findings of wide pulse pressure
  - Associated with a soft or absent S1 due to premature closure of the MV, soft A2
  - Normal or slightly widened pulse pressure that progressively narrows as HF progresses
- **Chronic severe:**
  - **Presentation**: asymptomatic and subtle symptoms (palpitation, CP) while cardiac compensation progresses, HF symptoms when LV dysfunction occurs
  - **Murmur**: high-pitched, blowing, decrescendo, early, mid or holodiastolic murmur
  - Wide pulse pressure (>100 mmHg) with evidence of peripheral findings of wide pulse pressure such as the Hill's sign or water hammer (Corrigan) pulses, Quincke's pulses (capillary pulsation in the fingernails); most of these signs are not very specific, the most specific sign is Hill's sign
  - Associated with reversed splitting of S2
  - Laterally displaced, diffuse, hyperdynamic apex if relatively normal LVEF, but a sustained impulse and an S3 gallop if reduced LVEF

Pulmonic Regurgitation
- High-pitched, blowing, decrescendo diastolic murmur at the upper left sternal border
- Usually due to annular enlargement from chronic PH (Graham Steell murmur) associated with an accentuated P2 or a history of a surgical repair of Tetralogy of Fallot (softer and lower-pitched)

■ Associated with signs of RV volume and pressure overload, with a midsystolic murmur from increased flow across PV (resulting in a to-and-fro murmur) in moderate to severe PR

Mitral stenosis
■ **Presentation**: insidious reduction of activity tolerance with dyspnea or hemoptysis in the setting of tachycardia or stress, resulting in increased cardiac output, atrial fibrillation, thromboembolism and evidence of PH and eventually RV failure
■ **Classic**: OS followed by a mid- to late diastolic low-pitched rumbling murmur at the apex with presystolic accentuation/murmur (an increase in the intensity of the murmur in late diastole following atrial contraction in sinus rhythm)
■ **Technique:** left lateral decubitus position with a bell
■ A2-OS interval inversely correlates with severity of MS and therefore the duration of the mitral diastolic murmur (more severe MS -> increased LA pressure -> decreased LA-LV pressure gradient -> earlier onset of OS and murmur -> longer duration of the murmur)
■ **Severe MS**

  – The murmur tends to be longer in duration, but can be short or silent in PH/RV failure
  – OS and S1/M1 can be soft or silent in severely calcific stenosis
  – A short A2-opening snap interval and longer duration of the murmur
  – Evidence of PH, RVH and RV failure: loud P2 or narrowly split/single S2 and RV lift, JVD, hepatomegaly, lower extremity edema
  – Reduced arterial pulse amplitude, vasoconstriction, resulting in pinkish-purple patches on the cheeks (mitral facies)

Tricuspid stenosis
■ An OS followed by a mid-to late diastolic rumble best heard along the LLSB, increasing in intensity with inspiration
■ Most frequently associated with MS, but can be primary TS
■ Associated with a prominent *a* wave and a slow *y* descent in the jugular venous pulse, presystolic hepatic pulsation and absence of RA gallop

Atrial septal defect
■ Usually asymptomatic, but can present with atrial arrhythmias (the most frequent presenting symptom), exercise intolerance, dyspnea and fatigue
■ No primary murmur, but associated with a midsystolic pulmonic ejection murmur and a mid-diastolic rumbling murmur (due to increased flow across TV in the setting of a large left-to-right shunt), hyperdynamic RV impulse, wide fixed splitting of the S2 while sitting or standing,
■ Can progress to PH and eventually Eisenmenger syndrome with associated findings.

Atrial myxoma
■ Often due to the obstruction of the mitral valve (or less commonly the tricuspid valve); findings similar to MS, difficult to distinguish between the MS and atrial myxoma murmur
■ A mid- to late diastolic murmur, presystolic crescendo murmur due to obstruction and tumor plop

Prosthetic valve (Table 1-11)
■ Dysfunction: a new or a change in the quality of an existing murmur, HF, new ECG abnormalities
■ Prosthetic valve thrombosis: shock, muffled heart sounds and soft murmurs

Continuous murmurs: murmurs that begin in systole and extend into diastole
■ **Blood flow from persistent pressure gradient between a higher pressure and a lower pressure system** throughout systole and diastole: PDA, aortopulmonary window, shunts, arteriovenous fistulas such as coronary, great vessel or hemodialysis lines [radiating to the infraclavicular area], ruptured sinus of Valsalva aneurysm (to-and-fro murmurs)

TABLE 1-11

NORMAL PROSTHETIC VALVE
SOUNDS

BIOPROSTHESIS		MECHANICAL		
Mitral valve	Aortic valve	Caged-ball (Starr-Edwards)	Single-tilting disk (Bjork-Shiley or Medtronic-Hall)	Bileaflet-tilting-disk (St. Jude Medical)
A midsystolic murmur and a soft, mid-diastolic murmur	A grade 2 or 3 midsystolic murmur at the base			
Closing sounds> opening sounds	Closing sounds> opening sounds	Opening=closing sounds	Closing sounds> opening sounds	Closing sounds> opening sounds

TABLE 1-12

MANEUVERS TO DIFFERENTIATE
DIASTOLIC MURMURS

VALVULAR DISEASE	THEORY	AR	MS
Inspiration		↓	↓
Handgrip or exercise	↑ Afterload, ↑ cardiac output	↑	↑
Squatting or passive leg raising	↑ Preload, ↑ afterload	↑	
Valsalva (Phase 2, the straining phase)	↓ Preload and ↓ afterload	↓	↓
First beat after a premature beat or after a long cycle length in atrial fibrillation	↑ Contractility>↑ preload	↑	
Amyl nitrite (Early)	↓ Afterload, Hypotension	↓	↑
Amyl nitrite (Late)	↑ Pulse, ↑ preload		↑

AR aortic regurgitation, MS mitral stenosis

- **Constriction in the systemic or pulmonary arteries**: coarctation of the aorta (best heard in the back)
- **Benign**: cervical venous hum best heard in the supraclavicular fossa that disappears when patient is supine or when internal jugular vein is compressed, mammary souffle of pregnancy (high-pitched, systolic or continuous murmur)

Patent ductus arteriosus
- Flow from the descending thoracic aorta to the pulmonary artery (Gibson's murmur)
- A machinery murmur with a maximal intensity at S2
- As pulmonary pressures increase, the diastolic component of the murmur becomes shorter until it disappears
- When right-sided pressures equalize with left-sided pressures (often associated with signs of PH and differential cyanosis), the murmur can become silent

Differentiating murmurs originating from the left and the right sided chambers of the heart
- In general, the intensity of the murmurs and sounds from the right-sided chambers of the heart increase with inspiration and decrease with expiration. An exception is the pulmonic ejection sound, which does not increase with inspiration. Murmurs and sounds from the left-sided chambers of the heart either remains stable or decrease with inspiration and increase with expiration.

In summary, understanding benefits as well as limitations of history and physical examination is important (Table 1-13). An isolated history or exam finding is neither sensitive nor specific. However when relevant findings are combined, the test performance improves significantly.

QUICK REVIEW (TABLE 1-14)

TABLE 1-13	PHYSICAL EXAMINATION BY BOARD-CERTIFIED CARDIOLOGISTS		HAND-HELD US BY TRAINED MEDICAL STUDENTS	
TEST PERFORMANCES OF ISOLATED PHYSICAL EXAMINATION BY CARDIOLOGISTS VS. HANDHELD ULTRASOUND BY TRAINED MEDICAL STUDENTS FOR MAJOR CARDIAC FINDINGS [25]	Sensitivity (%[a])	Specificity (%)	Sensitivity (%)	Specificity (%)
Valvular lesions	50	90	89	91
Systolic murmur	62	84	93	91
Diastolic murmur	16	93	75	91

[a]p<0.001 compared with hand-held ultrasound by trained medical students

TABLE 1-14		
QUICK REVIEW	**FINDING**	**ASSOCIATION**
	Hypotension, a diastolic murmur, CP and a new hemiplegia	Acute aortic dissection extending into the carotid and AV with AR
	Cough, heart block, CP, lupus pernio, erythema nodosum, granuloma	Sarcoidosis
	Central cyanosis	Significant right-to-left shunting at the level of the heart or lungs or hereditary methemoglobinemia
	Peripheral cyanosis	Small vessel constriction: severe HF, shock, peripheral vascular disease
	Differential cyanosis (cyanosis of the lower but not the upper extremities)	PDA, PH with right-to-left shunting at the great vessel level
	Tanned or bronze discoloration of the skin in unexposed areas, HF	Iron overload from hemochromatosis or repeated transfusion with CMP
	Xanthomas	Lipid disorders (palmer crease xanthoma is associated with type III hyperlipoproteinemia)
	Leathery, cobblestone, plucked-chicken appearance of the skin in the axial and skin folds of a young person with CP	Pseudoxanthoma elasticum with premature coronary artery disease
	High arched palate	Marfan syndrome and other connective tissue disease syndromes
	Large protruding tongue with parotid enlargement	Amyloidosis
	Bifid uvula and sudden onset CP radiating to the back	Loeys-Dietz syndrome with aortic aneurysm and/or dissection
	Orange tongue	Tangier disease (familial alpha-lipoprotein deficiency) with low HDL
	Ptosis, ophthalmoplegia, HF	Muscular dystrophies with CMP
	Hypertelorism, low-set ears, micrognathia, webbed neck	Congenital heart diseases: Noonan, Turner and Down syndromes
	Proptosis, lid lag, stare	Graves' hyperthyroidism
	Cutaneous venous collaterals over the anterior chest, asymmetric breast enlargement	Obstruction of the superior vena cava or subclavian vein, consider any indwelling catheter/leads related obstruction
	Pectus carinatum (pigeon chest) or pectus excavatum (funnel chest)	Connective tissue disorders
	Severe kyphosis of ankylosing spondylitis	Aortic regurgitation
	Elevated left external jugular vein	Persistent left-sided SVC or compression of the innominate vein from an intrathoracic structure such as a tortuous or aneurismal aorta
	Systolic pulsation near the right sternoclavicular joint or in the upper right parasternal region	Ascending aortic aneurysms
	A rise (or failure to decrease) in venous pressure with inspiration (Kussmaul sign)	Constrictive pericarditis, restrictive cardiomyopathy, pulmonary embolism, RV infarction, advanced systolic HF

REVIEW QUESTIONS

1. A 65-year-old man with a history of "heart murmur" and a "clean bill of health" on cardiac catheterization a year ago presented to an outpatient office for establishing cardiac care. He has been diagnosed with obesity, HTN and diabetes mellitus in the past. He denies any complaints, but his family states that he is sedentary.

    On physical examination, his blood pressure is 110/95 mmHg with a pulse of 90. His PMI is displaced laterally. He has an apical, high-pitched, blowing systolic murmur, a mid-diastolic filling complex and a widely split S2. The murmur increases with handgrip and passive leg raise.

    An echocardiogram shows a severely dilated LA and a moderately dilated LV with an LVEF of 50 % and LV end systolic dimension of 50 mm. There is a 20 mmHg mean gradient between the LV and the aorta. A moderate eccentric mitral regurgitation is seen with a regurgitant volume of 50 mL and a regurgitant fraction of 40 %. What is the next step?

    (a) Follow up in 1 year with an echocardiogram
    (b) Determine functional class and capacity and perform a transesophageal echocardiogram
    (c) Refer the patient for cardiac surgery
    (d) Refer the patient for an alcohol ablation

2. The above patient now presents emergently with acute onset dyspnea and orthopnea. His vitals are BP 95/80 mmHg, HR 120 bpm, respiratory rate of 25/min and O_2 saturation 85 % on room air (92 % on 2 L of oxygen). A brief physical examination reveals a soft, early, systolic murmur at the left axilla with an S3 and rales bilaterally. What is true concerning the test performance of these physical examination findings?

    (a) 75–80 % of the patients with chronic HF have rales & edema
    (b) Hearing S_3 in pregnancy is concerning for cardiomyopathy
    (c) S_3 has about 70 % sensitivity for the diagnosis of HF
    (d) In severe MR, the murmur is early systolic and soft, or absent.

ANSWERS

1. (b) Based on physical examination findings above, this patient has chronic MR. An apical systolic murmur can be due to MR, HCM or Gallavardin effect from AS and maneuvers can help to differentiate between these. Handgrip is best in differentiating MR from AS; the intensity of the murmur increases in MR while it decreases with AS. Increasing ventricular volume by passive leg raise or squatting increases the intensity of the murmur in MR while it decreases with HCM.

    In this patient with chronic MR, there is a disparity between findings on his physical examination and his echocardiography. His physical examination suggests severe MR with a mid-diastolic filling complex (which consists of S3 and a functional murmur simulating mitral stenosis due to increased volume of regurgitant jet flowing back into the LV) and a widely split S2 (suggestive of a premature closure of aortic value usually associated with a severe mitral regurgitation). There is also evidence of HF with a narrow pulse pressure (associated with a decreased cardiac index <2.2 L/min/m² [14]) and a displaced PMI (suggestive of a dilated heart). With an eccentric jet, echocardiography can underestimate the severity of mitral regurgitation.

    While this patient is without any complaints, his sedentary lifestyle may mask his symptoms. A thorough assessment of his functional class is needed in determining his symptom status [26] and exercise capacity. An exercise echocardiogram can determine exertional symptoms, exercise capacity and additional findings suggestive of pulmonary hypertension or severe mitral regurgitation (Class IIa recommendation). A transesophageal echocardiogram can assess the mitral regurgitation jet in the LA from a different angle for an accurate assessment of the MR, pulmonary pressures as well as details of the valve morphology, mechanism and potential for surgery

2. (d) The patient above is in acute HF due to acute severe MR, likely due to a papillary muscle or chordal rupture. Narrow pulse pressure (<25 % of the systolic pressure) is associated with low cardiac index and findings of orthopnea and rales combined have a high specificity and high positive predictive value for the diagnosis of HF. In acute severe MR, the murmur is often absent or short and early systolic as there is rapid equalization of pressures between the LA and the LV. An axillary murmur is most likely due to an anterior leaflet involvement with a regurgitant jet radiating towards axilla.

    About 75–80 % of the patients with chronic HF do not have rales and edema, but when found, these are predictive of HF diagnosis. S3 can be heard in high output states such as thyrotoxicosis or pregnancy and in young healthy patients <40 years old. S3 has sensitivity of 32–52 % and specificity of 87–92 % [22]. S3 can be heard in MR without HF and is thought to be due to the increased volume filling the ventricle during the early rapid filling phase.

REFERENCES

1. Myers J, Prakash M, Froelicher V, Do D, Partington S, Atwood JE. Exercise capacity and mortality among men referred for exercise testing. N Engl J Med. 2002;346(11):793–801.

2. Goldman L, Hashimoto B, Cook EF, Loscalzo A. Comparative reproducibility and validity of systems for assessing cardiovascular functional class: advantages of a new specific activity scale. Circulation. 1981;64(6):1227–34.

3. Weiner DA, Ryan TJ, McCabe CH, Kennedy JW, Schloss M, Tristani F, et al. Exercise stress testing. Correlations among history of angina, ST-segment response and prevalence of coronary-artery disease in the Coronary Artery Surgery Study (CASS). N Engl J Med. 1979;301(5):230–5.

4. Diercks DB, Boghos E, Guzman H, Amsterdam EA, Kirk JD. Changes in the numeric descriptive scale for pain after sublingual nitroglycerin do not predict cardiac etiology of chest pain. Ann Emerg Med. 2005;45(6):581–5.

5. Gupta M, Tabas JA, Kohn MA. Presenting complaint among patients with myocardial infarction who present to an urban, public hospital emergency department. Ann Emerg Med. 2002;40(2):180–6.

6. Canto JG, Shlipak MG, Rogers WJ, Malmgren JA, Frederick PD, Lambrew CT, et al. Prevalence, clinical characteristics, and mortality among patients with myocardial infarction presenting without chest pain. JAMA. 2000;283(24):3223–9.

7. Brieger D, Eagle KA, Goodman SG, Steg PG, Budaj A, White K, et al. Acute coronary syndromes without chest pain, an underdiagnosed and undertreated high-risk group: insights from the Global Registry of Acute Coronary Events. Chest. 2004;126(2):461–9.

8. Roy CL, Minor MA, Brookhart MA, Choudhry NK. Does this patient with a pericardial effusion have cardiac tamponade? JAMA. 2007;297(16):1810–8.

9. Klompas M. Does this patient have an acute thoracic aortic dissection? JAMA. 2002;287(17):2262–72.

10. Swap CJ, Nagurney JT. Value and limitations of chest pain history in the evaluation of patients with suspected acute coronary syndromes. JAMA. 2005;294(20):2623–9.

11. Thavendiranathan P, Bagai A, Khoo C, Dorian P, Choudhry NK. Does this patient with palpitations have a cardiac arrhythmia? JAMA. 2009;302(19):2135–43.

12. McDermott MM, Greenland P, Liu K, Guralnik JM, Criqui MH, Dolan NC, et al. Leg symptoms in peripheral arterial disease: associated clinical characteristics and functional impairment. JAMA. 2001;286(13):1599–606.

13. Hirsch AT, Criqui MH, Treat-Jacobson D, Regensteiner JG, Creager MA, Olin JW, et al. Peripheral arterial disease detection, awareness, and treatment in primary care. JAMA. 2001;286(11):1317–24.

14. Stevenson LW, Perloff JK. The limited reliability of physical signs for estimating hemodynamics in chronic heart failure. JAMA. 1989;261(6):884–8.

15. Khan NA, Rahim SA, Anand SS, Simel DL, Panju A. Does the clinical examination predict lower extremity peripheral arterial disease? JAMA. 2006;295(5):536–46.

16. Seth R, Magner P, Matzinger F, van Walraven C. How far is the sternal angle from the mid-right atrium? J Gen Intern Med. 2002;17(11):852–6.

17. Drazner MH, Hellkamp AS, Leier CV, Shah MR, Miller LW, Russell SD, et al. Value of clinician assessment of hemodynamics in advanced heart failure: the ESCAPE trial. Circ Heart Fail. 2008;1(3):170–7.

18. Butman SM, Ewy GA, Standen JR, Kern KB, Hahn E. Bedside cardiovascular examination in patients with severe chronic heart failure: importance of rest or inducible jugular venous distension. J Am Coll Cardiol. 1993;22(4):968–74.

19. Rohde LE, Beck-da-Silva L, Goldraich L, Grazziotin TC, Palombini DV, Polanczyk CA, et al. Reliability and prognostic value of traditional signs and symptoms in outpatients with congestive heart failure. Can J Cardiol. 2004;20(7):697–702.

20. Lederle FA, Simel DL. The rational clinical examination. Does this patient have abdominal aortic aneurysm? JAMA. 1999;281(1):77–82.

21. Magyar MT, Nam EM, Csiba L, Ritter MA, Ringelstein EB, Droste DW. Carotid artery auscultation – anachronism or useful screening procedure? Neurol Res. 2002;24(7):705–8.

22. Marcus GM, Gerber IL, McKeown BH, Vessey JC, Jordan MV, Huddleston M, et al. Association between phonocardiographic third and fourth heart sounds and objective measures of left ventricular function. JAMA. 2005;293(18):2238–44.

23. Bonow RO, Carabello BA, Chatterjee K, De Leon Jr AC, Faxon DP, Freed MD, et al. ACC/AHA 2006 guidelines for the management of patients with valvular heart disease: a report of the American College of Cardiology/American Heart Association Task Force on Practice Guidelines (writing Committee to Revise the 1998 guidelines for the management of patients with valvular heart disease) developed in collaboration with the Society of Cardiovascular Anesthesiologists endorsed by the Society for Cardiovascular Angiography and Interventions and the Society of Thoracic Surgeons. J Am Coll Cardiol. 2006;48(3):e1–148.

24. Munt B, Legget ME, Kraft CD, Miyake-Hull CY, Fujioka M, Otto CM. Physical examination in valvular aortic stenosis: correlation with stenosis severity and prediction of clinical outcome. Am Heart J. 1999;137(2):298–306.

25. Kobal SL, Trento L, Baharami S, Tolstrup K, Naqvi TZ, Cercek B, et al. Comparison of effectiveness of hand-carried ultrasound to bedside cardiovascular physical examination. Am J Cardiol. 2005;96(7):1002–6.

26. Bonow RO, Carabello BA, Chatterjee K, De Leon Jr AC, Faxon DP, Freed MD, et al. 2008 Focused update incorporated into the ACC/AHA 2006 guidelines for the management of patients with valvular heart disease: a report of the American College of Cardiology/American Heart Association Task Force on Practice Guidelines (Writing Committee to Revise the 1998 Guidelines for the Management of Patients With Valvular Heart Disease): endorsed by the Society of Cardiovascular Anesthesiologists, Society for Cardiovascular Angiography and Interventions, and Society of Thoracic Surgeons. Circulation. 2008;118(15):e523–661.

CHAPTER 2

Wai-Ee Thai, Bryan Wai, and Quynh A. Truong

Cardiac Noninvasive Imaging: Chest Radiography, Cardiovascular Magnetic Resonance and Computed Tomography of the Heart

CHAPTER OUTLINE

ABBREVIATIONS

ALARA	As Low As Reasonably Achievable
AP	Antero-posterior
bpm	Beats per minute
CABG	Coronary artery bypass graft
CAD	Coronary artery disease
CCS	Coronary calcium score
CHD	Coronary heart disease
CMR	Cardiac magnetic resonance
CT	Computed tomography
CTA	Computed tomography angiography
CXR	Chest X-ray
ECG	Electrocardiogram
Gd	Gadolinium
HR	Heart rate
LA	Left atrial
LV	Left ventricular
mSv	Millisievert
PA	Postero-anterior
RV	Right ventricular

INTRODUCTION

Non-invasive imaging plays an important role in the management of cardiac diseases. While chest radiography forms a standard part of the diagnostic work-up and follow-up of many cardiac patients, evolving technology related to cardiac computed tomography (CT) and cardiovascular magnetic resonance (CMR) imaging have contributed substantially to the diagnosis and prognosis of various cardiac pathologies. This chapter describes chest radiography findings of cardiopulmonary abnormalities and diseases, including recognition of valvular prostheses as well as pericardial and aortic abnormalities. This is followed by a section on cardiac CT and CMR where scan modes and sequences, indications specific to cardiology and safety issues are addressed.

CHEST RADIOGRAPHY

Advantages

Quick, portable, minimal radiation (0.02 millisieverts [mSv]), useful for serial follow-up

Normal Chest X-ray (CXR) Findings

Heart
- Normal cardiothoracic ratio of the heart width to the chest width is <50 % on postero-anterior (PA) projection

Diaphragm
- Normal chest expansion on CXR : 6±1 anterior ribs or 9±1 posterior ribs, right hemi-diaphragm higher than the left by up to 3 cm in 95 % of cases

Hila
- Left hilum usually higher by approximately 1 cm than the right hilum, equal density

Abnormal CXR Findings

Dextroposition
- In situs solitus, the position of the heart is on the right side secondary to a **non-cardiac abnormality** e.g. scoliosis, pneumonectomy, pulmonary agenesis, right pneumothorax, chronic volume loss or diaphragmatic hernia

Dextrocardia with situs inversus
- Heart on the right side with inverted abdominal viscera and lung morphology (Fig. 2-1). Thoracic situs is determined by the anatomy of the trachea and lungs, not the position of aortic arch or cardiac apex

Dextroversion
- Counter-clockwise rotation of a normally developed heart in the right hemithorax. On CXR, the apex is not evident as it lies behind the sternum, the left heart border is formed by the left atrium, the right border is formed by the right ventricle and the right atrium is in a posterior position. The aortic knob is in the normal left-sided position.

"Boot-shaped" heart
- Hallmark of Tetralogy of Fallot, due to right ventricular hypertrophy. The apical curvature of the left heart border is elevated "coeur en sabot" (Fig. 2-2a)

Mediastinal enlargement
- Technical factors causing width of mediastinum to appear exaggerated: patient positioning, antero-posterior (AP) projection or incomplete inspiration
- Pathological causes: aortic dissection, lymphadenopathy, thyroid, thymus, tumor

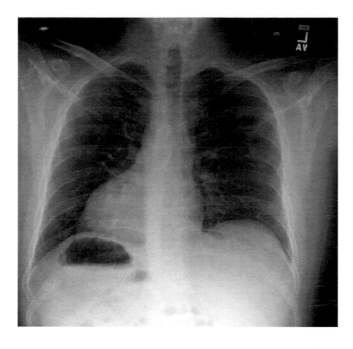

FIGURE 2-1

Dextrocardia with situs inversus. Frontal CXR demonstrating both the cardiac apical silhouette and gastric air bubble are on the *right side*. Note the "L" marker on the *upper right* hand corner signifying left

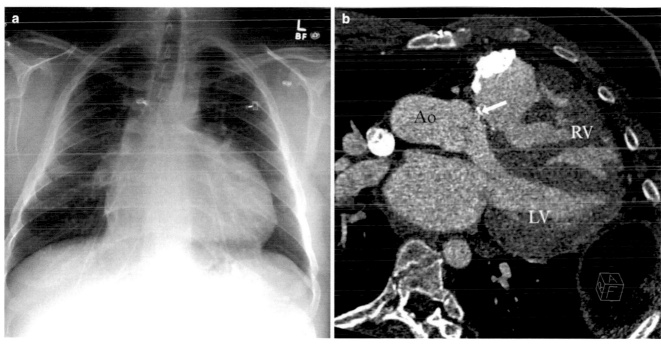

FIGURE 2-2

Tetralogy of Fallot. (**a**) CXR showing elevation of the apical curvature of the left heart border known as "coeur en sabot". (**b**) Cardiac CT showing an overriding aorta (*Ao*), ventricular septal defect patch (*arrow*), and right ventricular (*RV*) hypertrophy. The pulmonary stenosis is not shown on this CT slice. *LV* left ventricle

Enlarged cardiac silhouette
- Pericardial effusion, left ventricular (LV) dilatation, LV aneurysm

Unequal hilar densities
- Rotated film, lymph nodes, tumor

Hilar enlargement
- Pulmonary hypertension, lymphadenopathy (tuberculosis, sarcoid, lymphoma)

Elevated hemidiaphragm
■ Loss of lung volume, phrenic nerve palsy (e.g. post coronary artery bypass graft [CABG] surgery), subpulmonic effusion, subphrenic abscess, diaphragmatic rupture (e.g. post trauma), hepatomegaly

Increased translucency in lung fields
■ Pneumothorax (absent vascular markings with visible lung border), pulmonary hypertension, pulmonary emboli, hyperinflation and bullous changes in chronic obstructive pulmonary disease

Cardiopulmonary Abnormalities/Diseases on CXR

Heart Failure
■ Cardiomegaly
■ Kerley A lines: long (2–6 cm), unbranching lines seen coursing diagonally towards the hila caused by distension of anastomotic channels between peripheral and central lymphatics of the lungs. Kerley A lines are not seen without Kerley B or C lines.
■ Kerley B lines: thickened interlobular septa visible as short linear opacities (1 2 cm) in the subpleural regions indicative of interstitial pulmonary edema
■ Kerley C lines: seen as fine reticular opacities which may represent anastomotic lymphatics or superimposition of many Kerley B lines. Kerley C lines do not reach the pleura and do not course radially away from the hila
■ Peribronchial cuffing due to edema of the bronchial walls and peribronchial connective tissues
■ Poor distinction of lower lobe pulmonary vessels
■ Greater caliber of upper lobe vessels to lower lung zones
■ Pulmonary hila become enlarged and hazy
■ Bilateral patchy alveolar infiltrates (bat's wing appearance)

  – Pleural effusions
  – Chronic left atrial (LA) hypertension results in pulmonary hypertensive changes, right ventricular (RV) dilatation.

■ LA enlargement

  – Straightening of LA appendage segment between level of the main pulmonary artery and LV on the left heart border, double density to the right of the spine on PA CXR with increasing LA enlargement, splaying of carina >90°.

Pulmonary embolism
■ Oligemia
■ "Westermark sign" a dilatation of the pulmonary vessels proximal to an embolism along with collapse of distal vessels, sometimes with a sharp cutoff
■ Hampton hump, a triangular or rounded pleural-based infiltrate with the apex pointed toward the hilum, suggestive of pulmonary infarction

Pulmonary hypertension
■ Gradual taper of caliber between dilated central and hilar pulmonary arteries and smaller peripheral vessels (Fig. 2-3), if secondary to left-to-right shunting, the peripheral shunt vessels branch and extend towards the lung periphery

Reduced pulmonary blood flow
■ Small caliber central and hilar pulmonary arterial branches, reduced pulmonary vascular markings, seen in Tetralogy of Fallot, pulmonary atresia with ventricular septal defect, Ebstein's anomaly, tricuspid atresia

Right ventricular hypertrophy
■ Right ventricle is a midline and anterior structure and thus does not form a cardiac border in the PA projection, however in RV hypertrophy the apex may be elevated from the diaphragm and the left lower cardiac contour may become more rounded

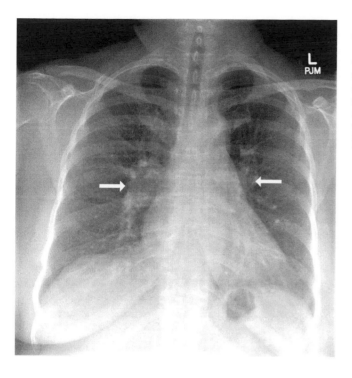

FIGURE 2-3

Pulmonary hypertension. CXR showing prominence of the main pulmonary artery and dilated left and right pulmonary arteries (*arrows*) associated with pruning of the peripheral pulmonary vasculature

Scimitar syndrome

■ Partial or total anomalous pulmonary venous return of the right lung veins to the inferior vena cava just above or below the diaphragm, frequently associated with right lung and right pulmonary artery hypoplasia

■ PA CXR: decrease in the size of the right thorax, shift of mediastinal structures and heart to the right, presence of anomalous vein "scimitar" as a vertical structure coursing towards the right cardiophrenic angle closely in parallel with the right atrial border

Pericardial Abnormalities

Pericardial Effusion

■ An abrupt asymmetrical change in the dimension of the cardiac silhouette without a change in the cardiac chamber size, larger effusions result in the appearance of a 'globular' shaped heart, 'fat pad' sign on lateral CXR is positive when an anterior pericardial stripe (separation by pericardial fluid between the pericardial fat posteriorly from the mediastinal fat anteriorly) is thicker than 2 cm

■ Echocardiography most commonly used to confirm the diagnosis

Pericardial calcification

■ Irregular calcification along the heart border, coexisting cardiac enlargement if large pericardial effusion (Fig. 2-4)

Pericardial cyst

■ Well demarcated, rounded mass more commonly near the right cardiophrenic border than the left cardiophrenic border, can have a pointed upper border, pericardial diverticulae changes contours and size during deep inspiration

Congenital absence of the pericardium

■ "Snoopy sign" with displacement of the LV and pulmonary artery towards the left side

Abnormalities of the Aorta

Calcification usually signifies degenerative intimal change, such as from atherosclerosis

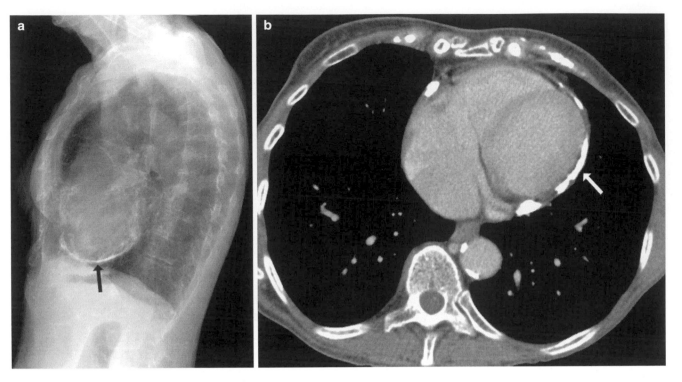

FIGURE 2-4

Pericardial calcification. (**a**) CXR and (**b**) CT image demonstrating calcification along the inferior cardiac border (*arrow*)

Coarctation
- "3" sign due to diminution of aortic arch segment with a concave notch in the proximal descending aorta and interruption of the descending aorta shadow distal to the coarctation, rib notching evident if retrograde collateral flow to the post-coarctation aorta by dilated intercostal arteries (Fig. 2-5a)

Thoracic aorta dilatation
- Increased curvature of the mid right heart border on PA projection or anterior aortic border on lateral projection suggest ascending aortic enlargement

Aortic dissection
- Prominent aortic arch from hypertension, atherosclerosis, connective tissue disorders, vasculitis, bicuspid aortic valve, blunt chest trauma or iatrogenic causes
- Abnormal if diameter >4 cm, focal pathological dilatation especially with widening of the arch beyond the origin of the left subclavian artery (Fig. 2-6a)
- Other CXR findings may include obliteration of the aortic knob, tracheal deviation, depression of the left main stem bronchus
- Pleural effusions, usually left sided, are associated with descending aortic dissection

Right-sided aortic arch
- The descending aorta typically runs parallel to the spine in continuity to the aortic arch on the left side on PA CXR, except in cases of a right sided aortic arch

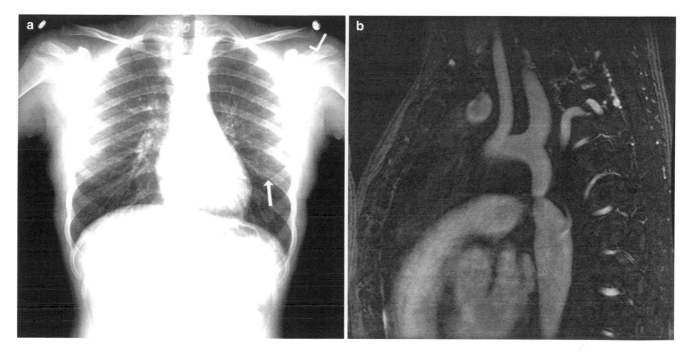

FIGURE 2-5

Aortic coarctation. (**a**) CXR showing left sided rib notching (*arrow*) due to retrograde collateral flow to the post-coarctation aorta by dilated intercostal arteries. (**b**) Cardiac Magnetic Resonance angiography demonstrating the aortic coarctation in the same patient

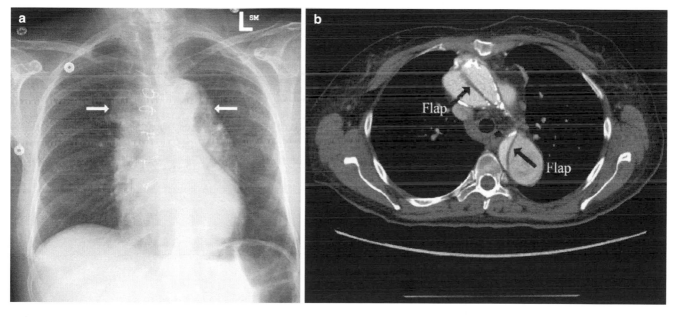

FIGURE 2-6

Aortic dissection. (**a**) CXR demonstrating a widened mediastinum (>4 cm, *white arrows*) in a patient with aortic dissection after blunt chest trauma. (**b**) Cardiac CT confirms a DeBakey Type 1 aortic dissection where the intimal tear/dissection flap (*black arrows*) originates in the ascending aorta and propagates to the aortic arch and descending aorta

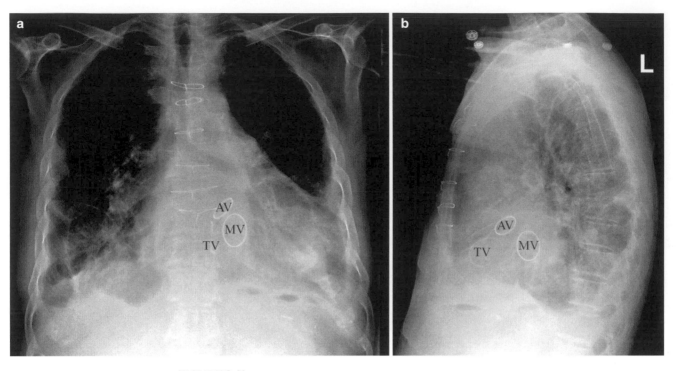

FIGURE 2-7

(**a**) Frontal and (**b**) Lateral CXR demonstrating the anatomic relationship of a patient with prosthetic aortic (*AV*) and mitral valve (*MV*) replacements and tricuspid valve (*TV*) annuloplasty ring. The AV is situated higher and is smaller and more anterior to the mitral valve on the lateral CXR. The TV annuloplasty ring is aligned medial-laterally and is positioned to the right of and below the AV

Identification of Valvular Prostheses on CXR (Fig. 2-7)

- Apart from homografts, prosthetic valves are radio-opaque
- Caged valves and heterografts: direction of flow is from the base ring to the struts
- Disc valves: the direction of flow is appreciated if the disc is seen in an open position

Aortic valve

- The opening of the valve ring is directed more vertically, facing obliquely and to the right, aortic valve is usually higher, smaller and more anterior to the mitral valve on lateral CXR, perceived direction of blood flow is towards the ascending aorta

Mitral valve

- Situated lower and more to the left than aortic valves, perceived direction of flow is towards the apex

Tricuspid valve

- Aligned in a medial-lateral direction, to the right of mitral valve and below the aortic valve

CARDIAC COMPUTED TOMOGRAPHY (CT)

Most current multi-detector CT scanners (64-, 256- and 320-slice scanners) have similar spatial resolution, however the increased detector slices and larger detector width allow more coverage of the heart in each heartbeat. Dual source CT scanners consist of two X-ray tube sources leading to improved temporal resolution to 75 ms. Spatial resolution is how close two objects can be discernible from each other. Temporal resolution is how fast an image could be acquired such that motion does not create image blurring, similar to the shutter speed of a camera.

ADVANTAGES OF CT	DISADVANTAGES OF CT
Rapid scan acquisition	Ionizing radiation
Excellent isotropic spatial resolution (XYZ plane)	Iodinated contrast complications e.g. extravasation, allergy, nephropathy
Compatible with metal devices	Metal devices causes beam hardening artifacts
Contrast able to be hemodialyzed	Diagnostic accuracy may be reduced by heart rate >70 beats per minute (bpm), irregular rhythm, severe coronary calcification, inability to sustain breath hold for at least 5–10 seconds
Allows arterial, venous and functional cardiac assessment	Less accurate assessment of coronary stents with diameter <3 mm

TABLE 2-1

ADVANTAGES AND DISADVANTAGES OF CARDIAC CT

CT SCAN MODE	SCAN TECHNIQUE	ADVANTAGES	DISADVANTAGES
Non-contrast enhanced scans			
Calcium score	Non-contrast scan where calcium (>130 Hounsfield Units) is detected	Non-contrast prognostic information	Does not assess stenosis severity or other plaque morphology (non-calcified or mixed plaques)
Contrast enhanced scans			
Non-ECG gated	Scan acquisition without ECG synchronization	More readily available scanners and technologists	Motion artifact
		Adequate for most aorta and pulmonary assessment	Not adequate for coronary or aortic root evaluation
Prospective ECG-triggered	Images acquired at a pre-defined set duration after the QRS complex	Radiation reduction as X-ray tube on only at pre-determined phase of the cardiac cycle	No functional assessment, potential for misregistration or slab artifacts if ectopy or heart rate variability
Retrospective ECG-gated	X-ray current continuously delivered throughout the cardiac cycle	Functional assessment Allows reconstruction at multiple points in the cardiac cycle	Higher radiation

TABLE 2-2

CT SCAN ACQUISITION MODES

Advantages and Disadvantages of Cardiac CT (Table 2-1)

CT Scan Acquisition Modes (Table 2-2)

Appropriate CT Indications

Appropriate CT indications: 2010 Appropriate use criteria for cardiac computed tomography [1].

A. **Indications for non-contrast coronary calcium score (CCS)**
    Risk assessment in _asymptomatic_ patients without known coronary artery disease (CAD):
    ■ At intermediate risk of CAD (correlates with 10-year absolute coronary heart disease [CHD] risk between 10 and 20 %)
    ■ At low risk of CAD (correlates with 10-year absolute CHD risk <10 %) with a family history of premature CAD

    – Patients with an Agatston score of >400 have a tenfold increased risk of cardiac events compared to a score of 0 [2]
    – The absence of calcium does not imply no significant coronary stenosis as 8–10 % of stenoses can be caused by non-calcified plaque.

FIGURE 2-8

Severe stenosis in the left anterior descending artery (*LAD*) due to non-calcified plaque (*arrow*). Curved multi-planar reformat cardiac CTA image in a patient presenting with acute chest pain and low-intermediate pre-test probability of acute coronary syndrome without elevated cardiac biomarkers or ischemic ECG changes

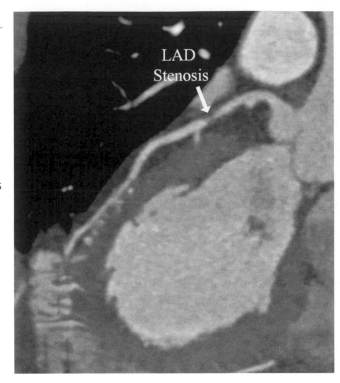

B. **Indications for CT angiography (CTA)**
    <u>Detection of CAD in *symptomatic* patients without known CAD who present with:</u>
    ■ **<u>Non acute symptoms</u>** (stable chest pain) possibly representing an ischemic equivalent with

    – intermediate pretest probability of CAD, or
    – low pretest probability of CAD with uninterpretable electrocardiogram (ECG) or unable to exercise

    ■ **<u>Acute symptoms</u>** with suspicion of acute coronary syndrome, low to intermediate pretest probability of CAD without high risk ECG changes or elevated cardiac biomarkers (Fig. 2-8)

    <u>Detection of CAD in other clinical scenarios</u>
    ■ Newly diagnosed clinical heart failure with no prior CAD and reduced LV ejection fraction (low to intermediate pretest probability of CAD)
    ■ Pre-operative coronary assessment prior to non-coronary cardiac surgery (intermediate pretest probability of CAD)

    <u>CTA in the setting of prior test results</u>
    ■ Prior normal ECG exercise testing with continued symptoms, prior Duke Treadmill score with intermediate risk findings
    ■ Discordant ECG exercise and imaging results, prior equivocal stress imaging procedure
    ■ Evaluation of new or worsening symptoms in the setting of past normal stress imaging study

    – Meta-analysis shows good diagnostic accuracy for detection of obstructive CAD (≥50 % stenosis) with sensitivity 98 % and specificity 88 % [3].
    – Due to high negative predictive values of 95–100 %, coronary CTA has been used to "rule out" obstructive CAD in chest pain patients with low to intermediate risk of CAD.
    – CT delayed enhancement: myocardial scar detectable on non-contrast delayed enhancement scans, good concordance regarding the presence of delayed

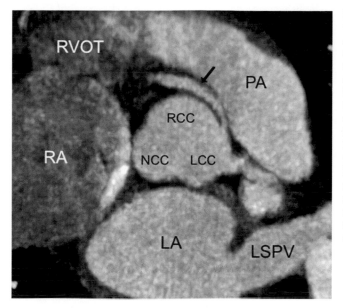

FIGURE 2-9

Anomalous right coronary artery with inter-arterial course. Cardiac CTA image demonstrating an anomalous right coronary artery (*arrow*) arising from the left coronary cusp (*LCC*) with an inter-arterial course between the aorta and pulmonary artery (*PA*). LA left atrium, *LSPV* left superior pulmonary vein, *NCC* non-coronary cusp, *RA* right atrium, *RCC* right coronary cusp, *RVOT* right ventricular outflow tract

enhancement in CT and cardiac magnetic resonance imaging (CMR) on a per-segment basis, though less accurate than CMR, and not clinical routine.

Post revascularization (coronary artery bypass graft surgery (CABG) or percutaneous coronary intervention)

■ Evaluation of graft patency after CABG in symptomatic patients

- CT ideal for graft assessment as high sensitivity (96 %), specificity (92 %) [4]
- Native coronary vessels are typically heavily calcified in this setting, limiting the diagnostic accuracy for stenosis evaluation

■ Localization of coronary bypass grafts and other retrosternal anatomy prior to reoperative chest or cardiac surgery
■ Evaluation of left main coronary stent (diameter >3 mm) in asymptomatic patients

Assessment of adult congenital heart disease

■ Coronary anomalies (Fig. 2-9)
■ Anomalies of thoracic arteriovenous or aortic vessels (aorto-venous fistulas, aortic coarctation)
■ Adult congenital heart disease (Figs. 2-2b and 2-10)

Assessment of ventricular morphology and function

■ If inadequate imaging from other noninvasive methods not requiring radiation (such as echocardiography or CMR):

- Evaluation of LV function following acute myocardial infarction or in heart failure patients
- Quantitative evaluation of RV size and function, assessment of RV morphology (focal aneurysm), in suspected arrhythmogenic RV dysplasia

Pre-procedural planning for electrophysiology procedures

■ Evaluation of pulmonary vein and LA anatomy (Fig. 2-11)

- Co-registration with electroanatomic mapping prior to pulmonary vein ablation
- Assessment for LA appendage thrombus (Fig. 2-12), but confirmation with transesophageal echocardiography still required

■ Evaluation of coronary vein anatomy such as prior to biventricular pacemaker implantation (Fig. 2-13)

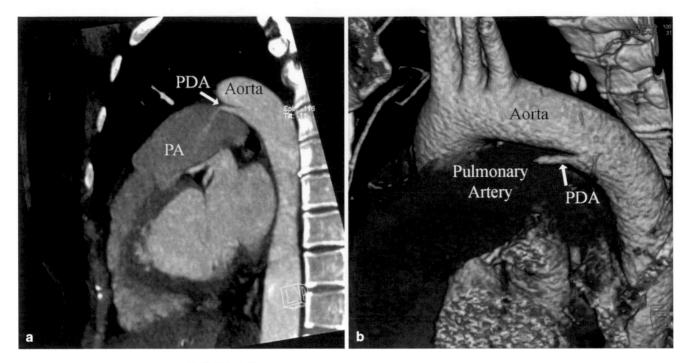

FIGURE 2-10

Patent ductus arteriosus (*PDA*). Cardiac CTA images (**a**, maximal intensity project; **b**, volume rendered image) demonstrating a PDA (*arrow*) with contrast traversing from the aorta to pulmonary artery (*PA*)

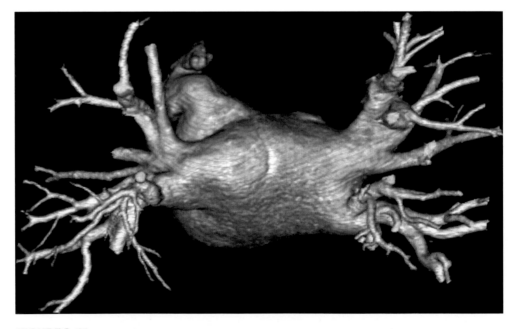

FIGURE 2-11

Pulmonary venous anatomy by CT prior to atrial fibrillation ablation. Volume rendered contrast-enhanced CT image showing the left atrium and pulmonary venous anatomy. This CT dataset is used to co-register with 3-dimensional electroanatomic map in the electrophysiology laboratory for atrial fibrillation ablation

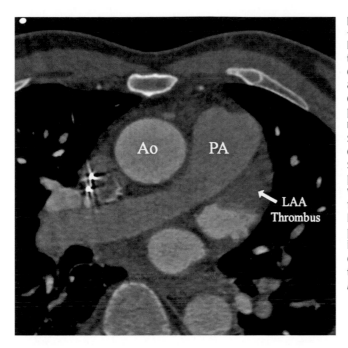

FIGURE 2-12

Left atrial appendage (*LAA*) thrombus. Contrast-enhanced cardiac CT shows a hypoattenuation filling defect in the LAA on arterial phase imaging, which may represent LAA thrombus or slow flow. A non-contrast delay scan (figure not shown) was subsequently performed within 1 min with persistence of the filling defect, suggesting a LAA thrombus. Transesophageal echocardiography is required for definitive confirmation of LAA thrombus. *Ao* aorta, *PA* pulmonary artery

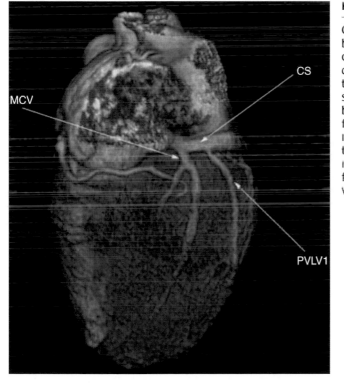

FIGURE 2-13

Coronary venous anatomy by contrast-enhanced cardiac CT. Volume rendered CT image showing the coronary venous system. CT venography may be used pre-procedurally to facilitate cardiac resynchronization therapy implantation. *CS* coronary sinus, *MCV* middle cardiac vein, *PVLV1* first posterior vein to the left ventricle

Evaluation of intra and extra cardiac structures

■ If other imaging techniques are inadequate, CT can be used for characterization of native and prosthetic cardiac valves, cardiac masses (tumors, thrombus)

  – CT is less sensitive for diagnosing valvular vegetations but useful for identifying paravalvular abscesses

■ Evaluation of pericardial anatomy

  – Pericardial effusions, thickening, fat, calcification (Fig. 2-4b), tumors, cysts
  – CMR and echocardiography for constrictive physiology assessment

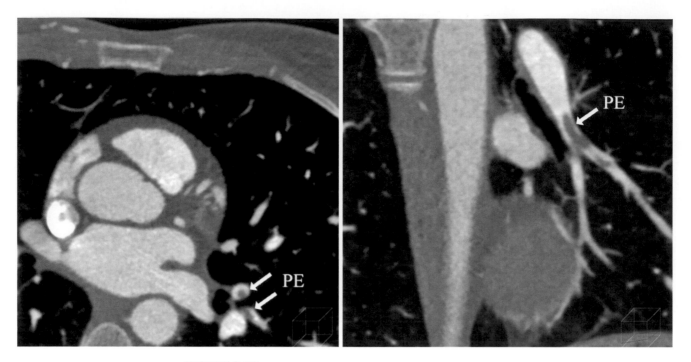

FIGURE 2-14

Pulmonary emboli (*PE*). Cardiac CTA images demonstrating the presence of PE (*arrows*) found incidentally in a patient presenting with acute chest pain

■ Diagnosis of other non-cardiac pathologies

– Thoracic aorta assessment: aortic aneurysm, dissection (Fig. 2-6b), thoracic trauma, tears, intramural hematoma, mediastinal hematomas
– Incidental findings: lung (pulmonary emboli (Fig. 2-14), pneumonia, nodules, effusion, atelectasis), liver (hemangiomas, cysts, tumor), bone (fractures, lytic lesions, degenerative disc disease), gastro-intestinal (hiatus hernia, esophageal thickening), mediastinal lymphadenopathy

Medications in CT

Beta-blockers
■ Given to reduce heart rate (HR), HR variability and ectopy to minimize motion artifact and allow accurate ECG-triggering (if HR >60–65 bpm)

Calcium channel blockers
■ Given if beta-blockers are contraindicated (in limited centers)

Sublingual nitroglycerin
■ If not contraindicated, it is administered for vasodilatory effects immediately prior to coronary CTA. Diagnostic accuracy is reduced if nitroglycerin is not given

Medications to avoid
■ Metformin due to small potential risk of lactic acidosis from acute kidney failure related to contrast dye administration. Hold for 48 hours following scan

CT Safety

Ionizing radiation
■ Adhere to the ALARA (As Low As Reasonably Achievable) principle regarding radiation with dose saving algorithms, minimization of repeated scans

■ **Stochastic effects**

– These effects occur by chance and are not dependent on the radiation dose received. An example is development of cancer in the future. There is also no lower threshold of radiation dose where it is certain that an adverse effect cannot occur.

■ **Non-stochastic or deterministic effects**

– These effects are directly related to the radiation dose received. For example, a large radiation dose may result in skin burns, hair loss, cataracts, sterility, gastrointestinal syndrome (e.g. ulcers), or hematopoietic syndrome (e.g. bone marrow suppression). There is a clear relationship between radiation dose and effect.

Side-effects related to iodinated contrast
■ **Tissue extravasation**

– Watch for compartment syndrome and infection

■ **Allergy**

– Resulting in skin reactions (itch, rash) or anaphylaxis – prior history of mild contrast reaction (hives or less) requires premedication with steroid and anti-histamine prior to contrast administration

■ **Contrast Induced Nephropathy**

– Occurs when there is a temporal relationship between deterioration of renal function and the administration of intravenous contrast, in the absence of any other etiology
– It can be defined as either a >25 % increase of serum creatinine or an absolute increase in serum creatinine of 0.5 mg/dL after a radiographic examination using a contrast agent
– This condition occurs in <2 % of patients, is very unlikely in patients with normal renal function (estimate Glomerular Filtration Rate >60 mL/min/1.73 m^2), typically occurs 48 hours post contrast, persists for 2–5 days and resolves by 7 10 days [5]

CARDIAC MAGNETIC RESONANCE (CMR) IMAGING

■ CMR imaging uses magnetic and radiofrequency fields to generate signals from hydrogen
■ The typical magnetic field strength used for clinical CMR are 1.0, 1.5 and 3.0 Tesla

Advantages and Disadvantages of CMR (Table 2-3)

ADVANTAGES OF CMR	DISADVANTAGES OF CMR
High spatial (XY plane) and temporal resolution	Scanner availability and imager expertise
Imaging less affected by body habitus	Claustrophobia
No ionizing radiation	Contraindicated in patients with foreign metallic objects in eye or brain, Starr-Edwards mechanical valve, and most pacemakers and implanted defibrillators
Images can be acquired in any tomographic plane	Long image acquisition time
	Gadolinium associated nephrogenic systemic fibrosis

TABLE 2-3

ADVANTAGES AND DISADVANTAGES OF CMR

CMR Scan Sequences

Dark Blood Imaging
- Flowing blood appears dark while slow moving structures such as myocardium is bright. T2 weighted images are sensitive to water content and will be represented as high signal in areas of acute injury such as myocarditis and infarction.

Bright blood Imaging
- Allows acquisition of cine images for assessment of cardiac function. Steady state free precession technique is commonly used for this purpose

Phase-contrast
- Allows measurement of velocity and quantification of blood flow

Perfusion
- Contrast agents such as gadolinium (Gd), which shortens T1 relaxation time, can be imaged as it transits through cardiac structures

MR angiography
- Allows 3-dimensional examination of complex cardiac and vascular structures

Late gadolinium enhancement
- Delayed hyperenhancement of Gd (~10 min after administration) is seen in areas of myocardial necrosis and fibrosis

CMR Indications [6]

Ischemic Heart disease
- Vasodilator perfusion or dobutamine stress function CMR in symptomatic patients with intermediate pre-test probability of CAD with uninterpretable ECG or cannot exercise
- Stress perfusion to detect CAD can be performed with first-pass Gd perfusion imaging
- Meta-analysis of 1,516 patients demonstrated perfusion imaging with CMR has a sensitivity 91 %, specificity 83 % in detecting CAD (≥50 % stenosis) [7]
- CMR parameters (LV ejection fraction, aortic flow, delayed enhancement) is incremental to perfusion data for predicting adverse outcomes [8]

Viability
- Degree of transmurality of late myocardial Gd enhancement is associated with the degree of myocardial viability [9]
- Myocardial segments with >50 % transmural enhancement have a low likelihood of functional recovery after revascularization [10]

Cardiomyopathy
- CMR can provide accurate measurements of biventricular function, volume, and tissue characterization for diagnosis, management, and prognosis
- It is appropriate to quantify LV function with CMR if echocardiographic imaging is technically limited or discordant with prior tests
- Ischemic cardiomyopathy: The pattern of late Gd enhancement is subendocardial and may be transmural with its location in a specific coronary artery distribution (Table 2-4)

Myocarditis
- The presence of two CMR criteria for myocarditis has a sensitivity of 67 % and specificity of 91 % for the diagnosis of myocarditis [11]

  - Late Gd enhancement is typically subepicardial (focal or widespread)
  - Increased T2 signal suggesting myocardial edema (regional or global, Fig. 2-15)
  - Early global relative Gd enhancement indicating myocardial hyperemia and capillary leakage (Fig. 2-16)

CARDIOMYOPATHY	LV DISTRIBUTION	REGION	PROGNOSIS
Ischemic	Subendocardial, extending to transmural	Coronary artery distribution	>50 % transmural=low likelihood of segmental functional recovery after revascularization
HCM	Midwall	Patchy, interventricular septum, interventricular junction	Independently associated with adverse outcome
Dilated	Midwall	Usually septal	Predicts death, CV hospitalization, VT
Myocarditis	Midwall, subepicardial	Variable Parvovirus B19: Lateral Herpes Virus 6: Septum	If lasting >4 weeks associated with poor outcome
Amyloidosis	Subendocardial	Global (if subendocardial), Patchy	Variable, predicts HF severity, ± death
Sarcoidosis	Any (frequently midwall at the RV insertion site at the LV inferoseptum)	Any pattern	9 fold ↑ adverse events 11.5 fold ↑ cardiac death
Anderson-Fabry	Epicardial/midwall	Basal Inferolateral	Unknown
Endomyocardial fibrosis	Subendocardial	Inflow tract, apex	Increased mortality Hazard Ratio 10.8
Chagas disease	Epicardial/midwall	Inferolateral/apex	Unknown

CV cardiovascular, *HCM* hypertrophic cardiomyopathy, *HF* heart failure, *LV* left ventricular, *RV* right ventricular, *VT* ventricular tachycardia

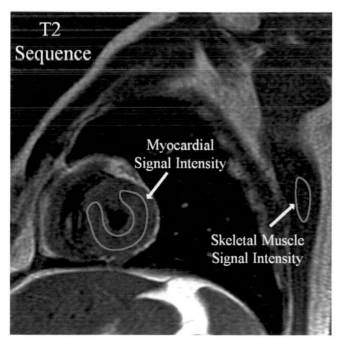

FIGURE 2-15

CMR T2 assessment for myocarditis. Offline measurement for increased global T2 myocardial enhancement corrected for skeletal muscle, which is one parameter for assessment of myocarditis

Sarcoidosis

- Presence of late Gd enhancement can be in any distribution (Fig. 2-17) and is associated with subsequent adverse cardiac events [12]
- CMR has a sensitivity of 100 % (78–100 %) and specificity of 78 % (64–89 %) with an overall accuracy of ~80 % in diagnosing cardiac sarcoidosis [13]

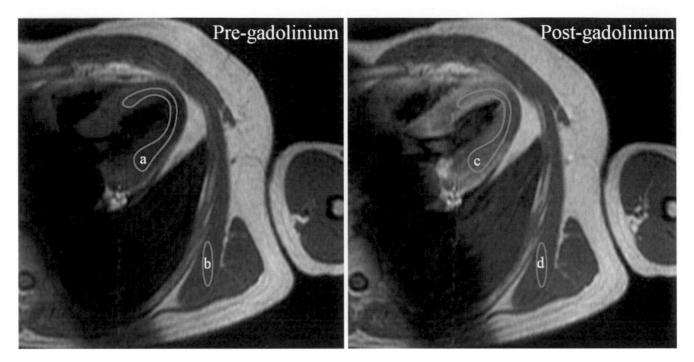

FIGURE 2-16

CMR early global relative gadolinium (Gd) assessment for myocarditis. Offline measurement comparing the pre- and post-Gd images. The ratios of pre-Gd myocardial: skeletal muscle (*a/b*) are compared to the post-Gd myocardial: skeletal muscle (*c/d*) signal intensities

FIGURE 2-17

Cardiac sarcoidosis. CMR delayed enhancement of the left ventricular short-axis at the mid-ventricular level showing patchy, myocardial scarring in the inferior septum (*arrow*) in a patient with known systemic sarcoidosis

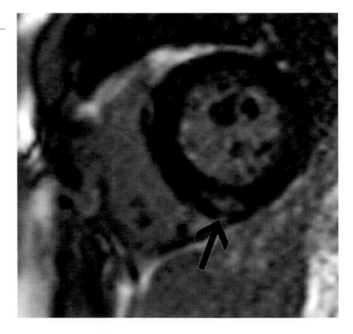

Amyloidosis
■ Global subendocardial left and right ventricular late Gd enhancement is the typical finding on CMR and is similar to the histological distribution of amyloid protein (Fig. 2-17) [14]

Hypertrophic cardiomyopathy
■ CMR able to identify increased regional wall thickness not appreciated on other imaging techniques as well as accurate quantification of LV mass
■ Various patterns of late Gd enhancement are identified in patients with hypertrophic cardiomyopathy (Fig. 2-18) and are shown to be associated with adverse prognosis [15]

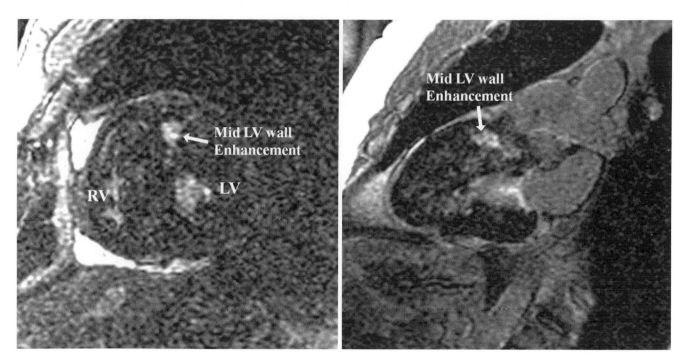

FIGURE 2-18

Hypertrophic cardiomyopathy with midwall delay gadolinium enhancement of the left ventricle (*LV*) which is associated with increased risk for sudden cardiac death. Note the thick myocardial wall. *RV* right ventricle

Hemochromatosis

■ T2* measurement of myocardium on CMR can be used to identify subjects with cardiac involvement in hemochromatosis, with a T2* of less than 20 ms is associated with LV systolic dysfunction [16]

Arrhythmogenic Right Ventricular Dysplasia

■ Quantitative evaluation of RV size and function, assessment of RV morphology (focal aneurysm) in suspected arrhythmogenic RV dysplasia

■ Fatty deposition and fibrosis in the RV by CMR are not part of the modified Task Force criteria [17]

Non-compaction cardiomyopathy

■ A diastolic ratio of non compacted to compacted myocardium of greater than 2.3 has a sensitivity of 86 % and specificity of 99 % for diagnosing non compaction cardiomyopathy [18]

Congenital Heart Disease

■ Quantification of LV and RV mass, volume and ejection fraction

■ Quantification of valvular disease

■ Assessment of great vessels, coronary anomalies, flow through surgical conduits

■ Specific indications for CMR in congenital heart disease

– Shunt size (Qp/Qs) calculation with phase contrast imaging

– Assessing anomalous pulmonary and systemic venous return

– Aortic abnormalities such as coarctation (Fig. 2-5b), aortic aneurysm

– Pulmonary artery abnormalities i.e. pulmonary atresia, stenosis

– Systemic to pulmonary collaterals

– Complex congenital disease assessment and follow-up post surgery i.e. post atrial/arterial switch operation for transposition of great arteries, Fontan operations and post-Tetralogy of Fallot repair

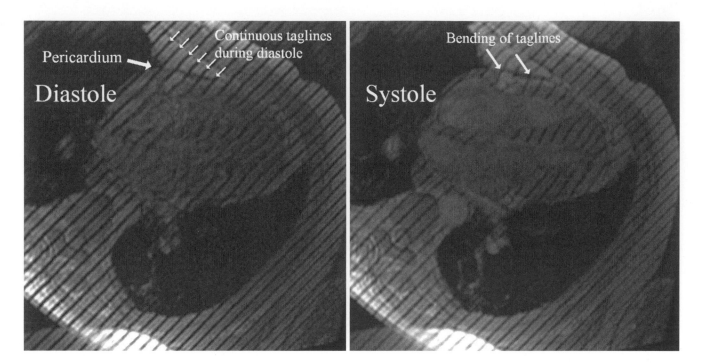

FIGURE 2-19

Pericardial constriction. Tagging CMR sequences showing unbroken taglines over the pericardium during ventricular diastole and *bending* of taglines over the pericardium during systole suggesting pericardial adhesions

Cardiac Tumors
- CMR is an excellent imaging modality for visualization and characterization of cardiac masses
- The main advantage of CMR includes better contrast resolution, multiplanar capability, ability to assess functional impact of the tumor, tissue characterization and detection of vascularity of the tumor with first pass perfusion imaging
- Differentiating intracardiac thrombus from tumor and benign from malignant cardiac masses is an important strength of CMR

Pericardial disease [19]
- Assessment of pericardial disease such as pericardial mass and pericardial constriction
- Features of pericardial constriction on CMR (thickened pericardium ≥4 mm, paradoxical motion of the interventricular septum, lack of normal breaking of tag lines on tagging sequence during cardiac contraction due to shear motion between visceral and parietal pericardium (Fig. 2-19), calcified pericardium)

Valvular heart disease
- If other forms of imaging such as echocardiography is technically limited, CMR can assess valvular function
- Qualitative assessment of regurgitant and stenotic jets can be seen on cine CMR
- Quantitative assessment of stenosis can be measured by planimetry or using phase contrast sequences to determine peak velocity across the valve
- Regurgitant volume and fraction can be assessed by phase contrast sequences (determining the forward and reverse flow) or by assessing the differences in RV and LV stroke volume.

Evaluation of pulmonary vein and left atrial (LA) anatomy
- Co-registration with electroanatomic mapping prior to pulmonary vein ablation

CMR Safety

- The use of Gd in end-stage renal patients is associated with a rare but serious complication of *nephrogenic systemic fibrosis*, which results in fibrosis of skin overlying the extremities and truck and deeper structures including muscle, lung and heart
- Ferromagnetic implants may lead to complications with CMR and should be screened prior to CMR [20]
- It is generally recommended a waiting period of about 6 weeks post implantation of weakly ferromagnetic devices such as cardiac valves and stents before CMR
- CMR in patients with pacemakers and implantable cardioverter-defibrillators can potentially lead to heating of the tip of the lead, inhibiting pacing output, activating tachyarrhythmia therapy or damage to the device
- CMR-compatible pacemaker systems have recently become available, although their use is currently limited

REVIEW QUESTIONS

1. **According to the 2010 appropriate use criteria for cardiac computed tomography; which of the following is false?**
   (a) It is appropriate to perform a CT calcium score in an asymptomatic patient with intermediate pretest probability of coronary artery disease
   (b) It is appropriate to perform CT angiography in an asymptomatic patient with intermediate pretest probability of coronary artery disease
   (c) It is appropriate to perform CT angiography in a patient with acute chest pain and intermediate pretest probability of coronary artery disease with normal ECG and cardiac biomarkers
   (d) It is appropriate to perform CT angiography for risk assessment in an asymptomatic patient with prior 3.5 mm left main stent
   (e) It is appropriate to perform CT angiography in a symptomatic patient with intermediate pretest probability of coronary artery disease with interpretable ECG and able to exercise

2. **What artificial valve is shown in this CXR (Fig. 2-20)?**
   (a) Mechanical mitral valve
   (b) Mechanic aortic valve
   (c) Bioprosthetic aortic valve
   (d) Mechanical tricuspid valve
   (e) Bioprosthetic mitral valve

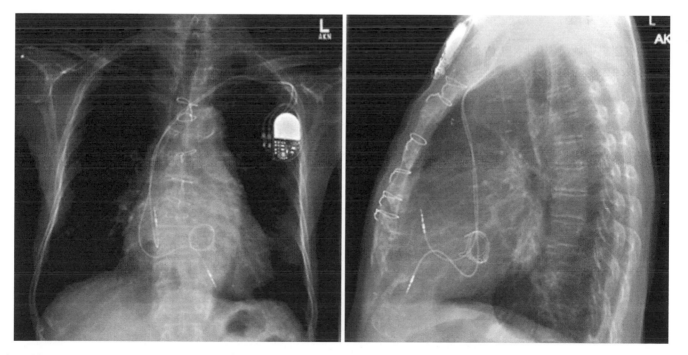

FIGURE 2-20

3. A 59 year old man who presented with symptoms of heart failure after mediastinal irradiation for Hodgkin lymphoma undergoes CMR. Which of the following feature is NOT consistent with pericardial constriction on CMR?
    (a) Pericardial thickness ≥4 mm
    (b) Left ventricular myocardial trabeculation ratio >2.3
    (c) Lack of normal breaking of tag lines during cardiac contraction
    (d) Pericardial calcification
    (e) Septal flattening on early diastolic filling

4. Which of the following complications does not occur with CT angiography?
    (a) Nephrogenic systemic fibrosis
    (b) Anaphylaxis
    (c) Compartment syndrome of the arm
    (d) Contrast induced nephropathy
    (e) Bradycardia

5. Which of the following is a stochastic effect from ionizing radiation?
    (a) Radiation burns
    (b) Cancer
    (c) Permanent sterility
    (d) Radiation sickness
    (e) Cataracts

6. A 52 year old woman with hypertension and dyslipidemia presents to the emergency department with worsening chest discomfort on minimal exertion. Her ECG was non-diagnostic and two sets of troponin were negative. She underwent coronary CTA. This image (Fig. 2-21) demonstrates:
    (a) Anomalous left coronary artery arising from the right Sinus of Valsalva with an interarterial course
    (b) Severe aortic regurgitation due to aortic dissection
    (c) Severe stenosis in the mid right coronary artery
    (d) Sinus venosus atrial septal defect
    (e) Unroofed coronary sinus

7. A 60 year old man with Type II diabetes on metformin and hypertension presents with dyspnea and impaired left ventricular systolic function on echocardiography. Based on the delayed gadolinium enhancement on CMR (Fig. 2-22), what is the most likely cause of the systolic dysfunction?
    (a) Myocarditits
    (b) Amyloid
    (c) Previous left anterior descending artery territory myocardial infarction
    (d) Previous right coronary artery territory myocardial infarction
    (e) Constrictive pericarditis

8. A 35 year old man with back pain has the above finding on CT (Fig. 2-24), which of the following is false?
    (a) He may have an autosomal dominant genetic disorder
    (b) He may have a diastolic and systolic murmur on examination

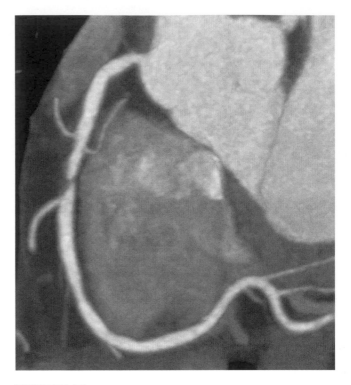

FIGURE 2-21

    (c) He requires urgent surgical consultation
    (d) He has non-compaction of the left ventricle
    (e) He may have a mutation of the transforming growth factor beta receptor 1

9. A 47 year old man presents for CTA to investigate first presentation of intermittent chest discomfort. He is a current smoker and has a past history of Type II diabetes on Metformin, dyslipidemia on Atorvastatin, erectile dysfunction on vardenafil and benign prostatic hypertrophy. On examination his heart rate is 79 bpm, he has a harsh ejection systolic murmur which becomes louder with the Valsalva maneuver and clear lung fields. Which of the following is not advised when performing CTA for this patient?
    (a) Withhold Metformin for 48 hours post CTA
    (b) Administration of metoprolol to achieve heart rate of 60–65 bpm
    (c) Administration of iodinated contrast for the coronary CTA
    (d) Administration of sublingual nitrates for coronary vasodilation to improve CTA accuracy
    (e) All the above can be advised or given

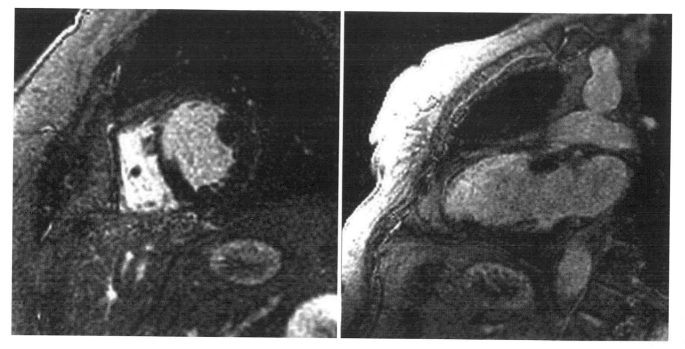

FIGURE 2-22

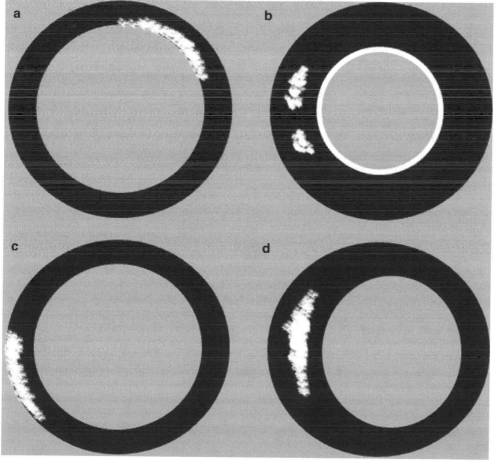

FIGURE 2-23

Distribution of late gadolinium enhancement in various cardiac conditions. (**a**) Ischemic (subendocardial enhancement), (**b**) Amyloid (global subendocardial enhancement), (**c**) Myocarditis (subepicardial enhancement), (**d**) Hypertrophic cardiomyopathy (mid wall enhancement)

19. Bogaert J, Francone M. Cardiovascular magnetic resonance in pericardial diseases. J Cardiovasc Magn Reson. 2009;11:14.

20. Levine GN, Gomes AS, Arai AE, Bluemke DA, Flamm SD, Kanal E, et al. Safety of magnetic resonance imaging in patients with cardiovascular devices: an American Heart Association scientific statement from the Committee on Diagnostic and Interventional Cardiac Catheterization, Council on Clinical Cardiology, and the Council on Cardiovascular Radiology and Intervention: endorsed by the American College of Cardiology Foundation, the North American Society for Cardiac Imaging, and the Society for Cardiovascular Magnetic Resonance. Circulation. 2007;116(24):2878–91.

CHAPTER 3

Pradeep Natarajan, Farouc A. Jaffer, and Marc S. Sabatine

Acute Coronary Syndrome

CHAPTER OUTLINE

ABBREVIATIONS

ACC	American College of Cardiology
ACE	Angiotensin-converting enzyme
ACS	Acute coronary syndrome
ADP	Adenosine diphosphate
AHA	American Heart Association
AKI	Acute kidney injury
aPTT	Activated partial thromboplastin time
ARB	Angiotensin receptor blocker
AS	Aortic stenosis
ASA	Aspirin
AV	Atrioventricular
BMS	Bare metal stent
CABG	Coronary artery bypass graft
CAD	Coronary artery disease
CCS	Canadian Cardiovascular Society
CHF	Congestive heart failure
CP	Chest pain
CPR	Cardiopulmonary resuscitation
CVA	Cerebrovascular accident
DAPT	Dual antiplatelet therapy
DES	Drug-eluting stent
DM	Diabetes mellitus
ECG	Electrocardiogram
GIB	Gastrointestinal bleeding
GP IIb/IIIa	Glycoprotein IIb/IIIa
HR	Heart rate
HTN	Hypertension
ICH	Intracranial hemorrhage
IV	Intravenous
LBBB	Left bundle branch block
LDL-C	Low density lipoprotein cholesterol
LMWH	Low molecular weight heparin
LV	Left ventricle
LVEF	Left ventricular ejection fraction
MACE	Major adverse cardiovascular events
MI	Myocardial infarction
MR	Mitral regurgitation
NSTEMI	Non-ST-elevation myocardial infarction
NTG	Nitroglycerin

OR	Odds ratio
PAD	Peripheral arterial disease
PCI	Percutaneous coronary intervention
PMN	Polymorphonuclear neutrophil
PO	Per os
PTCA	Percutaneous transluminal coronary angioplasty
RV	Right ventricle
SBP	Systolic blood pressure
SC	Subcutaneous
STEMI	ST-elevation myocardial infarction
TIA	Transient ischemic attack
Tn	Troponin
UA	Unstable angina
UFH	Unfraction heparin
VSR	Ventricular septal rupture
VT	Ventricular tachycardia

INTRODUCTION

Coronary artery disease is a major cause of mortality and morbidity in the United States and worldwide. In 2010, the American Heart Association reported that 17.6 million individuals in the United States had coronary artery disease and 8.5 million had a myocardial infarction.

DIAGNOSIS (See Table 3-1)

TABLE 3-1

LIKELIHOOD THAT SIGNS AND SYMPTOMS REPRESENT AN ACS SECONDARY TO CAD

FEATURE	HIGH LIKELIHOOD	INTERMEDIATE LIKELIHOOD	LOW LIKELIHOOD
	Any of the following:	Absence of high-likelihood features and presence of any of the following:	Absence of high- or intermediate-likelihood features but may have:
History	Chest or left arm pain, pressure, or tightness as chief symptom reproducing prior documented angina	Chest or left arm pain, pressure, or tightness as chief symptom Age >70 years	Possible ischemic symptoms in absence of any of the intermediate likelihood characteristics
	Known history of CAD, including MI	Male sex DM	Recent cocaine use
Exam	Transient MR murmur, hypotension, diaphoresis, pulmonary edema, or rales	Extracardiac vascular disease	Chest discomfort reproduced by palpation
ECG	New, or presumably new, transient ST-segment deviation (1 mm or greater) or T-wave inversion in multiple precordial leads	Fixed Q waves ST depression 0.5 to 1 mm or T-wave inversions >1 mm	T-wave flattening or inversion <1 mm in leads with dominant R waves Normal ECG
Cardiac markers	Elevated cardiac TnI, TnT, or CK-MB	Normal	Normal

Adapted from Anderson et al. [2]
ACS acute coronary syndrome, *CAD* coronary artery disease, *CK-MB* creatine kinase-MB, *DM* diabetes mellitus, *ECG* electrocardiogram, *MI* myocardial infarction, *MR* mitral regurgitation, *TnI* troponin I, *TnT* troponin T

History and Physical Examination (See Chap. 1)

■ There is often a broad range in the type of presenting pain and associated symptoms, particularly in women, older patients, young patients, diabetics, and those with renal insufficiency.

■ Substernal chest pain, pressure, or tightness typically occurs at rest or with increasing frequency for >20 min with often some relief to nitroglycerin. It may radiate to the neck, arms, shoulder, and/or jaws. Ischemic chest discomfort is often associated with dyspnea, diaphoresis, nausea, and/or vomiting [1–7].

■ Physical exam features that suggest a high likelihood of acute coronary syndrome (ACS) include diaphoresis, hypotension, transient mitral regurgitation (MR), and pulmonary edema.

■ Differential diagnosis of chest pain [1].

- Acute coronary syndrome
- Non-atherosclerotic coronary causes: dissection, spasm, embolism.
- Other cardiovascular: aortic dissection, pericarditis, myocarditis, stress-mediated cardiomyopathy, pulmonary embolism, pulmonary hypertension
- Gastrointestinal: esophageal (gastroesophageal reflux, esophageal spasm, esophagitis), gastric (gastritis, peptic ulcer disease), biliary (cholecystitis, cholelithiasis), pancreatitis
- Musculoskeletal: trauma, costochondritis, Tietze syndrome (inflammation of costal cartilages), fibromyalgia
- Pulmonary: pneumonia, malignancy, pneumothorax, pleuritis, pleural effusion
- Neuropathic: herpes zoster, postherpetic neurolagia, radiation, radiculopathy
- Psychiatric: panic disorder, hypochondriasis, malingering

Electrocardiogram

■ Normal ECG (electrocardiogram) carries a favorable prognosis but does not rule out ACS. Nearly 50 % of patients presenting with UA (unstable angina)/NSTEMI (non-ST-elevation myocardial infarction) have a normal or unchanged ECG [2].

■ UA/NSTEMI: new T wave inversions >0.2 mV and ≥0.05 mV ST depressions are suggestive [2].

■ STEMI (ST-elevation myocardial infarction): New ST elevations in ≥2 contiguous leads ≥0.2 mV in men or ≥0.15 mV in women in leads V2–V3 and/or ≥0.1 mV in other leads; new LBBB (left bundle branch block) is suggestive [6].

- Posterior MI (myocardial infarction): ST depression V1 and V2 (particularly if horizontal ST depression with upright T wave and tall R wave) and/or ST elevation V7–V9 (sensitivity 57 %, specificity 98 %) [8].

    ■ Approximately 4 % of acute MI patients have isolated posterior ST elevations; detecting the presence is important since it qualifies for acute reperfusion therapy.

- RV (right ventricular) MI: ST elevation ≥1 mm in V1 (sensitivity 28 %, specificity 92 %), and/or V_4R (sensitivity 93 %, specificity 95 %) [9].

Cardiac Biomarkers

■ Cardiac troponins are the preferred biomarker in an acute ACS [1, 10].

- A negative test early after symptom onset does not exclude an MI.
- A negative test by 6 h after symptom onset is often sufficient to exclude an MI but if the clinical suspicion is high, the test should be repeated at 8–12 h after symptom onset [11].
- High-sensitivity troponin assays: Improve early diagnosis and sensitivity particularly over the first 3 h at the potential expense of specificity (i.e. elevations due to non-ACS causes of myocyte injury) [12].

■ CK-MB (creatine kinase-MB) mass to CK (creatine kinase) activity ratio ≥2.5 indicates a myocardial source of CK-MB [10].

RISK STRATIFICATION

Estimating Risk

■ Early risk stratification, particularly in UA/NSTEMI, ensures prompt appropriate therapy. (see Table 3-2)

■ Risk-stratification models such as TIMI (see Table 3-3), GRACE, or PURSUIT models may be helpful in assisting with management strategies [13].

■ UA/NSTEMI acute coronary syndromes with increased risk (ie TIMI risk score ≥3), particularly those with ST depressions and/or elevated cardiac biomarkers, should be managed with an initial invasive approach (See section "Initial Conservative vs Invasive Strategy") [2, 3, 7].

TABLE 3-2

SHORT-TERM RISK OF DEATH OR NONFATAL MI IN PATIENTS WITH UA/NSTEMI (ACC/AHA 2007)

FEATURE	HIGH RISK	INTERMEDIATE RISK	LOW RISK
	At least 1 of the following features must be present:	*No high-risk features but must have 1 of the following:*	*No high- or intermediate-risk feature but may have any of the following features:*
History	Accelerating tempo of ischemic symptoms in preceding 48 h	Prior MI, PAD, CVA, or CABG Prior ASA use	
Character of pain	Prolonged ongoing (>20 min) rest pain	Prolonged (>20 min) rest angina, now resolved, with moderate or high likelihood of CAD Rest angina (>20 min) or relieved with rest or sublingual NTG Nocturnal angina New-onset or progressive CCS class III or IV angina in the past 2 weeks without prolonged (>20 min) rest pain but with intermediate or high likelihood of CAD	Increased angina frequency, severity, or duration Angina provoked at a lower threshold New onset angina with onset 2 weeks to 2 months prior to presentation
Clinical findings	Pulmonary edema, most likely due to ischemia New or worsening MR murmur S3 or new/worsening rales Hypotension, bradycardia, tachycardia Age >75 years	Age >70 years	
ECG	Angina at rest with transient ST-segment changes >0.5 mm Bundle-branch block, new or presumed new Sustained VT	T wave changes Pathological Q waves or resting ST-depression <1 mm in multiple lead groups	Normal or unchanged ECG
Cardiac markers	Elevated cardiac TnT, TnI, or CK-MB	Slightly elevated cardiac TnT, TnI, or CK-MB	Normal

Adapted from Anderson et al. [2]
ASA aspirin, *CABG* coronary artery bypass graft surgery, *CCS* Canadian Cardiovascular Society, *CK*-MB creatine kinase-MB, *CVA* cerebrovascular accident, *ECG* electrocardiogram, *MI* myocardial infarction, *MR* mitral regurgitation, *NTG* nitroglycerin, *PAD* peripheral arterial disease, *TnI* troponin I, *TnT* troponin T, *VT* ventricular tachycardia

[handwritten: TIMI]

TABLE 3-3

Risk factor (each worth 1 point)	
Age ≥65 years	
≥3 CAD risk factors	
Known CAD (stenosis ≥50 %)	
ASA use in past 7 days	
≥2 anginal episodes within past 24 h	
ST segment deviation ≥0.5 mm	
Elevated cardiac biomarkers	

TIMI RISK SCORE (UA/NSTEMI)

ASA aspirin, *CAD* coronary artery disease [13]

[handwritten notes: A = age >65; M = marker (+), mb/Tn-I; E = ECG Δ ≥.5 mm; R = Risk factors (≥3 RF); I = Ischemia (CP) ≥2 (24hr); h/o CAD (≥50% or h/o PCI); A = ASA use (last 7 days)]

GENERAL ANTI-ISCHEMIC THERAPIES

General

■ Bedrest, oxygen, morphine for analgesia [2–6].

Nitrates

■ These agents can treat initial or recurrent angina, improve symptoms of pulmonary congestion, and decrease blood pressure in hypertensive patients.
■ Caution in RV MI, severe AS (aortic stenosis), hypovolemia; contraindicated if concomitant phosphodiesterase inhibitor use [1].

Beta Blockers   *[handwritten: —only use ORAL, not IV]*

■ There is limited data for use in UA/NSTEMI but there is clear benefit in STEMI, recent MI, non-decompensated CHF (congestive heart failure), and stable angina so oral beta-blockers are recommended for all ACS unless there are clear contraindications (e.g. bradycardia, marked first or second degree AV block, active wheezing, signs of congestive heart failure or low-output state, or increased risk for cardiogenic shock (including SBP [systolic blood pressure] <100 mmHg, HR [heart rate] <60 bpm or >110 bpm, age >70 years, or delayed presentation) [2–6, 14].
■ Intravenous beta blockers may be used in hypertensive patients without contraindications.
■ Caution in the setting of cocaine toxicity.

[handwritten: BB uc/i: 1/2/3 HB, HypoTen'n, Decompensated CHF, low output state, shock.]

Calcium Channel Blockers *[handwritten: —Don't use IR. Dihydropyridine - Nifedipine (ok to use non-dihydropyridine like diltiazem-verapamil) (Do not use Nifedipine - Imm. Release Dihydropyridine)]*

■ When beta-blockers are contraindicated for non-cardiac reasons, a nondihydropyridine calcium channel blocker (e.g. diltiazem or verapamil) should be given instead [2, 5, 15, 16].
■ Immediate-release dihydropyridine calcium channel blockers (e.g. nifedipine) should not be administered [17].

UNSTABLE ANGINA/NSTEMI (See Fig. 3-1)

Initial Conservative vs Invasive Strategy

■ An initial conservative strategy involves maximizing medical therapy with anticoagulation, antiplatelets, beta-blockers, and nitrates and, if patients remain symptom-free, exercise testing is performed. Coronary angiography is limited to patients with persistence of symptoms, symptom recurrence, high risk stress test features, or systolic dysfunction [2, 3, 7].
■ An initial invasive strategy involves the same initial maximal medical therapy with prompt catheterization once the patient has stabilized, with revascularization as appropriate [2, 3, 7, 18].

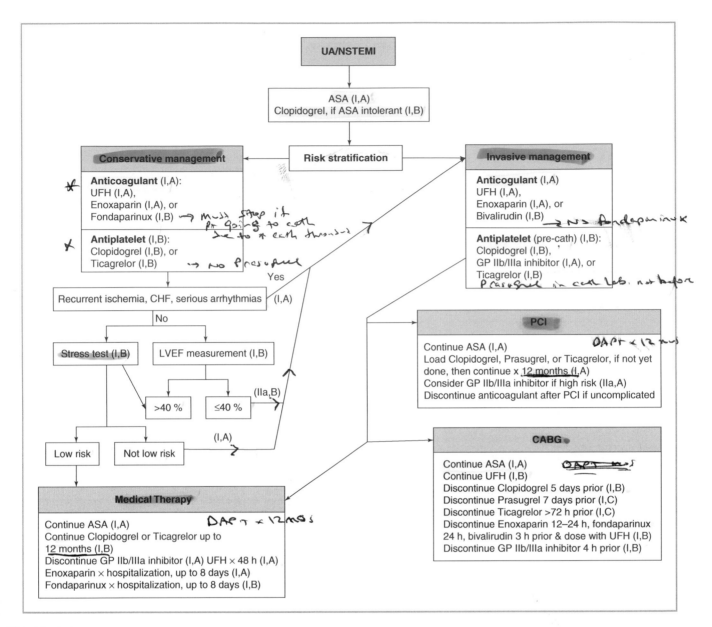

FIGURE 3-1

Algorithm for UA/NSTEMI management. Risk stratification assists in determining the major branchpoint is management strategy. Regardless of strategy, dual antiplatelet therapy in addition to an anticoagulant is recommended. Patients who are initially managed conservatively should undergo further non-invasive testing for additional risk stratification then referred for angiography if indicated and appropriate

■ An initial invasive is recommended in patients with intermediate to high risk of recurrent events (i.e. those with recurrent angina/ischemia, elevated cardiac biomarkers, new ST segment depression, CHF or new/worsening MR [mitral regurgitation], hemodynamic instability, sustained VT [ventricular tachycardia], LVEF [left ventricular ejection fraction]<0.40, PCI [percutaneous coronary intervention] within 6 months, or high risk score) barring contraindications.

■ For patients at high risk for clinical events, angiography within 24 h appears to be acceptable and others may go in 2–3 days unless there is a clinical change [18–20].

■ Low-risk patients without ischemia at low activity level for 12–24 h may undergo non-invasive stress testing. If there are subsequent high-risk findings, then proceed to coronary angiography barring contraindications [2, 3].

Antiplatelet Drugs

■ **Aspirin**

- ASA (aspirin) reduces MACE (major adverse cardiovascular events) by 46–51 % [21].
- Current U.S. guidelines recommend 162–325 mg crushed/chewed × 1 then 75–100 mg daily thereafter if medically managed [2–7].

    ■ Although prior guidelines recommended maintenance therapy of 162–325 mg for several months for patients with DES (drug-eluting stent), the latest guidelines note it is reasonable to use 81 mg daily [7, 22].
    ■ In those receiving ticagrelor, the ASA dosing should be 75–100 mg daily [7, 23]. Consider using non-enteric coated ASA to avoid "pseudoresistance".

■ **ADP (Adenosine Diphosphate) Receptor Blockers**

- An agent in this class should be given in addition to ASA regardless of whether the patient is medically managed or undergoes PCI. Given the risk of CABG (coronary artery bypass graft surgery)-related and non-CABG-related bleeding, the decision for ADP receptor blocker administration prior to coronary angiography must be weighed by the likelihood of emergency CABG and risk of bleeding [1, 3, 6, 7].

- **Clopidogrel**

    ■ Loading with 300 mg then administering 75 mg daily along with ASA results in a 20 % reduction in MACE by 9 months, with effects as early as 24 h [24, 25].
    ■ Compared to a 300 mg loading dose, a 600 mg loading dose achieves the greatest antiplatelet activity within 2-3 h and is recommended if angiography and revascularization is planned that day [7].

        - In CURRENT-OASIS 7, double-dose clopidogrel (600 mg load, 150 mg daily × 7 days, then 75 mg daily) compared to standard dosing in those undergoing PCI resulted in a decrease in MI and stent thrombosis but an increase in bleeding [22].

    ■ In medically treated patients, clopidogrel should be administered for at least 1 month, and ideally 12 months.
    ■ In PCI patients, clopidogrel should be administered for at least 12 months; 1 month is mandatory for BMS (bare metal stent) but 12 months is still preferred in the setting of the recent ACS.
    ■ In patients undergoing CABG, clopidogrel should be held for at least 5 days prior to surgery.
    ■ Although 20–25 % of patients are resistant to standard clopidogrel doses, optimal clopidogrel dosing based on individual genotyping and platelet reactivity testing has not yet been established, although studies show poorer outcomes in those with clopidogrel-resistance.

- **Prasugrel**

    ■ This agent has a more rapid onset of action with higher levels of platelet inhibition and more reliable inhibition compared to clopidogrel [1].
    ■ Since optimal clopidogrel dosing based on genotyping or platelet reactivity testing has not been validated, alternative ADP receptor blockade for those with clopidogrel resistance is reasonable.
    ■ The TRITON-TIMI 38 trial demonstrated that, compared with clopidogrel, prasugrel 60 mg loading and 10 mg daily thereafter resulted in decreased death/MI/stroke in ACS patients with planned PCI. However, there was increased non-surgical, surgical, and fatal bleeding [26].

S2 without extra heart sounds. CBC, LFTs, electrolytes, renal function, PT/INR, PTT are normal. Troponin is elevated at 0.1 ng/mL and ECG shows normal sinus rhythm and no notable abnormalities. Aspirin 325 mg, clopidogrel 300 mg, and UFH IV are administered. She ultimately proceeds to coronary angiography where she is found to have a focal 90 % mid-right coronary artery lesion with minimal left anterior descending artery and left circumflex artery luminal irregularities. She successfully undergoes stenting of the lesion with an everolimus-eluting stent. ASA is continued at 81 mg daily and clopidogrel is continued at 75 mg daily. Which of the following changes to her antiplatelet regimen would have further reduced her risk of cardiovascular mortality?

(a) Increase maintenance ASA to 325 mg daily.
(b) Increase clopidogrel regimen to 600 mg loading, 150 mg daily × 7 days, then 75 mg daily
(c) Change clopidogrel to ticagrelor 180 mg loading then 90 mg twice daily.
(d) Change to prasugrel 60 mg loading (when the decision for PCI was made) then 10 mg daily.
(e) None of the above.

3. A 36 year-old woman who is 36 weeks pregnant presents to the emergency department with chest pain. Her pregnancy thus far has only been complicated by gestational diabetes which she has been able to manage with diet. She reports just over 3 h of substernal chest pain without radiation but with associate dyspnea. Past medical history and family history are unremarkable. She is only taking a prenatal vitamin. Upon triage, her temperature is 37 °C, heart rate 92 bpm, blood pressure 152/90 mmHg (on both arms), respiratory rate 16/min, O_2 saturation 100 % on room air. Her chest discomfort has improved with nitroglycerin sublingual but it persists and she appears uncomfortable. Jugular venous pressure does not appear elevated and she has normal cardiac and lung sounds. Her triage ECG is shown below. Which of the following is correct regarding the next steps in management?

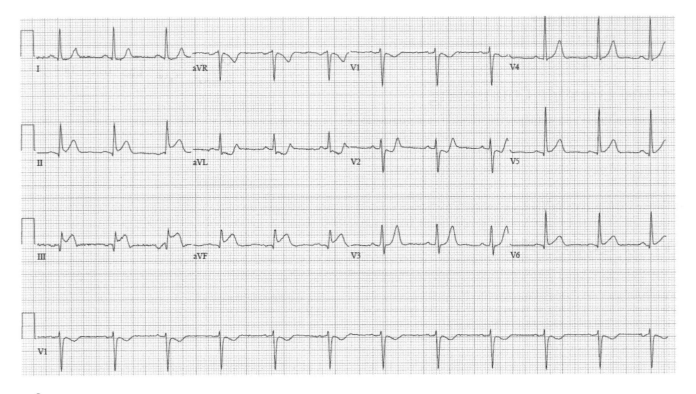

(a) She should be promptly taken to the cardiac catheterization with a planned <90 min door-to-balloon time.
(b) Alteplase should be immediately administered.
(c) An initial conservative approach without initial PCI or fibrinolysis is preferred.
(d) Aspirin should not be administered.
(e) The baby should be emergently delivered then the patient should immediately be taken to cardiac catheterization.

4. A 50 year-old man presents to the emergency department with chest pain. While having an emotional argument with his wife, he suddenly developed left-sided substernal chest pain that radiated to his left jaw with associated diaphoresis and shortness of breath. He took aspirin 325 mg at home and called emergency medical services. Upon arrival of emergency services, the patient's pain improved with two tablets of sublingual nitroglycerin but mild discomfort and dyspnea persisted. He has never seen a physician as an adult and takes no medications regularly. He smokes one pack of cigarettes daily for the past 25 years. Upon arrival to the emergency department, his temperature is 37.6 °C, heart rate 92 bpm, blood pressure 174/98 (similar in both arms), respiratory rate 20/min, and oxygen saturation 88 % on room air that corrects to 96 % with 4 L nasal cannula. He appears uncomfortable and mildly tachypneic. Jugular venous pressure is estimated at 10 cm H_2O. Lung fields are notable for crackles halfway up bilaterally. Cardiac exam reveals regular rate and rhythm, normal S1 and S2, and an S4 is heard without murmurs. Extremities reveal good distal pulses and are warm without peripheral edema.

ECG is shown below. He was promptly taken to the cardiac catheterization lab where he was found to have a 99 % mid-LAD lesion with TIMI-2 flow without other significant coronary artery disease. Prasugrel 60 mg was administered and a sirolimus-eluting stent was successfully placed. An echocardiogram showed a left ventricular EF of 45 % with mid-anterior, mid-anteroseptal, and anteroapical hypokinesis. Which of the following is NOT TRUE?

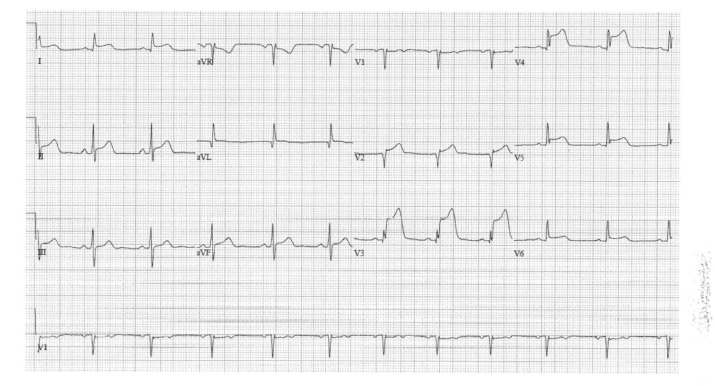

(a) An angiotensin converting enzyme (ACE) inhibitor should be started.

(b) Atorvastatin 80 mg daily is recommended.

(c) Smoking cessation counseling is recommended.

(d) He should remain on a thienopyridine for at least 12 months.

(e) A repeat TTE in 40 days is recommended to evaluate his candidacy for an ICD for primary prevention of sudden cardiac death.

ANSWERS

1. (c) This scenario depicts a gentleman who presents with an NSTEMI with frequent recurrent angina but currently without ongoing ischemic symptoms. His TIMI risk score of UA/NSTEMI is 3 and by the ACC/AHA 2007 classification, he is in the high risk category. Thus, the data supports an early invasive strategy, ideally within the first 24 h for high risk individuals according to the TIMACS trial. Fibrinolysis is not recommended for the management of NSTEMI. Since he will likely proceed to coronary angiography soon, fondaparinux would not be the best choice given the risk of catheter thrombosis and angiography/PCI should not proceed without the co-administration of UFH. In this scenario, clopidogrel should be administered; given his high risk presentation with recent recurrent rest angina, a load of 600 mg (as opposed to 300 mg) is reasonable given the potential for more urgent PCI of his ischemic symptoms recur on medical therapy before planned angiography so this is the correct answer. In the FRAXIS trial, nadroparin did not have an advantage compared to UFH with respect to MACE but there was increased major hemorrhage in those receiving nadroparin; the current data on LMWH for UA/NSTEMI does not support the use of agents other than enoxaparin in this class. Given the results of the ACUITY trial, bivalirudin should not be administered with a GP IIb/IIIa inhibitor given the increased risk of bleeding without a further reduction in ischemic events; however, bivalirudin alone is an appropriate alternative to the combination of UFH and GP IIb/IIIa inhibition given the reduced risk of bleeding.

2. (c) In this case, a woman with coronary artery disease risk factors presents with an NSTEMI and is found to have focal single-vessel coronary disease and undergoes successful PCI. The continuation of ASA 325 mg after the initial loading in patients with uncomplicated stenting is not required and does not contribute to significantly improved clinical outcomes. A strategy of double-dose clopidogrel as delineated in the CURRENT-OASIS 7 trial reduced MI and stent thrombosis in those undergoing PCI but there was no overall difference in MACE or mortality. The PLATO trial demonstrated a reduction in both cardiovascular and all-cause mortality with ticagrelor compared to clopidogrel and so this is the answer. Prasugrel, compared with clopidogrel, reduced MACE but a reduction in cardiovascular mortality was not demonstrated in the TRITON – TIMI 38 trial. due to ↑ bleed

3. (a) Risk factors for MI in pregnancy include age (>30 years), obesity, diabetes mellitus, hypertension, smoking, antiphospholipid antibody syndrome. The most common etiologies include underlying coronary atherosclerosis and associated thrombosis, and also coronary artery dissection. Coronary artery dissection is most common in the third trimester and within the first 1–2 month post-partum secondary to progesterone-mediated endothelial changes, increased eosinophil proteases, and diminished prostacyclin expression. The management of choice for STEMI in pregnancy is PCI. Given the relatively high rate of coronary artery dissection, coronary angiography should be performed very cautiously. Fibrinolytics are relatively contraindicated in pregnancy, particularly if labor and delivery are imminent or have happened recently. If possible, an initial conservative approach is preferred for NSTEMI with non-invasive evaluation but reperfusion therapy, similar to non-pregnant patients, is critical for STEMI management. Low doses (81–162 mg of aspirin, particularly in the second and third trimester have been found to be safe and antiplatelet therapy is important in the management of ACS in these patients. The patient would likely not tolerate the added physiologic stress of child birth in the setting of an STEMI and emergent delivery is not indicated for the purposes of managing her STEMI.

4. (e) This is a gentleman who presents with a STEMI and Killip class II symptoms. Given his systolic dysfunction and associated congestive heart failure, he meets indications for an ACE inhibitor. A high potency statin, such as atorvastatin 80 mg daily, should be administered for his acute coronary syndrome. Further risk factor management, such as smoking cessation, is critical prior to discharge. Current guidelines recommend dual antiplatelet therapy for a minimum of 12 months after the placement of a drug-eluting stent and there are ongoing studies that are evaluating this further. Given his current EF of >35 %, routine reassessment of his EF soon after discharge for the purposes of ICD placement for primary prevention is not recommended.

REFERENCES

1. Antman EM. ST-segment elevation myocardial infarction: pathology, pathophysiology, and clinical features. In: Libby P, Bonow RO, Mann DL, Zipes DP, editors. Braunwald's heart disease: a textbook of cardiovascular medicine. 8th ed. Philadelphia: Saunders; 2008. p. 1087–110.

2. Anderson JL, Adams CD, Antman EM, Bridges CR, Califf RM, Casey Jr DE, et al. ACC/AHA 2007 guidelines for the management of patients with unstable Angina/non-ST-Elevation myocardial infarction: a report of the American College of Cardiology/American Heart Association Task Force on Practice Guidelines (Writing Committee to Revise the 2002 Guidelines for the Management of Patients With Unstable Angina/Non-ST-Elevation Myocardial Infarction) developed in collaboration with the American College of Emergency Physicians, the Society for Cardiovascular Angiography and Interventions, and the Society of Thoracic Surgeons endorsed by the American Association of Cardiovascular and Pulmonary Rehabilitation and the Society for Academic Emergency Medicine. J Am Coll Cardiol. 2007;50(7):e1–157.

3. Wright RS, Anderson JL, Adams CD, Bridges CR, Casey Jr DE, Ettinger SM, et al. 2011 ACCF/AHA focused update of the Guidelines for the Management of Patients with Unstable Angina/Non-ST-Elevation Myocardial Infarction (updating the 2007 guideline): a report of the American College of Cardiology Foundation/American Heart Association Task Force on Practice Guidelines developed in collaboration with the American College of Emergency Physicians, Society for Cardiovascular Angiography and Interventions, and Society of Thoracic Surgeons. J Am Coll Cardiol. 2011;57(19):1920–59.

4. Antman EM, Anbe DT, Armstrong PW, Bates ER, Green LA, Hand M, et al. ACC/AHA guidelines for the management of patients with ST-elevation myocardial infarction–executive summary: a report of the American College of Cardiology/American Heart Association Task Force on Practice Guidelines (Writing Committee to Revise the 1999 Guidelines for the Management of Patients With Acute Myocardial Infarction). Circulation. 2004;110(5):588–636.

5. Antman EM, Hand M, Armstrong PW, Bates ER, Green LA, Halasyamani LK, et al. 2007 Focused Update of the ACC/AHA 2004 Guidelines for the Management of Patients With ST-Elevation Myocardial Infarction: a report of the American College of Cardiology/American Heart Association Task Force on Practice Guidelines: developed in collaboration With the Canadian Cardiovascular Society endorsed by the American Academy of Family Physicians: 2007 Writing Group to Review New Evidence and Update the ACC/AHA 2004 Guidelines for the Management of Patients With ST-Elevation Myocardial Infarction, Writing on Behalf of the 2004 Writing Committee. Circulation. 2008;117(2):296–329.

6. American College of Emergency Physicians; Society for Cardiovascular Angiography and Interventions, O'Gara PT, Kushner FG, Ascheim DD, Casey DE Jr, et al. 2013 ACCF/AHA guideline for the management of ST-elevation myocardial infarction: a report of the American College of Cardiology Foundation/American Heart Association Task Force on Practice Guidelines. J Am Coll Cardiol. 2013;61(4):e78–140.

7. Levine GN, Bates ER, Blankenship JC, Bailey SR, Bittl JA, Cercek B, et al. 2011 ACCF/AHA/SCAI Guideline for Percutaneous Coronary Intervention: a report of the American College of Cardiology Foundation/American Heart Association Task Force on Practice Guidelines and the Society for Cardiovascular Angiography and Interventions. Circulation. 2011;124(23):e574–651.

8. Brady WJ, Erling B, Pollack M, Chan TC. Electrocardiographic manifestations: acute posterior wall myocardial infarction. J Emerg Med. 2001;20(4):391–401.

9. Roth A, Miller HI, Kaluski E, Keren G, Shargorodsky B, Krakover R, et al. Early thrombolytic therapy does not enhance the recovery of the right ventricle in patients with acute inferior myocardial infarction and predominant right ventricular involvement. Cardiology. 1990;77(1):40–9.

10. Zimmerman J, Fromm R, Meyer D, Boudreaux A, Wun CC, Smalling R, et al. Diagnostic marker cooperative study for the diagnosis of myocardial infarction. Circulation. 1999;99(13):1671–7.

11. Reichlin T, Irfan A, Twerenbold R, Reiter M, Hochholzer W, Burkhalter H, et al. Utility of absolute and relative changes in cardiac troponin concentrations in the early diagnosis of acute myocardial infarction. Circulation. 2011;124(2):136–45.

12. Keller T, Zeller T, Ojeda F, Tzikas S, Lillpopp L, Sinning C, et al. Serial changes in highly sensitive troponin I assay and early diagnosis of myocardial infarction. JAMA. 2011;306(24):2684–93.

13. Antman EM, Cohen M, Bernink PJ, McCabe CH, Horacek T, Papuchis G, et al. The TIMI risk score for unstable angina/non-ST elevation MI: a method for prognostication and therapeutic decision making. JAMA. 2000;284(7):835–42.

14. Chen ZM, Pan HC, Chen YP, Peto R, Collins R, Jiang LX, et al. Early intravenous then oral metoprolol in 45,852 patients with acute myocardial infarction: randomised placebo-controlled trial. Lancet. 2005;366(9497):1622–32.

15. The effect of diltiazem on mortality and reinfarction after myocardial infarction. The Multicenter Diltiazem Postinfarction Trial Research Group. N Engl J Med. 1988;319(7):385–92.

16. Effect of verapamil on mortality and major events after acute myocardial infarction (the Danish Verapamil Infarction Trial II--DAVIT II). Am J Cardiol. 1990;66(10):779–85.

17. Goldbourt U, Behar S, Reicher-Reiss H, Zion M, Mandelzweig L, Kaplinsky E. Early administration of nifedipine in suspected acute myocardial infarction. The Secondary Prevention Reinfarction Israel Nifedipine Trial 2 Study. Arch Intern Med. 1993;153(3):345–53.

18. Boden WE, O'Rourke RA, Crawford MH, Blaustein AS, Deedwania PC, Zoble RG, et al. Outcomes in patients with acute non-Q-wave myocardial infarction randomly assigned to an invasive as compared with a conservative management strategy. Veterans Affairs Non-Q-Wave Infarction Strategies in Hospital (VANQWISH) Trial Investigators. N Engl J Med. 1998;338(25):1785–92.

19. Mehta SR, Granger CB, Boden WE, Steg PG, Bassand JP, Faxon DP, et al. Early versus delayed invasive intervention in acute coronary syndromes. N Engl J Med. 2009;360(21):2165–75.

20. Montalescot G, Cayla G, Collet JP, Elhadad S, Beygui F, Le Breton H, et al. Immediate vs delayed intervention for acute coronary syndromes: a randomized clinical trial. JAMA. 2009;302(9):947–54.

21. Antithrombotic Trialists' Collaboration. Collaborative meta-analysis of randomised trials of antiplatelet therapy for prevention of death, myocardial infarction, and stroke in high risk patients. BMJ. 2002;324(7329):71–86.

22. CURRENT-OASIS 7 Investigators. Dose comparisons of clopidogrel and aspirin in acute coronary syndromes. N Engl J Med. 2010; 363(10):930–42.

23. Wallentin L, Becker RC, Budaj A, Cannon CP, Emanuelsson H, Held C, et al. Ticagrelor versus clopidogrel in patients with acute coronary syndromes. N Engl J Med. 2009;361(11):1045–57.

24. Yusuf S, Zhao F, Mehta SR, Chrolavicius S, Tognoni G, Fox KK, et al. Effects of clopidogrel in addition to aspirin in patients with acute coronary syndromes without ST-segment elevation. N Engl J Med. 2001;345(7):494–502.

25. Mehta SR, Yusuf S, Peters RJ, Bertrand ME, Lewis BS, Natarajan MK, et al. Effects of pretreatment with clopidogrel and aspirin followed by long-term therapy in patients undergoing percutaneous coronary intervention: the PCI-CURE study. Lancet. 2001;358(9281): 527–33.

26. Wiviott SD, Braunwald E, McCabe CH, Montalescot G, Ruzyllo W, Gottlieb S, et al. Prasugrel versus clopidogrel in patients with acute coronary syndromes. N Engl J Med. 2007;357(20):2001–15.

27. Inhibition of platelet glycoprotein IIb/IIIa with eptifibatide in patients with acute coronary syndromes. The PURSUIT Trial Investigators. Platelet Glycoprotein IIb/IIIa in Unstable Angina: Receptor Suppression Using Integrilin Therapy. N Engl J Med. 1998;339(7):436–43.

28. Inhibition of the platelet glycoprotein IIb/IIIa receptor with tirofiban in unstable angina and non-Q-wave myocardial infarction. Platelet Receptor Inhibition in Ischemic Syndrome Management in Patients Limited by Unstable Signs and Symptoms (PRISM-PLUS) Study Investigators. N Engl J Med. 1998;338(21):1488–97.

29. Cohen M, Demers C, Gurfinkel EP, Turpie AG, Fromell GJ, Goodman S, et al. A comparison of low-molecular-weight heparin with unfractionated heparin for unstable coronary artery disease. Efficacy and Safety of Subcutaneous Enoxaparin in Non-Q-Wave Coronary Events Study Group. N Engl J Med. 1997;337(7):447–52.

30. Antman EM, McCabe CH, Gurfinkel EP, Turpie AG, Bernink PJ, Salein D, et al. Enoxaparin prevents death and cardiac ischemic events in unstable angina/non-Q-wave myocardial infarction. Results of the thrombolysis in myocardial infarction (TIMI) 11B trial. Circulation. 1999;100(15):1593–601.

31. Blazing MA, de Lemos JA, White HD, Fox KA, Verheugt FW, Ardissino D, et al. Safety and efficacy of enoxaparin vs unfractionated heparin in patients with non-ST-segment elevation acute coronary syndromes who receive tirofiban and aspirin: a randomized controlled trial. JAMA. 2004;292(1):55–64.

32. Ferguson JJ, Califf RM, Antman EM, Cohen M, Grines CL, Goodman S, et al. Enoxaparin vs unfractionated heparin in high-risk patients with non-ST-segment elevation acute coronary syndromes managed with an intended early invasive strategy: primary results of the SYNERGY randomized trial. JAMA. 2004;292(1):45–54.

33. Stone GW, McLaurin BT, Cox DA, Bertrand ME, Lincoff AM, Moses JW, et al. Bivalirudin for patients with acute coronary syndromes. N Engl J Med. 2006;355(21):2203–16.

34. Fifth Organization to Assess Strategies in Acute Ischemic Syndromes Investigator. Comparison of fondaparinux and enoxaparin in acute coronary syndromes. N Engl J Med. 2006;354(14):1464–76.

35. Mega JL, Braunwald E, Wiviott SD, Bassand JP, Bhatt DL, Bode C, et al. Rivaroxaban in patients with a recent acute coronary syndrome. N Engl J Med. 2012;366(1):9–19.

36. Bär FW, Verheugt FW, Col J, Materne P, Monassier JP, Geslin PG, et al. Thrombolysis in patients with unstable angina improves the angiographic but not the clinical outcome. Results of UNASEM, a multicenter, randomized, placebo-controlled, clinical trial with anistreplase. Circulation. 1992;86(1):131–7.

37. Hochman JS, Sleeper LA, Webb JG, Sanborn TA, White HD, Talley JD, et al. Should we emergently revascularize occluded coronaries for cardiogenic shock. N Engl J Med. 1999;341(9):625–34.

38. Svilaas T, Vlaar PJ, van der Horst IC, Diercks GF, de Smet BJ, van den Heuvel AF, et al. Thrombus aspiration during primary percutaneous coronary intervention. N Engl J Med. 2008;358(6):557–67.

39. Randomised trial of intravenous streptokinase, oral aspirin, both, or neither among 17,187 cases of suspected acute myocardial infarction: ISIS-2. ISIS-2 (Second International Study of Infarct Survival) Collaborative Group. Lancet. 1988;2(8607):349–60.

40. Thrombolysis in Myocardial Ischemia (TIMI 3A) investigators. Early effects of tissue-type plasminogen activator added to conventional therapy on the culprit coronary lesion in patients presenting with ischemic cardiac pain at rest. Results of the Thrombolysis in Myocardial Ischemia (TIMI IIIA) Trial. Circulation. 1993;87(1):38–52.

41. Gershlick AH, Stephens-Lloyd A, Hughes S, Abrams KR, Stevens SE, Uren NG, et al. Rescue angioplasty after failed thrombolytic therapy for acute myocardial infarction. N Engl J Med. 2005;353(26):2758–68.

42. Assessment of the Safety and Efficacy of a New Treatment Strategy with Percutaneous Coronary Intervention (ASSENT-4 PCI) investigators. Primary versus tenecteplase-facilitated percutaneous coronary intervention in patients with ST-segment elevation acute myocardial infarction (ASSENT-4 PCI): randomised trial. Lancet. 2006;367(9510): 569–78.

43. Sabatine MS, Cannon CP, Gibson CM, López-Sendón JL, Montalescot G, Theroux P, et al. Effect of clopidogrel pretreatment before percutaneous coronary intervention in patients with ST-elevation myocardial

infarction treated with fibrinolytics: the PCI-CLARITY study. JAMA. 2005;294(10):1224–32.

44. Sabatine MS, Cannon CP, Gibson CM, López-Sendón JL, Montalescot G, Theroux P, et al. Addition of clopidogrel to aspirin and fibrinolytic therapy for myocardial infarction with ST-segment elevation. N Engl J Med. 2005;352(12):1179–89.

45. Chen ZM, Jiang LX, Chen YP, Xie JX, Pan HC, Peto R, et al. Addition of clopidogrel to aspirin in 45,852 patients with acute myocardial infarction: randomised placebo-controlled trial. Lancet. 2005; 366(9497):1607–21.

46. Mehilli J, Kastrati A, Schulz S, Früngel S, Nekolla SG, Moshage W, et al. Abciximab in patients with acute ST-segment-elevation myocardial infarction undergoing primary percutaneous coronary intervention after clopidogrel loading: a randomized double-blind trial. Circulation. 2009;119(14):1933–40.

47. Stone GW, Witzenbichler B, Guagliumi G, Peruga JZ, Brodie BR, Dudek D, et al. Bivalirudin during primary PCI in acute myocardial infarction. N Engl J Med. 2008;358(21):2218–30.

48. Antman EM, Morrow DA, McCabe CH, Murphy SA, Ruda M, Sadowski Z, et al. Enoxaparin versus unfractionated heparin with fibrinolysis for ST-elevation myocardial infarction. N Engl J Med. 2006;354(14):1477–88.

49. Cohen M, Gensini GF, Maritz F, Gurfinkel EP, Huber K, Timerman A, et al. The safety and efficacy of subcutaneous enoxaparin versus intravenous unfractionated heparin and tirofiban versus placebo in the treatment of acute ST-segment elevation myocardial infarction patients ineligible for reperfusion (TETAMI): a randomized trial. J Am Coll Cardiol. 2003;42(8):1348–56.

50. Yusuf S, Mehta SR, Chrolavicius S, Afzal R, Pogue J, Granger CB, et al. Effects of fondaparinux on mortality and reinfarction in patients with acute ST-segment elevation myocardial infarction: the OASIS-6 randomized trial. JAMA. 2006;295(13):1519–30.

51. Pfeffer MA, Braunwald E, Moyé LA, Basta L, Brown Jr EJ, Cuddy TE, et al. Effect of captopril on mortality and morbidity in patients with left ventricular dysfunction after myocardial infarction. Results of the survival and ventricular enlargement trial. The SAVE Investigators. N Engl J Med. 1992;327(10):669–77.

52. Effect of ramipril on mortality and morbidity of survivors of acute myocardial infarction with clinical evidence of heart failure. The Acute Infarction Ramipril Efficacy (AIRE) Study Investigators. Lancet. 1993;342(8875):821–8.

53. Pfeffer MA, McMurray JJ, Velazquez EJ, Rouleau JL, Køber L, Maggioni AP, et al. Valsartan, captopril, or both in myocardial infarction complicated by heart failure, left ventricular dysfunction, or both. N Engl J Med. 2003;349(20):1893–906.

54. Pitt B, Remme W, Zannad F, Neaton J, Martinez F, Roniker B, et al. Eplerenone, a selective aldosterone blocker, in patients with left ventricular dysfunction after myocardial infarction. N Engl J Med. 2003;348(14):1309–21.

55. Schwartz GG, Olsson AG, Ezekowitz MD, Ganz P, Oliver MF, Waters D, et al. Effects of atorvastatin on early recurrent ischemic events in acute coronary syndromes: the MIRACL study: a randomized controlled trial. JAMA. 2001;285(13):1711–8.

56. Cannon CP, Braunwald E, McCabe CH, Rader DJ, Rouleau JL, Belder R, et al. Intensive versus moderate lipid lowering with statins after acute coronary syndromes. N Engl J Med. 2004;350(15):1495–504.

CHAPTER 4

RODRIGO M. LAGO AND THOMAS A. LAMATTINA

Chronic Coronary Artery Disease

CHAPTER OUTLINE

ABBREVIATIONS

ACE	Angiotensin converting enzyme
ACS	Acute coronary syndromes
ARB	Angiotensin receptor blockers
CABG	Coronary artery bypass graft
CAD	Coronary artery disease
CCB	Calcium channel blockers
CCS	Canadian Cardiovascular Society
CTA	Computed tomography angiography
EBCT	Electron beam CT
ECG	Electrocardiographic
FFR	Fractional flow reserve
HCTZ	Hydrochlorothiazide
IVUS	Intravascular ultrasound
LAD	Left anterior descending
LBBB	Left bundle branch block
LM	Left main
LV	Left ventricular
MI	Myocardial infarction
MRI	Magnetic resonance imaging
PCI	Percutaneous coronary intervention
SPECT	Single photon emission computed tomography
WPW	Wolff–Parkinson–White

INTRODUCTION

Over the last two decades, due to improvement in the management of acute coronary syndromes (ACS), the increasing aging of the population, and the epidemics of diabetes and obesity, the management of patients with chronic coronary artery disease (CAD) has become an increasingly common and important part of clinical practice. The spectrum of chronic ischemic heart disease includes patients who have asymptomatic myocardial ischemia, stable angina pectoris, unstable angina, or prior myocardial infarction (MI) with residual ischemia. Mortality from ischemic heart disease increases in all age groups as blood pressure, vascular stiffness and endothelial dysfunction become more prevalent. New insights into the mechanisms underlying chronic stable coronary disease have led to the emergence of new anti-ischemic treatments and the role for revascularization has been reformulated.

EPIDEMIOLOGY

- The prevalence of angina in patients with CAD in epidemiological studies increases with age in both sexes [1].

  - After development of stable angina, the 2-year incidence of non-fatal MI and cardiovascular death were 14.3 and 5.5 % in men and 6.2 and 3.8 % in women
  - Prognosis can vary considerably dependent on baseline clinical, functional, and anatomical factors.

- Prognostic assessment and risk stratification is an important part of the management of patients with chronic CAD.

  - It is important to select those patients who could potentially benefit from revascularization, in contrast to those in whom medical therapy may be appropriate.

- The presence of conventional cardiovascular risk factors for the development of CAD (hypertension, hypercholesterolemia, diabetes, family history of premature CAD, and smoking) can adversely influence prognosis in patients with established stable CAD.

  - Treatment aiming on reducing these risk factors can positively influence outcomes in these patients.

- Left ventricular (LV) function is the strongest predictor of survival in patients with chronic stable CAD followed by the distribution and severity of coronary artery stenosis.

  - Left main (LM) disease, three-vessel disease, and the proximal involvement of the left anterior descending (LAD) coronary artery are common predictors of poor outcome and increase the risk of ischemic events [2, 3].

PATHOPHYSIOLOGY

- Cardiac ischemia results from an imbalance between myocardial oxygen supply and demand.

  - Cardiac ischemia can cause either an acute coronary syndrome (ACS) (ST elevation MI, Non-ST elevation MI, or unstable angina) or chronic stable angina.

    - A sudden reduction in myocardial oxygen supply caused by atherosclerotic plaque injury and thrombosis is usually the mechanism of ACS.

- In contrast, an increase in myocardial oxygen demand in the setting of inadequate coronary perfusion and a limited ability to increase myocardial oxygen supply is usually the mechanism of ischemia in chronic stable CAD.
- Ischemia-induced sympathetic activation can further increase the severity of myocardial ischemia through a further increase of myocardial oxygen consumption and coronary vasoconstriction.

NATURAL HISTORY

- As coronary atherosclerosis progresses, there is deposition of atherosclerotic plaque beneath the intima [4]. Plaque extends eccentrically and outward without significantly compromising luminal diameter (Fig. 4-1).

  – In this stage, stress testing or angiography may not identify obstructive CAD even in the presence of significant atherosclerosis.

- As atherosclerosis progress, encroachment of the atherosclerotic plaque into the lumen can result in hemodynamic obstruction and angina

  – Either stress testing or coronary angiography can detect these abnormalities.

    - In this situation, the functional nature of the obstructive coronary lesion can be also detected by fractional flow reserve measured during cardiac catheterization.

- The ischemic cascade is characterized by a sequence of events, resulting in metabolic abnormalities, perfusion mismatch, regional and then global diastolic and systolic dysfunction, electrocardiographic (ECG) changes, and angina.

  – Adenosine released by ischemic myocardium has been shown to be the main mediator of angina through stimulation of A1 receptors located on cardiac nerve endings.

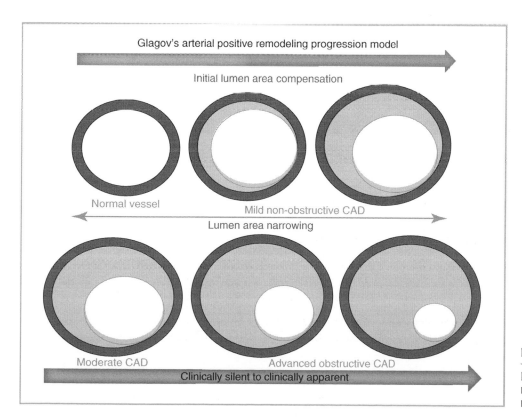

FIGURE 4-1

Progression of CAD and arterial remodeling (The Glagov's arterial remodeling model)

■ Myocardial ischemia may also be silent.

  – In patients who exhibit painless ischemia, dyspnea and palpitation may represent anginal equivalents.

    ■ Dyspnea in these cases may also be due to ischemic LV systolic or diastolic dysfunction, or due to ischemic mitral regurgitation.

■ When luminal obstruction is less than 40 %, maximal flow during exercise can usually be maintained. But luminal diameter reduction of more than 50 % may be associated with ischemia when coronary blood flow becomes inadequate to meet cardiac metabolic demand during exercise or stress.

  – For a similar degree of stenosis, the ischemic threshold is influenced by other factors including the degree of development of collateral circulation and coronary vascular tone.

■ Patients with stable angina are at risk of developing an ACS [4].

  – The hemodynamic severity of the atherosclerotic plaque prior to destabilization is frequently mild, and the plaques are lipid-rich and vulnerable to rupture or erosion [5].

    ■ Activation of inflammatory cells within the atherosclerotic plaque appears to play an important role in atherosclerotic plaque destabilization, ultimately leading to plaque erosion, fissure, or rupture.

CLINICAL PRESENTATION, DIAGNOSIS, AND RISK STRATIFICATION

Signs and Symptoms

■ The diagnosis of angina pectoris in patients with chronic coronary disease includes reproducible left-sided anterior chest discomfort triggered by physical activity or emotional stress.

■ Location, character, duration, and relation to exertion and other exacerbating or relieving factors may define the characteristics of discomfort related to myocardial ischemia.

  – These symptoms are typically worse in cold weather or after meals and are relieved by rest or sublingual nitroglycerin.

  – Typical features of stable angina include complete reversibility of the symptoms and repetitiveness of the anginal symptoms over time.

  – In stable angina, the angina threshold may vary considerably due to a variable degree of vasoconstriction at the site of stenosis and distal coronary vessels, depending on environmental factors such as temperature, mental stress, and individual neurohormonal influences [6, 7].

■ William Heberden first introduced the term 'angina pectoris' in 1772 although its pathological etiology was not recognized until years later [8, 9].

  – Chest pain is characterized as typical angina, atypical angina, and non-cardiac chest pain.

    ■ Angina is a syndrome that includes discomfort in the chest, jaw, shoulder, back, epigastric area or arm. The chest pain is aggravated by exertion or emotional stress and relieved by rest and/or nitroglycerin.

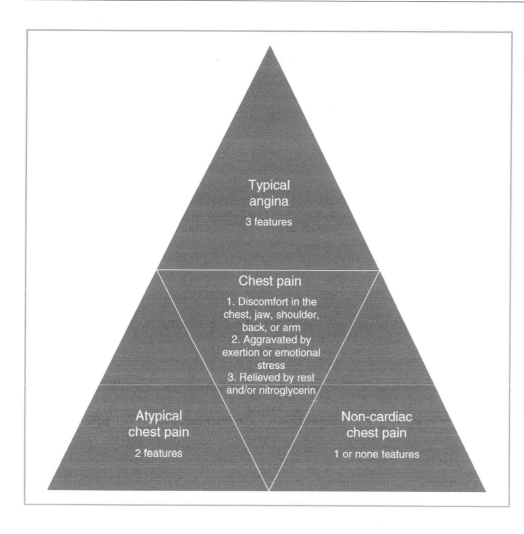

FIGURE 4-2

Differential diagnosis of chest pain

- ■ Atypical angina is generally defined by two of the above three features, and non-cardiac chest pain is generally defined as chest pain that meets 1 or none of the above criteria (Fig. 4-2)
- ■ In order to classify the severity of symptoms based on the threshold at which symptoms occur in relation to physical activities, the Canadian Cardiovascular Society (CCS) Classification (Table 4-1) is an useful tool to determine the functional impairment of the patient and to quantify response to therapy [10].

- – Alternative classification systems such as the Seattle angina questionnaire [11] may also be used to determine the functional status of the patient and to quantify response to therapy and may offer superior prognostic information.

■ Physical signs in patients with angina pectoris are non-specific.

- – During or immediately after an episode of myocardial ischemia, a third or fourth heart sound may be heard.
- – A new murmur of mitral regurgitation may be apparent.
- – Other signs that can be present include xanthelasma in patients with dyslipidemia, lung crackles and elevated jugular venous pressure in patients with heart failure, and other signs of vascular disease such as diminished peripheral pulses and vascular bruits.

TABLE 4-1	CLASS I	CLASS II	CLASS III	CLASS IV
GRADING OF ANGINA PECTORIS BY THE CANADIAN CARDIOVASCULAR SOCIETY (CCS) CLASSIFICATION SYSTEM	Ordinary physical activity does not cause angina, such as walking, climbing stairs. Angina occurs with strenuous, rapid, or prolonged exertion at work or recreation	Slight limitation of ordinary activity. Angina occurs on walking or climbing stairs rapidly, walking uphill, walking or stair climbing after meals or in cold, or in wind, or under emotional stress. Angina occurs on walking more than two blocks on the level and climbing more than one flight of ordinary stairs at a normal pace and in normal condition	Marked limitations of ordinary physical activity. Angina occurs on walking 1–2 blocks on the level and climbing 1 flight of stairs in normal conditions and at a normal pace	Inability to carry on any physical activity without chest discomfort. Anginal symptoms may be present at rest

From Campeau [10]. Copyright 1976 American Heart Association, Inc.

Laboratory Testing

■ Laboratory tests are of low utility in chronic stable angina and therefore are not recommended routinely in patients with chronic coronary disease.

– Classical cardiac biochemical markers of myocardial injury such as troponin or CKMB are usually negative, however highly-sensitive troponins may be elevated in those with stable coronary disease.
– Natriuretic peptides such as BNP or NT-proBNP may be mildly elevated in those with stable angina.

■ Fasting plasma glucose [12, 13] and lipid profile [14] should be evaluated in all patients with suspected coronary disease to establish the patient's cardiovascular risk profile.

■ Renal function should be initially evaluated in patients with chronic coronary disease.

– Renal dysfunction may occur due to associated vascular comorbidities and has a negative impact on prognosis in patients with CAD [15].

■ Additional laboratory testing, including cholesterol subfractions (ApoA and ApoB) [16], homocysteine [17], lipoprotein (a) (Lpa), coagulation profile, NT-proBNP [18], and markers of inflammation (hs-C-reactive protein) [19, 20], have been used to improve risk prediction in selected patients, but presently lack a defined therapeutic response if found to be elevated.

Non-Invasive Diagnostic Testing

■ **Resting electrocardiogram**

– All patients with suspected stable coronary artery disease should have a resting 12-lead ECG recorded.

- A normal or non-specific ECG is not uncommon and does not exclude the diagnosis of chronic myocardial ischemia.

  - Patients with normal baseline ECG have better prognosis since that usually implies normal LV function.

- The resting ECG may show signs of CAD such as previous MI or an abnormal ST-T segment with ST depression and/or T wave inversion.
- Other ECG findings may include left ventricular hypertrophy, bundle branch blocks, AV node block, atrial fibrillation, and frequent ventricular ectopy, all which can predict worse prognosis in patients with CAD.

- **ECG stress testing**

  - Exercise ECG is more sensitive and specific than the resting ECG for detecting myocardial ischemia and is the test of choice to identify inducible ischemia in patients with suspected stable angina.

    - Horizontal or down-sloping ST segment depression of more than 1 mm defines a positive test with a sensitivity and specificity for the detection of significant coronary disease of 68 and 77 %, respectively [21].

  - Exercise ECG testing is not of diagnostic value in the presence of left bundle branch block (LBBB), paced rhythm, and Wolff–Parkinson–White (WPW) syndrome, in which cases, the ECG changes cannot be evaluated. Other confounders are the use of digoxin, resting ECG depression greater than 1 mm, and the presence of LV hypertrophy.
  - ECG changes associated with myocardial ischemia when accompanied by chest pain suggestive of angina during exercise, especially when these changes occur at a low workload and persist during the recovery period further increases the specificity of the test.
  - A fall in systolic blood pressure or lack of increase of blood pressure during exercise, the appearance of a systolic murmur of mitral regurgitation, or the presence of ventricular arrhythmias during exercise may reflect more severe CAD and increase the probability of severe myocardial ischemia.
  - The Duke treadmill score is a well-validated score that combines exercise time, ST-deviation, and angina during exercise to calculate the patient's risk (Fig. 4-3) [22, 23].
  - Interpretation of stress testing requires a Bayesian approach (Fig. 4-4).

    - This dictates that the post test probability of a true positive result is based on the pre-test probability of disease presence.
    - Diagnosis using the Bayes' formula is a probabilistic assessment and not a binary decision (true or false).

Duke treadmill score

Exercise time (min) – 5 × ST deviation (mm) – 4 × Exercise angina*
*Exercise angina: 0 = none; 1 = non-limiting; 3 = exercise limiting

	1-year mortality
Low risk: ≥ 5	0.25 %
Intermediate risk: 4 to −10	1.25 %
High risk: ≤ −11	5.25 %

FIGURE 4-3

Duke Treadmill Score

FIGURE 4-4

Bayes' Theorem diagram. The post-test probability of disease after a test is influenced not only by the sensitivity and specificity of the test but also by the pre-test probability of disease. In patients with a low pre-test probability of disease (A), a positive test result will minimally increase the post-test probability and therefore have a low discrimination power. Similarly, in patients with high pre-test probability (B), a positive test will only confirm the presence of disease and therefore have a low discrimination power. The higher discrimination power of the test occurs in patients with intermediate pre-test probability of disease (C). For a given pre-test probability, the post-test probability becomes progressively higher as the test becomes more abnormal. As the sensitivity of the test increases, the negative test curve shifts further away from the line of identity. As the specificity of the test increases, the positive test curve shifts away from the line of identity

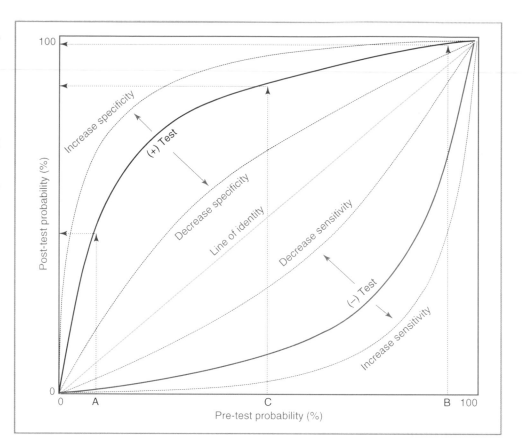

TABLE 4-2

PRE-TEST PROBABILITY OF CAD BY AGE, GENDER, AND SYMPTOMS

AGE (YEARS)	GENDER	TYPICAL ANGINA	ATYPICAL CHEST PAIN	NON-CARDIAC CHEST PAIN	ASYMPTOMATIC
30–39	Men	Intermediate	Intermediate	Low	Very low
	Women	Intermediate	Low	Very low	Very low
40–49	Men	High	Intermediate	Intermediate	Low
	Women	Intermediate	Low	Very low	Very low
50–59	Men	High	Intermediate	Intermediate	Low
	Women	Intermediate	Intermediate	Low	Very low
60–69	Men	High	Intermediate	Intermediate	Low
	Women	High	Intermediate	Intermediate	Low

High, greater than 90 % pretest probability; *Intermediate*, between 10 and 90 % pretest probability; *Low*, between 5 and 10 % pretest probability; *Very low* less than 5 % pretest probability

■ Once the presence of symptoms that may represent obstructive CAD is identified, the pretest probability of CAD should be assessed. The pre-test probability can be determined by an established risk score, such as the Framingham Risk Score and further modified by the nature of symptoms at an individual patient level.

– Diamond and Forrester described the relationship between clinical symptoms and angiographically significant CAD (Table 4-2) [24].

■ Patients with symptoms of angina and intermediate pre-test probability of coronary disease based on age, gender, and symptoms, unless unable to exercise or have ECG changes that make ECG non-evaluable are candidates for ECG stress testing as the initial assessment tool for diagnosis and risk stratification.

■ **Imaging stress testing**

– Stress imaging offers superior diagnostic performance over conventional exercise ECG testing for the detection of obstructive CAD.

■ The ability to quantify and localize areas of ischemia makes stress-imaging techniques often preferred in patients with previous revascularization.

– Myocardial perfusion scintigraphy using [201]Th and ^{99m}Tc radiopharmaceuticals are the most commonly used methods of imaging employing single photon emission computed tomography (SPECT) in association with an exercise test on either a stationary bicycle or a treadmill.

■ Reported sensitivities and specificities are approximately 90 and 90 % respectively.

– The SPECT myocardial perfusion imaging Appropriateness Criteria recommends:

■ For patients without symptoms:

– Use of radionuclide stress imaging only in high cardiovascular risk patients.
– In those asymptomatic patients with intermediate cardiovascular risk with a non-interpretable ECG, the use of radionuclide imaging was considered of uncertain benefit.

■ In symptomatic patients:

– Radionuclide imaging is considered appropriate if patients had an intermediate or high likelihood for CAD by pre-test assessment. Imaging test was also considered appropriate for symptomatic patients at low likelihood of CAD if they were unable to exercise or had a non-interpretable ECG.

– Pharmacological stress testing with either perfusion scintigraphy or echocardiography may be employed and is indicated in patients who are unable to exercise adequately.
– Other potential imaging modality that can be used to detect functional CAD is stress cardiac magnetic resonance imaging (MRI) or echocardiography with dobutamine infusion.

■ **Non-invasive techniques to assess coronary calcification and coronary anatomy**

– Cardiac computed tomography angiography (CTA) using electron beam CT (EBCT) and multi-detector CT (MDCT) has been validated for the detection and quantification of the extent of coronary disease and calcification [25–27].

■ The extent of coronary calcification correlates with the overall burden of coronary atherosclerotic plaque.
■ The use of CT angiography in stable angina is indicated in patients with a low pre-test probability of disease, with a non-conclusive exercise ECG or stress imaging test.
■ The strength of CT angiography is its strong *negative predictive value*. A negative scan excludes significant atherosclerosis.

■ **Non-invasive risk stratification of stable angina**

– Risk stratification of patients with stable angina is important to determine the need for invasive testing and to identify those patients at highest risk, and therefore most likely to benefit from more aggressive treatment (Table 4-3).

TABLE 4-3	HIGH-RISK (>3 % ANNUAL MORTALITY RATE)	INTERMEDIATE RISK (1–3 % ANNUAL MORTALITY RATE)	LOW-RISK (<1 % ANNUAL MORTALITY RATE)
NON-INVASIVE RISK STRATIFICATION OF CHRONIC STABLE CAD	Severe resting left ventricular dysfunction (LVEF <35 %)	Mild/moderate resting left ventricular dysfunction (LVEF 35–49 %)	Low-risk treadmill score (score>5)
	High-risk treadmill score (score<−11)	Intermediate-risk treadmill score (−11<score<5)	Normal or small myocardial perfusion defect at rest or with stress[a]
	Severe exercise left ventricular dysfunction (exercise LVEF <35 %)	Stress-induced moderate perfusion defect without LV dilation or increased lung intake (thallium-201)	Normal stress echocardiographic wall motion or no change of limited resting wall motion abnormalities during stress[a]
	Stress-induced large perfusion defect (particularly if anterior) Stress-induced multiple perfusion defects of moderate size Large, fixed perfusion defect with LV dilation or increased lung uptake (thallium-201) Stress-induced moderate perfusion defect with LV dilation or increased lung uptake (thallium-201) Echocardiographic wall motion abnormality (involving greater than two segments) developing at low dose of dobutamine (less than or equal to 10 mg/kg/min) or at a low heart rate (<120 beats/min) Stress echocardiographic evidence of extensive ischemia	Limited stress echocardio-graphic ischemia with a wall motion abnormal-ity only at higher doses of dobutamine involving less than or equal to two segments	

[a]Patients with these findings will probably not be at low risk in the presence of either a high-risk treadmill score or severe resting left ventricular dysfunction (LVEF<35 %)

- The clinical evaluation, the response to stress testing, the LV systolic function, and the extent of CAD are elements used to add incremental prognostic value.
- The incremental benefit of stress imaging test has been validated particularly in patients with stable angina and intermediate-risk Duke Treadmill Scores (AHA/ACC Class I indication for stress imaging).
- The negative predictive value of imaging stress test is high and a normal stress perfusion study is associated with a subsequent rate of cardiac death and MI of less than 1 % per year [28].

Invasive Diagnostic Testing

■ **Coronary angiography**

- Despite the limitations of coronary angiography to identify vulnerable atherosclerotic plaques that are likely to cause acute coronary events, the extent, severity, and location of CAD have been demonstrated to be important prognostic indicators in patients with stable angina.
- Invasive assessment of coronary anatomy in patients with stable angina is indicated when there is a high-likelihood of severe obstructive CAD, particularly if symptoms are severe (Class three or greater of CCS Classification) and inadequately responding to optimal medical treatment.

- Other indications for coronary angiography include:

  - Symptoms of angina and heart failure
  - High-risk criteria on stress testing
  - Survivors of cardiac arrest
  - Ventricular arrhythmias
  - Prior myocardial revascularization (either percutaneous coronary intervention (PCI) or coronary artery bypass graft (CABG)) who develop recurrence of angina
  - Inconclusive or conflicting diagnosis on non-invasive testing who have an intermediate to high risk pre-test probability of CAD.

- **Intravascular ultrasound (IVUS)**

  - IVUS allows for accurate measurement of coronary luminal diameter, assessment of atherosclerotic lesions, and quantification of atheroma and calcium deposition. It is also an important tool to assess for interventional target lesions and stent placement. This technique offers excellent qualitative and quantitative assessment of coronary anatomy with additive benefit when used in conjunction with coronary angiography, particularly as an adjunct to coronary intervention.

- **Fractional flow reserve (FFR)**

  - Invasive assessment of functional severity of coronary lesions can be performed by measuring intracoronary FFR.
  - It is an attractive option to allow assessment of functional severity of an atherosclerotic lesion of indeterminate importance at the time of angiography,
  - This technique involves inducing hyperemia through intracoronary injection of a vasodilator. FFR is calculated as the ratio of distal coronary pressure to aortic pressure measured during maximal hyperemia. A normal value for FFR is 1.0 regardless of the status of the microcirculation, and an FFR less than 0.75 is deemed pathological [29, 30].

TREATMENT OF CHRONIC ISCHEMIC HEART DISEASE

Medical Treatment

The goals of pharmacological treatment of stable angina are to improve quality of life by reducing the severity and/or frequency of symptoms and to improve prognosis reducing the risk of MI and cardiac death.

- Medical therapy is a viable alternative for the treatment of most patients with stable angina, reserving an invasive treatment strategy for patients at high-risk or with symptoms that are poorly controlled by medical treatment.

  - Co-existing disorders such as diabetes and/or hypertension in patients with stable angina should be well controlled, dyslipidemia should be corrected, anemia treated, and smoking cessation attempted.

    - Patients with stable angina should be started on at least two classes of anti-anginal therapies as a minimum standard for medical therapy.
    - Triple anti-anginal therapy can be considered when optimal two drug regimens are insufficient to control symptoms.
    - Patients whose symptoms are poorly controlled on double therapy should be assessed for the need for revascularization.

Revascularization for Chronic Ischemic CAD

■ Revascularization should be considered for those at high-risk based on noninvasive testing or with continued symptoms despite optimal medical therapy.

– PCI is considered appropriate in patients with 2-vessel CAD without involvement of the proximal LAD and uncertain in patients with 3-vessel disease.

– In patients with LM stenosis and/or LM stenosis and multivessel CAD, CABG is appropriate and likely to improve cardiovascular outcomes and survival. On the contrary, PCI is considered unlikely to improve the outcomes in this group of patient according to the ACCF/SCAI/STS/AATS/AHA/ASNC 2009 Appropriateness criteria for coronary revascularization.

■ Revascularization is also preferred over medical therapy among patients with three vessel CAD and reduced LV systolic function if the risk of procedural complications is not prohibitive.

■ PCI is more effective than medical therapy in treating symptoms and improving exercise capacity.

– There is no study to date that showed a benefit in cardiovascular outcomes of death and MI with PCI over optimal medical therapy, especially in the lower risk group of patients. [45–48] though patients who underwent PCI in comparative effectiveness trials of medical therapy versus PCI did have a significant reduction in symptoms and the burden of ischemia.

– The BARI-2D trial [49] enrolled patients with both diabetes and stable CAD that were assigned to either PCI or CABG and then randomized to revascularization or medical therapy.

■ At 5 years there was no overall significant difference in the primary end points of death and major cardiovascular events between study groups.

– Patients who were assigned to CABG had fewer events as compared with optimal medical therapy

– The SYNTAX trial comparing CABG with PCI in multivessel and left main disease, demonstrated that the rates of events at 12 months were overall significantly higher in the PCI group due to an increased rate of repeat revascularization.

■ Using a risk score to predict hazard, the primary outcome was particularly frequent in those with high SYNTAX scores randomized to PCI

■ Similar outcomes between PCI and CABG were observed in patients with lower SYNTAX scores.

– Thus, taken together, data would argue for optimal medical therapy for all patients, reserving revascularization for those failing aggressive medical programs.

■ When revascularization is performed, the choice of strategy should be dictated by patient specific factors.

■ Stable ischemic heart disease without prior CABG

– The presence of high-risk findings on noninvasive testing, higher severity of symptoms, or an increasing burden of CAD lowers the threshold for revascularization in patients with stable angina.

- Revascularization is considered appropriate in patients with 1- or 2-vessel CAD with or without involvement of the proximal LAD and class III or IV angina regardless of the level of medical therapy.
- In patients with intermediate severity coronary stenosis, additional evaluations using FFR or IVUS to identify significant stenosis beyond their appearance by angiography is warranted.

■ Stable ischemic heart disease with prior CABG

- Similar to the pattern seen in patients without prior CABG, the presence of high-risk findings on noninvasive testing, higher severity of symptoms, or an increasing burden of disease in either the bypass grafts or native coronaries tends to increase the likelihood of an appropriate rating for revascularization.
- The only inappropriate criteria for revascularization in patients with prior CABG is in patients receiving no or minimal anti-ischemic therapy or having low-risk findings on noninvasive testing.

SUMMARY AND CONCLUSIONS

■ The diagnosis of chronic stable angina is made on the basis of symptoms, a noninvasive stress test demonstrating myocardial ischemia, and documentation of coronary atherosclerosis on coronary angiography.

■ Medical treatment should be started early, and management of patients with chronic CAD should include lifestyle modifications, smoking cessation, weight control, regular exercise, and aggressive control of cardiovascular risk factors. Drugs to slow the progression of atherosclerosis, including statins are indicated.

■ Coronary angiography and revascularization is indicated if symptoms continue despite medical

REVIEW QUESTIONS

1. **A 59 year old non-smoker man with hypertension, dyslipidemia, and family history of premature coronary artery disease presents to the cardiology outpatient clinic with a history of exertional chest pain that occurred for the past month a few times while he was playing basketball with friends. More recently, the chest pain occurs at lower levels of exertion while he was washing his car. The chest pain is located in the left-sided chest and radiates to his left arm, resolves after stop exercising and never occurs at rest. His baseline ECG was within normal limits and there were no ST-T abnormalities or pathological Q waves noticed. His current medical regimen includes a beta-blocker, diltiazem, hydrochlorothiazide (HCTZ), and a statin. A treadmill exercise stress test was obtained. The patient exercised in a standard Bruce protocol for 12 min and achieved 10 METS with a** normal blood pressure response to exercise at 88 % of his maximal predicted heart rate. During the test he developed reproducible chest pain at peak exercise that resolved at rest. His exercise EKG showed 2 mm horizontal ST segment depressions in leads II, III, aVF, V5, and V6 during peak exercise that also resolved in the recovery phase. SPECT Myocardial perfusion images showed a moderate size reversible defect in the anterior and apical walls of the left ventricle during the stress phase of the test. The left ventricular systolic function was normal with an ejection fraction of (65 %) and there were no wall motion abnormalities, ischemic LV dilation or increase lung uptake. He was then referred for invasive coronary angiography. The angiographic images are shown here (Fig. 4-5): What is a true statement?

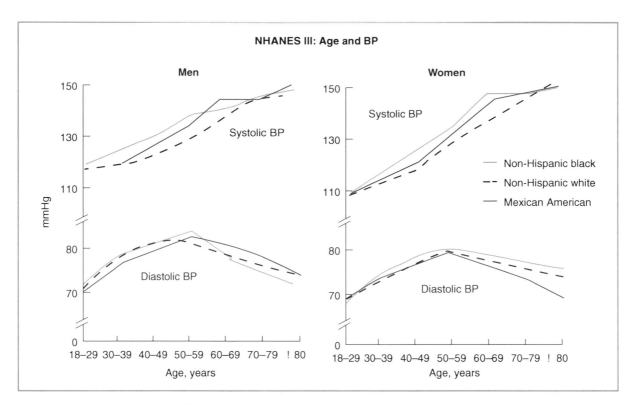

FIGURE 5-1

Changes in systolic and diastolic blood pressure with age (Used with permission from Burt et al. [5])

- High pulse wave velocity, which results in the reflected pulse waves arriving at the central aorta during systole rather than after the dicrotic notch (as occurs in younger individuals)
- Endothelial dysfunction, which results in impaired flow-mediated arterial dilation

■ These physiologic and pathologic effects of aging are modulated to a significant extent by behavioral and environmental influences including physical activity, diet (e.g. caloric and sodium intake, low potassium intake, atherogenic diet, etc.) [8, 9].

Additional Differences with Aging

■ The autonomic nervous system undergoes significant changes with aging

- Downregulation and decreased responsiveness of beta-receptors and increased ambient catecholamine concentrations
- The increased norepinephrine concentrations common in older individuals may be due to homeostatic mechanisms counterbalancing decreased responsiveness of the adrenergic receptors [10]

■ Elderly hypertensives usually have low renin, low aldosterone, salt-sensitive hypertension because of decreased natriuretic activity of the nephrosclerotic kidney and increased sodium reabsorption [11]

■ Renal function declines with age

- Between the ages of 30 and 85, approximately one quarter of the cortex is lost due to glomerulosclerosis and interstitial fibrosis with impairment of renal hemodynamics [12]

  ■ Renal changes from nephrosclerosis and changes of the juxtaglomerular apparatus result in low renin and aldosterone levels. This may be related to expansion of total body water and suppression of renin activity [13]

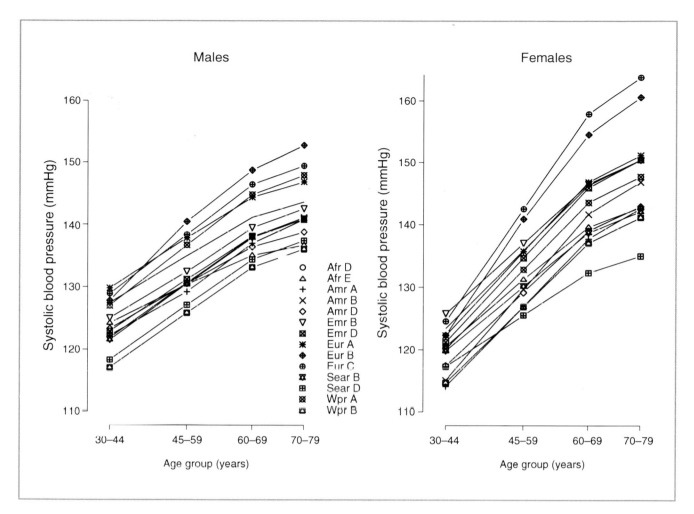

FIGURE 5-2

SBP by gender, age, and World Health Organization (WHO) subregion (Used with permission from Lawes et al. [6])

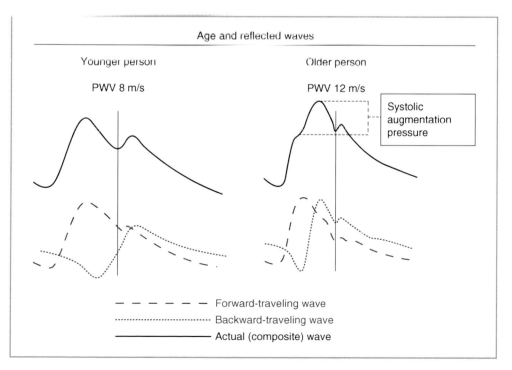

FIGURE 5-3

Effect of arterial stiffening on pulse wave velocity, reflected pressure waves and central arterial pressure in younger and older persons. *PWV* pulse wave velocity (Modified from Asmar [7])

- ■ The decreased renal function in hypertension may impair excretion of medications or their metabolites, especially in the elderly with polypharmacy and associated comorbidities (e.g. coronary heart disease (CHD), diabetes, dyslipidemia, and osteoarthritis)

  – Renal dysfunction predicts cardiovascular (CV) outcomes and mortality in older hypertensives [14]

- ■ Polypharmacy

  – Polypharmacy and cost result in decreased adherence to therapy
  – Polypharmacy in combination with decreased renal function increases the probability of drug interactions and adverse events

- ■ Non-steroidal anti-inflammatory agents (NSAIDs)

  – There is increased use of NSAIDs among older patients (see Drug-Induced Hypertension)

- ■ Orthostatic hypotension

  – Related to impaired baroreflex function (probably also related to stiffening of the carotid arteries [15]), venous insufficiency, varicosities, and diabetic neuropathy
  – A significant problem, especially in older hypertensives
  – Orthostatic hypotension is a predictor of poor outcomes in older individuals, and when compounded by changes in skeletal health and impaired equilibrium, may cause falls

Secondary Hypertension

Acute Kidney Disease

- ■ Acute glomerular disease may result in volume retention and hypertension due to increased sodium reabsorption
- ■ Acute vascular injury due to vasculitis or connective tissue disease (e.g. SLE, scleroderma) may induce hypertension by increased activation of the RAAS triggered by ischemia

Chronic Kidney Disease (CKD)

- ■ Many causes of CKD may lead to hypertension through sodium retention and volume expansion, increased activity of the RAAS due to ischemia, and enhanced sympathetic tone

Renovascular Hypertension

- ■ Most common form of secondary hypertension
- ■ Usually related to renal artery stenosis (RAS) due to atherosclerosis of the large renal arteries or their ostia

  – When stenosis exceeds 70 % of the diameter (about 90 % reduction in cross-sectional area), a hemodynamically significant decrease in blood flow results in decrease of intraglomerular pressure with subsequent activation of the RAAS and increased sodium reabsorption

- ■ RAS is a manifestation of widespread atherosclerosis that may involve other arterial beds (cerebrovascular, coronary, peripheral)

  – Patients with these conditions are more likely to have RAS [16, 17]

- ■ Stenoses of renal arteries, detected by invasive or non-invasive diagnostic modalities are not uncommon in the elderly, but these may be incidental and non-hemodynamically-significant
- ■ In addition to controlling hypertension, revascularization of significant RAS should improve GFR or slow the decline of renal function if the stenosis is the primary cause of renal dysfunction, which is not always the case [18]

  – In clinical trials of patients with RAS, there has not been a marked clinical benefit from revascularization procedures

Primary Aldosteronism (PA)

■ Relatively common cause of resistant hypertension (hypertension despite the use of at least three antihypertensives)

■ Usually associated with adrenal hyperplasia (usually bilateral) or an adrenal adenoma

■ May also be caused by familial hyperaldosteronism, adrenal carcinoma, or ectopic aldosterone-producing tumors

■ Diagnostic clues include suppressed plasma renin activity, high aldosterone, and hypokalemia (may not be present) in a hypertensive patient [19]

■ Diagnostic approach includes measurement of

  – Plasma renin activity (PRA), plasma renin concentration (PRC), and plasma aldosterone concentration (PAC), as well as random plasma aldosterone concentration-to-plasma renin activity (PAC/PRA) ratio

  – PAC/PRA ratio >25 suggests PA, while normal and hypertensives without PA have ratios <10

■ If PAC/PRA ratio suggests PA, one or more confirmatory tests should be performed, including [20]

  – Measurement of urinary aldosterone excretion after oral sodium chloride loading (>12 mg/24 h after 200 mmol/day (~6 g/day) sodium intake suggests PA)

  – Measurement of PAC after IV sodium chloride loading (PAC > 10 ng/dL) after infusion of 2 L normal saline over 4 h suggests PA

  – Fludrocortisone suppression test (upright PAC > 6 ng/dL after 4 days suggests PA)

  – Captopril challenge (PAC, normally suppressed by 25–50 mg of captopril, remains elevated in PA, while PRA remains low)

  – Certain medications (e.g. aldosterone receptor antagonists (ARA)) must be held during testing

■ If confirmatory tests are positive, patients should undergo adrenal CT

■ Selective adrenal vein sampling may be used to distinguish unilateral from bilateral adrenal involvement in cases where surgery (unilateral adrenalectomy) is an option

■ For unilateral adrenal involvement or for extra-adrenal lesions, surgical resection is often primary therapy

■ Medical treatment (e.g. for bilateral adrenal hyperplasia) is based on the use of ARAs

Thyroid Disease

■ Both hyperthyroidism and hypothyroidism may be associated with hypertension.

Cushing's Syndrome

■ Increased ACTH levels, whether iatrogenic, from adrenal tumors, or from other paraneoplastic activity, can lead to hypertension, which may be severe

Pheochromocytomas

■ Rare catecholamine-producing tumors that can cause paroxysmal hypertension

Aortic Coarctation

■ Relatively common congenital abnormality that leads to predominately upper-extremity hypertension secondary to mechanical obstruction (typically distal to the brachiocephalic circulation)

Obstructive sleep apnea (OSA)

■ Associated with an increased incidence of hypertension

■ OSA should be treated due to a variety of sequelae, including fatigue, systemic and pulmonary hypertension, and all-cause and CAD-related mortality

  – May be related to other conditions (e.g. obesity and dyslipidemia) and to morbid events (e.g. HF and stroke) [21]

Drug-Induced Hypertension

■ Medication use is an important cause of secondary hypertension

- Causes include NSAIDs, stimulants, and sympathomimetic decongestant agents and oral contraceptive pills.

  ■ NSAIDs exert anti-inflammatory activity by inhibiting the production of prostaglandins that mediate inflammation. This inhibition, however, may result in decreased renal function, sodium and water retention, BP elevation, and HF
  ■ NSAIDs may impair the BP-lowering effect of ACE inhibitors, ARBs, and diuretics [22, 23]

DIAGNOSIS OF HYPERTENSION

Techniques

■ Blood pressure, especially SBP in elderly individuals, exhibits variability with successive BP measurements and environmental changes such as temperature and emotional state
■ It is important to measure the pressure several times in a comfortable position after sitting for 5 min

- Orthostatic changes should be ascertained by measuring the pressure after standing for 1–3 min

■ Pseudohypertension, a measurement of a high BP value in the presence of normal intraluminal BP because of noncompressible arteries

- May occur in older individuals, but is uncommon
- The Osler maneuver (palpable radial or brachial artery when the cuff is inflated above SBP), may be used, although sensitivity and specificity are not very high
- Definitive diagnosis requires intraarterial measurement

■ Home BP monitoring

- Should be performed using a reliable automated device
- Measurements made three times in the morning and three times in the evening for seven consecutive days
- An inexpensive and reliable method of monitoring antihypertensive therapy

■ Ambulatory BP is a predictor of target organ damage as well as outcomes that surpasses office BP [24]
■ Ambulatory BP measurement is now recommended in the National Institute for Health and Clinical Excellence (UK) guidelines to confirm the diagnosis following an initial elevated BP measurement in the clinic [25]

Association with Risk

■ Data from the Framingham Study have shown that in younger ages, DBP is more important in determining risk of CHD while in older individuals, the risk primarily is determined by SBP ([26], Fig. 5-4)
■ In older patients, lower DBP is associated with higher risk
■ Studying persons aged 50–79 years without clinical evidence of CHD, the investigators reported that CHD risk increased with lower DBP for a given SBP, suggesting that higher pulse pressure determines the risk in older individuals ([27], Fig. 5-5)
■ This relationship could be explained by

- Decreased coronary flow
- A stiffer aortic reservoir related to older age
- Comorbidities (e.g. diabetes)
- Lifestyle factors (e.g. smoking)

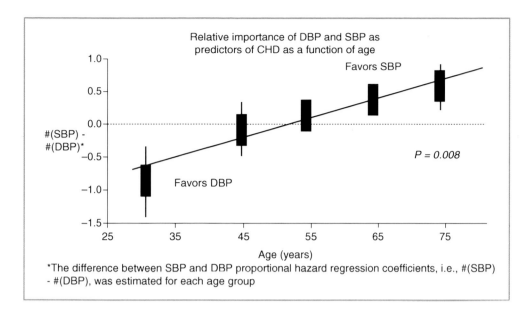

FIGURE 5-4

Relative importance of DBP and SBP as predictors of CHD as a function of age. *CHD* coronary heart disease (Used with permission from Franklin et al. [26])

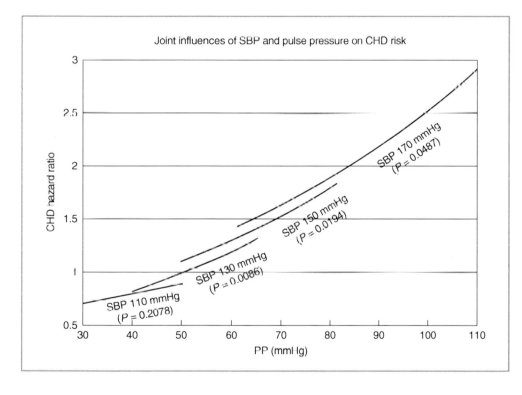

FIGURE 5-5

Joint influences of SBP and pulse pressure on CHD risk (Used with permission from Franklin et al. [27])

SEQUELAE OF HYPERTENSION

Target Organ Damage

- Hypertension results in damage to the arterial system, brain, heart, eyes, and kidneys.
- Peripheral arterial disease (PAD) is frequently associated with hypertension

    - PAD is likely to occur in the same patients who have cerebrovascular disease and CHD and is associated with a marked increase in the occurrence of acute myocardial infarction (MI) and stroke

FIGURE 5-6

Elevated SBP is a strong risk
factor for cardiovascular mortality (Used with permission from
Flack et al. [33])

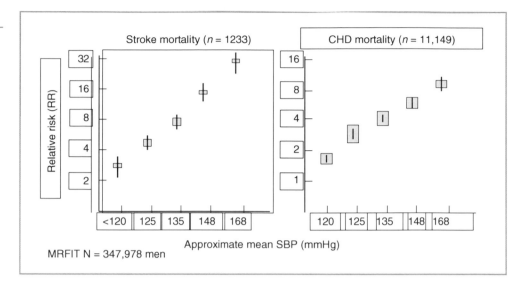

- Hypertension is an important risk factor for the development of abdominal and thoracic aortic aneurysm and aortic dissection

  - The probability is increased among smokers and those with connective tissue disorders
  - BP control is very important and surgery is necessary when the aneurysms reach specific dimensions since mortality following rupture is extremely high

- Hypertensive retinopathy with arteriovenous nicking, arteriolar narrowing, and in some cases hemorrhages, exudates, and papilledema increases in frequency with age and SBP [28]
- Diabetes mellitus (DM), a current worldwide epidemic, increases the risk in hypertensive patients and interacts with hypertension in causing CV events, CKD, and HF [29, 30]

  - Obesity, another public health issue, is related to and may be causative of diabetes, with the majority of the population being either obese (BMI >30) or overweight (BMI > 25) [31]

Morbid and Mortal Events

- Hypertension accounts for more attributable deaths worldwide than any other risk factor, whereas smoking and high cholesterol are second and third, respectively [32]
- The causes of death related to hypertension are CHD, stroke, HF, and CKD, especially when hypertension coexists with diabetes ([33], Fig. 5-6)
- Age is a major determinant of risk for both stroke and CHD events

  - BP tends to increase with age and the relative risk imposed by a given BP level decreases with age
  - However, because of the higher baseline risk (risk at SBP of 110 mmHg), the absolute increase in risk due to a given level of hypertension is much higher at older ages

    - For patients aged 50–59, the relative risk for fatal stroke is approximately 16 for patients with SBP of 180 mmHg compared to those with SBP of 110 mmHg, while for patients aged 80–89, the relative risk is approximately 2
    - On the other hand, the increase in absolute risk for mortality from stroke is 15 (from 1 to 16) for the younger age group and about 75 for the older age group ([34], Fig. 5-7, left panel). Similar increases in mortality from CHD are seen with increasing age and BP (Fig. 5-7, right panel). These linear-log plots demonstrate the exponential relationship of a given SBP to risk.

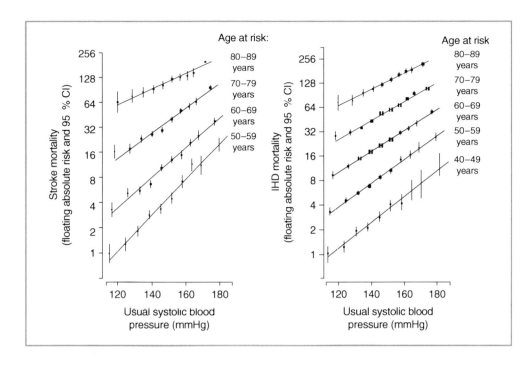

FIGURE 5-7

Cardiovascular disease mortality with increasing SBP by age (Used with permission from Lewington et al. [34])

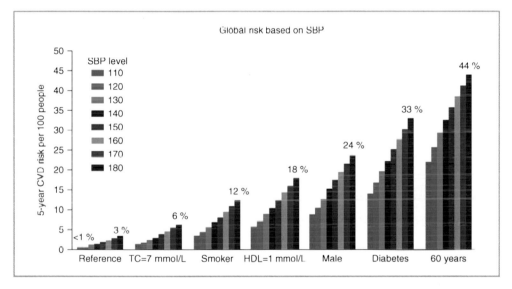

FIGURE 5-8

Global risk as a function of SBP interacting with other risk factors (Used with permission from Jackson et al. [35])

■ Similarly, the relationship of age to mortality risk for any given level of BP can be redrawn with other risk factors (e.g. total cholesterol, LDL), alone or in combination, substituted for age

- Hypertension, when it is the only risk factor (usually in a young person), imparts a small or moderate risk of cardiovascular and renovascular events
- It is the combined presence of additional risk factors interacting with age that increase the risk ([35], Fig. 5-8)

■ Among risk factors, obesity and diabetes have become an epidemic in the U.S. and worldwide

- There are 285 million people with diabetes worldwide. This number will increase to 438 million by the year 2030 [36]

- The great majority have type 2 diabetes that is related to obesity and frequently coexists with hypertension
- Diabetes markedly increases the risk of CV events at any level of BP [37]
- One way to visualize the effect of diabetes is presented in Fig. 5-9 (modified from [38])

HYPERTENSION AND HEART FAILURE

- Left ventricular systolic dysfunction (LVSD) and HF are common complications of aging and hypertension, in part because of increased survival after MI
- Hypertension may result in HF via two pathways:

    - The development of acute MI leading to HF with impaired LV systolic function
    - The development of left ventricular hypertrophy (LVH) leading to HF with preserved EF (HFPEF), probably related to diastolic dysfunction

        - Patients with HFPEF tend to have concentric left ventricular (LV) remodeling with high LV mass/volume ratio as well as cardiomyocyte hypertrophy
        - Those with HF with reduced EF (HFREF) tend to have eccentric LV remodeling with low LV mass/volume ratio with loss of myofibers [39]

- Hypertension, when untreated, results in increased LV wall thickness and decreased diastolic function causing impaired early diastolic filling due to delayed myocardial relaxation and decreased passive mid-diastolic filling due to a stiffer left ventricle

    - Decreased diastolic filling and afterload mismatch may cause HFPEF. The impedance mismatch can result in flash acute pulmonary edema.

- Treatment of ISH with chlorthalidone-based stepped therapy resulted in marked decrease in the occurrence of HF in the Systolic Hypertension in the Elderly Program (SHEP) [40]

    - The occurrence of HF was related to SBP, as expected, but also to pulse pressure, after accounting for SBP.
    - This may be due to concomitant and parallel decreases in both large artery and left ventricular compliance or potentially to a decrease in coronary flow related to low DBP [41].

- Uncontrolled hypertension and aging interact to exacerbate the development of HF, especially in the presence of obesity or diabetes, which further contribute to increased LV mass, LV wall thickness, and abnormal diastolic LV filling patterns

    - Impairment of systolic function is initially compensated for by increased LV thickness, but ultimately, LV remodeling associated with neurohormonal activation, increased wall tension, apoptosis, myocyte loss, fibrosis, chamber dilatation, and depressed systolic function leads to HF
    - In the Cardiovascular Health Study, LVSD in the absence of HF was associated in a graded fashion with higher incidence of future clinical HF, as well as with higher mortality [42]

- Prevention of HF is a major objective of antihypertensive therapy.

    - Controlling hypertension prevents LV hypertrophy and acute MI, both of which reduce the incidence of HF

- HF is associated with neurohormonal activation involving the sympathetic, endothelin, vasopressin, and renin-angiotensin systems, which maintain and worsen the myocardial changes described above, while at the same time contribute to inadequate peripheral circulatory adaptation

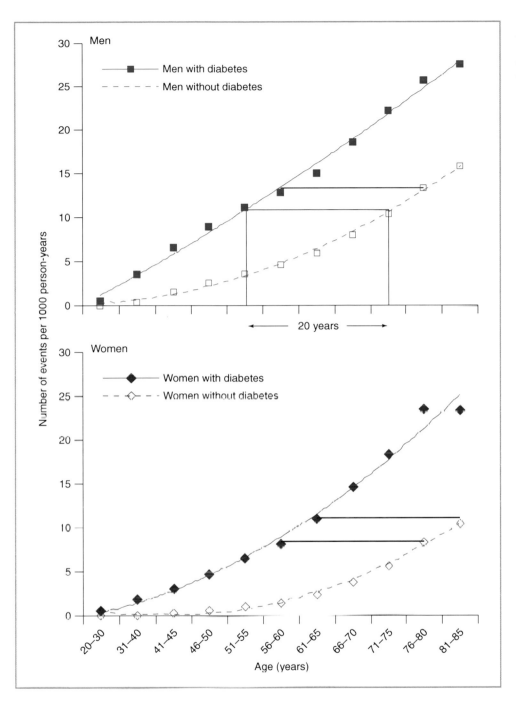

FIGURE 5-9

Effect of diabetes and age on risk of cardiovascular events (Modified from Booth et al. [38])

TREATMENT OF HYPERTENSION

General Guidelines

■ Nonpharmacologic therapy and lifestyle modification are important in treating hypertension

– Nonpharmacologic therapy may delay the need for pharmacologic therapy in some and may facilitate control of BP with lower doses or lower number of medications in most patients [43, 44]

■ Weight loss, sodium reduction, and their combination were found useful in controlling hypertension without pharmacotherapy in older hypertensive patients who needed one or two medications for control in TONE

FIGURE 5-10

Odds ratio of stroke based on SBP difference achieved between randomized groups (Used with permission from Turnbull et al. [47])

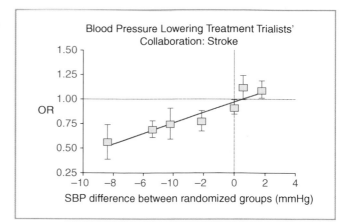

- The combination was more effective than either of the two interventions alone [45]
- Patients randomized to sodium restriction maintained their improved dietary habits even 5 years after discontinuing contact with the clinical trial center, while this was not true for caloric restriction and weight loss [46]
- Excessive alcohol consumption is associated with increased BP, probably resulting from sympathetic activation and cortisol increase

- The effect of antihypertensive therapy in decreasing cardiovascular events is more pronounced when the BP drop is bigger ([47], Fig. 5-10)

Differing Patient Subsets

- Among the medications approved for control of hypertension, diuretics, calcium channel blockers (CCBs), ACE inhibitors (ACEI), and beta blockers (BB) may be used as a first line drug in patients with hypertension (Table 5-1)
- A number of coexisting conditions as well as demographic differences may alter the preferred agents used to treat hypertension and the BP targets to be achieved
- Adverse effects of medications become important in different patient subsets (e.g. bronchospastic disease for beta-blockers)

  - The use of diuretics in treating hypertension in older people is associated with hyperglycemia, compared to CCBs, which have a neutral effect, and to agents affecting the renin angiotensin system which are associated with lower glucose concentrations [48, 49]

    - The hyperglycemia associated with chlorthalidone in the Systolic Hypertension in the Elderly Program (SHEP) was not associated with impaired outcomes compared to patients who had diabetes at baseline at 14-year follow-up [50]
    - Thiazide-type diuretics produce hyperglycemia in part by impaired insulin release related to hypokalemia rather than through insulin resistance, the common mechanism of diabetes in older adults [51, 52]

  - Gout is another adverse effect associated with thiazide diuretics and both hypertension and diuretic use increase the chance of developing this condition [53]

- Treatment targets

  - The Seventh Report of the Joint National Commission (JNC), JNC 7 guidelines for antihypertensive treatment targets [43] include:

    - General: <140/90 mmHg
    - DM or CKD: 130/80 mmHg
    - CHD or CVA: There is no unanimity on different BP targets in these populations

COEXISTENT DISEASE	TARGET BP (MMHG)	PREFERRED DRUGS	CONTRAINDICATED DRUGS
Coronary heart disease	<130/80	BB; CCB[a]; ACEI	
Left ventricular hypertrophy	140/80[c]	ACEI/ARB	
Heart failure	<130/80	BB; Diuretics; ACEI; ARA	Non-dihydropyridine CCB
Cerebrovascular disease	140/80	Diuretics; ACEI, CCB	
Diseases of the aorta and PVD	<135–145/60–90	BB+ACEI/ARB	
Diabetes mellitus	<130/80 140/80[b]	ACEI/ARB; CCB	
Primary aldosteronism	140/80	ARA, potassium-sparing diuretics	
Renovascular disease	140/80[c]	ACEI or ARB and diuretics	Caution with ACE or ARB in patients with bilateral RAS (monitor GFR)
Chronic kidney disease	<130/80	ACEI or ARB	(Aliskerin if already on ACEI/ARB)

[a]If normal left ventricular systolic function
[b]No benefit observed for SBP 120 mmHg versus 140 mmHg; increase in mortality noted if SBP <115 mmHg and DBP <65 mmHg
[c]140/90 mmHg refers to the blood pressure target for the general population, but lower targets have been suggested for this group

- The ACCF/AHA 2011 expert consensus document suggests a comprehensive approach to treatment ([54], Fig. 5-11)
- Special considerations

  - In the U.S., older Black Americans have more severe hypertension and have high rates of stroke, LVH and CKD [43]

    - Blacks in NHANES III were less likely to have their BP controlled. They are also more likely to have diabetes and increased BMI.
    - Blacks are more likely high-volume/low-renin hypertensives, and hence diuretics as well as CCB may be reasonable agents to start with, however responsiveness to ACEI and ARB remains in this patient subgroup, so their use should not be discouraged.

  - Controlling hypertension alone is not sufficient since other risk factors (e.g. hypercholesterolemia, diabetes, and smoking) have an additive and possibly multiplicative effect in causing cardiovascular disease

    - In the TNT clinical trial, the best outcomes were observed among patients in the lowest SBP and lowest LDL tertiles [55]

  - While tight blood pressure control is desirable in advanced CKD, the use of ACEI plus ARBs, or ACE (or ARB) plus aliskerin (a direct renin inhibitor) is to be avoided, given the risk of hypotension, hyperkalemia, and risk for progressive renal failure.

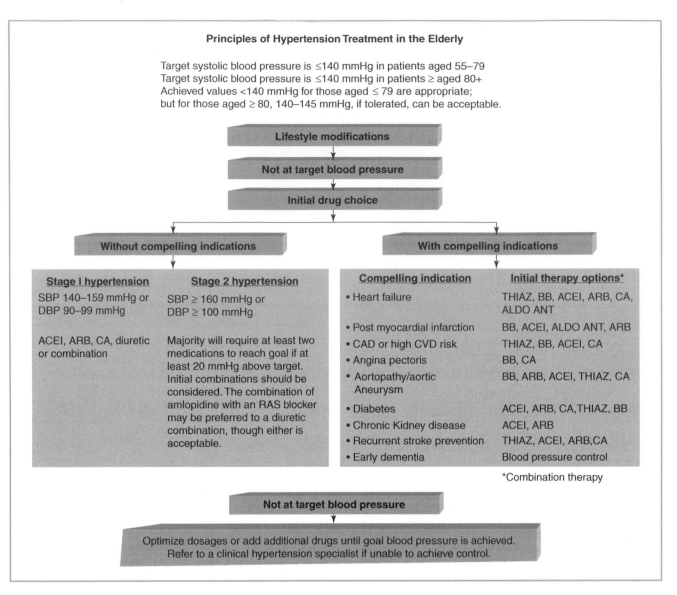

FIGURE 5-11

Algorithm for treatment of hypertension in the elderly (Used with permission from Aronow et al. [54])

Resistant Hypertension

■ BP above goal despite the concurrent use of 3 antihypertensive medications of different classes
■ Occurs in about 20–30 % of patients

  – Causes include secondary hypertension, such as renal artery stenosis, as well as medication induced hypertension

■ More common in older and obese patients
■ Carries high CV risk as it is associated with severe hypertension, DM, CKD.
■ Pseudoresistance refers to lack of control due to poor adherence, white coat hypertension, lack of appropriate medication dose titration, etc.

■ Clinical evidence suggests that addition of a thiazide diuretic and/or ARA in those with resistant hypertension is an effective intervention
■ Additional antihypertensive classes that may be helpful as third-fifth line agents include

- Aldosterone receptor antagonists (ARA) (e.g. spironolactone, eplerenone), with particular benefit in HF
- Centrally-acting alpha-2 agonists (e.g. clonidine, alpha-methyldopa (also useful during pregnancy or for pregnancy-induced hypertension due to lack of teratogenicity))
- Alpha-blocking agents (e.g. doxazosin (had higher incidence of HF in ALLHAT), phentolamine (for hypertensive emergency))
- Hydralazine, a peripheral vasodilator, has been shown to be especially effective in combination with BB or spironolactone
- Minoxidil (another peripheral vasodilator) is also used to prevent hair loss

Severe/Malignant Hypertension and Hypertensive Crises

■ Hypertensive crisis refers the sudden or rapid development of severe hypertension (SBP ≥180 mmHg and/or DBP ≥120 mmHg)
■ Hypertensive crises tend to occur among patients with poor medication adherence, acute sodium load
■ A hypertensive crisis constitutes a hypertensive emergency when the patient develops acute complications, including

- Retinal hemorrhages, exudates, or papilledema.
- Renal involvement (malignant nephrosclerosis, proteinuria, hematuria)
- Hypertensive encephalopathy with cerebral edema; may cause headache, nausea vomiting, confusion, seizures, coma

  ■ This may predominantly affect the posterior circulation, presenting with a reversible leukoencephalopathy

- Stroke (ischemic or hemorrhagic)
- Myocardial ischemia or infarction
- Aortic dissection

■ Management of hypertensive emergency involves immediate control of BP using sodium nitroprusside, clevidipine, nicardipine, or labetalol

- Lower DBP initially by up to 25 %
- Aim for DBP 100–105 mmHg within 6–8 h
- Avoid lowering SBP below 160 mmHg in the acute setting (given change in cerebral autoregulation)
- Exception: aortic dissection, where goals are SBP 120 mmHg, MAP 80 mm, achieved over 5–10 min
- Reduce blood pressure to goal on oral medications, gradually over 2–3 months

■ Hypertensive urgency refers to a hypertensive crisis without symptoms or the above acute target organ damage

- Reduce blood pressure more gradually, over 24–48 h

FIGURE 6-2

Schematic of intestinal pathway. Chylomicrons (*CM*) are assembled in intestinal epithelial cells and secreted into the circulation, where they undergo lipolysis by lipoprotein lipase (*LPL*). CM-remnants are taken up by the liver. *LRP* lipoprotein receptor-related protein

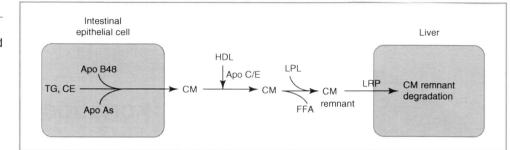

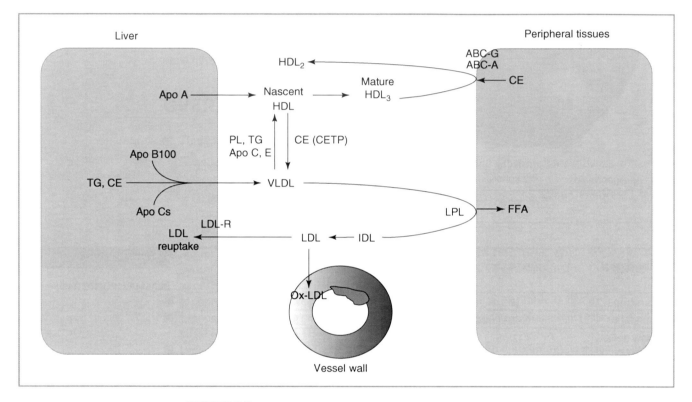

FIGURE 6-3

Schematic of hepatic pathway. TG-rich VLDL are assembled in the liver and secreted into the circulation. Cholesteryl ester transfer protein (*CETP*) facilitates transfer of TG from VLDL to HDL in exchange for cholesterol. VLDL is hydrolyzed by LPL to release FFA that are taken up by peripheral tissues (fat, muscle). LDL generated from LPL action can enter the vessel wall, where its oxidation and uptake by macrophages leads to foam cell formation, a key step in atherogenesis. Nascent HDL secreted from the liver play an important role in reverse cholesterol transport

■ Hepatic Pathway (Fig. 6-3):

- Coordinates the transport of TG and cholesterol between the liver and target peripheral tissues
- Hepatocytes package TG with Apo B100 to form VLDL
- In the circulation, VLDL interacts with HDL to [1]: acquire additional lipoproteins (Apo C and E), and [2] exchange TG for CE
- Like CM, VLDL undergoes lipolysis by LPL to produce FFA
- VLDL hydrolysis yields IDL, which undergoes further hydrolysis by hepatic lipase to form LDL, the main courier of FC and CE
- LDL is taken by the liver, a process mediated by the LDL receptor (LDL-R)
- LDL modification in the vessel wall and uptake by macrophages leads to foam cell formation, a key step in atherogenesis

LIPOPROTEIN DISORDERS AND CHD RISK

- Several lipid and lipoprotein variables have been reported to confer an increased risk of CHD:

  - Elevated total cholesterol (TC) and LDL cholesterol (LDL-C) [6, 7]
  - Low HDL-C and high TG [6, 8]
  - Elevated non-HDL cholesterol (a measure of the total burden of Apo-B containing atherogenic lipoprotein particles) [9]
  - Apo B lipoprotein levels [9]
  - Elevated Lp(a) [10]
  - Small, dense LDL particles [11]

- NCEP-ATPIII guidelines identify LDL-C as the primary lipid target for intervention [4, 5]
- A continuous log-linear relationship exists between LDL-C and CHD risk [5]:

  - a decrease of 1 mg/dL in LDL-C results in a 1 % decrease in CHD relative risk
  - a given mg/dL change in LDL-C produces the same change in relative risk of CHD at any level of LDL-C

- Although LDL-C is the primary lipid target, other parameters such as low HDL-C, non-HDL-C, and Apo B appear to be stronger predictors of CHD risk [9, 12, 13]
- An increase of 1 mg/dL in HDL-C is associated with a 2–3 % decrease in CHD risk [8], but to date there is no RCT to support targeting HDL-C
- ATPIII identified non-HDL-C, a surrogate marker of Apo B levels, as a secondary target in patients with TG > 200 mg/dL (Non-HDL-C = TC - HDL-C)
- NCEP ATPIII guidelines did not recommend routine testing for emerging lipid risk markers

DIAGNOSIS AND SCREENING

- The most common lipoprotein disorders encountered clinically are related to age, physical inactivity, diet, obesity, and lifestyle factors (smoking)
- Recent classification systems from WHO and NCEP focus on thresholds and cut points for serum lipoprotein lipids to diagnose and treat lipoprotein disorders (Table 6-3)
- Plasma levels of lipids (cholesterol and triglycerides) and lipoprotein cholesterol (LDL-C and HDL-C) define three general patterns of lipoprotein disorders commonly encountered in clinical settings:

  - Hyperlipidemia refers to an elevation in LDL-C (and TC)
  - Hypertriglyceridemia refers to an elevation in TG
  - Dyslipidemia refers to a combination of hypertriglyceridemia and low HDL-C with either a normal or elevated TC or LDL-C (commonly seen in insulin resistant states)

- Fasting lipid profile (FLP), which provides direct measurement of TC, TG, HDL-C and calculated LDL-C, is the preferred initial test, rather than measurement of non-fasting TC and HDL-C alone.

LIPID	OPTIMAL (MG/DL)	BORDERLINE ELEVATION (MG/DL)	ELEVATED/HIGH RISK (MG/DL)
TC	<200	200–239	>240
LDL-C	<100 (100–129-near optimal)	130–159	>160
HDL-C	≥60	40–59 (men) 50–59 (women)	<40 (men) <50 (women)
TG	<150	150–199	>200

TABLE 6-3

SERUM LIPID CONCENTRATIONS

- The Friedewald formula [14] (below) is used to calculate LDL-C, because direct measurement of LDL-C is time consuming and costly

$$LDL\text{-}C = TC - (HDL + TG / 5)$$

- The LDL-C calculated from the Friedewald formula is inaccurate at higher TG levels [15], and direct measurement of LDL should be considered if TG > 400 mg/dL [4, 15]
- ATP III screening guidelines: FLP at least once every 5 years for individuals older than 20 years of age, with consideration for more frequent testing in older individuals with risk factors [4]
- Significant elevations in LDL-C (> 190 mg/dL) can indicate a genetic disorder that warrants further consideration and family testing
- Patients admitted with MI should have a FLP within 24 h of admission (levels drawn later will be spuriously low due to hepatic stress response or medications)

MANAGEMENT OF LIPOPROTEIN DISORDERS

Drugs that Modulate Lipid Metabolism

Hyroxymethylglutaryl-Coenzyme A Reductase Inhibitors (Statins)
- Statins inhibit HMG-CoA reductase, the rate-limiting enzyme in sterol synthesis
- Statins increase expression of LDL-R and decrease CE formation, leading to enhanced LDL-C clearance from plasma and reduced VLDL production
- Statins are the drugs of choice for reducing LDL-C (20–55 % reduction)
- Statins also modestly decrease TG (5–30 %) and increase HDL-C (2–10 %)
- Data support efficacy of statins in primary and secondary prevention across age groups, in men and women, and in type 2 diabetes (T2D) [3, 4]
- Starting statin dose should be sufficient to decrease the LDL-C by 30–40 % [4] (Table 6-4)
- Doubling the dose of any of the statins yields a further 6 % decrease in LDL-C
- Starting doses should be lower in smaller patients, the elderly, and patients of East Asian ancestry, in whom starting doses of rosuvastatin should be 5 mg
- Statins are relatively safe with low rates of liver toxicity (1.4 %) and myopathy (0.2 %) [3]
- The risk of myopathy is significantly higher with 80 mg of simvastatin and doses higher than 40 mg of simvastatin should be avoided
- The risk of myositis is increased if statins are used with niacin or fibrates (especially gemfibrozil)
- Lower doses of potent statins (atorvastatin and rosuvastatin) are associated with lower rates of myositis and transaminitis
- Lovastatin, simvastatin, and atorvastatin are metabolized by CYP 3A4 and should be used with caution with other drugs that are metabolized using the same pathway

TABLE 6-4			
	STATIN	DOSE (MG/DL)	LDL-C REDUCTION (%)
DOSES OF AVAILABLE STATINS REQUIRED TO ATTAIN 30–40 % REDUCTION IN LDL-C	Fluvastatin	40–80	25–35
	Lovastatin	40	31
	Pravastatin	40	34
	Simvastatin	20–40	35–41
	Atorvastatin	10	39
	Rosuvastatin	5–10	39–45
	Pitavastatin[a]	2–4	38–45

[a]Most recently approved statin (FDA approval in 8/2009)

(macrolides, antifungals, cyclosporine, verapamil, amlodipine, ranolazine, or large quantities of grapefruit juice)

- Statins are contraindicated in pregnancy (Class X for known teratogenic effects) and other alternatives such as bile acid sequestrants (Class B) and fibrates (Class C) should be used

Fibrates

- Fibrates activate peroxisome proliferator-activated receptor alpha (PPARα) which increases apo A-I and represses apo B and VLDL production
- Lower TG 20–35 % and increase HDL-C by 6–18 % with modest effect on LDL-C (~20 % reduction)
- Drugs of choice for severe hypertriglyceridemia
- Helsinki Heart Study [16] and VA-HIT [17] trials showed fibrate monotherapy reduces CV events
- However the recent FIELD [18] and ACCORD [19] trials raise questions regarding clinical benefits of combined fibrate therapy in T2D patients with modest TG and HDL-C abnormalities
- ATPIII recommends considering adding fibrates to statins in high risk patients with TG and HDL-C abnormalities [4], although trial data for this strategy is lacking
- Gemfibrozil can inhibit glucurodination and elimination of statins, thereby significantly increasing the risk of statin-myotoxicity

Niacin

- Niacin has multiple effects including suppression of lipolysis, reduced hepatic synthesis of TG and VLDL secretion, increased apo B degradation, and decreased catabolism of HDL
- Most potent HDL-raising agent (10–35 %) that also lowers TG (20–30 %) and LDL-C (10–25 %)
- The CDP (coronary drug project) [20] showed niacin monotherapy decreased CV events by ~30 %
- ATPIII guidelines recommend addition of Niacin to statins in high risk patients with low HDL-C and high TG to address residual risk [4], although trial data for this strategy is lacking
- Recent AIM-HIGH trial investigating addition of niacin to patients on simvastatin and controlled LDL showed no benefit [21]
- Side effects include cutaneous flushing, hyperuricemia, transaminitis, and hyperglycemia

Bile Acid Sequestrants

- Interrupt reabsorption of cholesterol-containing bile acids
- Mainly used as an adjunctive therapy in patients with severe elevations in LDL-C
- Modest decreases in LDL-C (15–30 %) and small increases in HDL-C (5–15 %)
- Frequent GI side effects and occasionally results in hypertriglyceridemia

Cholesterol Absorption Inhibitors (Ezetimibe)

- Inhibits intestinal cholesterol absorption via cholesterol transport interference
- Reduces LDL-C (10–25 %) but may have beneficial effects on TG, apo B, and HDL-C
- Addition of ezetimibe to statins decreases LDL-C by an additional 25–30 %
- ENHANCE trial showed that addition of ezetimibe to simvastatin did not affect the surrogate marker of carotid intimal thickness [22]
- SHARP trial showed simvastatin/ezetimibe safely reduced LDL-C and CV events in patients with CKD compared to placebo [23] (Table 6-5)

Core concepts from NCEP ATPIII treatment guidelines

- Risk assessment and categorization using non-LDL risk factors (RF) and risk modifiers (Table 6-6) and Framingham Risk Score (FRS) are the first steps
- Evaluation of secondary causes of lipoprotein disorders
- Individualized LDL-C goals (primary target) and non-HDL-C goals (secondary target if TG > 200) based on risk stratification (Table 6-7)
- Therapeutic lifestyle changes (TLC) for all patients
- Appropriate initiation and intensity of pharmacologic therapy based on risk
- Treatment of non-lipid risk factors and secondary causes of dyslipoproteinemia
- Management considerations in genetic disorders

TABLE 6-5			
PRIMARY LIPID-MODIFYING DRUG CLASSES	**DRUG CLASS**	**METABOLIC EFFECTS**	**CLINICAL CONSIDERATIONS**
	Statins	↓LDL-C 20–55 % ↑HDL-C 2–10 % [a] ↓TG 5–30 %	↓CV events, CHD deaths, need for PCI, CVA, total mortality Liver and muscle toxicity (monitor CK, LFTs) Potential drug interactions between some statins[b] and CYP450 3A4 inhibitors (macrolides, antifungals, cyclosporine, grapefruit juice) Use with caution with fibrates (avoid gemfibrozil) and niacin Avoid simvastatin at 80 mg (ok to continue if tolerated>1 year) Absolute contraindications: active or chronic liver disease Relative contraindications: concomitant use of some drugs
	Fibrates: Gemfibrozil Fenofibrate	↓TG 20–35 % ↑HDL-C 6–20 % ↓TC/LDL-C 20–25 %[c]	Reduced CV events (monotherapy) in 1° and 2° prevention No benefit observed in statin-treated DM patients with dyslipidemia GI side effects, transaminitis, muscle injury, elevation in creatine (not related to reduction in GFR) Absolute contraindications: severe renal/ hepatic disease Relative contraindications: statins (avoid gemfibrozil)
	Nicotinic acid: Multiple OTCs Prescription: Slo-Niacin Niaspan	↓TG 20–30 % ↑HDL-C 10–35 % ↓LDL-C 10–20 %	Reduced CV events as monotherapy Recent trial data show no benefit in statin-treated patients with well controlled LDL-C and persistent low HDL-C Frequent side effects: cutaneous flushing, hyperuricemia, hypertriglyceridemia, hepatotoxicity, gastritis Absolute contraindications: hepatic disease, severe gout Relative contraindications: DM, hyperurice-mia, Peptic ulcer disease
	Bile acid sequestrants: Cholestyramine Colestipol Colesevam	↓LDL-C 15–25 %	Mainly used as adjunctive therapy for LDL-C lowering Frequent GI side effects and may increase TG Many potential drug interactions Interferes with absorption of other drugs (administer 1 h after or 3 h before other medications) Absolute contraindications: TG>400 mg/dL Relative contraindications: TG>200 mg/dL
	Cholesterol absorption inhibitor: Ezetimibe	↓LDL-C 10–20 % ↓LDL-C additional 25 % with statin	Used primarily as adjunctive therapy with statin for LDL-C lowering No trial data to support incremental clinical benefit over statin alone Rarely causes myopathy

[a]Less consistent than LDL effects
[b]Lovastatin, simvastatin>atorvastatin
[c]May increase LDL-C in patients with elevated TGs ("beta-shift")

Risk factor

1. Cigarette smoking
2. Hypertension (BP≥140/90 mmHg or treatment for hypertension)
3. Low HDL (< 40 mg/dL for men and<50 mg/dL for women)[a]
4. Family history of premature CAD[b]
5. Age (≥45 years for men and ≥55 years for women)

[a]HDL-C>60 mg/dL represents a protective factor (removes 1 risk factor)
[b]CHD in male 1st degree relative<55 years and female 1st degree relative<65 years

TABLE 6-6

MAJOR NON-LDL RISK FACTORS

TABLE 6-7

LDL-C AND NON-HDL-C GOALS
BASED ON RISK STRATIFICATION

RISK CATEGORY	LDL-C GOAL (MG/DL)	NON-HDL-C[A] GOAL (MG/DL)	DRUG THERAPY FOR LDL-C (MG/DL)
High risk: CHD or CHD equivalents (10-years risk>20 %) (<100 mg/dL-consider drugs)	<100 <70 (for very high risk)[b]	<130	≥100
Moderately-high risk: 2+ RF (10 years-risk 10–20 %)	<130	<160	≥130
Moderate risk: 2+ RF (10 years-risk <10 %)	<130	<160	≥160
Low risk: 0–1 RF (10 years-risk <10 %)	<160	<190	≥190

[a]Non-HDL-C=TC-HDL-C
[b]Optional target for very high risk patients: established CHD and (1) history of ACS, (2) T2D or MetS, (3) multiple RF, (4) severe or poorly controlled RF

■ Step 1- Risk assessment:

– ATPIII recommends classification of risk into four groups:

1. High Risk (10 years risk >20 %)
2. Moderately High Risk (2+ RF and 10 years risk 10–20 %)
3. Moderate Risk (2+ RF and 10 years risk <10 %)
4. Low risk (10 years risk >10 %)

– Classify patients with established CHD, other forms of atherosclerotic disease (peripheral and cerebrovascular disease, abdominal aneurysms), and T2D as "high risk"
– Classify CHD patients as "very high risk" if [1]: history of acute coronary syndrome (ACS) [2], multiple RF including T2D or metabolic syndrome (MetS), or [3] severe or poorly controlled RF
– If no established CHD or CHD equivalents, count major non-LDL risk RF (Table 6-6)
– If 0–1 RF, classify as low risk
– If 2+ RF, calculate FRS and classify patients as follows:

1. FRS 10 years risk >20 % classify as "high risk"
2. FRS 10 years risk 10–20 % classify as "moderately-high risk"
3. FRS 10 years risk <10 % classify as "moderate risk"

■ Step 2: Rule out and treat secondary causes of lipoprotein disorders (T2D, thyroid disorders, drugs, nephrosis)

■ Step 3: Establish LDL-C goal based on risk:

  – LDL-C is the primary target (Table 6-7)
  – For CHD and CHD equivalents, target LDL-C is <100 mg/dL (optional LDL-C goal of <70 mg/dL in very high risk patients)
  – For moderately-high risk and moderate risk patients, LDL-C goal is <130 mg/dL
  – For low risk patients, LDL-C goal is <160 mg/dL
  – If TG > 500 mg/dL (imminent risk of pancreatitis), treat hypertriglyceridemia first

■ Step 4: Establish secondary goals (non-HDL-C and MetS):

  – Non-HDL-C is a marker of the total burden of atherogenic TG-rich lipoproteins
  – Non-HDL-C is a secondary goal when TG >200 mg/dL
  – Non-HDL-C goals are 30 mg/dL higher than LDL-C goals for each risk group
  – Interventions to decrease non-HDL-C include:

    1. Increase statin dose
    2. Add second agent (fibrate/niacin)
    3. TLC

  – ATPIII also identifies MetS as a secondary target for aggressive treatment

■ Step 5: Initiate TLC in all patients and pharmacologic therapy in selected patients (Table 6-7):

  – All patients with lipoprotein disorders should be encouraged to undertake TLC:

    1. Decrease intake of dietary saturated fats (< 7 % total calories) and cholesterol (< 200 mg/dL)
    2. Exercise
    3. Increase plant phytosterol (2 g/day) and fiber (10–25 g/day) intake

  – Initiating pharmacologic therapy in high risk patients:

    1. Statins are drugs of choice for LDL-C lowering in patients with hyperlipidemia and dyslipidemia
    2. Start drug therapy if LDL-C >100 mg/dL
    3. If baseline LDL-C <100 mg/dL, starting drug therapy to attain an LDL-C <70 mg/dL is a therapeutic option
    4. Initial statin dose should achieve a 30–40 % decrease in LDL-C
    5. If TG >200 mg/dL or HDL-C levels are low, consider niacin or fibrate

  – Initiating pharmacologic therapy in moderately-high risk patients:

    1. Start drug therapy if LDL-C >130 mg/dL
    2. Consider drug options if LDL-C is 100–130 mg/dL
    3. Initial statin dose should achieve a 30–40 % decrease in LDL-C

  – Initiating pharmacologic therapy in moderate risk patients:

    1. Start drug therapy if LDL-C >160 mg/dL
    2. Consider drug options if LDL-C is 130–160 mg/dL

  – Initiating pharmacologic therapy in low risk patients: recommended threshold LDL-C > 190 mg/dL (starting drug for LDL-C 160–190 mg/dL is an option)

■ Follow-up after initiating therapy:

  – Repeat FLP 6 weeks after initiation of therapy and again at 6 weeks intervals until at goal (LDL-C and any appropriate secondary targets)
  – If LDL-C not at goal, consider increasing statin dose, switching to a more potent statin, or adding adjunctive agent (niacin, fibrate, bile acid sequestrant, ezetimibe)
  – After LDL-C is at goal, patients should be tested every 6–12 months

- Baseline LFTs should be checked prior to initiation of therapy with statin, niacin, or fibrate, and then again 3 months after start of treatment, and then every 6–12 months
- CKs should be checked if patient complains of myalgias

Management of Genetic Dyslipidemias

Familial Hypercholesterolemia (FH)
- Autosomal co-dominant disorder due to mutation in LDL-R
- Heterozygous form (prevalence 1 in 500 people) results in LDL-C twice normal (190–350 mg/dL)
- Homozygous form (prevalence 1 in 1.1 million) results in LDL-C in 400–1,000 mg/dL range
- Tendon xanthoma, corneal arcus senilis usually present
- Premature CHD is common in the third decade in men and in the fourth decade in women
- LDL- lowering therapy initiated in teenage years with statin (1st line), bile acid sequestrant, or multi-drug regimen
- Homozygous FH patients often need plasma apheresis
- Family testing indicated

Familial Defective apolipoprotein B (FDB)
- Autosomal dominant disorder due to mutation in Apo B100 gene (prevalence of 1 in 1,000)
- Results in 1.5–2 fold elevations in LDL-C (160–300 mg/dL)
- Xanthomas as well as premature CHD and aortic valve disease are common
- As with heterozygous FH, combination LDL-lowering therapy is effective
- Family testing indicated

Polygenic Hypercholesterolemia
- Due to complex interactions between environmental factors and multiple genetic factors
- LDL-C > 190 mg/dL but generally milder than heterozygous FH
- Relatively common (prevalence 1 in 20)
- Only ~10 % of 1st degree relatives of affected individuals have elevated LDL-C
- Increased risk of CHD but xanthomas are absent
- TLC, LDL-lowering therapy with statins or bile acid sequestrants or combination therapy are indicated

Familial Hypertriglyceridemia
- Genetic defect undefined
- Affected individuals have normal or mildly elevated TC and LDL-C, but significant hypertriglyceridemia (200–500 mg/dL fasting and greater than 1,000 mg/dL after meals)
- Xanthoma usually absent and the relationship with CAD is not as strong as with FH
- Treatment based on dietary modifications, exercise, and drug therapy

Familial Combined Hyperlipidemia (FCH)
- Common familial lipoprotein disorder (prevalence of 1 in 50 people)
- Lipid abnormalities in FCH include elevated TC and LDL-C (>190 mg/dL) and TG (>300 mg/dL)
- Few clinical signs are present, but there is an increased risk of premature CAD
- Management is similar to other genetic dyslipidemias: TLC and statin, and consideration for addition of niacin or fibrate if indicated

Genetic Disorders Affecting HDL
- Hypoalphalipoprotenemia-low HDL levels due to mutation of Apo A-1, but only a subset of these patients have an increased risk of CHD
- Tangier's Disease- Low HDL-C due to ABCA-1 mutation with no clear increased risk of CHD

■ Lecithin cholesterolacyl transferase (LCAT) Deficiency– Absent LCAT activity leads to decreased CE formation in circulating HDL particles and low HDL-C, without a clear increase in CHD risk
■ CETP Deficiency- Absence of CETP leads to accumulation of cholesterol in HDL, leading to high HDL-C levels but no clear protection against CHD

QUICK REVIEW

■ Disorders of lipoproteins are important targets in primary and secondary prevention of CHD
■ Recent classification systems from WHO and NCEP focus on cut points for serum and lipoprotein lipids to diagnose and treat lipoprotein disorders
■ FLP is the initial screening test of choice
■ NCEP ATPIII guidelines advocate a step-wise approach to the diagnosis and management of lipoprotein disorders (Fig. 6-4)
■ LDL-C is the primary target, but non-HDL-C and MetS are secondary targets in select populations
■ TLC should be encouraged in all patients with lipoprotein disorders
■ Statins are drugs of choice for LDL-lowering therapy

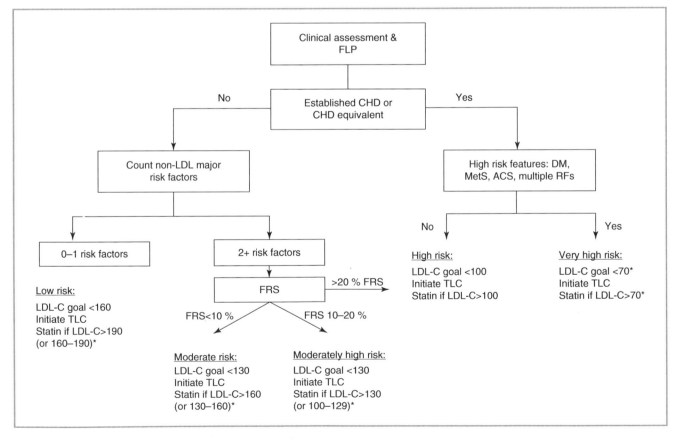

FIGURE 6-4

Summary of NCEP ATPIII guidelines for management of hyperlipidemia. Management strategy emphasizes individual risk assessment and establishing LDL-C (primary target) goals based on risk. * Optional targets based on 2004 ATPIII update

- Fibrates are most effective in treating hypertriglyceridemia, which should be the addressed first if TG elevations are severe (>500 mg/dL) and risk of pancreatitis is imminent
- Reassess FLP in 6 weeks intervals until LDL-C and secondary targets are at goal, then annually
- Marked elevations of LDL-C suggest a genetic disorder such as FH

REVIEW QUESTIONS

1. **A 58 year-old Asian man with no prior cardiac history presents to your office for evaluation. He has not seen in a doctor "in over 20 years." The patient smokes a half a pack of cigarettes daily and is not currently on any medications. He reports that his father suffered a heart attack at the age of 53. In the clinic, his BP is 154/93 with a HR of 78, and his BMI is 28. The patient's physical examination is notable only for the presence of an S4. An ECG shows sinus rhythm and evidence of LVH. A FLP and baseline labs show:**

Total cholesterol – 220 mg/dL	AST – 32 IU/L
Triglycerides – 286 mg/dL	ALT – 24 IU/L
HDL-C – 34 mg/dL	CK – 55 IU/L
LDL-C – 131 mg/dL	Fasting glucose – 103 mg/dL

You see the patient in follow-up 2 weeks later. At that time, his BP is 158/89. His Framingham 10-years risk score is 28 %. You initiate treatment for his HTN and outline a plan for dietary changes, exercise, and smoking cessation. The next best step in your management is:
   - (a) No further therapy is needed at this time
   - (b) Start 10 mg of lovastatin daily
   - (c) Start 80 mg of simvastatin daily
   - (d) Start 20 mg of atorvastatin daily
   - (e) Start 600 mg of gemfibrozil twice daily

2. **The above patient is seen in follow up 6 weeks later. He has quit smoking and his BP is now well controlled at 132/80. A repeat FLP shows the following:**

Total cholesterol – 188 mg/dL	Triglycerides – 268 mg/dL
HDL-C – 40 mg/dL	LDL-C – 94 mg/dL

The next best step in your management is:
   - (a) No further therapy is needed since LDL-C is less than 100 mg/dL
   - (b) Increase atorvastatin to 40 mg daily
   - (c) Discontinue atorvastatin and start gemfibrozil 600 mg twice daily
   - (d) Add eztimibe 10 mg to the current dose of atorvastatin
   - (e) Add gemfibrozil 600 mg twice daily to the current dose of atorvastatin

3. **A 17 year-old female is referred to your office for consultation after a recent abnormal fasting lipid panel. She is healthy and her family history is notable for hyperlipidemia and premature CHD in her father, who suffered an MI in his 30s. A screening fasting lipid panel showed the following:**

Total cholesterol – 267 mg/dL	Triglycerides – 90 mg/dL
HDL-C – 55 mg/dL	LDL-C – 194 mg/dL

In clinic, her BP is 118/67 and a HR of 66 with a BMI of 19. She was noted to have a nodular, mobile 0.5 cm mass over the right Achilles tendon. The ECG was within normal limits. The next best step in her treatment is to:
   - (a) Advise her to undertake therapeutic lifestyle modifications and defer drug therapy since statins are not safe in teenagers
   - (b) Calculate her 10 years risk score and start therapy if she is classified as moderate risk
   - (c) Calculate her 10 years risk score and start therapy if she is classified as high risk
   - (d) Calculate her 10 years risk score and start therapy if she is classified as very risk
   - (e) Initiate therapy with a statin after checking a pregnancy test

ANSWERS

1. (d) According to NCEP ATPIII, patients with two or more risk factors with a FRS 10 years risk score of >20 % should be classified as high risk with a goal LDL-C of less than 100 mg/dL. Drug therapy is recommended for LDL-C levels greater than 130 mg/dL. This patient likely has metabolic syndrome with an atherogenic dyslipidemia characterized by mild elevations in TC and LDL-C, low HDL-C, and elevated triglycerides. Based on these issues and his baseline LDL-C, initiation of LDL-C lowering drug therapy is indicated. Although the Helsinki Heart Study [16] and VA-HIT [17] suggest that this patient would benefit from fibrate therapy, statins are considered the drugs of choice for LDL-lowering in patients with dyslipidemia. Starting doses of statins should be sufficient to lower LDL-C 30–40 %. Among the choices presented, 20 mg of atorvastatin represents the best selection. A dose of 10 mg of lovastatin is unlikely to achieve a 30–40 % reduction in LDL-C. Simvastatin 80 mg daily will likely decrease the LDL-C by >40 %; however, based on a recent FDA review, the 80 mg dose of simvastatin should not be started based on a significantly

higher risk of myotoxicity compared to other statins and lower doses of simvastatin. This is a particularly important issue in older patients and individuals of Asian ancestry.

2. (b) In patients with the atherogenic dyslipidemia of the metabolic syndrome and TG>200 mg/dL, NCEP ATPIII recommends establishing a secondary non-HDL-C goal of <130 mg/dL. Non-HDL-C is a surrogate marker of apo B lipoprotein levels that predicts CV events and is calculated by subtracting HDL-C from TC. Although the LDL-C is at goal (<100 mg/dL), the non-HDL-C is still elevated at 148 mg/dL. Therefore, further intervention is required. NCEP ATPIII recommend two strategies to address non-HDL-C [1]: intensifying statin therapy and [2] adding either a fibrate or niacin to the statin. Based on current available evidence, intensifying statin therapy represents the best first option. This patient may not reach his non-HDL-C goal with just intensification of statin therapy, and at that time, it would be reasonable to consider addition of niacin or fibrates, but current evidence has not established that this offers additional clinical benefit [19, 21]. As discussed above, since LDL-C is the primary target, discontinuing atorvastatin in favor of fibrate monotherapy is not indicated.

3. (e) This patient likely has heterozygous familial hypercholesterolemia. The typical features in this patient include an LDL-C>95th percentile for age (190–350 mg/dL), a 1st degree relative with severe hypercholesterolemia, and the Achilles tendon xanthoma. Patients with FH are at a risk for premature CHD and should be treated with LDL-C lowering therapy. Several studies demonstrate that statins, which are first line therapy for reducing LDL-C in these patients, are safe in children as young as 8 years of age [24, 25]. There is no role for the FRS calculation in the treatment-decision analysis in these patients because the expert consensus is that traditional risk scores significantly underestimate their CV risk.

REFERENCES

1. Yusuf S, Hawken S, Ounpuu S, Dans T, Avezum A, Lanas F, et al. Effect of potentially modifiable risk factors associated with myocardial infarction in 52 countries (the INTERHEART study): case-control study. Lancet. 2004;364(9438):937–52.

2. Fruchart JC, Sacks FM, Hermans MP, Assmann G, Brown WV, Ceska R, et al. The residual risk reduction initiative: a call to action to reduce residual vascular risk in dyslipidaemic patient. Diab Vasc Dis Res. 2008;5(4):319–35.

3. Baigent C, Keech A, Kearney PM, Blackwell L, Buck G, Pollicino C, et al. Efficacy and safety of cholesterol-lowering treatment: prospective meta-analysis of data from 90,056 participants in 14 randomised trials of statins. Lancet. 2005;366(9493):1267–78.

4. Expert Panel on Detection, and Treatment of High Blood Cholesterol in Adults. Third Report of the National Cholesterol Education Program (NCEP) Expert Panel on Detection, Evaluation, and Treatment of High Blood Cholesterol in Adults (Adult Treatment Panel III) final report. Circulation. 2002;106(25):3143–421.

5. Grundy SM, Cleeman JI, Merz CN, Brewer Jr HB, Clark LT, Hunninghake DB, et al. Implications of recent clinical trials for the national cholesterol education program adult treatment panel III guidelines. Circulation. 2004;110(2):227–39.

6. Wilson PW, D'Agostino RB, Levy D, Belanger AM, Silbershatz H, Kannel WB. Prediction of coronary heart disease using risk factor categories. Circulation. 1998;97(18):1837–47.

7. Pekkanen J, Linn S, Heiss G, Suchindran CM, Leon A, Rifkind BM, et al. Ten-year mortality from cardiovascular disease in relation to cholesterol level among men with and without preexisting cardiovascular disease. N Eng J Med. 1990;322(24):1700–7.

8. Gordon DJ, Probstfield JL, Garrison RJ, Neaton JD, Castelli WP, Knoke JD, et al. High-density lipoprotein cholesterol and cardiovascular disease. Four prospective American studies. Circulation. 1989;79(1):8–15.

9. Sniderman A, McQueen M, Contois J, Williams K, Furberg CD. Why is non-high-density lipoprotein cholesterol a better marker of the risk of vascular disease than low-density lipoprotein cholesterol? J Clin Lipidol. 2010;4(3):152–5.

10. Stubbs P, Seed M, Lane D, Collinson P, Kendall F, Noble M. Lipoprotein(a) as a risk predictor for cardiac mortality in patients with acute coronary syndromes. Eur Heart J. 1998;19(9): 1355–64.

11. Lamarche B, Tchernof A, Moorjani S, Cantin B, Dagenais GR, Lupien PJ, et al. Small, dense low-density lipoprotein particles as a predictor of the risk of ischemic heart disease in men. Prospective results from the Quebec Cardiovascular Study. Circulation. 1997;95(1):69–75.

12. Pischon T, Girman CJ, Sacks FM, Rifai N, Stampfer MJ, Rimm EB. Non-high-density lipoprotein cholesterol and apolipoprotein B in the prediction of coronary heart disease in men. Circulation. 2005;112(22):3375–83.

13. Ridker PM, Rifai N, Cook NR, Bradwin G, Buring JE. Non-HDL cholesterol, apolipoproteins A-I and B100, standard lipid measures, lipid ratios, and CRP as risk factors for cardiovascular disease in women. JAMA. 2005;294(3):326–33.

14. Friedewald WT, Levy RI, Fredrickson DS. Estimation of the concentration of low-density lipoprotein cholesterol in plasma, without use of the preparative ultracentrifuge. Clin Chem. 1972;18(6):499–502.

15. Nauck M, Warnick GR, Rifai N. Methods for measurement of LDL-cholesterol: a critical assessment of direct measurement by homogeneous assays versus calculation. Clin Chem. 2002;48(2): 236–54.

16. Frick MH, Elo O, Haapa K, Heinonen OP, Heinsalmi P, Helo P, et al. Helsinki Heart Study: primary-prevention trial with gemfibrozil in middle-aged men with dyslipidemia. Safety of treatment, changes in risk factors, and incidence of coronary heart disease. N Eng J Med. 1987;317(20):1237–45.

17. Rubins HB, Robins SJ, Collins D, Fye CL, Anderson JW, Elam MB, et al. Gemfibrozil for the secondary prevention of coronary heart disease in men with low levels of high-density lipoprotein cholesterol. Veterans Affairs High-Density Lipoprotein Cholesterol Intervention Trial Study Group. N Eng J Med. 1999; 341(6):410–8.

18. Keech A, Simes RJ, Barter P, Best J, Scott R, Taskinen MR, et al. Effects of long-term fenofibrate therapy on cardiovascular events in 9795 people with type 2 diabetes mellitus (the FIELD study): randomised controlled trial. Lancet. 2005;366(9500):1849–61.

19. Ginsberg HN, Elam MB, Lovato LC, Crouse 3rd JR, Leiter LA, Linz P, et al. Effects of combination lipid therapy in type 2 diabetes mellitus. N Eng J Med. 2010;362(17):1563–74.

20. Coronary Drug Project Research Group. Clofibrate and niacin in coronary heart disease. JAMA. 1975;231(4):360–81.

21. Boden WE, Probstfield JL, Anderson T, Chaitman BR, Desvignes-Nickens P, Koprowicz K, et al. Niacin in patients with low HDL cholesterol levels receiving intensive statin therapy. N Eng J Med. 2011;365(24):2255–67.

22. Kastelein JJ, Akdim F, Stroes ES, Zwinderman AH, Bots ML, Stalenhoef AF, et al. Simvastatin with or without ezetimibe in familial hypercholesterolemia. N Eng J Med. 2008;358(14): 1431–43.

23. Baigent C, Landray MJ, Reith C, Emberson J, Wheeler DC, Tomson C, et al. The effects of lowering LDL cholesterol with simvastatin plus ezetimibe in patients with chronic kidney disease (Study of Heart and Renal Protection): a randomised placebo-controlled trial. Lancet. 2011;377(9784):2181–92.

24. de Jongh S, Ose L, Szamosi T, Gagne C, Lambert M, Scott R, et al. Efficacy and safety of statin therapy in children with familial hypercholesterolemia: a randomized, double-blind, placebo-controlled trial with simvastatin. Circulation. 2002;106(17):2231–7.

25. McCrindle BW, Ose L, Marais AD. Efficacy and safety of atorvastatin in children and adolescents with familial hypercholesterolemia or severe hyperlipidemia: a multicenter, randomized, placebo-controlled trial. J Pediatr. 2003;143(1):74–80.

CHAPTER 7

Paul L. Huang

Diabetes Mellitus and the Metabolic Syndrome

CHAPTER OUTLINE

ABBREVIATIONS

3VD	3 vessel disease
ACS	Acute coronary syndrome
ADA	American Diabetes Association
AHA	American Heart Association
ATPIII	Adult Treatment Panel III
BMI	Body mass index
BS	Blood sugar
CAD	Coronary artery disease
CABG	Coronary artery bypass graft
CHF	Congestive heart failure
Cr	Creatinine
CVD	Cardiovascular disease
DES	Drug eluting stent
DM	Diabetes mellitus
DM1	Diabetes mellitus Type 1
DM2	Diabetes mellitus Type 2
DPP4	Dipeptidyl protease-4
GI	Gastrointestinal
GLP-1	Glucagon-like peptide-1
GTT	Glucose tolerance test
GWAS	Genome-wide association studies
HbA1c	Hemoglobin A1c
IFG	Impaired fasting glucose
IGT	Impaired glucose tolerance
LM	Left main
MI	Myocardial infarction
NCEP	National Cholesterol Education Program
NHLBI	National Heart Lung Blood Institute
PCI	Percutaneous coronary intervention
PPAR	Peroxisome proliferator-activated receptor
STEMI	ST-segment elevation myocardial infarction
TG	Triglyceride

INTRODUCTION

Diabetes mellitus (DM) significantly increases risk for atherosclerotic cardiovascular disease, and cardiovascular disease (CVD) is the most frequent cause of death in patients with DM. Coronary disease in diabetic patients is often more complex, more widespread, and more diffuse, making revascularization options complicated. Patients with DM also suffer from an array of microvascular and macrovascular complications. However, the increased cardiovascular risk seen in these patients can be modified by lifestyle interventions, as evidenced by several large clinical trials. The cardiologist needs to be familiar with medical therapy for diabetes, as well as how DM affects management of established cardiovascular disease and cardiovascular risks.

DEFINITIONS AND CLASSIFICATIONS

Classification of DM

Diabetes can be separated into four major classes based on causes and mechanisms:

- **Type 1 diabetes (DM1)** results from destruction of pancreatic beta-cells, which make insulin. Often, this is due to autoimmune response following a viral infection. Because the cause of diabetes is absolute lack of insulin, type 1 diabetics generally require insulin.
- **Type 2 diabetes (DM2)** results from a combination of insulin resistance and impaired beta-cell function. Historically, insulin resistance had been considered the primary defect in DM2. However, recent genome-wide association studies (GWAS) have identified genetic variants associated with DM2 that appear to affect beta cell function, suggesting the importance of the insulin secretory response in DM2.
- **Gestational diabetes** is diagnosed during pregnancy. Gestational diabetes generally resolves following pregnancy, but women who have had it are more likely to develop DM2 later in life than those who have not.
- **Other medical causes** include pancreatic tissue destruction (for example, from cystic fibrosis, pancreatic tumors, or surgery), medications (particularly for HIV-1 infection and organ transplantation), and genetic defects (in beta cell function or insulin secretion or action).

Diagnosis of DM2

According to the American Diabetes Association (ADA), a person can be diagnosed with DM2 in any one of four ways [1].

1. **Classic symptoms**
   Classic symptoms include polyuria, polydipsia, and unexplained weight loss. Because these are nonspecific, these symptoms need to be associated with a random blood glucose >200 mg/dL. Other symptoms include increased appetite, fatigue, and blurry vision.
2. **Fasting glucose (Table 7-1)**
   A fasting glucose level after at least an 8 h fast >125 mg/dL on more than one occasion
3. **Glucose tolerance test (Table 7-2)**
   In an oral glucose tolerance test (GTT), fasting blood glucose is measured after an overnight (8 h) fast. 75 g glucose, usually provided in a standardized flavored solution, is administered, and blood sugar is again measured at 2 h. If the 2 h blood sugar is over 200, the result is consistent with DM2.
4. **Hemoglobin A1c (Table 7-3)**
   Glycosylated hemoglobin, or hemoglobin A1c, reflects the average blood sugar of the past two to three months. In 2010, the ADA added HbA1c criteria for the diagnosis of DM2. HbA1c of 6.5 % or higher is consistent with DM2.

TABLE 7-1	FASTING PLASMA GLUCOSE (MG/DL)	DIAGNOSIS
FASTING GLUCOSE LEVELS	≤100	Normal
	100–125	Impaired fasting glucose (IFG)
	>125	Consistent with diabetes[a]

[a]Confirmed by repeating test on a different day

TABLE 7-2	2-H GLUCOSE (MG/DL)	DIAGNOSIS
ORAL GLUCOSE TOLERANCE TEST RESULTS	<140	Normal
	140–200	Impaired glucose tolerance (IGT)
	≥200	Consistent with diabetes[a]

[a]Confirmed by repeating test on a different day

TABLE 7-3	HBA1C (%)	DIAGNOSIS
HbA1c LEVELS	≤5.7	Normal
	5.7–6.5	Prediabetes (by HbA1c)
	≥6.5	Consistent with diabetes[a]

[a]Confirmed by repeating test on a different day

Generally, the diagnosis of diabetes is not based on a single blood test on one occasion, and is most confidently made when two tests, done on separate occasions, are both consistent with DM2.

Prediabetes

Prediabetes is an imprecise term, which reflects increased risk for diabetes, or an intermediate step in the progression to diabetes. Using the same tests listed above for diabetes, there are diagnostic criteria that can be used to define prediabetes.

1. **Fasting glucose**
    A normal fasting glucose is ≤100 mg/dL. A fasting glucose >125 mg/dL is consistent with DM2. The intermediate range, 100–125 mg/dL is neither normal nor diagnostic for DM2. The precise term for these intermediate values is impaired fasting glucose (IFG).
2. **Glucose tolerance**
    On a GTT, a two hour glucose <140 mg/dL is considered normal. A two hour glucose of 200 mg/dL is consistent with DM2. The intermediate range, 140–200 mg/dL is neither normal nor diagnostic for DM2, The precise term for these intermediate values for the two hour glucose in a GTT is impaired glucose tolerance (IGT).
3. **Hemoglobin A1c (HbA1c)**
    HbA1c of ≤5.7 % is considered normal. HbA1c ≥6.5 % is consistent with DM2. A value between 5.7 and 6.5 % is neither normal, nor consistent with DM2, and may be considered a sign of prediabetes.

These three definitions are based on different tests. A person could have both IFG and IGT, IFG but not IGT, or IGT but not IFG. Similarly, intermediate HbA1c values suggestive of prediabetes may or may not be associated with IFG or IGT. To be precise, the test that indicates someone has prediabetes should be specified.

Metabolic Syndrome

Definition
The metabolic syndrome refers to the co-occurrence of several known cardiovascular risk factors, including hyperglycemia/insulin resistance, obesity, atherogenic dyslipidemia, and hypertension [2]. There are several overlapping definitions for the metabolic syndrome. The National Cholesterol Education Program (NCEP) Adult Treatment Panel III (ATPIII) devised a definition for the metabolic syndrome, which was updated by the American Heart Association (AHA) and National Heart Lung Blood Institute (NHLBI) in 2005. According to this definition, metabolic if *three or more of the following five criteria* are met [3]:

- **waist circumference** over 40 in. (men) or 35 in. (women)
- **blood pressure** over 130/85 mmHg
- **fasting triglyceride (TG) level** over 150 mg/dL
- **fasting HDL cholesterol** less than 40 (men) or 50 (women) mg/dL
- **fasting blood sugar** over 100 mg/dL

Medical therapy for any of the above meets the criteria, even if the current treated value of the patient does not. Thus, a person taking an antihypertensive medication meets the blood pressure criteria, even though his blood pressure may be less than 130/85. Similarly, a person taking gemfibrozil for hypertriglyceridemia meets the TG criteria even if her treated value may be less than 150 mg/dL.

Importantly, atherogenic dyslipidemia is represented twice in these five criteria, once for low HDL and once for high TG. Furthermore, the definition of metabolic syndrome does not include specific values of LDL cholesterol. People with overt DM2 by definition meet the blood sugar criteria, but may not have metabolic syndrome if they do not meet at least two additional criteria.

Epidemiology
Over 50 million in the US have metabolic syndrome
Prevalence increases with age; prevalence is 24 % over age 20, and >30 % over age 50

Clinical importance
The metabolic syndrome is important for several reasons. First, it identifies patients who are at high risk of developing atherosclerotic CVD and overt DM2. Metabolic syndrome increases risk for CVD by twofold [4–6], and risk of DM2 fivefold [7]. Second, by considering the relationships between the components of metabolic syndrome, we may better understand the pathophysiology that links them with each other and with the increased risk of CVD [2, 8].

PREVENTION OF DIABETES

Finnish Diabetes Prevention Study (DPS) [9]

Question:	effectiveness of lifestyle intervention
Subjects:	522 non-diabetic overweight/obese subjects with mean body mass index (BMI) of 31 and IGT
Design:	randomization to intervention (dietary and exercise counseling) vs. control
Follow-up:	4 years
Result:	Incidence of DM2 was 11 % in intervention group as compared with 23 % in control group (*p* < 0.001), a 58 % reduction
Conclusion:	dietary and exercise counseling reduces the development of DM2 (and or slows the progression to DM2) in people at risk (overweight and IGT)

Diabetes Prevention Program [10]

Question:	lifestyle intervention vs. metfomin vs. placebo (Fig. 7-1)
Subjects:	3,234 non-diabetic subjects with mean BMI of 34 and IFG or IGT

FIGURE 7-1

Lifestyle intervention compared with metformin and placebo in the prevention of DM2.

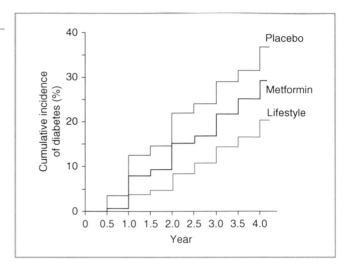

Design: randomization to placebo, metformin, or lifestyle modification (>7 % wt loss and >150 min exercise/week)

Follow-up: 3 years

Result: Lifestyle modification was associated with 58 % reduction in development of diabetes (4.8 cases per 100 person-years), and metformin was associated with 31 % reduction (7.8 cases per 100 person-years) as compared with placebo (11.0 cases per 100 person-years).

Conclusion: lifestyle modification was more effective than metformin, though both reduced development of DM2 in people at risk (weight and IFG or IGT).

Effectiveness of Medications in Preventing DM2

Several studies show effectiveness of specific medications in preventing DM2.

STOP NIDDM [11] showed that acarbose resulted in a 25 % relative risk reduction in development of diabetes compared with placebo

TRIPOD [12] showed that troglitazone resulted in a 56 % risk reduction in development of DM2

DREAM –Ramipril [13] showed that rosiglitazone was associated with 60 % reduction in new DM2 in subjects with IGT, though ramipril did not have an effect

ACT-NOW [14] showed benefit of pioglitazone.

TREATMENT OF HYPERGLYCEMIA

Treatment Targets

HbA1c

The most important endpoint for assessing glycemic control is the HbA1c, since it integrates long term glycemic control, does not vary moment to moment, and does not depend on fasting state. While a normal HbA1c is less than 5.5, most physicians aim for a target HbA1c of 7.0 in patients with DM2. In the ACCORD study (see below), intensive glycemic control targeting a HbA1c of 6.4 or below resulted in higher morbidity and mortality, in part due to hypoglycemia. Thus, HbA1c of 7.0 serves as a reasonable goal for glycemic control in most patients, with the exception of extremely motivated patients and those who are better able to manage possible hypoglycemic episodes.

ACCORD (Action to Control Cardiovascular Risk in Diabetes) [15]

Question:	compare intensive glycemic control with conventional therapy, and effects of statins and fibrates
Subjects:	10,251 DM2 subjects with HbA1c >7.5 % and existing coronary artery disease (CAD)
Design:	randomized to intensive treatment (target HbA1c <6 %) vs. standard treatment (target HbA1c = 7.0–7.9 %); both groups could be treated with insulin, metformin, sulfonylureas, or other medications. Additional design studied effects of statins and fibrates.
Follow-up:	5.6 years
Result:	Intensive therapy reduced HbA1c to 6.4 %, as compared with 7.5 % in the conventional therapy group. Intensively treated group showed 10 % lower composite endpoint of death, MI, and stroke, but excess of all-cause mortality. Study prematurely terminated (17 months early) because of excess deaths in the intensively treated group.
Conclusion:	Intensive therapy resulting in HbA1c of 6.4 % is associated with increased mortality.

Additional targets

Additional targets include fasting glucose or post-prandial glucose levels, particularly for fine adjustments of insulin regimens. These targets show more variability, and may not reflect long term glycemic control, so they are less useful for management of other medical treatments for hyperglycemia.

Medications for Diabetes

Metformin

- a biguanide
- limits release of glucose by the liver
- also reduces peripheral insulin resistance
- low risk of hypoglycemia
- has gastrointestinal (GI) side effects and is best taken with meals
- caution in renal failure (Creatinine (Cr) of 1.4–1.5)
- rare side effect of lactic acidosis
- reduces HbA1c by 1–2 %, which is among most potent oral medications

Sulfonylureas

- examples include glyburide, glimeride, glipizide
- act as insulin secretagogues (stimulate pancreatic beta cells to secrete insulin)
- side effects of hypoglycemia, weight gain, and rash
- metabolized by liver and excreted by kidneys, so caution in liver and renal failure
- reduces HbA1c by 1–2 %, considered potent

Thiazolidinediones

- peroxisome proliferator-activated receptor (PPAR)-gamma agonists
- examples include rosiglitazone, pioglitazone
- act by binding to PPAR-gamma, which is involved in peripheral insulin signaling
- side effects include weight gain, fluid retention, and increased risk of bone fracture
- not associated with hypoglycemia
- caution in congestive heart failure (CHF) due to fluid retention
- rosiglitazone associated with increased risk of myocardial infarction (MI)
- metabolized by liver
- reduces HbA1c by 1–2 % but takes up to 12 weeks to work

Glucagon-like peptide-1 (GLP-1) agonists

- examples include exenatide, liraglutide
- must be given by injection once or twice a day

- GLP-1 agonists are longer acting than GLP-1, which lasts minutes
- bind to GLP-1 receptors to increase post-prandial insulin secretion and reduce glucagon
- causes weight loss
- slows GI motility
- can cause nausea and vomiting
- exenatide is excreted by kidneys
- reduces HbA1c by ~1 %

Dipeptidyl protease-4 (DPP4) inhibitors
- examples include sitagliptin, saxagliptin, linagliptin
- block DPP4, the enzyme that breaks down GLP-1
- once daily, oral
- low risk of hypoglycemia
- no effect on weight, no GI side effects
- renal metabolism

Meglitinides
- examples include nateglitanide and rapaglitinide
- increase pancreatic insulin secretion, effect similar to sulfonylureas
- short-acting peptides, lasting minutes to hours
- given by injection
- take with meals, TID injections
- gemfibrozil increases rapaglitinide levels eightfold; avoid combination
- liver metabolism (CYP 3A4)

Alpha glucosidase inhibitors
- examples include acarbose and miglitol
- block the enzymes that break down complex carbohydrates
- taken with meals
- may cause GI side effects: abdominal pain, diarrhea
- reduces HbA1c by 0.5 %

Amylin analogs
- examples include pramlintide
- analog of amylin, a pancreatic peptide that increases potency of insulin
- injected with meals
- may cause severe hypoglycemia
- associated with weight loss

Insulin (Table 7-4)
- examples include insulin lispro, insulin regular, insulin glargine (from shortest to longest lasting formulation)
- SC or IV
- its ability to reduce HbA1c is unlimited
- can cause severe hypoglycemia
- associated with weight gain

Approach

Evaluation:
- Determine current HbA1c level and how much it differs from target is important
- For most, target HbA1c of 7.0 % is reasonable
- Knowing how much each medication is likely to reduce HbA1c will guide therapy (Table 7-5).

TABLE 7-4

INSULIN THERAPY
FOR DM

INSULIN TYPE (BRAND NAME)	ROUTE	ONSET	PEAK	DURATION	USE
Rapid					
Lispro (Humalog)	SC	30 min	30–90 min	<6 h	At the same time as the meal
Aspart (Novolog)	SC	15 min	1–3 h	3–5 h	
Glulisine (Apidra)	SC	30 min	30–90 min	<6 h	
Short					
Regular (Humulin R, Novolin R)	SC	30–60 min	2–4 h	6–12 h	30–60 min before meals
Regular (Humulin R, Novolin R)	IV	15 min	15–30 min	30–60 min	
Intermediate					
NPH (Humulin N, Novolin N)	SC	1–2 h	4–14 h	10–24 h	BID or overnight
Long					
Glargine (Lantus)	SC	1 h	No peak	24 h	Daily
Detemir (Levemir)	SC	1 h	No peak	6–23 h	
Pre-mixed					
Novolog Mix 70/30 (aspart protamine/aspart)	SC	15 min	1–4 h	12–24 h	BID before mealtime
Humalog Mix 50/50 or 75/25 (lispro protamine/lispro)	SC	30 min	30 min–2 h	6–12 h	
Humulin Mix 50/50 or 70/30 (NPH/regular)	SC	30 min	2–4 h	16–24 h	

TABLE 7-5

APPROACH TO MEDICAL THERAPY
FOR DM2

INTERVENTION	EXPECTED DECREASE IN HBA1C (%)	ADVANTAGES	CONCERNS
Initial approach:			
Lifestyle modifications to lose weight and increase physical activity	1–2	Effective Low cost Additional benefits	Difficult to maintain
Metformin	1–2	Low risk of hypoglycemia Low risk of weight gain Inexpensive	Lactic acidosis Avoid in renal failure GI side effects
Additional therapy:			
Sulfonylureas	1–2	Inexpensive	Weight gain Hypoglycemia
Thiazolidinediones	1–2	Pio improves lipid profile	Increased MI risk Avoid in CHF (wt gain, fluid retention)
Insulin	Unlimited	No dose limit Inexpensive Improved lipid profile	Injections Hypoglycemia Weight gain Fingerstick monitoring
Other medications:			
GLP-1 agonists (aka incretins)	0.5–1	Weight loss Low risk of hypoglycemia	Injections GI side effects
DPP4 inhibitors	0.5–1	Once a day dosing Low risk of hypoglycemia No effect on weight	
Meglitinides	1–1.5	Short acting	Injections Take with meals
Amylin analog	0.5–1		Injections Hypoglycemia Weight loss
Alpha glucosidase inhibitors	0.5		GI side effects

GLYCEMIC CONTROL

Microvascular Complications

Microvascular complications of diabetes include retinopathy, nephropathy, and neuropathy. The results of two large clinical trials, the DCCT and the UKDPS, established a clear relationship between degree of glycemic control and microvascular complications.

DCCT (Diabetes Control and Complications Trial) [16]

Question:	effect of intensive vs. conventional glycemic control on diabetic complications
Subjects:	1,441 type 1 diabetic subjects on insulin therapy
Design:	intensive (target HbA1c ≤6 %) vs. conventional insulin therapy
Follow-up:	6.5 years
Result:	Intensive therapy reduced retinopathy by 76 %, microalbuminuria by 39 %, albuminuria by 54 %, and neuropathy by 60 % as compared with conventional insulin therapy Intensive therapy was associated with 2- to 3-fold increase in sever hypoglycemia
Conclusion:	Intensive therapy delays onset and slows progression of diabetic retinopathy, nephropathy, and neuropathy in DM1 patients on insulin

UKPDS (UK Prospective Diabetes Study) [17]

Question:	effect of intensive vs. conventional glycemic control on diabetes-related endpoints
Subjects:	5,102 DM2 subjects
Design:	randomized to intensive treatment with insulin, intensive treatment with sulfonylurea, or conventional treatment with diet
Follow-up:	up to 13 years
Result:	Intensive therapy reduced diabetes-related endpoints by 12 %, mainly because of a 25 % risk reduction in microvascular endpoints. Risk of diabetes-related death was reduced by 10 % (and all cause mortality by 6 %) but these differences did not reach significance. Intensive therapy was associated with more hypoglycemic episodes. No significant differences were found between insulin or oral medications in intensive therapy.
Conclusion:	Intensive therapy, either with insulin or sulfonylureas, reduces risk of microvascular diabetic complications, but only tended to be associated with decreased mortality.

Macrovascular Complications

In contrast to microvascular complications, macrovascular complications (coronary disease, MI, stroke) are less consistently associated with degree of glycemic control.

UKPDS follow-up [18]

Question:	follow-up of DM2 patients in UKPDS randomized to intensive glucose control for additional 10 years
Subjects:	3,277 DM2 subjects originally randomized to intensive glucose control
Design:	followed for 10 years, no requirement to continue intensive glucose control
Follow-up:	10 years
Result:	Sulfonylurea-insulin treatment was associated with 13 % reduction in all-cause mortality and 15 % reduction in MI compared with conventional therapy. Metformin was associated with 27 % risk reduction in all cause mortality and 33 % reduction in MI compared with conventional therapy.
Conclusion:	Patients originally randomized to intensive therapy showed reductions in mortality and MI during 10 year follow up.

EDIC-DPP follow up (Epidemiology of Diabetes Interventions and Complications) [19]

Question:	follow up of DCCT subjects for additional 10 years
Subjects:	1,441 DM1 subjects
Design:	originally randomized to intensive treatment with insulin vs. conventional treatment; treatment assignment not extended
Follow-up:	10 years beyond original 6.5 year period
Result:	The group originally randomized to intensive therapy showed 42 % risk reduction in cardiovascular events compared with the group originally randomized to conventional therapy.
Conclusion:	Patients originally randomized to intensive therapy showed reductions in MI, stroke, and death during additional 10 year follow up.

Several large meta-analyses of these and other results suggest that glycemic control is associated with reduction in CV events.

TREATMENT OF HYPERLIPIDEMIA

Atherogenic Dyslipidemia

Seen in many patients with DM2, metabolic syndrome, polycystic ovary disease
■ elevated TG
■ low HDL
■ small, dense LDL particles

DM2 as a CVD Risk Equivalent

■ In the NCEP ATP III and 2005 AHA/ACC update, DM2 is considered to be a CVD risk equivalent [20].
■ The goal for the LDL cholesterol is 70–100 in persons with established CVD, or those with DM2, regardless of whether they have established CVD
■ Pathophysiologic reason: smaller, denser LDL particles are more atherogenic

Goals

■ Primary goal for atherogenic dyslipidemia: reduce the LDL to 70–100 mg/dL
■ Secondary goal: reduce the triglyceride level to 150 mg/dL or less

Studies on Treatment of Hyperlipidemia in DM2

CARDS (Collaborative Atorvastatin Diabetes Study) [21]

Question:	effect of atorvastatin on cardiovascular events and death in DM2 patients with LDL cholesterol <160 mg/dL
Subjects:	2,838 DM2 subjects without known CVD
Design:	randomized to atorvastatin 10 mg/day vs. placebo
Follow-up:	3.9 years
Result:	Atorvastatin reduced relative risk for cardiac events (including MI, CVD death, and stroke) by 37 % Study terminated 2 years earlier than scheduled because of significantly lower rate of events in treated group
Conclusion:	Patients with DM2 without known CVD benefit from reduced CVD risk from statin treatment

HPS (Heart Protection Study) [22]

Question:	effect of simvastatin and antioxidants on cardiovascular events and death
Subjects:	5,963 subjects with DM2 in total of 20,536 subjects,
Design:	randomized to simvastatin 40 mg/day vs. placebo; additional design looked at effect of antioxidant vitamins, in 2×2 factorial study

Follow-up: 6 years
Result: In subjects with DM2, simvastatin reduced CVD events by 28 %, regard-
              less of starting cholesterol level
Conclusion: Patients with DM2 benefit from reduced CVD risk from statin treatment

Additional studies

Meta-analyses confirm that statin therapy reduces CVD events and mortality in patients with DM2, including those without known CVD and throughout a range of starting LDL cholesterol levels.

Individual studies show that DM2 patients benefit from statins (4S-DM, ASPEN1, ASPEN2, CARE-DM, TNT-DM, and ASCOT-DM), fibrates (VA-HIT, DAIS), and niacin (ADMIT, ADVENT) in terms of reduction in CVD events.

DIABETES AND HEART DISEASE

Thiazolidinediones, CHF, and MI

- Both rosiglitazone and pioglitazone are associated with weight gain and fluid retention, and should be used with caution in CHF
- Meta-analyses suggest that rosiglitazone is associated with excess risk for nonfatal MI with RR of 1.43 [23]; similar findings have not been demonstrated for pioglitazone
- FDA issued a "black box" warning for rosiglitazone in 2007
- Rosiglitazone is associated with increased TG levels, increased LDL levels, and less increase in HDL than pioglitazone

Revascularization vs. Medical Therapy

DM2 is associated with

- more diffuse and complex CAD
- increased CV events

BARI 2D (Bypass Angioplasty Revascularization Investigation) [24]

Question: effect of (1) revascularization (PCI or surgery) vs. medical therapy alone
              and (2) method of glycemic control (insulin-sensitization vs. insulin pro-
              viding), on mortality
Subjects: 2,368 DM2 subjects with known CVD (coronary angiogram with >50 %
              stenosis or documented ischemia)
Design: 2 × 2 factorial design, randomized to (1) elective revascularization with
              percutaneous coronary intervention (PCI) or coronary artery bypass graft
              (CABG), as opposed to initial medical therapy, and (2) insulin-sensitiza-
              tion or insulin providing treatment for diabetes
Follow-up: 5 years
Result: No significant difference in 5 year mortality or major CV events between
              elective revascularization vs. initial medical therapy. No significant differ-
              ence between the two methods of glycemic control. In patients with DM2,
              mortality was lower with CABG than multi-vessel PCI.
Conclusion: There is no clear benefit from early elective revascularization with PCI or
              CABD as compared with optimal medical therapy. Patients with DM2 and
              known CVD showed lower mortality with CABG than multi-vessel PCI.

SYNTAX (Synergy Between Percutaneous Coronary Intervention with Taxus and Cardiac Surgery) [25, 26]

Question: effectiveness of CABG vs. PCI with drug eluting stent (DES) in patients
              with 3 vessel disease (3VD) or left main (LM) disease
Subjects: 1,800 subjects with 3VD or LM disease amenable to both CABG and PCI

Design: randomized to CABG vs. PCI with DES (Taxus)
Follow-up: 1year
Result: Overall, major adverse cardiac or cerebrovascular events at 12 months were lower in CABG arm (12.4 %) than PCI arm (17.8 %). In subjects with DM2, major adverse events in CABG arm was 14.2 % as compared with 26.0 % in PCI arm. Differences in non-diabetic subjects were not significant.
Conclusion: Patients with DM2 and 3VD or LM disease have better outcome with CABG than PCI

Acute Coronary Syndrome (ACS) and Glucose Control

■ Most of the randomized trials used intensive insulin along with exogenous glucose infusion (±potassium) in patients with ACS and showed initial promise in intensive insulin+glucose±potassium therapy – for example, DIGAMI trial showed decreased mortality with insulin+glucose therapy [27]. However large scale trials such as CREATE-ECLA study did not show benefit with insulin+glucose+potassium therapy [28].

■ Less data exists on insulin therapy to normalize blood glucose to a target level.

■ Based on evidence from large scale noncardiac intensive care unit trials such as NICE-SUGAR trial [29], which showed increased mortality with intensive insulin regimen, ACC/AHA 2009 focused updates downgraded their recommendation on insulin from Class I to Class IIa.

■ ACC/AHA 2009 focused updates state that it is reasonable to give insulin based regimen to achieve and maintain glucose levels less than 180 mg/dL while avoiding hypoglycemia for patients with ST-segment elevation MI (STEMI) with either a complicated or uncomplicated course (Class IIa, Level of Evidence: B)

Transplants

Diabetes in cardiac transplant patients

■ up to 20 % of cardiac transplant recipients have DM2 at the time of transplantation
■ 15 % of cardiac transplant recipients develop new DM2 within 5 years
■ incidence of DM2 is higher with tacrolimus as compared with cyclosporine for immunosuppression
■ incidence of DM2 goes up with higher doses of steroids
■ management of DM2 in transplant patients, including target HbA1c levels and medical therapy, is same as non-transplant patients.

REFERENCES

1. American Diabetes Association. Diagnosis and classification of diabetes mellitus. Diabetes Care. 2010;33 Suppl 1:S62–9.

2. Huang PL. A comprehensive definition for metabolic syndrome. Dis Model Mech. 2009;2(5–6):231–7.

3. Grundy SM, Cleeman JI, Daniels SR, Donato KA, Eckel RH, Franklin BA, et al. Diagnosis and management of the metabolic syndrome: an American Heart Association/National Heart, Lung, and Blood Institute Scientific Statement. Circulation. 2005;112(17): 2735–52.

4. Ford ES. Risks for all-cause mortality, cardiovascular disease, and diabetes associated with the metabolic syndrome: a summary of the evidence. Diabetes Care. 2005;28(7):1769–78.

5. Galassi A, Reynolds K, He J. Metabolic syndrome and risk of cardiovascular disease: a meta-analysis. Am J Med. 2006;119(10):812–9.

6. Gami AS, Witt BJ, Howard DE, Erwin PJ, Gami LA, Somers VK, et al. Metabolic syndrome and risk of incident cardiovascular events and death: a systematic review and meta-analysis of longitudinal studies. J Am Coll Cardiol. 2007;49(4):403–14.

7. Ford ES, Li C, Sattar N. Metabolic syndrome and incident diabetes: current state of the evidence. Diabetes Care. 2008;31(9): 1898–904.

8. Huang PL. eNOS, metabolic syndrome and cardiovascular disease. Trends Endocrinol Metab. 2009;20(6):295–302.

9. Lindstrom J, Louheranta A, Mannelin M, Rastas M, Salminen V, Eriksson J, et al. The Finnish Diabetes Prevention Study (DPS): lifestyle intervention and 3-year results on diet and physical activity. Diabetes Care. 2003;26(12):3230–6.

10. Knowler WC, Barrett-Connor E, Fowler SE, Hamman RF, Lachin JM, Walker EA, et al. Reduction in the incidence of type 2 diabetes with lifestyle intervention or metformin. N Engl J Med. 2002;346(6):393–403.

11. Chiasson JL, Josse RG, Gomis R, Hanefeld M, Karasik A, Laakso M. Acarbose for prevention of type 2 diabetes mellitus: the STOP-NIDDM randomised trial. Lancet. 2002;359(9323):2072–7.

12. Snitker S, Watanabe RM, Ani I, Xiang AH, Marroquin A, Ochoa C, et al. Changes in insulin sensitivity in response to troglitazone do not differ between subjects with and without the common, functional Pro12Ala peroxisome proliferator-activated receptor-gamma2 gene variant: results from the Troglitazone in Prevention of Diabetes (TRIPOD) study. Diabetes Care. 2004;27(6):1365–8.

13. DREAM Trial Investigators. Incidence of diabetes following ramipril or rosiglitazone withdrawal. Diabetes Care. 2011;34(6):1265–9.

14. DeFronzo RA, Tripathy D, Schwenke DC, Banerji M, Bray GA, Buchanan TA, et al. Pioglitazone for diabetes prevention in impaired glucose tolerance. N Engl J Med. 2011;364(12):1104–15.

15. Gerstein HC, Miller ME, Byington RP, Goff Jr DC, Bigger JT, Buse JB, et al. Effects of intensive glucose lowering in type 2 diabetes. N Engl J Med. 2008;358(24):2545–59.

16. The Diabetes Control and Complications Trial Research Group. The effect of intensive treatment of diabetes on the development and progression of long-term complications in insulin-dependent diabetes mellitus. N Engl J Med. 1993;329(14):977–86.

17. UK Prospective Diabetes Study (UKPDS) Group. Intensive blood-glucose control with sulphonylureas or insulin compared with conventional treatment and risk of complications in patients with type 2 diabetes (UKPDS 33). Lancet. 1998;352(9131):837–53.

18. Holman RR, Paul SK, Bethel MA, Matthews DR, Neil HA. 10-year follow-up of intensive glucose control in type 2 diabetes. N Engl J Med. 2008;359(15):1577–89.

19. Nathan DM, Cleary PA, Backlund JY, Genuth SM, Lachin JM, Orchard TJ, et al. Intensive diabetes treatment and cardiovascular disease in patients with type 1 diabetes. N Engl J Med. 2005;353(25):2643–53.

20. Grundy SM, Cleeman JI, Merz CN, Brewer Jr HB, Clark LT, Hunninghake DB, et al. Implications of recent clinical trials for the National Cholesterol Education Program Adult Treatment Panel III Guidelines. J Am Coll Cardiol. 2004;44(3):720–32.

21. Colhoun HM, Betteridge DJ, Durrington PN, Hitman GA, Neil HA, Livingstone SJ, et al. Primary prevention of cardiovascular disease with atorvastatin in type 2 diabetes in the Collaborative Atorvastatin Diabetes Study (CARDS): multicentre randomised placebo-controlled trial. Lancet. 2004;364(9435):685–96.

22. Collins R, Armitage J, Parish S, Sleigh P, Peto R. MRC/BHF Heart Protection Study of cholesterol-lowering with simvastatin in 5963 people with diabetes: a randomised placebo-controlled trial. Lancet. 2003;361(9374):2005–16.

23. Nissen SE, Wolski K. Effect of rosiglitazone on the risk of myocardial infarction and death from cardiovascular causes. N Engl J Med. 2007;356(24):2457–71.

24. Frye RL, August P, Brooks MM, Hardison RM, Kelsey SF, MacGregor JM, et al. A randomized trial of therapies for type 2 diabetes and coronary artery disease. N Engl J Med. 2009;360(24):2503–15.

25. Serruys PW, Morice MC, Kappetein AP, Colombo A, Holmes DR, Mack MJ, et al. Percutaneous coronary intervention versus coronary-artery bypass grafting for severe coronary artery disease. N Engl J Med. 2009;360(10):961–72.

26. Banning AP, Westaby S, Morice MC, Kappetein AP, Mohr FW, Berti S, et al. Diabetic and nondiabetic patients with left main and/or 3-vessel coronary artery disease: comparison of outcomes with cardiac surgery and paclitaxel-eluting stents. J Am Coll Cardiol. 2010;55(11):1067–75.

27. Malmberg K. Prospective randomised study of intensive insulin treatment on long term survival after acute myocardial infarction in patients with diabetes mellitus. DIGAMI (Diabetes Mellitus, Insulin Glucose Infusion in Acute Myocardial Infarction) Study Group. BMJ. 1997;314(7093):1512–5.

28. Mehta SR, Yusuf S, Diaz R, Zhu J, Pais P, Xavier D, et al. Effect of glucose-insulin-potassium infusion on mortality in patients with acute ST-segment elevation myocardial infarction: the CREATE-ECLA randomized controlled trial. JAMA. 2005;293(4):437–46.

29. Finfer S, Chittock DR, Su SY, Blair D, Foster D, Dhingra V, et al. Intensive versus conventional glucose control in critically ill patients. N Engl J Med. 2009;360(13):1283–97.

CHAPTER 8

IMAD AHMADO, GAURAV A. UPADHYAY, AND HENRY GEWIRTZ

Nuclear Cardiology and Exercise Stress Testing

CHAPTER OUTLINE

ABBREVIATIONS

ACC	American College of Cardiology
AHA	American Heart Association
Bq	Becquerel
^{11}C	Carbon
CABG	Coronary artery bypass graft surgery
CAD	Coronary artery disease
Ci	Curie
CKD	Chronic Kidney disease
COPD	Chronic obstructive pulmonary disease
CORE	Center of Rotation Error
DBP	Diastolic blood pressure
^{18}F	Fluorine
ECG	Electrocardiogram
EF	Ejection fraction
G	Gray
HR	Heart rate
IC	Internal conversion
IT	Isomeric transition
IVCD	Intraventricular conduction delay
LAD	Left anterior descending
LBBB	Left bundle branch block
LMCA	Left main coronary artery
LV	Left ventricular
LVEF	Left ventricular ejection fraction
MET	Metabolic equivalents of task
MI	Myocardial infarction
mph	Miles per hour
^{99}Mo	Molybdenum
MPI	Myocardial perfusion imaging
^{13}N	Nitrogen
^{15}O	Oxygen
PET	Positron emission tomography
PVC	Premature ventricular complexes
R	Roentgen
RAD	Radiation absorbed dose
^{82}Rb	Rubidium
RMR	Resting metabolic rate
SBP	Systolic blood pressure

SDS   Summed Difference Score
SPECT   Single-photon emission computed tomography
SRS   Summed Rest Score
SSS   Summed Stress Score
ST60/ST80 ST-segment is assessed at the J-point and 60/80 ms
Sv   Sievert
^{99m}Tc Technetium-99m
^{201}TI Thallium-201
TID   Transit ischemic dilatation
VO$_2$ Estimated oxygen uptake

INTRODUCTION

Exercise stress testing and radionuclide myocardial perfusion imaging (MPI) are commonly performed in order to provide medical diagnosis of coronary artery disease (CAD) and to assist with risk stratification and clinical management for patients with established CAD. Exercise stress testing also provides an objective, standardized measure of the patient's functional capacity, which is important prognostically and also an essential component of any cardiac rehabilitation program.

MPI is performed in the context of stress testing to determine the presence and extent of myocardial ischemia. Either treadmill exercise or a pharmacologic 'stress' with adenosine, regadenoson, or dobutamine is employed. Next, an objective method is utilized to assess the degree of ischemia induced. Commonly used single-photon emission computed tomography (SPECT) MPI tracers include technetium-99m-sestamibi or tetrofosmin, and in some labs thallium-201, for rest imaging. All of these determine relative regional myocardial flow in order to assess for ischemia. However, positron emission tomography (PET) can assess absolute regional myocardial flow and the availability of new tracers for PET will greatly expand the use of PET for MPI.

This chapter presents a general frame work for MPI stress test selection and also reviews American College of Cardiology (ACC)/American Heart Association (AHA)/American Society of Nuclear Cardiology (ASNC) guidelines and appropriateness criteria regarding indications for such testing.

PHYSICS, RADIATION SAFETY, AND INSTRUMENTATION

A basic background in nuclear physics and radiation is essential for better understanding of nuclear cardiology, and in order to provide protection for oneself and others from radiation.

A. **Basic nuclear physics**
  ■ **Background**: Radionuclides commonly used for SPECT myocardial perfusion imaging include technetium-99m (^{99m}Tc) and thallium-201 (^{201}TI). Positron emission tomography (PET) utilizes Rubidium (^{82}Rb), oxygen (^{15}O), nitrogen (^{13}N), carbon (^{11}C), and fluorine (^{18}F) to label a wide variety of tracer molecules in order to assess myocardial blood flow and metabolism. In addition, PET can reveal important information about molecular signaling and responses of the myocardium to pathological states as ischemia and heart failure (HF). In sharp contrast to SPECT imaging, which can assess relative differences in tracer distribution, PET is capable of absolute quantitative measurement of myocardial tracer content. Thus PET can differentiate between normal and abnormal regions of the heart with better accuracy and allows direct quantitative comparison between patients.
  ■ Commonly used tracers (Table 8-1)

RADIONUCLIDES	GENERATION	HALF-LIFE	GAMMA RAYS/X-RAYS (KEV)	MYOCARDIAL EXTRACTION FRACTION (%)	COMMENTS
SPECT					
Technetium-99m (^{99m}Tc)-Sestamibi	On-site generator	6 h	140 (ideal photopeak)	60	Most commonly used for medical procedures
Thallium-201 (^{201}Tl)	Cyclotron	73 h	80	75	Active, Na/K ATPase-dependent
PET					
Rubidium (^{82}Rb)	Cyclotron	76 s	511	60	Greater spatial and temporal resolution compared with SPECT
					Absolute quantization of myocardial blood flow possible

TABLE 8-1

TRACERS COMMONLY USED FOR MYOCARDIAL PERFUSION IMAGING

B. Radiation Exposure, Units, and Dose Limits
■ **Radiation exposure**

- In the United States, ionizing radiation from medical procedures make up almost 50 % of radiation exposure, while in other parts of the world, natural background comprises the majority of radiation exposure.
- The linear no-threshold model: there is a linear dose response relationship in future risk of cancer but any exposure to ionizing radiation, can induce a future risk of malignancy.

■ **Units of radiation dose**

- Radiation exposure: ionizing radiation concentration in air, measured in Roentgen (R)
- Absorbed dose: how much is absorbed in a specific tissue, measured in radiation absorbed dose (RAD) or Gray (Gy). Gy = 100 RAD
- Effective dose: equivalent whole body dose taking into consideration the organ irradiated, usually used in assessing risk of radiation, measured in Sievert (Sv) or radiation equivalent dose (REM). Sv = 100 REM

■ **Average effective radiation dose in common cardiac procedures** (Table 8-2)
■ **Radiation Dose Limits**

- Guiding principle: **ALARA** – As Low As Reasonably Achievable.
- Three factors to achieve this goal

  ■ *Decrease time.*
  ■ *Increase distance*: Radiation exposure diminishes in an inverse square relative to distance from radiation source.
  ■ *Use shielding*

- Non-occupational dose limit: 5 mSv per year
- Occupational dose limit: 50 mSv per year

TABLE 8-2

AVERAGE EFFECTIVE RADIATION
DOSE IN COMMON CARDIAC
PROCEDURES [43]

PROCEDURE	AVERAGE EFFECTIVE DOSE (mSv)
CXR, posteroanterior	0.02
CXR, posteroanterior and lateral	0.1
CT coronary calcium score	3
Coronary angiogram	7
CT chest	8
Nuclear cardiac stress test (Rest/Stress Tc-99m-MIBI exam)	15–20
Cardiac (dose is tracer and protocol dependent: stress only 30 mCi 13-N-ammonia)	2.5
CTA, pulmonary embolism protocol	15
Coronary angioplasty or stent	15
CT coronary angiogram (with current 128 slice CT and dedicated coronary protocol)	2–5

STRESS TESTING AND PROTOCOLS

Induction of Myocardial Ischemia

Exercise

■ **Types of exercise testing**: commonly treadmill or bicycle. Arm ergometry or rowing machine available.

■ **Subject preparation**

– *Medications*:

■ Diagnosis of CAD: negative inotropic medications, particularly β-blockers are usually held so that a maximal heart rate (HR) response may be achieved.

■ Known CAD, ischemic threshold or efficacy of antianginal therapy: take usual cardiovascular medications

■ **Exercise protocols**

– *Standard Bruce Protocol*: the most widely used and validated protocol. A multi-stage test in which successive stages increase estimated oxygen uptake (VO$_2$) and myocardial demand [1]

■ Stage I is roughly equivalent to four metabolic equivalents of task

– *Modified Bruce Protocol*: in assessment of patients soon after myocardial infarction (MI) or in those who are elderly or sedentary [2]. The protocol adds two stages prior to Stage I of the Standard Bruce Protocol:

– *Other protocols* include the *Cornell, Naughton,* and *Balke* protocols, all of which offer the ability to begin at a lower workload and assess at more stages.

■ **Test termination and adequacy**

– **Test termination**: based on perceived exertion, anginal symptoms, electrocardiogram (ECG) assessment, and clinical symptoms [3]

■ *Absolute indications for terminating exercise testing* include (from the 2001 AHA Exercise Standards for Testing and Training) [3]:

– ST-segment elevation (>1.0 mm) in leads without diagnostic Q-waves
– Drop in systolic blood pressure (SBP) of >10 mmHg from baseline , despite an increase in workload, when accompanied by other evidence of ischemia
– Moderate-to-severe angina that is intolerable
– Central nervous system symptoms (e.g., ataxia, dizziness, or
– near-syncope)
– Signs of poor perfusion (cyanosis or pallor)

TABLE 8-3

Absolute

Acute MI (within 2 days)
High-risk unstable angina
Uncontrolled cardiac arrhythmias
Severe aortic stenosis
Uncontrolled symptomatic HF
Acute pulmonary embolus or pulmonary infarction
Acute aortic dissection
Acute myocarditis or pericarditis
Unstable patient for non-cardiac reason
Patient is unable to give consent

Relative

Left main coronary stenosis
Moderate stenotic valvular heart disease
Electrolyte abnormalities
Severe arterial hypertension
Significant arrhythmias
Hypertrophic cardiomyopathy and other forms of outflow tract obstruction
High-degree atrioventricular block
Mental or physical impairment leading to inability to exercise adequately

- Sustained ventricular tachycardia (VT)
- Technical difficulties in monitoring ECG or SBP
- Subject's desire to stop

■ *Relative indications for terminating exercise testing* [3] include:

- ST or QRS changes such as excessive ST depression (>2 mm of horizontal or downsloping ST-segment depression) or marked axis shift
- Drop in SBP of >10 mmHg from baseline , despite an increase in workload, *in the absence* of other evidence of ischemia
- Increasing chest pain
- Fatigue, shortness of breath, wheezing, leg cramps, or claudication
- Arrhythmias in addition to sustained ventricular tachycardia, others, such as multifocal premature ventricular complexes (PVC), triplets of PVCs, supraventricular tachycardia, heart block, or bradyarrhythmias
- General appearance of exhaustion or poor tissue perfusion
- Hypertensive response (SBP>250 mmHg or diastolic blood pressure (DBP)>than 115 mmHg)
- Development of bundle-branch block or intraventricular conduction delay (IVCD) that cannot be distinguished from VT

- **Adequate** if the patient can achieve at least 85 % of her or his maximal predicted HR [4]

■ *Maximal predicted HR* = 220 – age (in years)
■ *Peak double product* or *rate pressure product (RPP)* = $HR \times SBP$

- RPP of apparently healthy males (n > 700; ages 25–54) was between 25,000 (10th percentile) and 40,000 (90th percentile) [3]

■ **Contraindications to exercise stress testing** (Table 8-3)

- Exercise stress testing is associated with a small risk of death (0.5 per 10,000), MI (3.6 per 10,000) and serious arrhythmia (4.8 per 10,000) [3].
- When the patient is unable to exercise or ECG will be uninterpretable for ischemia (e.g.; LBBB, LVH, WPW), pharmacological stress testing is employed. In patients unable to exercise long term prognosis may be somewhat worse, due to the fact that inability to exercise is a marker of poorer functional status [5].

Vasodilators

- **Background**: induce coronary vasodilatation and hyperemia. Regional flow differences between diseased (less hyperemic) and normal vessels (more hyperemic) are visualized as perfusion defects using MPI
- **Vasodilator stress agents**: adenosine, regadenoson and dypridamole are the most commonly used agents in the US [6],

  – Adenosine: is an endogenously present purine nucleoside molecule which produces dose-dependent myocardial hyperemia through activation of adenonsine A_{2A} receptors in the coronary vasculature [7]

    - *Mechanism*: nonselective agonist of A_1, A_{2A}, A_{2B}, A_3, and A_4 receptors (throughout the body) with half-life of < 10 s
    - *Side effects*: flushing, headache, nausea, mild fall in arterial blood pressure (BP), bradyarrhythmia, bronchospasm, and transient A-V block including complete heart block
    - *Protocol*: IV adenosine at 140 µg/kg/min for 5–6 min. Radiotracer is injected after 2–3 min of infusion.

  – Regadenoson: recently approved selective A_{2A} agonist [8]

    - *Mechanism*: high affinity selective A_{2A} agonism, peak of 1–4 min and half-life of 30 min
    - *Side effects*: similar to adenosine but at lower overall incidence than for adenosine.
    - *Protocol*: Regadenoson is administered as a single bolus of a pre-filled intravenous syringe of 0.4 mg (in 5 mL) over 10 s. The radiotracer is subsequently injected before the end of the first minute after infusion

  – Dipyridamole: produces coronary hyperemia by impairing the cellular reuptake of adenosine [9]

    - *Mechanism*: inhibits nucleoside transporter and causes an accumulation of adenosine in the interstitial space. It has a substantially longer half-life than adenosine or regadenoson.
    - *Side effects*: similar to those of adenosine and regadenoson, but usually longer lasting
    - *Protocol*: infused at 0.56 mg//kg over 4 min. The radionuclide tracer is injected 7–9 min after initiation. Aminophylline is also required 1–2 min after radiotracer in order to reverse effects

- **Subject preparation**

  – *Medications*: aminophylline is used as an antidote to adenosine, regadenoson, and dipyridamole, and cannot be used within the 24 h preceding the test with vasodilator compounds (Table 8-4)

- **Contraindications**: patients at a greater chance for suffering the known side effects to vasodilator agents (Table 8-4)

Dobutamine

- **Background**: inotropic/chronotropic stimulation with synthetic catecholamine, when exercise or vasodilator-stressing is not feasible or is contraindicated [10].
- **Mechanism**: β-1 adrenoreceptor agonist (increase inotropy and chronotropy) but also with β-2 effects (can cause hypotension). Atropine can also be added to achieve target HR.
- **Side effects**: arrhythmia is common. Nonsustained VT and sustained atrial fibrillation are not uncommon among patients with history of left ventricular dysfunction. Hypotension, angina, nonspecific chest pain, and dyspnea also occur in a minority of patients. Headache, paresthesias, and nausea have also been reported
- **Protocol**: dobutamine infusion is escalated in scheduled doses, beginning with 5–10 µg/kg per min, up to 40 µg/kg with attention to maximal HR. Indications to terminate dobutamine infusion are similar as to those for exercise stress testing.
- **Subject preparation**: All β-blocking medications must be held for a 24–48 h period
- **Contraindications**: in patients in whom enhanced contractility, increased dP/dT are harmful and patients who are at high risk of side effects (Table 8-4)

ADENOSINE/REGADENOSON/DIPYRIDAMOLE	DOBUTAMINE
Severe asthma, chronic obstructive pulmonary disease (relative contraindication for regadenoson)	Unstable angina
SBP<90	Recent MI (within 1–3 days)
HR<40 bpm	SBP<90
Xanthines: e.g., caffeine, tea, dark chocolate, aminophylline or theophylline within 24 h of testing	SBP>200
High degree atrioventricular block/sick sinus syndrome	Significant history of ventricular tachyarrhythmias
Less than 2 days after MI	Severe aortic stenosis Hypertrophic cardiomyopathy Large aortic aneurysm or aortic dissection

TABLE 8-4

CONTRAINDICATIONS FOR PHARMACOLOGICAL STRESS TESTING

Detection of Myocardial Ischemia

Electrocardiogram

- **Background**: a broad spectrum of ECG changes during exercise are considered normal. Myocardial ischemia, in particular, manifests on the ECG stress testing with ST segment changes
- **Physiologic ECG changes with stress** [3]

  - *P-wave*: magnitude increases, particularly in the inferior leads
  - *PR segment*: shortens and slopes downward, particularly in the inferior leads. The 'Ta wave,' or repolarization of the atrial *p-wave* is thought to drive the downward sloping of the *PR segment*
  - *QRS complex*: a decrease in the *R-wave* amplitude is noted in the apical leads (V_5, V_6), associated with an increasing S-wave depth
  - *J-point depression*: The *J-point* (or *J-junction*) is depressed during exercise, particularly in the apicolateral leads (V_4-V_6). This is felt to be due to atrial repolarization (i.e., the 'Ta' wave) and often leads to 'upsloping' ST depressions of <2 mm
  - *T-wave*: decrease in T-wave amplitude seen in early in exercise, resolves within 1 min into recovery

- **Baseline ECG abnormalities which make it difficult to diagnose ischemia from ECG** (Table 8-5)
- **Abnormal ECG responses during stress testing** (See Fig. 8-1)

  - *ST-segment depression*: single most common manifestation of myocardial ischemia

    - Measured relative to the P-R segment, which serves as the isoelectric baseline for practical purposes (true isoelectric point is T-P segment)
    - At least three consecutive beats in the same lead should be assessed
    - The ST-segment is assessed at the J-point and 60 ms (ST60) or 80 ms (ST80) afterwards. ST80 is the norm in most labs. ST60 may be preferred with ventricular rates>130 beats/min [3]
    - Horizontal or downsloping ST-segment depression which is>0.10 mV (1 mm) in magnitude persisting for 80 ms is considered abnormal and a risk factor for future events [3]

      - Time of appearance of ST-segment shifts, associated workload, and duration of ST-depression into recovery are all associated with severity of CAD [11]
      - Intensification of minor pre-exercise ST-segment depression to levels ≥1 mm may also predict future events [12]

TABLE 8-5	Complete LBBB
BASELINE ECG ABNORMALITIES WHICH MAKE IT DIFFICULT TO DIAGNOSE ISCHEMIA FROM THE ELECTROCARDIOGRAM	Preexcitation syndrome
	Left ventricular hypertrophy
	Digoxin therapy
	Greater than 1 mm of resting ST-segment depression
	Electronically paced ventricular rhythm

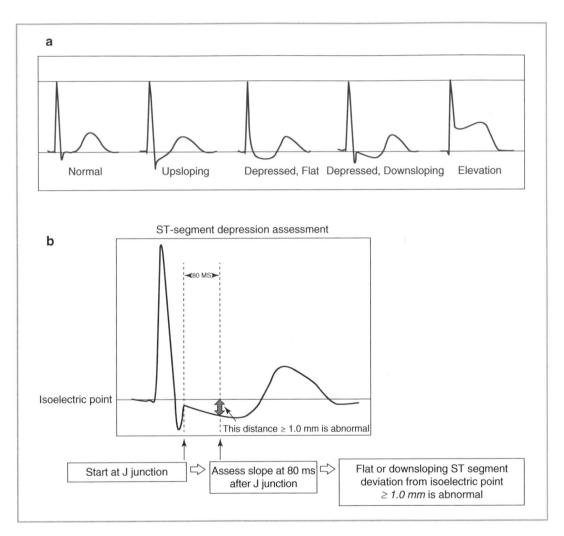

FIGURE 8-1

Abnormal and borderline ECG changes during exercise stress testing (Courtesy of Dr. Hanna Gaggin) (**a**) ST Segment Patterns (**b**) Measurement of ST Segment Depression

- *ST-segment elevation*: may occur in territories where Q-waves are present (in which case they are associated with wall motion abnormality or aneurysm and not necessarily new ischemia) or in a noninfarcted territory (in which case it is suggestive of transmural ischemia) [3]

   ■ Persistent J-point elevation > 0.10 mV (1 mm) in three consecutive beats is considered abnormal
   ■ Prinzmetal's or variant angina is associated with coronary artery spasm which may manifest with significant 'tombstone-like' ST-segment elevation [13]
   ■ Isolated ST-segment elevation in a VR has been associated with proximal left anterior descending (LAD) and left main coronary artery (LMCA) stenosis [14]

- *U-wave inversion*: uncommon, observed in recovery after stress testing. Associated with LAD or LMCA disease [15]
- *Arrhythmia*: exercise-induced ventricular ectopy after MI may be associated with increased mortality [16]. In asymptomatic, apparently healthy volunteers, however, exercise-induced repetitive monomorphic ventricular ectopy is not associated with adverse outcomes [17]. In addition, exercise-induced atrial arrhythmia is not associated with worse prognosis.
- *Intraventricular block*: rate-related intraventricular blocks are common and are not necessarily a marker of underlying ischemia. While exercise-induced right bundle branch block (RBBB) may be a benign finding , exercise-induced left bundle branch block (LBBB) appears to be associated with increased risk of mortality and future cardiac events

■ Blood pressure response during exercise

- Along with ECG monitoring, regular blood pressure monitoring is essential during exercise-ECG testing
- SBP normally rises during testing while DBP usually decreases with exercise
- A lack of rise in SBP or fall in DBP with exercise and angina is suggestive of significant underlying ischemia, and should be monitored carefully during testing [18]

Radionuclide tracers used for MPI
■ Thallium-201

- *Background*: It is a potassium analog, in which the initial uptake of thallium is highly dependent on coronary blood flow; later thallium redistribution is largely independent of coronary blood flow [19]
- *General Protocol*: injection of tracer at peak exercise or with pharmacologic stress agent followed by immediate imaging and subsequent redistribution images 3–4 h later
- *Strengths*: redistribution of tracer over time may be used for differentiating viable tissue (which may be 'hibernating') from scar

  - ■ Infarcted myocardium is characterized by a fixed dense thallium defect on both the initial and delayed images
  - ■ Hibernating myocardium has a an initial defect similar to infarcted myocardium, but shows uptake in the delayed images (i.e.; rest redistribution [20]) Viable myocardium has activity more than 50 % of that in a normal segment.

- *Limitations*: relatively low energy of emitted Hg X-rays makes thallium-201 imaging more susceptible to scatter and soft tissue attenuation which reduces overall resolution

■ Technetium-99m

- *Background*: Two technetium-99m agents are commercially available:

  - ■ ^{99m}Tc-sestamibi (Cardiolite™, also called 'MIBI'): is an isonitrile compound which is a lipophilic cation which is concentrated within the mitochondria due to the negative charge across the mitochondrial membrane, maintenance of which is a complex, active energy (ATP) requiring process and thus an indicator of cellular viability. There is minimal redistribution, and ECG-gated functional assessment is also possible
  - ■ ^{99m}Tc-tetrofosmin (Myoview™): is another lipophilic cationic compound with minimal redistribution and tracer washout and which provides similar clinical utility as ^{99m}Tc-sestamibi

- *General Protocol*: typically requires two injections of technetium 99m labeled tracer in order to obtain rest and stress imaging. Most common protocols include
  - ■ One-day single isotope imaging: rest and stress images are obtained on a single day
  - ■ One-day dual isotope imaging: patient receives thallium-201 at rest and immediately after rest images can undergo stress, during which technetium-99m labeled tracer is administered at peak stress

TABLE 8-6	Higher resolution (temporal and spatial)
ADVANTAGES OF CARDIAC PET AND PET/CT VERSUS CONVENTIONAL PLANAR OR SPECT IMAGING	Enhanced attenuation correction (depth independent)
	Peak-stress ejection fraction assessment
	Quantitation of myocardial blood flow
	Myocardial metabolism assessment
	Cardiac and coronary anatomy correlation with simultaneous CT scan

TABLE 8-7	**Myocardial perfusion**
COMMONLY EMPLOYED CARDIAC PET RADIOTRACER ELEMENTS	Rubidium-82 (potassium analogue, short half life of 76 s, used with pharmacological stress test)
	O-15 water
	F-18 (longer half life of 110 min)
	N-13 ammonia
	Myocardial metabolism
	Glucose metabolism: F-18 (FDG) (glucose analogue, used to assess myocardial viability)
	Fatty acid metabolism: C-11 palmitate (on site cyclotron and generally not used clinically)
	Oxidative metabolism: C-11 acetate (on site cyclotron and generally not used clinically)

- ■ Two-day single isotope imaging: allows for larger doses of technetium-99m labeled tracer on successive days

  – *Strengths*: overall, technetium-99m labeled tracers offer higher quality imaging data (versus thallium), and are less prone to soft tissue attenuation artifact. In addition, functional assessment of left ventricular ejection fraction (LVEF) is achievable through ECG-gated imaging.
  – *Limitations*: spatial resolution still limited to approximately 1 cm.

- ■ **Cardiac positron emission tomography (PET) tracers**

  – *Background*: PET utilizes higher-energy, dual photon emissions tracers which provide technically superior, quantitative images in comparison with that of conventional technetium 99m labeled tracers employed in SPECT (Table 8-6) [21, 22]. Commonly used myocardial perfusion tracers include Rubidium-82 (CardioGen-82™) and 13-N ammonia (requires on site cyclotron). Fluorine-18 (flurpiridaz) is in clinical trials and has not yet been FDA approved for clinical use. Myocardial glucose metabolism clinically is assessed with Fluoro-2-deoxyglucose (FDG) (Table 8-7).

IMAGE ACQUISITION, PROCESSING, AND INTERPRETATION

Image Acquisition and Processing

- ■ **SPECT**: a series of planar images usually are obtained over a 180° arc to reconstruct the heart in a three dimension view.
- ■ **ECG-gated perfusion imaging**: R-wave gated perfusion imaging slices are reconstructed in space and time to create an endless loop movie spanning one cardiac cycle [23].

  – Usually done by dividing the cardiac cycle to 8 or 16 frames. 8-frame gated images underestimate ejection fraction but give better counts density.
  – Typically, beats with R-R interval within ± 40 % of the average are accepted. In certain cases (e.g., atrial fibrillation, frequent ventricular beats) it may be necessary to open the window even wider to obtain adequate counts. However, ejection fraction measurement may be less reliable especially if large count drop off in late frames which manifests as a "blinking" cine loop.

Interpretation

■ **Review unprocessed (raw) data**
Evaluate for patient motion, lung uptake (stress thallium images), count density, possible attenuation artifacts, and look for any extracardiac uptake [24]

■ **Review individual myocardial slices**
Assess the orientation, alignment, intensity, cavity size, and defects. Defects are described by location, size and degree of reversibility. Defects typically are scored in the context of a 17-segment tomographic model (Figs. 8-2 and 8-3) [25]

Gauging Extent and Severity of Ischemia

■ **Qualitative severity analysis**

– Mild: decrease in counts compared to adjacent activity without the appearance of wall thinning
– Moderate: wall thinning
– Severe: defects that approach background activity

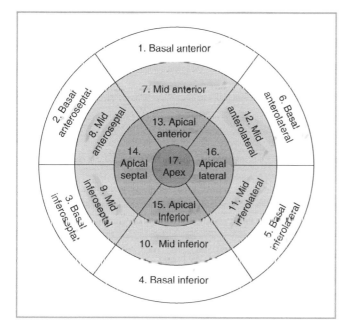

FIGURE 8-2

Circumferential polar plot of the 17 myocardial segments and the recommended nomenclature for tomographic imaging of the heart (Courtesy of Dr. Hanna Gaggin)

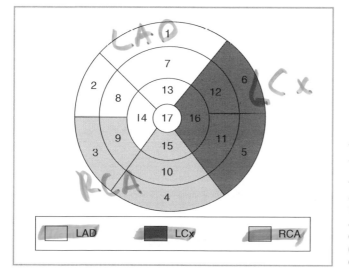

FIGURE 8-3

Assignment of the 17 myocardial segments to the territories of the left anterior descending (*LAD*), right coronary artery (*RCA*), and the left circumflex coronary artery (*LCX*) (Courtesy of Dr. Hanna Gaggin)

- **Semi-quantitative severity analysis**: utilizes 17-segment tomographic model (Fig. 8-2). Scores are attributed to each segment according to its perfusion :

  - Normal Perfusion: 0
  - Mild reduction in counts: 1
  - Moderate reduction in counts: 2
  - Severe reduction in counts: 3
  - Absent uptake: 4
  - Calculate overall scores:

    - **Summed Stress Score (SSS)**: Extent and severity of CAD

      $$SSS = \sum Stress\ segmental\ scores$$

    - **Summed Rest Score (SRS)**: Extent and severity of infarction.

      $$SRS = \sum Rest\ segmental\ scores$$

    - **Summed Difference Score (SDS)**: Extent and severity of ischemia/reversibility

      $$SDS = SSS - SRS$$

Evaluating ECG-Gated SPECT Data

- **General areas of evaluation:**

  - Evaluate myocardial thickening
  - Evaluate wall motion
  - Calculate LVEF

- **Discrepancies between perfusion data and functional data**

  - Normal Perfusion with abnormal Contractile function:

    - Non-ischemic cardiomyopathies (sometimes, the heart walls are thin secondary to cardiac dilatation)
    - Conduction abnormalities such as LBBB and Dual chamber Pacemaker (abnormal septal contraction with septal normal perfusion)
    - S/P coronary artery bypass graft (CABG) (abnormal septal contraction with septal normal perfusion)
    - Right ventricle abnormalities (volume or pressure overload)

  - Abnormal perfusion with normal contractile function:

    - Image artifacts
    - Exercise or pharmacological stress-induced ischemia (in case of severe ischemia one may see corresponding contractile abnormalities of varying severity)
    - perfusion defect in patient who had recent revascularization (secondary to endothelial dysfunction)

- **Differences between Scar and image attenuation artifact**:

  - Scar has decreased or absent wall motion and thickening
  - Attenuation artifact has normal wall motion and wall thickening

Review of Common Artifacts

- **Instrumentation and tracers related artifacts** include increased background noise (obscures the heart), misalignment of the head of the camera and wrong slice selection [26]. Two major artifacts are:

  1. Center of Rotation Error (CORE): Two heads of SPECT camera and each head rotate on different center points leading to disruption to the borders of the heart.

2. Ramp filter artifact: computer generated artifact due to efforts to correct for star artifact. Star artifact is inherent to the filtered back projection algorithm for image reconstruction. The ramp artifact results when extra cardiac activity projects into the plane of reconstruction, is mistaken for back projected cardiac rays and erroneously subtracted from the slice, leaving an spurious defect behind.

■ Patient related artifacts

1. Patient motion – common cause of "hurricane" artifact (break in short axis images which cause them to look like hurricane sign on weather map)
2. Soft tissue attenuation leading to falsely low counts (breast, left hemi-diaphragm, and lateral chest wall fat) [27]
3. Septum wall artifact (short septum, decrease tracer in septum during exercise SPECT secondary to LBBB)
4. The "Eleven O'clock" defect: The etiology generally thought to be related to the site of right ventricle insertion to LV septal region

■ Gating images errors and artifacts:

1. Arrhythmia with excessive beat rejection
2. Incorrect gating (T-R wave gating, P-R wave gating, etc.)
3. Software errors: caused by inability of the software to correctly identify the borders of the heart, like in case of big scar or significant extra-cardiac activity.

PROGNOSIS AND RISK STRATIFICATION BASED ON TESTING

A. **Treadmill Exercise testing prognosis:** This is the preferred method of stress testing in most but not all patients. There are number of variables associated with an increased risk of an adverse outcome in patients with CAD. These include:

- ■ Poor exercise capacity (<5 METs) [28]
- ■ Anginal chest pain, especially if it occurs at low workload in association with other evidence of myocardial ischemia (See below)
- ■ Fall in BP during exercise [29]
- ■ Impaired HR response to exercise [30]
- ■ Significant ischemic ST depression at a low workload
- ■ Multiple leads with ST depression
- ■ ST segment elevation (in leads without pathological Q waves)
- ■ Ventricular ectopy at a low workload or during early recovery [31]

B. **The Duke Treadmill Score:** $= Ex_{min} - (5 \cdot ST\downarrow) - (4 \cdot Ang\,Index)$

[handwritten margin note:] Anginal Index 0 = No Angina 1 = non-limiting CP 2 = limiting CP

- ■ The most common indicator used for exercise stress test prognosis.

- ■ It can be determined by the following equation [32]: Treadmill score=duration of exercise in minutes on the Bruce protocol - 5× maximal mm ST depression - 4× treadmill angina index. Treadmill Angina Index: 0 if no angina, 1 if non-limiting angina, 2 if limiting angina. Patients are classified as low, moderate, or high risk according to the score:

  - Low Risk=treadmill score greater than or equal to +5, 99 % four-year survival.
  - Moderate Risk=treadmill score −10 to +4, 95 % four-year survival
  - High Risk=treadmill score less than −10, 79 % four-year survival

- ■ There were a number of important exclusions in Duke Score study:

  - Significant valvular or congenital heart disease.
  - An uninterpretable ECG.
  - Coronary revascularization procedure in the past.
  - Recent MI.

[handwritten margin note:] } Excluded from Duke TST score

C. **The Myocardial Perfusion Imaging Test Prognosis:**

■ The risk of death or myocardial infarction in patients with normal MPI has been shown to be <1 % per year [33].
■ Factors that predict poor prognosis

– Inability to exercise [34]
– Extensive perfusion defect
– Large Reversible defect
– Multivessel defect distribution
– LV dysfunction
– Abnormal perfusion with transit ischemic dilatation (TID)
– Post infarct ischemia

■ The risk of death or MI in patients with normal MPI has been shown to be slightly >1 % per year (vs <0.5 % for normal ETT MIBI) if they have one of these:

– Diabetes: the risk is 1–2 % with normal images, and if the images abnormal the risk is significantly is higher [35].
– Pharmacological stress: inability of exercise is indicative of worse prognosis.
– Chronic Kidney disease (CKD): Very high prevalence of CAD in patient of CKD.
– Elderly patient [36].

■ The outcome of abnormal MPI is related to extent and severity of perfusion defects. Many studies found that high SSS predicts death and non-fatal MI; while SDS predicts MI. Also low LVEF in gated SPECT predicts death [37].
■ MPI also help to predict benefit of therapy: patients with >10 % ischemic myocardium and <10 % scar, have shown greater benefit of early revascularization in retrospective observational studies [38]. Good prospective randomized clinical trial data are lacking.
■ TID: ratio of the heart cavity size in the stress (dilated LV) to rest (normal LV) images >1.20, and under certain conditions is a prognostic indicator [39]:

– TID with abnormal perfusion has adverse prognosis
– TID with normal perfusion is not associated with adverse prognosis and may be a normal variant.

■ Ischemic ECG with vasodilator SPECT:

– Patients with ischemic ECG have abnormal MPI >90 % of the time. Patient should be evaluated for balanced ischemia with severe three vessels disease when SPECT is normal
– Few studies showed that patient with ischemic ECG and normal vasodilator SPECT carry slightly worse prognosis compared to normal ECG and normal vasodilator SPECT [40].

ACC/AHA GUIDELINES FOR EXERCISE AND MYOCARDIAL PERFUSION IMAGING

A. ACC/AHA recommendations for exercise tests are shown in Tables 8-8, 8-9, 8-10, and 8-11 [4].
B. ACC/AHA recommendations for MPI are shown in Tables 8-12, 8-13, 8-14, 8-15, and 8-16 [41].

(TST)Stress testing in USA

Class I

1. Patients undergoing initial evaluation with suspected or known CAD, including those with complete right bundle-branch block or less than 1 mm of resting ST depression. Specific exceptions are noted below in Class IIb
2. Patients with suspected or known CAD, previously evaluated, now presenting with significant change in clinical status
3. Low-risk unstable angina patients 8–12 h after presentation who have been free of active ischemic or HF symptoms
4. Intermediate-risk unstable angina patients 2–3 days after presentation who have been free of active ischemic or HF symptoms

Class IIa

1. Intermediate-risk unstable angina patients who have initial cardiac markers that are normal, a repeat ECG without significant change, and cardiac markers 6–12 h after the onset of symptoms that are normal and no other evidence of ischemia during observation

Class IIb

1. Patients with the following resting ECG abnormalities
   Pre-excitation (Wolff-Parkinson-White) syndrome
   Electronically paced ventricular rhythm
   Greater than 1 mm of resting ST depression
   Complete left bundle-branch block or any interventricular conduction defect with a QRS duration greater than 120 ms

Class III

1. Patients with severe comorbidity likely to limit life expectancy and/or candidacy for revascularization
2. High-risk unstable angina patients

	TABLE 8-8
	ACC/AHA GUIDELINES FOR THE USE OF EXERCISE TESTING IN RISK STRATIFICATION IN PATIENTS WITH UNSTABLE ANGINA

(TST) Stress testing MI

Class I

1. Before discharge for prognostic assessment, activity prescription, evaluation of medical therapy (submaximal at about 4–6 days)
2. Early after discharge for prognostic assessment, activity prescription, evaluation of medical therapy, and cardiac rehabilitation if the predischarge exercise test was not done (symptom limited; about 14–21 days)
3. Late after discharge for prognostic assessment, activity prescription, evaluation of medical therapy, and cardiac rehabilitation if the early exercise test was submaximal (symptom limited; about 3–6 weeks)

Class IIa

1. After discharge for activity counseling and/or exercise training as part of cardiac rehabilitation in patients who have undergone coronary revascularization

Class IIb

1. Patients with the following ECG abnormalities:
   Complete left bundle-branch block
   Pre-excitation syndrome
   Left ventricular hypertrophy
   Digoxin therapy
   Greater than 1 mm of resting ST-segment depression
   Electronically paced ventricular rhythm
2. Periodic monitoring in patients who continue to participate in exercise training or cardiac rehabilitation

Class III

1. Severe comorbidity likely to limit life expectancy and/or candidacy for revascularization
2. At any time to evaluate patients with acute myocardial infarction who have uncompensated congestive HF, cardiac arrhythmia, or noncardiac conditions that severely limit their ability to exercise
3. Before discharge to evaluate patients who have already been selected for, or have undergone, cardiac catheterization. Although a stress test may be useful before or after catheterization to evaluate or identify ischemia in the distribution of a coronary lesion of borderline severity, stress imaging tests are recommended

	TABLE 8-9
	ACC/AHA GUIDELINES FOR THE USE OF EXERCISE TESTING IN MANAGEMENT OF PATIENTS WITH ACUTE MYOCARDIAL INFARCTION

40. Abbott BG, Afshar M, Berger AK, Wackers FJ. Prognostic significance of ischemic electrocardiographic changes during adenosine infusion in patients with normal myocardial perfusion imaging. J Nucl Cardiol. 2003;10(1):9–16.

41. Klocke FJ, Baird MG, Lorell BH, Bateman TM, Messer JV, Berman DS, et al. ACC/AHA/ASNC guidelines for the clinical use of cardiac radionuclide imaging–executive summary: a report of the American College of Cardiology/American Heart Association Task Force on Practice Guidelines (ACC/AHA/ASNC Committee to Revise the 1995 Guidelines for the Clinical Use of Cardiac Radionuclide Imaging). J Am Coll Cardiol. 2003;42(7):1318–33 [Guideline Practice Guideline].

42. Hendel RC, Berman DS, Di Carli MF, Heidenreich PA, Henkin RE, Pellikka PA, et al. ACCF/ASNC/ACR/AHA/ASE/SCCT/SCMR/SNM 2009 appropriate use criteria for cardiac radionuclide imaging: a report of the American College of Cardiology Foundation Appropriate Use Criteria Task Force, the American Society of Nuclear Cardiology, the American College of Radiology, the American Heart Association, the American Society of Echocardiography, the Society of Cardiovascular Computed Tomography, the Society for Cardiovascular Magnetic Resonance, and the Society of Nuclear Medicine. Circulation. 2009;119(22):e561–87 [Practice Guideline].

43. Lee CI, Elmore JG. Radiation-related risks of imaging studies. 2012. Available from: http://www.uptodate.com/contents/radiation-related-risks-of-imaging-studies?source=search_result&search=radiation&selectedTitle=2%7E150. Updated 13 Feb 2012; Cited 11 June 2012.

CHAPTER 9

FARHAD ABTAHIAN AND IK-KYUNG JANG

Cardiac Catheterization, Coronary Arteriography and Intravascular Diagnostics

CHAPTER OUTLINE

ABBREVIATIONS

ACS	Acute coronary syndrome
AI	Aortic insufficiency
AP	Anterior posterior
AS	Aortic stenosis
AV	Aortic valve
AVA	Aortic valve area
BSA	Body surface area
CABG	Coronary artery bypass graft
CAD	Coronary artery disease
CIN	Contrast induced nephropathy
CO	Cardiac output
CVA	Cerebrovascular accident
CVP	Central venous pressure
DFP	Diastolic flow period
DM	Diabetes mellitus
FFR	Fractional flow reserve
HF	Heart failure
HOCM	Hypetrophic obstructive cardiomyopathy
HR	Heart rate
IVC	Inferior vena cava
IVUS	Intravascular ultrasound
LA	Left atrium
LAD	Left anterior descending artery
LAP	Left atrial pressure
LAO	Left anterior oblique
LCx	Left circumflex artery
LIMA	Left internal mammary artery
LM	Left main
LVEDP	Left ventricular end diastolic pressure
MAP	Mean arterial pressure
MR	Mitral regurgitation
MV	Mitral valve
MVA	Mitral valve area
MVO_2	Mixed venous oxygen saturation

NSTEMI	Non-STE-elevation myocardial infarction
OCT	Optical coherence tomography
PA	Pulmonary artery
PAO_2	Pulmonary artery oxygen saturation
PAWP	Pulmonary artery wedge pressure
PBF	Pulmonary blood flow
PCI	Percutaneous coronary intervention
PDA	Posterior descending artery
PHT	Pulmonary hypertension
PVO_2	Pulmonary venous oxygen saturation
PVR	Pulmonary vascular resistance
RA	Right atrium
RAO	Right anterior oblique
RCA	Right coronary artery
RV	Right ventricle
RVEDP	Right ventricular end diastolic pressure
SBP	Systemic blood flow
SCD	Sudden cardiac death
SEP	Systolic ejection period
STEMI	ST-elevation myocardial infarction
SVC	Superior vena cava
SVG	Saphenous vein graft
VO_2	Oxygen consumption

INTRODUCTION

Cardiac catheterization is currently the gold standard diagnostic procedure for assessing cardiac function and coronary anatomy. It is also a platform for the treatment of coronary artery disease, peripheral vascular disease and, increasingly, structural heart disease.

CARDIAC CATHETERIZATION

- 1.3 million percutaneous coronary interventions (PCI) and 1.1 million diagnostic catheterizations performed in annually in U.S.
- Contraindications (all relative): active gastrointestinal bleeding, coagulopathy (INR >1.8), acute renal failure, acute stroke, untreated infection, anemia, anaphylactoid contrast allergy, intracranial hemorrhage.

RADIATION SAFETY [1]

- Dose dependent effects of radiation: skin injury, cataracts, hair loss
- Typical dose 3–5 mSv. Goal dose is as low as reasonably achieved
- Stochastic effect: cancer, genetic defects.
- Operator exposure is predominantly from scatter off of patient.
- Energy of radiation decreases with square root of distance.

ARTERIAL ACCESS

- Femoral artery most common access site in U.S. 3 % performed from radial artery but increasing rapidly [2].

    - Advantage of radial access: ↓70 % in major bleeding versus femoral; ↑ambulation time and ↑patient comfort. Possible ↓ in mortality with ST-elevation myocardial infarction (STEMI) [3].

– Limitations of radial access: technically challenging, ↑procedure time (↑radiation and contrast). Two percent procedure failure rate.

■ Brachial access: similar complication rate as femoral access. Rarely used.

LEFT HEART CATHETERIZATION

■ Use of anticoagulation indicated for prolonged cases (e.g. previous coronary artery bypass graft (CABG) and when crossing stenotic aortic valve (AV)).

(A) Coronary angiography (see below):

(B) Left Ventriculography (Figs. 9-1–9-4):

■ Left ventriculography by power injection of 30–40 ml of contrast at 10–15 mL/s:

– Right anterior oblique (RAO) shows anterior, anterolateral, apical and inferior/posterior walls
– Left anterior oblique (LAO) shows anterior, lateral, inferior and septal walls
– Left ventriculogram contraindicated if left ventricular end diastolic pressure (LVEDP) >25 mmHg or in presence of critical left main coronary artery stenosis (LMCA) stenosis.

■ Findings

– Wall motion assessment
– Ejection fraction
– Presence of ventricular septal defect
– Presence of aneurysm

■ True left ventricular (LV) aneurysms have broad neck and are associated with akinetic wall. Pseudoaneurysms have narrow necks.

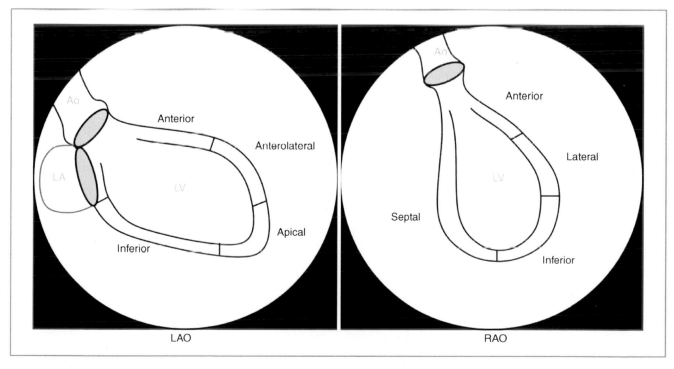

FIGURE 9-1

Left ventriculogram. *Ao* aorta, *LA* left atrium, *LV* left ventricle

– Assessment of valvular regurgitation

■ Sellar's criteria: (1) partial filling of proximal chamber, (2) complete filling of proximal chamber but less dense than distal chamber, (3) equal opacification of proximal chamber in 4–5 beats, (4) equal opacification of proximal chamber in ≤3 beats.

(C) Pressure assessment in left heart catheterization

■ AV gradient assessed by simultaneous aortic and LV pressures (e.g. double lumen pigtail catheter). Indicated when non-invasive results inconclusive or discordant with clinical assessment (Class I recommendation). Not indicated when non-invasive results are conclusive (Class III)

■ Mitral valve (MV) gradient assessed by simultaneous LV and pulmonary capillary wedge pressure (PCWP) or left atrial (LA) pressure

(D) Transseptal Catheterization:

■ Indications: assessment of native or prosthetic mitral valve stenosis (PCWP overestimates transmitral gradient), mitral valve commissurotomy, pulmonary vein isolation (electrophysiology), percutaneous mitral valve valvuloplasty, assessment of LVEDP in presence of mechanical AV, hypertrophic obstructive cardiomyopathy (Fig. 9-2).

■ Complications: puncture of atrial free wall, aortic root, coronary sinus, or pulmonary artery (PA).

(E) Complications of Left Heart Catheterization [4]:

■ Most commonly access site related (<1 % of diagnostic procedures versus 5–20 % of PCIs).

■ Risk factors for access site complications: age, female sex, smaller body surface area, emergent procedures, multi-vessel coronary artery disease (CAD), anti-platelet therapy, coagulopathy, renal dysfunction, liver dysfunction, pre-existing peripheral arterial disease and use of larger sheaths [5].

■ Vascular complications: hematomas, retroperitoneal bleeding, pseudoaneurysm, atriovenous fistula, infection.

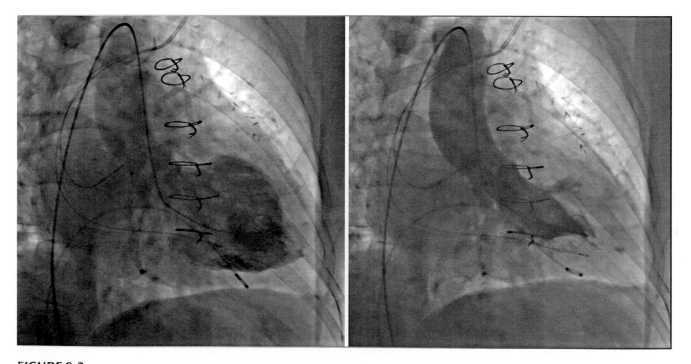

FIGURE 9-2

Apical hypertrophic cardiomyopathy in RAO view

■ Retroperitoneal bleed: hypotension or back pain post procedure

  - CT scan is recommended diagnostic modality

■ Pseudoaneurysm

  - Treated with manual compression (small) or ultrasound guided thrombin injection (large)

■ Cerebrovascular Accident (0.07 %): MRI shows cerebral embolic events in 22 % of patients after crossing severe aortic valve→majority asymptomatic [6].
■ Other: contrast induced nephropathy (CIN), myocardial infarction (0.05 %), arrhythmia, perforation of cardiac chamber or PA, death.

CONTRAST AGENTS

■ Nonionic low-osmolar contrast agents preferred.

  - Significantly lower osmolality associated with lower risk of adverse reactions (arrhythmia, hypotension, nausea, increased LVEDP, pulmonary edema).
  - All agents have equal risk of contrast induced nephropathy (CIN).

■ CIN [7] is defined as rise in creatinine >0.5 mg/dL or 25 % above baseline within 48 h.

  - Incidence 2 %.
  - Increased risk in patient with chronic renal insufficiency, diabetes mellitus (DM), anemia and the elderly.
  - Progression to end stage renal disease is very rare.
  - Prehydration can reduce the risk of CIN.

■ Contrast allergy [8]

  - Severe reactions in ~1 % of patients.
  - Prophylaxis: 60 mg prednisone or 100 mg hydrocortisone 12 h and immediately prior to procedure, diphenhydramine 25–50 mg IV immediately prior.

CLOSURE DEVICES

■ Four types: suture, collagen plug, passive hemostatic patch, metallic clips.
■ Allow for sheath removal in anti-coagulated patients and earlier ambulation (1–2 h versus 4–6 h).
■ No difference in risk of access site complications versus manual compression [9].

ENDOMYOCARDIAL BIOPSY

■ Indications for endomyocardial biopsy [10]:

  - New onset heart failure (HF) <2 weeks with dilated LV and hemodynamic compromise
  - New onset HF 2 weeks to 3 months with dilated LV and ventricular arrhythmia or heart block or failure to respond to therapy
  - Diagnosis of infiltrative cardiomyopathy (e.g. amyloid and sarcoid)
  - Monitoring of transplanted heart for rejection.

■ Complications of endomyocardial biopsy:

  - Cardiac perforation
  - Ventricular arrhythmia
  - Heart block
  - Tricuspid injury (risk reduced with use of longer sheath).

RIGHT HEART CATHETERIZATION (RHC)

■ Indications for RHC:

- – Cardiogenic shock
- – Discordant right and left heart failure
- – Complicated myocardial infarction (MI)
- – Severe chronic HF requiring supportive therapy
- – Diagnosis and assessment of pulmonary hypertension
- – Differentiation of septic vs. cardiogenic shock
- – Pericardial disease
- – Diagnosis and assessment of intracardiac shunts
- – Congenital heart disease

■ Complications

- – Infection
- – Pneumothorax
- – Arrhythmia
- – Carotid artery cannulation
- – Right atrium (RA)/right ventricle (RV)/PA rupture
- – Pulmonary infarction
- – Complete heart block (esp. with baseline left bundle branch block).

(A) Pressure measurement (Fig. 9-5):

■ Zero reference pressure is established at the level of the atria
■ Atrial pressure: three waves

- – (a) atrial systole
- – (c) closing of AV valve
- – (v) RV systole

■ Two descents

- – (x) atrial relaxation with open AV valve
- – (x') continued atrial relaxation with closed AV valve
- – (y) tricuspid valve opening

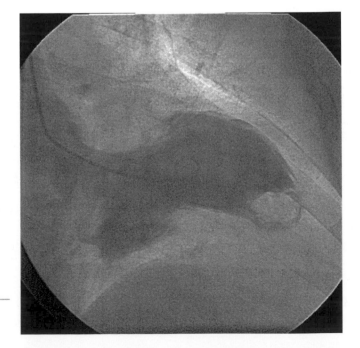

FIGURE 9-3

A calcified clot in apex in RAO view

Diastole   Systole

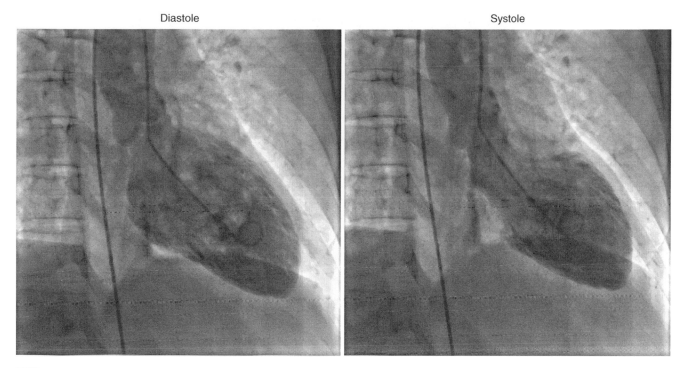

FIGURE 9-4

Apical ballooning in takotsubo cardiomyopathy (RAO view)

- Spontaneous respirations: pressure decreases with inspiration and increases with exhalation

    This is reversed with mechanical respiration.

- PCWP gives good estimate of mean LA pressure but is delayed and blunted compared to direct LA pressure [11] (Fig. 9-6, Table 9-1)

(B) Cardiac output (CO):

- Thermodilution

    - Tends to underestimate CO with aortic regurgitation (AR), mitral regurgitation (MR) or tricuspid regurgitation (TR)
    - Inaccurate in low CO state (CO <2.5 L/min), shunt or irregular rhythm.

- Fick Method

$$CO_{Fick}\,(L/min) = \frac{O_2\,consumption(mL/min)}{Arteriovenous\,O_2\,difference(vol\,\%) \times 1.36(mLO_2/gmHgb) \times Hgb(mg/dL) \times 10}$$

    - O_2 consumption (VO_2) 125 mL/min/m² (elevated in HF, fevers, sepsis, lung infections)
    - Largest source of error is oxygen consumption especially if assumed.
    - Not affected by TR or low output state.
    - Should not be used with severe MR or AI to calculate valve area since CO is not equivalent to transvalvular flow in the setting of severe regurgitation.
    - Must be in steady state

- Angiographic Method: tracing end diastolic and end systolic images

$$CO_{Angio} = (end\,diastolic\,volume - end\,systolic\,volume) \times heart\,rate$$

FIGURE 9-5

Normal right heart catheterization tracings. *LA* left atrium, *LV* left ventricle, *MV* mitral valve, *PA* pulmonary artery, *PCWP* pulmonary capillary wedge pressure, *RA* right atrium

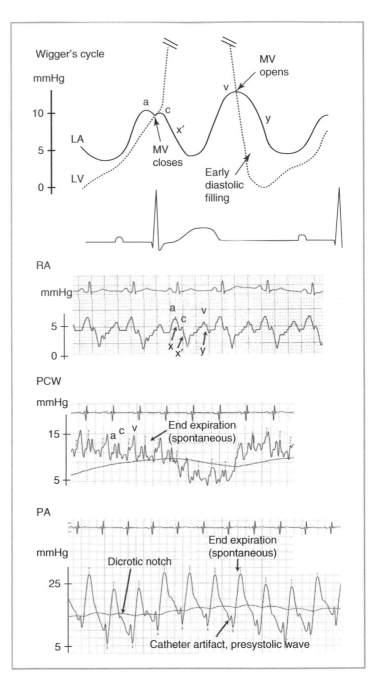

(C) Shunts:

■ Screening for shunts by measuring oxygen saturation in superior vena cava (SVC) and PA

 – Considered positive if difference >7 %
 – If positive, a full shunt run including SVC, vena cava (IVC), high-mid-low RA, RV inflow and outflow, main PA, right and left PA, pulmonary vein, LA, LV, and Aorta is performed.

■ Qp: Qs calculation

$$\text{Pulmonary blood flow (Qp)} = \frac{O_2 \text{ consumption (mL / min/ m}^2)}{\text{Pulmonary venous} O_2 - \text{Pulmonary arterial } O_2}$$

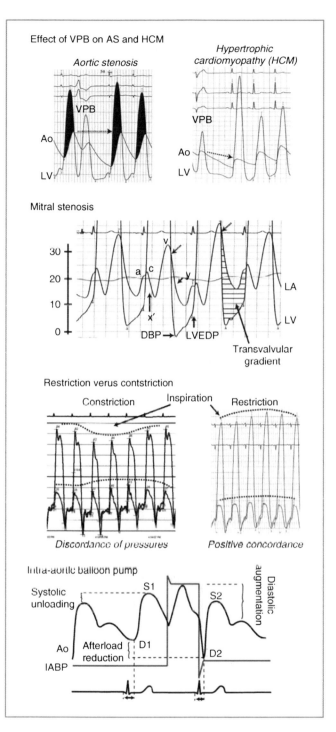

FIGURE 9-6

Common abnormal pressure tracings. *Ao* aorta, *AS* aortic stenosis, *DBP* diastolic blood pressure, *HCM* hypertrophic cardiomyopathy, *IABP* intraaortic baloon pump, *LA* left atrium, *LV* left ventricle, *LVEDP* left ventricular end diastolic pressure, *VPB* ventricular premature beat

$$\text{Systemic blood flow (Qs)} = \frac{O_2 \text{ consumption (mL / min / m}^2)}{\text{Systemic arterial } O_2 - \text{Mixed venous } O_2}$$

$$\text{Shunt Fraction} = Q_p / Q_s = \frac{SAO_2 - MVO_2}{PVO_2 - PAO_2}$$

$$MVO_2 = \text{Saturation in the chamber proximal to the shunt} = \frac{3(SVC\,O_2) + (IVC\,O_2)}{4}$$

TABLE 9-1	MEASURE	NORMAL RANGE	COMMENT
RHC NORMAL VALUES	Right atrium	1–6 mmHg	Equivalent to CVP and RVEDP in absence of TV disease
	Right ventricle	15–25/1–8 mmHg	
	Pulmonary artery	15–25/4–12 mmHg	
	PCWP	4–12 mmHg	Equivalent to LAP and LVEDP in absence of MV disease
	Left atrium	2–12 mmHg	
	Left ventricle	90–140/5–12 mmHg	
	Cardiac output	4–6 L/min	
	Cardiac index	2.4–4 L/min/m²	CO/BSA
	Systemic vascular resistance (SVR)	700–1,600 dyn×s/cm⁵	SVR(Woods)=(MAP − RA)/CO1 Wood=80 dyn×s/cm⁵
	Pulmonary vascular resistance (PVR)	20–130 dyn×s/cm⁵	PVR (Woods)=(Mean PA − PCWP)/CO>240 dyn×s/cm⁵ limit heart transplant eligibility

BSA body surface area, *CO* cardiac output, *CVP* central venous pressure, *MAP* mean arterial pressure, *MV* mitral valve, *LAP* left atrial pressure, *LVEDP* left ventricular end diastolic pressure, *PA* pulmonary artery, *PCWP* pulmonary capillary wedge pressure, *RA* right atrium, *RVEDP* right ventricular end diastolic pressure, *TV* tricuspid valve

SAO_2 = Systemic arterial O_2, MVO_2 = Mixed venous O_2, PVO_2 = Pulmonary venous O_2 (systemic O_2 saturation can substitute for PVO_2), PAO_2 = Pulmonary arterial O_2

(D) Calculation of Stenotic Valve Area (Gorlin Formula):

■ Based on relationship between flow velocity, pressure gradient and area of stenotic valve

– AV area (AVA) calculated based on flow during systole only (systolic ejection period (SEP))
– Mitral valve area (MVA) is calculated based on flow during diastole (diastolic flow period (DFP)).

$$AVA(cm^2) = \frac{Cardiac\,output(L/min) \times 1000mL/L}{44.3 \times Heart\,rate\,(beats/min) \times SEP(s) \times \sqrt{mean\,gradient(mmHg)}}$$

$$MVA\,(cm^2) = \frac{Cardiac\,output(L/min) \times 1000\,mL/L}{37.7 \times Heart\,rate\,(beats/min) \times DEP(s) \times \sqrt{mean\,gradient(mmHg)}}$$

Simplified Hakki formula:

$$AVA(cm^2) = \frac{Cardiac\,output(L/min)}{\sqrt{mean\,gradient\,(mmHg)}}$$

■ Limitations of the Gorlin formula:

– Errors in CO measurement are more important than errors in the pressure gradient measurement, because square root of the mean gradient is used in the formula
– May underestimate the valve area in low CO states
– May be inaccurate in mixed valvular disease (stenosis and regurgitation)
– Does not apply to mechanical valves

INTRA-AORTIC BALLOON PUMP (IABP) [12]

■ Indications

– Cardiogenic shock
– Refractory angina

– Support during high risk PCI
– Refractory HF
– Refractory ventricular arrhythmia

■ Hemodynamic effects (See Fig. 9-5D)

– Assisted systolic pressure (S2)<unassisted (S1)
– Assisted diastolic pressure (D2)<unassisted (D1)
– Augmented diastolic pressure>systolic pressure (S1 and S2)
– Mean arterial pressure is increased.

CORONARY ANGIOGRAPHY

■ Gold standard diagnostic test for diagnosing coronary artery disease and determining treatment options.

(A) Indications for coronary angiography are listed in Table 9-2 [13–18]

■ Other Indications:

– Stable Coronary Artery Disease:
– Patients with class I or II angina despite medical therapy (Class IIa)
– Patients with progression of stress test abnormalities (Class IIa)
– Patients with high risk occupations and abnormal but not high risk stress tests (Class IIa)
– Periodic evaluation after heart transplantation (Class IIb)
– Prior to ascending aorta surgery or surgical correction of congental heart disease
– Unexplained cardiac arrest in a young patient.
– Patients with hypertrophic cardiomyopathy with angina despite medical therapy or if heart surgery is planned
– Prior to cardiac transplantation (donor)
– Heart failure without explained cause

(B) Contraindications (non-emergency situations only):

■ Coagulopathy
■ Severe anemia
■ Severe electrolyte abnormalities
■ Recent deterioration in renal function
■ Uncontrolled severe hypertension
■ Infection at planned access site.

(C) Normal Coronary Anatomy (Fig. 9-7):

■ LMCA arises above the left aortic sinus and the right coronary artery (RCA) above the right coronary sinus. Best viewed in antero-posterior (AP) projection.
■ LMCA courses divides in to left anterior descending (LAD) and left circumflex (LCx) (30 % of population have a ramus intermedius branch).

– Ramus courses similarly to diagonal or obtuse marginal artery.

■ LAD gives rise to 1–3 diagonal arteries (supplying anterior wall, anterolateral papillary muscle, and anterior RV wall) and septal arteries (supplying apical and anterior two-thirds of septum). Best viewed with cranially angulated projections.

– Diagonal arteries define margin of heart in RAO projection.
– LAD comes straight down in LAO projections

■ LCx gives rise to 1–3 obtuse marginal arteries supplying the lateral wall. Best viewed with caudally angulated projections.
■ RCA gives rise to conus branch, marginal arteries (supply RV free wall), posterior descending artery (PDA) (supply posterior third of septum), and posterolateral

TABLE 9-2

INDICATIONS FOR CORONARY ANGIOGRAPHY

	CLASS I	CLASS III
Nonspecific chest pain (CP)	High risk finding on noninvasive testing	No high-risk finding on non-invasive testing or repeat hospitalizations for chest pain
Stable coronary artery disease (CAD)	Survivors of sudden cardiac death (known or suspected CAD)	Patients with severe comorbidity where risks outweigh benefits
	Canadian Cardiovascular Society (CCS) class III and IV symptoms despite medications	CCS I or II with response to medical therapy and no evidence of ischemia on non-invasive testing
	High-risk criteria on non-invasive testing: LVEF<35 %; ST depressions >1 mm with low exercise capacity; hypotension with exercise; moderate to large area of ischemia (especially anterior wall).	Patient does not desire revascularization
	Heart failure symptoms and angina	
	Serious ventricular arrhythmia	
	Clinical characteristics indicate high likelihood of severe CAD	
Monitoring of symptoms in stable CAD	Marked limitation of ordinary activity despite maximal medical therapy	
ST-elevation MI	Candidates for primary PCI or rescue PCI	Patients not considered to be candidates for revascularization due to extensive comorbidities
	Cardiogenic shock and candidate for PCI	
	Prior to surgical repair of VSD or MR	
	Persistent hemodynamic or electric instability	
Post-STEMI hospitalization	Continued ischemia either spontaneous or with minimal exertion	Patients not considered to be candidates for revascularization
	Intermediate or high risk findings on non-invasive testing	
	Prior to definitive therapy for mechanical complications if sufficiently stable.	
	Persistent hemodynamic instability	
Unstable angina/NSTEMI (management)	Early invasive strategy in high risk patients: recurrent angina despite maximal medical therapy, positive biomarkers, HF symptoms (S3, pulmonary edema, MR), depressed LV function, hemodynamic or electrical instability, PCI in prior 6 months, prior CABG	Patients in whom risks of revascularization outweigh benefits
	High risk finding on non-invasive testing	Patients with chest pain but low probability of acute coronary syndrome (ACS)
UA/NSTEMI post discharge	Patients initially treated conservatively but with recurrent UA or CCS class III/IV angina despite medical therapy.	Repeat angiography not indicated in absence of change in symptoms or results of non-invasive testing
Printzmetal angina	Episodic chest pain with ST elevations that resolve with nitroglycerin or CCB	Provocative testing should not be done in patients with high-grade obstructive lesions
Cardiac syndrome X	If no ECGs are available from CP episodes, provocative testing to rule out coronary spasm	Routine angiography is not indicated in asymptomatic patients post CABG
Post-CABG	Low threshold for angiography if patients have recurrent symptoms of ischemia	
Post-PCI	Suspected stent thrombosis	Routine angiography is not indicated in asymptomatic patients post PCI
	Recurrent ischemia or high risk non-invasive testing within 9 months of PCI	

Prior to valvular surgery	Patients at risk of having CAD, reduced LV function, noninvasive testing consistent with ischemia Patient with mild to moderate valvular disease but with symptoms of ischemia (CCS>1)	Not indicated in patients younger than 35 years old without risk factors for or symptoms suggestive of ischemia.
Prior to non cardiac surgery	Angina not responsive to medical therapy High risk finding on non-invasive testing Unstable angina/NSTEMI Equivocal non-invasive testing in high risk patient undergoing high risk surgery	Known CAD but low risk non-invasive testing Asymptomatic patients post PCI or CABG Mild angina with preserved LV function and no high risk features on non-invasive testing Patients older than 40 as part of evaluation for non-cardiac transplantation if non-invasive testing shows no high risk features.

CABG coronary artery bypass graft, *CCB* calcium channel blocker, *HF* heart failure, *LV* left ventricle, *LVEF* left ventricular ejection fraction, *MI* myocardial infarction, *MR* mitral regurgitation, *NSTEMI* non-ST segment elevation MI, *PCI* percutaneous coronary intervention, *VSD* ventricular septal defect, *UA* unstable angina

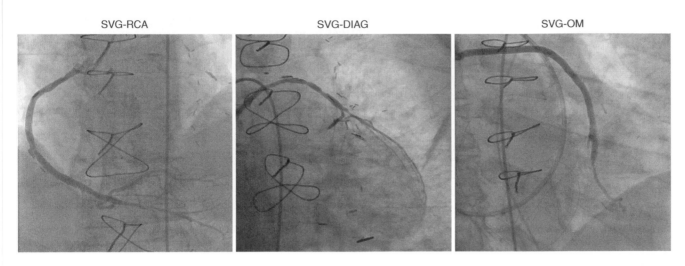

FIGURE 9-9

Saphenous vein grafts

- ■ Bypass grafts: Important to obtain prior operative reports to guide search for grafts (Fig. 9-9).

  - – Saphenous vein grafts (SVG) to RCA system typically arise in anterolateral aortic wall superior to native RCA.
  - – SVG to LAD or Diagonal artery is usually above the RCA graft from the anterior aorta.
  - – SVG to LCx system is typically superior to the SVG to LAD/diagonal artery and arise from anterolateral aorta.
  - – LIMA graft: must rule out significant subclavian artery stenosis. Left lateral view to assess the anastomosis of the LIMA to the LAD.

(E) Anomalous Coronary Arteries: (Table 9-4)

- ■ Occur in up to 5 % of population

  - – Majority are discovered incidentally and are of no clinical significance (also see Chap. 21).

(F) Collateral Circulation (Fig. 9-10):

- ■ Can form within hours after STEMI
- ■ Rentrop classification

  - – 0=no filling
  - – 1=side branch filled
  - – 2=partial filling occluded artery
  - – 3=complete filling of occluded artery.

(G) Assessing Coronary Lesions:

- ■ Type A: Discrete (<10 mm), concentric, nonangulated segment, smooth contour, minimal calcium, non-ostial, no thrombus, no significant side branch involvement.
- ■ Type B: Tubular (<20 mm), eccentric, moderate angulation (45–90°), irregular, calcified, ostial, bifurcation, thrombus present, total occlusion <3 months.
- ■ Type C: Diffuse (>20 mm), angulated >90°, bifurcation but unable to protect side branch, total occlusion >3 months, degenerated SVG.
- ■ Flush occlusion or hazy stump and dye hang-up are consistent with thrombus (typically in patients presenting with acute coronary syndrome (ACS))

TABLE 9-4

CLASSIFICATION OF THE
ANOMALOUS CORONARY ARTERY

Anomaly of origin and course

Absence of left main trunk (Separate LAD and LCx ostia)

Anomalous location of coronary ostium, from pulmonary artery: must be corrected usually at birth

Anomalous origination of coronary ostium from opposite coronary sinus, or non-cusped (posterior) sinus: course between aorta and RVOT associated with increased risk of SCD. Treat with CABG or PCI

Single coronary artery

Myocardial bridging: maybe associated with ischemia. Five percent of general population but 30–50 % of patients with HCM. Treatment with medication versus PCI versus CABG not established

Anomaly of intrinsic coronary artery anatomy

Congenital ostial stenosis or atresia: often associated with other congenital disease

Coronary ectasia or aneurysm: Kawasaki disease, connective tissue disease, arteritis → risk thrombosis and embolism

Coronary hypoplasia

Intramural coronary artery (myocardial bridging): abrupt narrowing of vessel during systole

Intercoronary communication

Anomaly of coronary termination

Coronary artery fistula → terminate in RV (40 %), RA (25 %), PA (17 %), coronary sinus or SVC. Asymptomatic in 50 %. Associated with continuous murmur. Maybe cause ischemia, HF, arrhythmia. Treat with surgical closure or coil embolization

CABG coronary artery bypass graft, *HCM* hypertrophic cardiomyopathy, *HF* heart failure, *LAD* left anterior descending, *LCx* left circumflex, *PA* pulmonary artery, *PCI* percutaneous coronary intervention, *RA* right atrium, *RV* right ventricle, *RVOT* right ventricular outflow track, *SCD* sudden cardiac death, *SVC* superior vena cava

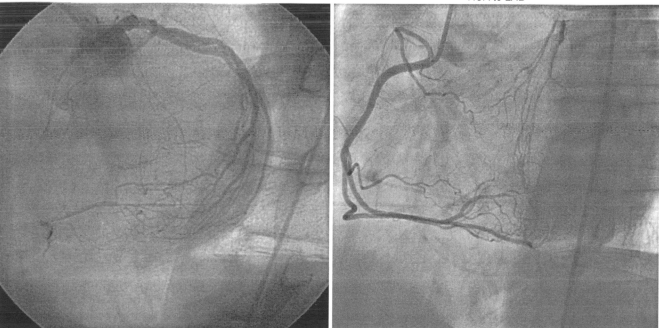

Lcx to RCA   RCA to LAD

FIGURE 9-10

Collateral vessels visualized by angiography

CAROTID ARTERY DISEASE

- Symptomatic Disease – Transient ischemic attack or stroke within 6 months

    - Endarterectomy (CEA) or Stenting (CAS) for angiographic lesions greater than 50 % or those judged to be greater than 70 % on non-invasive testing
    - No intervention on patients with stenoses less than 50 %
    - Proceed early to revascularization (<2 weeks) after TIA/stroke

- Aysmptomatic Disease

    - Controversy exists regarding medical management vs. revascularization
    - Can consider revascularization in stenoses >70 % if low risk of procedure-related complications and long-term expected survival

        - Octagenerians are high-risk for revascularization by both CEA and CAS

- CREST trial: No difference in stroke/MI/death for CAS vs. CEA in broad group of patients [10].

    - Slightly increased risk of minor stroke with CAS.
    - Slightly increased risk of NSTEMI with CEA.

MESENTERIC VASCULAR DISEASE

- Prevalence

    - Angiographic stenosis may be present in over half of patients with known systemic atherosclerosis
    - Causes

        - Atherosclerosis – etiology in >90 % of cases
        - Median arcuate ligament syndrome (compression of celiac artery or SMA by median arcuate ligament)
        - FMD
        - Vasculitis

    - Angiographic stenoses may not be associated with symptoms

        - Significant disease in two vessels often necessary to provoke symptoms due to rich collateral networks in the gut

    - IMA stenosis/occlusion usually well tolerated due to hypogastric, meandering mesenteric, and Marginal artery of Drummond collaterals

- Presentation

    - Symptoms of chronic mesenteric ischemia: post-prandial abdominal pain (intestinal angina), "food fear", weight loss

- Diagnosis

    - Non-invasive testing: Doppler ultrasonography, CTA, MRA

- Treatment

    - Percutaneous stenting is a viable treatment strategy in patients with atherosclerotic disease and no evidence of an arterial compression syndrome (such as median arcuate ligament syndrome)

- Acute mesenteric ischemia

    - Often due to thromboembolism or hypotension with insufficiency at watershed territories
    - Usually a surgical emergency requiring urgent laparotomy
    - Adjunctive endovascular techniques are sometimes used

DEEP VENOUS THROMBOSIS (DVT)

Incidence

- 1–2 per 1,000 patient years
- Incidence increases tenfold after age 50

Risk Factors

- Malignancy
- Pregnancy
- Prior DVT
- Oral contraceptives
- May-Thurner syndrome (left common iliac vein compression by the right common iliac artery)
- Virchow's triad

  - Hypercoaguability
  - Stasis
  - Endothelial injury

Presentation

- Painful, swollen lower extremity
- Upper extremity DVT (<10 % of all DVT) are usually associated with indwelling catheters or pacemaker/defibrillators

Diagnosis (Table 10-3)

See Fig. 10-3.

Treatment

- Provoked proximal DVT: 3–6 months anti-coagulation (INR = 2–3 with warfarin)
- Unprovoked proximal DVT receives 6 months to indefinite anti-coagulation

  - LMWH preferred in patients with malignancy
  - Catheter-directed lysis reduces post-thrombotic syndrome in iliofemoral DVT

CLINICAL FEATURE	SCORE
Active cancer (treatment ongoing or within 6 months or palliative)	1
Paralysis, paresis or recent plaster immobilization of the lower extremities	1
Recent bedridden for more than 3 days or major surgery within 4 weeks	1
Localized tenderness along the distribution of the deep venous system	1
Entire leg swollen	1
Calf swelling by more than 3 cm when compared with the asymptomatic leg (measured 10 cm below the tibial tuberosity)	1
Pitting edema (greater in the symptomatic leg)	1
Collateral superficial veins (non-varicose)	1
Alternative diagnosis as likely as or greater than that of DVT	−2

TABLE 10-3

WELL'S SCORE FOR DVT DIAGNOSIS [11]

Courtesy of Well et al. [11]
Interpretation: High probability >3; Moderate probability 1–2; Low probability <0
In patients with bilateral symptoms, the more symptomatic leg is used

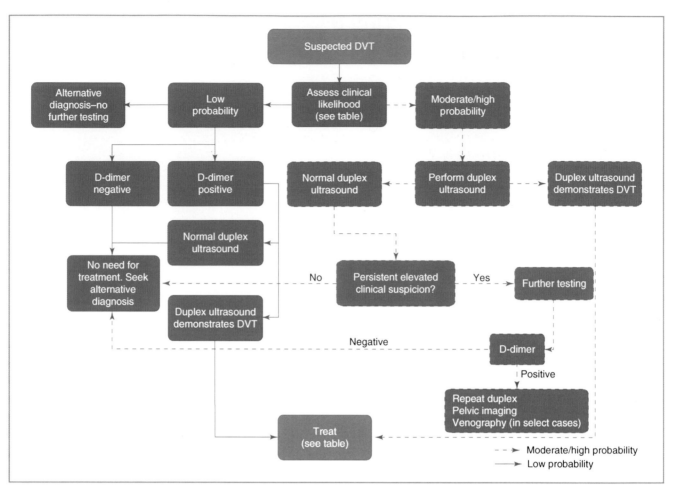

FIGURE 10-3

Diagnostic algorithm for DVT (Courtesy of Weinberg and Jaff [14])

■ Calf DVT: typically 3 months anti-coagulation for symptomatic pts vs. no anti-coagulation and serial ultrasonography (4–6 ultrasounds over 2–4 weeks) to monitor for proximal extension,

■ Superficial venous thrombosis: non-steroidal anti-inflammatory drugs and warm compresses.

– Consider anti-coagulation for proximal clot (i.e.: near saphenofemoral junction).

■ Catheter-Associated DVT: remove catheter, anti-coagulation for 3 months or less

Complications

■ Post-thrombotic syndrome (PTS)

– Persistent long-term swelling in the lower extremity that may be associated with skin changes (stasis dermatitis)
– Leg may feel fatigued, heavy and weak
– Is a common consequence of proximal iliofemoral DVT
– Prevention

■ Consider early catheter-directed lysis for newly diagnosed iliofemoral DVT
■ Use 20–40 mmHg graduated compression stockings for long term prevention of venous insufficiency and PTS

– Treatment

■ Compression therapy
■ Angioplasty/stenting of proximal occluded deep veins
■ Rarely open surgical bypass procedures

■ Phlegmasia Dolens

– Massive thrombosis of a limb with patent collaterals (phlegmasia alba dolens) or obstructed collaterals with resultant compartment syndrome, arterial compromise and venous gangrene (phlegmasia cerulea dolens)
– Risk factors include post-operative states, malignancy, hypercoaguability, and May-Thurner Syndrome
– Mortality rates are up to 25 % with PE causing at least 1/3 of deaths and amputations are common
– Presents as pain, swelling, and cyanosis of the affected limb
– Treatment includes leg elevation, anticoagulation, catheter-directed thrombolysis, and open surgical thrombectomy

PULMONARY EMBOLISM (PE)

Incidence

■ 400,000–600,000 cases per year diagnosed in the USA

Risk Factors Are Identical to DVT

See section "Risk Factors."

Presentation

■ Sudden onset of pleuritic chest pain
■ Dyspnea
■ Cough
■ Hemoptysis
■ Tachycardia + hypotension

Diagnosis

■ History – assess for risk factors and presenting symptoms above
■ Physical exam – tachypnea, tachycardia, hypoxia, accentuated P2 component of S2, RV heave
■ Electrocardiogram – sinus tachycardia, RBBB, anterior precordial repolarization abnormalities
■ D-dimer – highly sensitive but poorly specific test that is useful to rule out DVT
■ Chest radiography – most commonly unremarkable, may see Westermark sign (oligemic focus distal to PE) or Hampton's hump (wedge-shaped consolidation representing infarction)
■ Echocardiography – increased RVSP, right ventricular dilation and hypokinesis
■ Well's criteria (Table 10-4)

– For moderate or high probability proceed to CT angiogram or ventilation/perfusion (V/Q) scan:

Treatment

■ Immediate parenteral anticoagulation

– Transition to long-term agents (warfarin vs. LMWH/fondaparinux)

TABLE 10-4	CLINICAL FEATURE	SCORE
	Clinical signs and symptoms of DVT (minimum of leg swelling and pain with palpation of the deep veins)	3
WELL'S SCORE FOR PE DIAGNOSIS [12]	An alternative diagnosis is less likely than PE	3
	Heart rate greater than 100	1.5
	Immobilization or surgery in the previous 4 weeks	1.5
	Previous DVT/PE	1.5
	Hemoptysis	1
	Malignancy (on treatment, treated in the last 6 months or palliative)	1

Courtesy of Wells et al. [12]
Interpretation: High probability >6; Moderate probability >2 and <6; Low probability <2. If the D-dimer is negative a cutoff point of four points or less makes a PE unlikely

■ Provoked PE (status post trauma, prolonged immobilization, or recent surgery) should be treated for a minimum of 3 months
■ Unprovoked PE should be treated for 6–12 months with treatment extension considered
■ Second unprovoked PE is an indication for lifelong anti-coagulation
■ IVC filter for select indications

– VTE with contraindication to anticoagulation
– Recurrent VTE despite adequate anti-coagulation

MASSIVE PE: PE ASSOCIATED WITH HEMODYNAMIC INSTABILITY (SYSTOLIC BP <90 MMHG)

■ International Cooperative Pulmonary Embolism Registry showed a 4.5 % incidence and greater than 50 % 90-day mortality [13]
■ Diagnostic studies

– Massive PE often associated with acute RV strain pattern on ECG ("S1Q3T3")
– Transthoracic echocardiography reveals akinesia of the RV free wall with apical sparing (McConnell's sign)

■ Treatment

– Consider peripheral IV or catheter-directed thrombolysis

■ Absolute contraindications to thrombolysis are:

– active internal bleeding or severe coagulopathy
– cerebrovascular event, neurosurgical procedure, cerebral trauma in the past 3 months
– history of hemorrhagic stroke
– active intracranial malignancy
– aortic dissection

– Consider surgical or catheter based embolectomy strategies for those not eligible for thrombolysis.

REVIEW QUESTIONS

1. **A 44 year old woman with a history of hypertension presents to the Emergency Room with complaints of severe headaches for several days. Her outpatient medication list includes amlodipine 10 mg daily, lisinopril 40 mg daily, and hydrochlorothiazide 25 mg daily. Vital signs revealed blood pressure of 185/95 and a heart rate of 78. Examination is significant for an abdominal bruit and bilateral carotid bruits. A CT (head) does not show any signs of intracranial hemorrhage. The treatment most likely to benefit this patient is:**
   (a) Addition of metoprolol XL 50 mg daily to her regimen
   (b) Surgical revascularization of her carotid arteries
   (c) Angiography and balloon angioplasty of the renal arteries
   (d) Carotid angiography with consideration of stent placement
   (e) Angiography and stenting of the renal arteries

2. **A 56 year old man with a history of tobacco use, hypertension, and diabetes presents to you with complaints of right calf pain after walking two blocks. His medication regimen includes aspirin, cilostazol, ramipril, atenolol, and metformin. He has been advised to walk daily and, for 6 months, he has adhered to a regimen of 30–45 min of walking on a treadmill at his house but has to stop frequently due to right calf pain. He had a recent CTA that revealed a focal 3 cm high-grade 80 % stenosis of the right external iliac artery. The next most appropriate step in management is:**
   (a) Addition of clopidogrel 75 mg daily to his regimen
   (b) Addition of warfarin to his regimen with goal INR=2–3.

   (c) Discontinuation of atenolol.
   (d) Percutaneous right external iliac artery revascularization.
   (e) Continue current regimen including daily walking program with follow-up in 6 months.

3. **A 75 year old patient is hospitalized with a hip fracture. Their past medical history is notable for hypertension, colon cancer treated with hemi-colectomy 2 months prior to presentation, and diabetes mellitus. Their medications include metoprolol, lisinopril, metformin, and aspirin. On hospital day 2, the patient undergoes an open reduction and internal fixation of the hip, which is uneventful. On hospital day 3, however, the leg contralateral to the surgical repair is edematous, painful, and indurated.**

   A venous thrombosis of the proximal femoral venous system is identified using Doppler ultrasound and systemic anticoagulation is begun.

   All of the following are true EXCEPT
   (a) Treatment should last for 3–6 months at a minimum
   (b) The development of post-thrombotic syndrome may be minimized with the use of graduated compression stockings after anticoagulation is begun
   (c) Placement of a permanent filter for the inferior vena cava will reduce the risk of complications in this patient
   (d) Painful venous plethora of the leg should be treated as a vascular emergency
   (e) Thrombosis of the left leg may be due to a congenital anomaly of the venous drainage of the limb.

ANSWERS

1. (c) The patient's demographic information, resistant hypertension, and abdominal/carotid bruits should raise suspicion for fibromuscular dysplasia.

   Given resistant hypertension on three medications including a diuretic, renal angiography with angioplasty is indicated in this case. In FMD, stent placement is often unnecessary as good long-term results have been noted with angioplasty alone. There is no clear indication to intervene on her carotid arteries given her absence of neurologic symptoms currently. Addition of metoprolol XL to her regimen is unlikely to normalize her blood pressure.

2. (d) The patient is on optimal medical therapy and a structured walking program. He continues to have life-limiting symptoms despite this so endovascular revascularization of the right external iliac artery is indicated.

   Neither dual anti-platelet therapy nor warfarin have not been shown to have benefit in this clinical circumstance. There is no need to discontinue his beta-blocker.

3. (c) Vena cava filters have very specific indications for patients with venous thrombosis, and should be removed as soon as the risk period has passed. Permanent implantation of filters not only does not appear to reduce risk in the long run, but in fact may increase the risk for vascular complications.

   All other statements are true: anticoagulation, though individualized for each patient, should continue a minimum of 3 months, and probably longer. Compression stockings may reduce the risk for painful edema of the limb after resolution of the DVT, while phlegmasia cerulea dolens is a vascular emergency, due to risk of venous gangrene. Lastly, the May-Thurner anomaly is a congenital compressive syndrome of the left-sided iliac vein, which increases the risk for spontaneous and recurrent venous thrombosis of this vessel.

REFERENCES

1. Hirsch AT, Haskal ZJ, Hertzer NR, American Association for Vascular Surgery, Society for Vascular Surgery, Society for Cardiovascular Angiography and Interventions, Society for Vascular Medicine and Biology, Society of Interventional Radiology, ACC/AHA Task Force on Practice Guidelines, American Association of Cardiovascular and Pulmonary Rehabilitation, National Heart, Lung,and Blood Institute, Society for Vascular Nursing, TransAtlantic Inter-Society Consensus, Vascular Disease Foundation, et al. ACC/AHA 2005 guidelines for the management of patients with peripheral arterial disease (lower extremity, renal, mesenteric, and abdominal aortic): executive summary a collaborative report from the American Association for Vascular Surgery/Society for Vascular Surgery, Society for Cardiovascular Angiography and Interventions, Society for Vascular Medicine and Biology, Society of Interventional Radiology, and the ACC/AHA Task Force on Practice Guidelines (Writing Committee to Develop Guidelines for the Management of Patients with Peripheral Arterial Disease) endorsed by the American Association of Cardiovascular and Pulmonary Rehabilitation; National Heart, Lung, and Blood Institute; Society for Vascular Nursing; TransAtlantic Inter-Society Consensus; and Vascular Disease Foundation. J Am Coll Cardiol. 2006;47(6):1239–312.
2. Norgren L, Hiatt WR, Dormandy JA, et al. Inter-society consensus for the management of peripheral arterial disease (TASC II). J Vasc Surg. 2007;45(Suppl S):S5–67.
3. CAPRIE Steering Committee. A randomised, blinded, trial of clopidogrel versus aspirin in patients at risk of ischaemic events (CAPRIE). Lancet. 1996;348(9038):1329–39.
4. Bhatt DL, Fox KA, Hacke W, et al. Clopidogrel and aspirin versus aspirin alone for the prevention of atherothrombotic events. N Engl J Med. 2006;354:1706–17.
5. Anand S, Yusuf S, Xie C, et al. Oral anticoagulant and antiplatelet therapy and peripheral arterial disease. N Engl J Med. 2007;357(3):217–27.
6. Adam DJ, Beard JD, Cleveland T, et al. Bypass versus angioplasty in severe ischaemia of the leg (BASIL): multicentre, randomised controlled trial. Lancet. 2005;366:1925–34.
7. van Jaarsveld BC, Krijnen P, Pieterman H, et al. The effect of balloon angioplasty on hypertension in atherosclerotic renal-artery stenosis. N Engl J Med. 2000;342:1007–14.
8. Bax L, Woittiez AJ, Kouwenberg HJ, Mali WP, Buskens E, Beek FJ, et al. Stent placement in patients with atherosclerotic renal artery stenosis and impaired renal function: a randomized trial. Ann Intern Med. 2009;150:840–8.
9. Wheatley K, Ives N, Gray R, Kalra PA, Moss JG, Baigent C, et al. Revascularization versus medical therapy for renal-artery stenosis. N Engl J Med. 2009;361(20):1953–62.
10. Brott TG, Hobson 2nd RW, Howard G, et al. Stenting versus endarterectomy for treatment of carotid-artery stenosis. N Engl J Med. 2011;363:11–23.
11. Wells PS, Anderson DR, Bormanis J, Guy F, Mitchell M, Gray L, et al. Value of assessment of pretest probability of deep-vein thrombosis in clinical management. Lancet. 1997;350(9094):1795–8.
12. Wells PS, Anderson DR, Rodger M, Ginsberg JS, Kearon C, Gent M, et al. Derivation of a simple clinical model to categorize patients probability of pulmonary embolism: increasing the models utility with the SimpliRED D-dimer. Thromb Haemost. 2000;83(3):416–20.
13. Kucher N, Rossi E, De Rosa M, Goldhaber SZ. Massive pulmonary embolism. Circulation. 2006;113(4):577–82.
14. Weinberg I, Jaff M. Venous thromboembolism. Textbook of cardiovascular intervention. Philadelphia: Springer; 2013.

CHAPTER 11

David M. Dudzinski and Eric M. Isselbacher

Diseases of the Aorta

CHAPTER OUTLINE

ABBREVIATIONS

AAA	Abdominal aortic aneurysm
ACC/AHA	American College of Cardiology/American Heart Association
ACEI	Angiotensin converting enzyme inhibitor
ACS	Acute coronary syndrome
AI	Aortic insufficiency
AS	Aortic stenosis
AV	Aortic valve
AVR	Aortic valve replacement
BAV	Bicuspid aortic valve
BP	Blood pressure
bpm	Beats per minutes
CABG	Coronary artery bypass graft
cm	Centimeter
CT(A)	Computed tomogram (angiography)
CXR	Chest x-ray
dP/dt	Change in pressure over change in time which is a measure of left ventricle ejection impulse, an index of shear stress on the aortic wall
DTAA	Descending thoracic aortic aneurysm
EVAR	Endovascular aortic aneurysm repair
GCA	Giant cell arteritis
HF	Heart failure
HR	Heart rate
IMA	Inferior mesenteric artery
IMH	Intramural hematoma of the aorta
IRAD	International Registry of Acute Aortic Dissection
LDL	Low density lipoprotein
LR	Likelihood ratio
M:F	Male to female ratio
mmHg	Millimeters of mercury
MMP	Matrix metalloproteinase
MR	Magnetic resonance
PAD	Peripheral artery disease
PAU	Penetrating atherosclerotic ulcer of the aorta

SBP	Systolic blood pressure
SD	Standard deviation
SMA	Superior mesenteric artery
STS	Society of Thoracic Surgeons
SVC	Superior vena cava
TAA	Thoracic aortic aneurysm
TAAA	Thoracoabdominal aortic aneurysm
TEE	Transesophageal echocardiography
TEVAR	Thoracic endovascular aortic repair
TGF	Transforming growth factor
TIA	Transient ischemic attack
TTE	Transthoracic echocardiography
USPSTF	United States Preventive Services Task Force

INTRODUCTION

The aorta is the largest artery in the body and diseases of the aorta, such as aneurysms, typically remain asymptomatic and undetected until either discovered incidentally on an imaging study or the development of an acute complication. When detected, both thoracic and abdominal aortic aneurysms should be followed carefully on serial imaging studies until large enough to merit intervention. In recent years, endovascular approaches have offered important alternatives to traditional open surgical techniques. Various classes of cardiac medications may have salutary effects on the aorta and can be used to reduce stress on the aorta and even improve vascular remodeling. The aorta is also affected by a number of congenital conditions as well as autoimmune vasculitides. For aortic coarctation, please refer to Chap. 21.

AORTIC ANATOMY

■ The largest artery in the body; muscular
■ Histologically contains three layers:

 – Intima (endothelium supported by internal elastic lamina)
 – Media (smooth muscle cells and numerous elastic fibers that give the aorta remarkable tensile strength)
 – Adventitia (collagenous support matrix with external elastic lamina, and site of entry of the vasa vasorum externae)

■ The segments of the aorta are differentiated by their anatomic location, size, and branch vessels (Table 11-1). Dimensions in males are slightly larger than in females, and the aortic diameters generally increase with age.

TABLE 11-1			
AORTA ANATOMY			

AORTIC SEGMENTS	DIVISIONS	APPROXIMATE DIAMETERS (CM)	MAJOR BRANCH ARTERIES
Ascending	Root (sinuses of Valsalva)	≤4.0	Right and left main coronary arteries
	Ascending aorta	≤3.5	None
Arch		≤3.0	Brachiocephalic (innominate), left subclavian, and left common carotid arteries
Descending		≤2.5	Intercostal, spinal, bronchial arteries
Abdominal	Suprarenal	≤2.0	Celiac axis, SMA, and renal arteries
	Infrarenal	≤2.0	IMA, common iliac arteries

GENERAL HISTORY AND PHYSICAL EXAMINATION

■ **Relevant history**:

- Due to aorta: Chest, back, abdominal, flank pain or discomfort.
- Due to complications of aortic disease

  ■ Depends on the segment of the aorta affected and branch vessels and distal organ territories that are impacted.
  ■ Look for neurological symptoms, syncope, heart failure, myocardial infarction, renal failure, thromboembolic disease, compression of adjacent structures such as nerves, esophagus or tracheobronchial tree.

■ **Past medical history** aortic disease, vascular disease, hypertension (HTN), thromboembolic events, trauma
■ **Family history**: aortic disease
■ **Physical examination**:

- Bilateral blood pressure (BP) and pulses (radial, carotid, femoral), pulsus paradoxus
- Look for evidence of aortic insufficiency (AI), tamponade, heart failure and neurological deficit, pulsatile abdominal mass

IMAGING MODALITIES

Chest Radiography (CXR)

■ CXR has overall limited sensitivity (~30–60 %) for thoracic aortic aneurysm, and alone cannot be used to exclude acute or chronic aortopathy.
■ Calcification or tortuosity of the ascending, arch, and descending thoracic aorta may be visualized, but this is a non-specific finding in the elderly.
■ Opacification of the aorticopulmonary window, enlargement of the thoracic aorta, increased mediastinal width, displacement of trachea from midline, or obscured/irregular aortic margin may indicate thoracic aortic aneurysm, dissection, or rupture. Displaced intimal calcium and pleural effusion may indicate dissection.

Echocardiography and Ultrasonography

■ Portable, avoids radiation and contrast media, and can be deployed intra-operatively.
■ **Transthoracic Echocardiography (TTE)**

- TTE cannot provide a comprehensive exam of the aorta, but certain regions can be visualized: aortic valve and root, ascending aorta, arch, descending, and abdominal aorta
- TTE is reasonable for assessing aortic valve disorders and monitoring aortic root and ascending aortic dilatation (e.g. especially in Marfan syndrome). It is not sensitive enough to rule out thoracic aortic dissection (sensitivity 70 %).

■ **Transesophageal Echocardiography (TEE)**

- TEE can visualize the ascending aorta, transverse arch, and entire descending thoracic aorta. The distal ascending aorta and proximal aortic arch may be obscured by the trachea.
- TEE, in contrast to other modalities, can provide functional information such as flow dynamics in true and false lumens, detection of AI, detection of cardiac tamponade, and assessment of left ventricular function.

■ **Abdominal ultrasonography** is the technique of choice for screening for infrarenal abdominal aortic aneurysm (AAA), but is less accurate as applied to the suprarenal aorta or branch vessels.

Computed Tomography (CT)

■ CT is a highly accurate, rapid, reproducible, and readily available technique for detecting and sizing aortic aneurysms and for the diagnostic evaluation of suspected aortic dissection.

■ CT is also helpful at mapping branch vessels, and for detecting mimics of aortic disease (e.g. pericardial disease, gastrointestinal disease).

Magnetic Resonance (MR) Imaging

■ MR is also a highly accurate technique for aortic imaging. However, the study time is lengthy and the patient is relatively inaccessible, making this modality unsuitable for acute or unstable patients.

■ MR is most often performed with intravenous gadolinium as a contrast agent, but the "black-blood" technique with spin-echo sequences can provide satisfactory images without the need for gadolinium.

Aortography

■ Catheter-based aortography is an invasive technique that can demonstrate the full extent of aneurysmal disease and dissection, map branch vessel involvement, and demonstrate the presence of AI.

■ However, aortography is not readily available in most settings, requires an expert physician operator, and requires that potentially unstable patients undergo a prolonged procedure.

AORTIC ANEURYSMS

Definitions

■ Aneurysm=dilatation of the aorta involving all three vessel wall layers. Pseudoaneurysm=contained leak of blood in communication with vessel.

■ Fusiform=symmetric circumferential bulging of the aorta. Saccular=asymmetric localized bulging of the aortic wall.

Abdominal Aortic Aneurysms (AAA)

■ **Epidemiology**: up to 3 % prevalence >50 years, and 5 %>65 years, with M:F ratio up to 10:1 [1].

  – Infrarenal AAA represents the most common location.

■ **Etiology** [2]:

  – Chief pathophysiologic factors are atherosclerosis and smoking. Male gender, advanced age, dyslipidemia, and family history also contribute.

  – Inflammation, both primary or secondary to atherosclerosis, is increasingly recognized as a key factor that results in oxidative stress in the aortic media, deterioration of aortic tensile properties, and apoptosis of smooth muscle cells.

  – There is an increased prevalence of AAA among first-degree relatives of affected individuals. Genetic basis still unclear (may include structural proteins, proteases such as matrix metalloproteinases (MMP), or immunomodulatory genes).

  – Bacteria and mycobacteria can generate infectious (also known as mycotic) aneurysms.

■ **History and Examination** [3, 4]

  – Most AAA are asymptomatic, and diagnosed on physical examination or incidentally on imaging.

- Patients may have persistent pain in the lower abdomen or lower back, with a "gnawing" character.
- New or worsening pain may herald AAA expansion or rupture.
- Classic triad of AAA rupture=pain, hypotension, and pulsatile abdominal mass.
- Space-occupying effects of AAA include extremity ischemia, gastrointestinal or ureteral obstruction.
- Palpation of a pulsatile mass may help detect AAAs large enough to merit repair (sensitivity 68 %, positive predictive value 43 %), but alone is not sufficient to exclude AAA.

    - Sensitivity correlates with AAA diameter (61 % for 3.0–3.9 cm, 82 % for >5.0 cm), but sensitivity decreases with obesity.
    - Palpation maneuvers for AAA are not believed to cause rupture.

- Auscultation of bruits does not help diagnose AAA.

■ **Screening and Diagnosis**

- Screening by exam and ultrasound is recommended by American College of Cardiology (ACC)/American Heart Association (AHA) (class I in 2006 guidelines) for males above age 60 who are siblings or offspring of parents with AAA.
- The United States Preventive Services Task Force (USPSTF) recommends abdominal ultrasonography screening for infrarenal AAA in all males age 65–74 who have ever smoked (ACC/AHA 2006 guidelines IIa recommendation)
- There are no recommendations for screening females or older males.

■ **Prognosis**: Risk of rupture varies with size. Annual risks are 0.3 % for AAA diameter <4.0 cm, 1.5 % for 4.0–4.9 cm, and 6.5 % for 5.0–5.9 cm [5].

- Females with AAA have a greater risk of rupture than males, and experience rupture at smaller AAA diameters.
- Overall mortality from AAA rupture >50–80 %.
- Mural thrombus within an AAA is associated with increased rates of growth and cardiovascular events.

■ **Medical Treatment**

- Smoking cessation and lipid control (LDL goal <70 mg/dL) is essential.

    - Studies of statins in AAA suggest possible reduction in AAA growth.

- Aspirin, reduction in BP, and reduction of dP/dt are reasonable.
- Beta-blockers carry a IIa recommendation for reducing the rate of AAA growth. For repair of atherosclerotic AAA, perioperative beta-blockade has a class I indication.
- Angiotensin converting enzyme inhibitors (ACEI) may, in addition to BP reduction, reduce rate of AAA rupture.
- Several studies have hinted a role for macrolide and tetracycline antibiotics based on a possible effect on *Chlamydophila* (previously thought to be important in AAA pathogenesis), and for anti-inflammatory and anti-metalloproteinase properties. However, such therapies are not yet recommended for clinical use.

■ **AAA Repair** [3]:

- **Indications**: given high mortality from ruptured AAA, **prophylactic repair should be undertaken when infrarenal AAA ≥5.5 cm in males and 5.0 cm in females. Infrarenal AAA of 4.0–5.4 cm should be re-imaged every 6–12 months**.

    - Size threshold smaller in females, in those with small body habitus, or those with family history of AAA or rupture.
    - Growth velocity >0.5 cm/year may be an indication for repair.
    - Symptoms always constitute an indication for repair.
    - Suprarenal AAA (or thoracoabdominal aneurysms, see below) may be repaired at sizes of 5.5–6.0 cm.

- **Surgical repair of AAA**

  ■ Resection of aneurysm and replacement with a synthetic graft.

- **Endovascular aortic aneurysm repair (EVAR)** [6–9]

  ■ Percutaneous fluoroscopically-guided deployment of an expanding endovascular stent inside the aneurysm and attached to the aorta at the proximal and distal aneurysm margins, thereby excluding the aneurysm from aortic blood flow.
  ■ Only about half of AAA patients have anatomy suitable for EVAR: anatomic considerations include aneurysm length, proximal and distal landing zones, tortuosity, aneurysm thrombus or calcium, iliac artery diameter.
  ■ EVAR reduces peri- and immediate post-procedure morbidity and mortality and post-operative hospitalization, but whether the long-term outcomes are improved or are as durable as open surgical repair remains under investigation. Randomized trials suggest no difference in long-term mortality (EVAR-1, DREAM and OVER trials), although a single retrospective Medicare analysis from 2012 suggests higher all-cause mortality at 2.5 years from open repair vs. EVAR [9].
  ■ Endoleak: EVAR is associated with endoleak, or persistent blood flow into the aneurysm sac due to inability to completely exclude it from circulation.
  ■ Post-EVAR patients require imaging surveillance at 1, 6, and 12-months, in order to monitor for endoleaks, assess graft position, check aneurysm sac size, and gauge need for reintervention (class I).
  ■ Repair endoleaks that leak into aneurysm sac around an imperfect seal at proximal and/or distal anastomosis of stent graft OR structural defect, e.g. tear, stent fracture, etc.
  ■ EVAR patients have an approximately 10 % higher reintervention rate at 6 years compared to open repair.

- The 2011 ACC/AHA guidelines on peripheral artery disease (PAD) give a class I recommendation for "open or endovascular repair of infrarenal AAAs" in "good surgical candidates."

  ■ There is a class IIa recommendation for open AAA repair in good surgical candidates who could not comply with surveillance imaging post-EVAR.

- Due to short-term advantages, EVAR has been considered for higher risk patients (e.g. older, high perioperative risks). However, the EVAR-2 trial studied patients deemed "physically ineligible" to undergo open repair and found no improvement in all-cause mortality versus medical therapy alone.

  ■ The 2011 ACC/AHA PAD guidelines give EVAR a class IIb recommendation in high risk surgical patients (uncertain benefit in this group).

Thoracic Aortic Aneurysm (TAA)

■ **Epidemiology**: TAA is believed to be about one-third as common as AAA. Because TAA is a clinically silent disease, the incidence is estimated from autopsy series at 3–4%.

- TAA is most commonly seen >age 50; the age of onset is earlier than for AAA.
- Male:Female ratio is ~2:1, as compared to AAA which has a much higher ratio.

■ **Anatomic location**:

- Ascending aorta: 60 %

  ■ Root aneurysms are associated with Marfan syndrome, and ascending aortic aneurysms with bicuspid aortic valve or sporadic aneurysms.

- Arch: 10 %
- Descending thoracic aorta: 40 %

–   Thoracoabdominal (see below): <10 %
–   Multiple aneurysms: <10 %

■ **Etiology** [10–12]:

–   HTN and atherosclerosis are the primary risk factors for non-syndromic descending and thoracoabdominal aneurysms.
–   For root and ascending aneurysms, medial degeneration is the final common etio-pathologic pathway.

   ■ Medial degeneration may be acquired (e.g. HTN) or congenital (e.g. Marfan syndrome).
   ■ Medial degeneration (previously called cystic medial necrosis), involves smooth muscle cell apoptosis, elastic fiber degeneration (particularly important in Marfan syndrome), and infiltration of subintimal spaces with mucoid proteoglycan.
   ■ MMP's are also implicated.

–   Bicuspid aortic valve (AV) is the most common cardiac congenital anomaly (~1–2 % population prevalence; Male:Female ration is 3:1), and is associated with TAA, dissection, and coarctation [13].

   ■ BAV is associated with aortic medial degeneration.

–   Genetic TAA syndromes:

   ■ *Marfan syndrome*: Besides thoracic aortopathy, manifestations include valvular, skeletal, and ocular pathology. The etiology is an autosomal dominant defect in fibrillin-1, a structural glycoprotein in the extracellular matrix of the aorta media. Fibrillin-1 is also involved in downregulating the activity of TGF-beta.

      –   Aortic root dilatation is present in 80 % of Marfan adults. Aneurysms may also appear in carotid/other cerebral arteries and the abdominal aorta.

   ■ *Loeys-Dietz syndrome*: Mutations in the TGF-beta receptor cause a syndrome of arterial tortuosity with hypertelorism, bifid uvula, and cleft palate.
   ■ *Ehlers-Danlos syndrome, type IV*. This autosomal dominant defect in type III pro-collagen affects large and medium arteries, causing carotid and vertebral dissec-tions. It also causes characteristic facial features and also marked weakness of skin, gastrointestinal, and uterine structures.
   ■ *Familial thoracic aortic aneurysm syndrome*: These are found in 20 % of those with unexplained TAAs. There is no one genetic defect to screen for.

–   Syphilis, once a common infectious cause of saccular TAA, is now a rarity.
–   Autoimmune conditions may be associated with aortitis and secondary TAA (see below).

■ **History and Examination** [11, 12]

–   TAAs are in general asymptomatic, but patients may have chronic back or chest pain, with the location of pain related to anatomic location of TAA. A pulsating sensation may be reported.
–   The space-occupying TAA can cause symptoms depending on location and the structure affected (Table 11-2)

TABLE 11-2

SPACE-OCCUPYING SYMPTOMS OF TAA

AFFECTED STRUCTURE	RESULTANT SYMPTOMS
Coronary arteries	Chest pain
Trachea, bronchioles	Dyspnea, stridor, wheeze, cough
Esophagus	Dysphagia
Superior vena cava (SVC)	SVC syndrome
Recurrent laryngeal nerve	Hoarseness (Ortner's syndrome)
Spinal cord compression	Horner's syndrome, paraplegia

- Aortic root or ascending aortic aneurysms may present with AI or even HF.
- TAA may erode into the spine or esophagus.
- TAA may present with thromboembolic phenomena, e.g. to cerebral, spinal, visceral, or extremity arteries.
- Acute pain may herald dissection or impending rupture.

   ■ Location of pain has some correlation with anatomy: anterior pain with ascending TAAs, neck pain with arch aneurysms, interscapular pain with DTAA.

■ **Screening and Diagnosis**:

- Most TAA are recognized incidentally on CXR, CT, or TTE.
- TTE is recommended as the first test for assessment of the ascending aorta in known or suspected connective tissue disorders, or genetic conditions that predispose to TAA (2011 ACC/AHA Appropriate Use Criteria for Echocardiography) [14]
- There are no consensus guidelines on population screening for TAA.
- For first-degree relatives of patients with TAA, screening with echocardiography or CT is recommended.
- In patients with BAV, ACC/AHA 2006 valve guidelines give a class I recommendation for an initial TTE for assessment of aortic root and ascending aortic dimensions [15].

   ■ If the TTE is insufficient to document morphology and dimensions, or ascending aortic dilatation is present, then CT or MR is reasonable.
   ■ BAV patients with root or ascending aorta >4.0 cm should have yearly imaging (though the size cutoff can be reduced for smaller stature patients).

■ **Prognosis** [10–12]:

- Growth velocity of TAA is variable but approximated at 0.5–5 mm/year; growth rates are higher for larger aneurysms and DTAA.
- Annual risks of dissection or rupture vary with TAA size, from <2 % for diameter <5.0 cm, 3 % for 5.0–5.9 cm, and 6.9 % for >6.0 cm.

   ■ Patients with underlying connective tissue disease such as Marfan, Loeys-Dietz, and Ehlers-Danlos syndromes experience rupture at smaller sizes.

- TAA rupture causes ~75 % mortality at 24 h.

■ **Surveillance imaging**

- Once thoracic aortic pathology is detected, a full imaging evaluation of the thoracic aorta should be performed to document extent of disease and baseline aortic diameters.
- ACC/AHA guidelines recommend annual imaging for following most aneurysms

   ■ It is also reasonable to obtain the first follow-up imaging exam at 6 months after diagnosis to exclude rapid growth (as may be seen in aortitis).
   ■ Once a TAA growth trajectory is stable, ACC/AHA guidelines consider imaging every 2–3 years for smaller TAA in older patients.

- Re-imaging should be considered for a change in clinical status or physical exam.

■ **Medical management** [12]

- The primary goals are to reduce dP/dt and BP in order to reduce aortic wall tension and reduce the risk of aortic dissection or rupture
- Goal heart rate <60 beats per minute (bpm) and systolic BP<110–120 mmHg.
- Trial data is limited

   ■ Beta-blockers have been the mainstay of medical treatment for TAA. While beta-blockers have been demonstrated to reduce the rate of aneurysm growth in Marfan patients with large aneurysms, their efficacy in aneurysms of other etiologies has not been proven.

- Losartan, an angiotensin receptor blocker, is also a TGF-beta antagonist and has been proven to dramatically reduce the rate of aneurysm growth in a mouse model of Marfan syndrome. Angiotensin receptor blockers have also been shown to slow aneurysm growth in a small non-randomized study of children with Marfan syndrome. A large multicenter randomized placebo-controlled trial of losartan is underway [16].

- Burst Precautions

    - Patients should avoid activity or exertion that can acutely raise aortic wall stress.
    - Guidelines suggest avoiding heavy lifting or straining, i.e., isometric activities that would require the Valsalva maneuver.

- **TAA Repair** [11, 12]

    - **Indications**: Suggested criteria for elective TAA repair based on ACC/AHA guidelines include the following diameter thresholds:

        - **Repair of ascending TAA at a diameter of ≥5.5 cm, but at a lower diameter of ≥5.0 cm for those with Marfan syndrome, BAV, or a familial thoracic aortic aneurysm syndrome, and at a diameter of ≥4.2–4.4 cm for Loeys-Dietz syndrome.**

            - For those with Marfan syndrome and BAV who have either a small or large body habitus, surgery is recommended when the ratio of the maximal root or ascending aortic cross-sectional area (in square centimeters) to patient height (in meters) is >10.

        - Arch diameter ≥5.5 cm
        - Descending TAA diameter ≥5.5–6.0 cm
        - Rapid growth rate of a TAA >0.5 cm/year
        - In patients undergoing cardiothoracic surgery for another indication (e.g., coronary artery bypass graft (CABG), AVR), an aortic root or ascending aortic diameter >4.5 cm may be repaired.
        - TAA symptoms are an indication for repair.

    - **Open surgical approach**

        - Ascending and arch TAA require median sternotomy, while descending TAA and thoracoabdominal aortic aneurysms (TAAA) are approached via left thoracotomy.

            - Surgical repair of descending TAA and TAAA are associated with significant morbidity, including risk of spinal cord ischemia and paraplegia. Various neuroprotective strategies help reduce spinal cord ischemia.

        - Repair of arch aneurysms is usually performed with insertion of prefabricated branched graft and supported by antegrade cerebral perfusion.
        - Root aneurysms used to require sacrificing the aortic valve and insertion of a valved-conduit (composite aortic graft or Bentall procedure). Now the aortic valve can usually be preserved and resuspended within the prosthetic graft (valve-sparing root repair or David procedure).
        - In recent decades, overall surgical mortality has declined from 10 to 20 % to approximately 5 %.

    - **Thoracic endovascular aortic repair (TEVAR)**

        - For descending TAA, TEVAR is an alternative to open repair when anatomy is conducive.
        - Akin to EVAR for AAA, TEVAR provides an upfront reduction in morbidity and mortality, but long-term mortality benefits are not proven.
        - Although there are no randomized trials of TEVAR versus open repair, large registry and metaanalysis data (a mix aneurysms and dissections) have been favorable. TEVAR is therefore now recommended for descending TAA ≥5.5 cm; the Society

- Blood pressure

  - At presentation, approximately one third of patients are hypertensive, while one seventh are hypotensive and one seventh are in shock.
  - Hypertensive is a more common presentation for Type B dissections.
  - Hypotension in a type A dissection suggests severe AI, tamponade, or coronary ischemia.
  - BP must be measured in both arms, and frequently needs to measured in both arms and both legs, in order to recognize pseudohypotension, or a spuriously low BP measurement due to dissection affecting the a branch artery.
  - A BP differential of >20 mmHg is considered significant.

- Syncope is seen commonly in type A dissection (19 %) and uncommonly in type B (3 %).
- Focal neurologic deficit is present in ~1/6 cases of thoracic aortic dissection.
- Whenever a constellation of cardiovascular, neurologic, and abdominal symptoms is otherwise unexplained, an acute aortic syndrome must be considered as a potential unifying diagnosis.

■ **Sequelae of Aortic Dissection**

- Hemopericardium resulting in pericardial effusion and potentially cardiac tamponade and shock.
- Acute AI, potentially causing heart failure or shock.
- Acute myocardial infarction (inferior more common than anterior, due to predilection of dissection to extend into right coronary artery)
- Dissection involving other branch arteries: Carotid (stroke or transient ischemic attack), spinal (paraplegia), renal (acute renal insufficiency), mesenteric (abdominal pain, mesenteric ischemia), or iliac arteries (lower extremity pain, ischemia).

■ **Diagnosis** [11, 18, 20]

- ECG and CXR are quick tests (especially for patients at low and intermediate risk of dissection) that may reveal an alternate explanation for the presenting symptoms. However, they cannot be used to rule in or out aortic dissection.
- To definitively diagnose or exclude aortic dissection, one should obtain a CT angiogram, a TEE, or an MR angiogram. In most settings CT is preferred. The ultimate choice of diagnostic tests depends on which modalities are readily available at a given institution and the expertise with which a test can be performed and interpreted.
- When clinical suspicion for dissection is quite high, one negative imaging modality (CT, TEE, or MR) may not be sufficient to fully exclude the diagnosis, and the evaluation should include a second confirmatory test (ACC/AHA guideline, class I).
- Biomarkers: D-dimer alone cannot be used to exclude aortic dissection as the negative predictive value is only ~97 %. The D-dimer can be normal in causes of intramural hematoma.

■ **Prognosis**

- Type A

  - Immediate death rate may be as high as 40 %.
  - Mortality is estimated at 1–2 % per hour after dissection.
  - Death is commonly related to hemopericardium and tamponade, rupture, or propagation of dissection. Survival can be improved with early recognition and treatment.

- Type B

  - Overall 30-day mortality is 10 % for uncomplicated patients managed medically but rises to 30 % among patients with complications who require surgical treatment.

■ **Treatment of type A dissection** [11, 21]

- Urgent surgical repair is indicated for acute type A dissections.
- The goal of surgery is to replace the dissected ascending aorta, in order to prevent death from aortic rupture.

- The aortic arch is typically not repaired in the acute setting, unless the arch is significantly dilated or the intimal tear is located within the arch.
- Preoperative coronary angiography is typically not indicated as it causes an unnecessary delay in aortic repair.
- Medical therapy should be instituted while awaiting operative repair.
- dP/dt reduction and HR goal <60 represent primary goals, with secondary goal SBP <100–120 mmHg (or to the minimum level that preserves perfusion).
- IV beta-blockade should be started first, so as to avoid reflex tachycardia (and thus increased dP/dt) from vasodilator therapy. Propranolol, metoprolol, esmolol, or labetalol are all reasonable; when beta-blockers are contraindicated, IV diltiazem or verapamil should be considered.
- Sodium nitroprusside can also be used for rapid reduction and careful titration of BP.
- Analgesia is necessary to blunt pain-related increases in HR and BP.
- Hypotension: If due to tamponade, the treatment is volume resuscitation and emergent surgery; pericardiocentesis is not helpful and in fact associated with increased mortality (and should only be considered en route to the operating room or after cardiopulmonary bypass is established, unless the patient is in arrest).

■ **Treatment of type B dissection**

- Uncomplicated type B dissection is managed medically with reduction of dP/dt and BP, as detailed above.
- Intervention is indicated for complications, including malperfusion syndromes, refractory pain, refractory HTN, enlarging aneurysms, or rupture.
- Endovascular intervention is now generally preferred over open surgical repair to treat complicated type B dissections because they are associated with a significant lower 30-day mortality.

    ■ However, the long term impact of stent-grafting an acutely dissected descending aorta remains unknown.
    ■ In has been theorized that early stent-grafting of uncomplicated type B dissections might serve to prevent potential late complications or aneurysm expansion and a randomized trial is underway, but at present there are no data to support such a strategy.

■ **Late complications**: Patients are at risk and must be followed for aneurysm formation, recurrent dissection, rupture, AI (for those involving the root or ascending aorta), and endoleak (following TEVAR procedures).

- The highest risk is in the first 1–2 years.
- Medications to reduce dP/dt and control HTN can reduce the rate of complications. The goals are a HR of <60 and a SBP of <120.

    ■ Beta-blockers have been shown to improve late outcomes and therefore represent the mainstay of chronic therapy.
    ■ Calcium channel blockers, ACE inhibitors, and angiotensin receptor blockers may also be of benefit but the data are unclear.

- Because of the risk of progressive aortic growth following acute aortic dissection, patients should undergo serial surveillance imaging at intervals of 1, 3, 6, and 12-months and then annually thereafter, if stable.

Intramural Hematoma [22]

■ **Definition**: Bleeding contained within the media of the aortic wall but without communication with the aortic lumen
■ **Etiology**: Some may be due to rupture of the vasa vasorum within the aortic wall, whereas others appear secondary to microscopic intimal tears.
■ **Epidemiology**: The risk factors are similar to those of aortic dissection, although it is less commonly seen among those with Marfan syndrome.

- IMH accounts for 6–10 % of acute aortic syndromes
- The descending aorta is affected in 60 % of cases.

■ **History and Examination**: clinical presentation is similar to classic aortic dissection.
■ **Diagnosis**: IMH is diagnosed using CT, MR, or TEE.

– Unlike classic aortic dissection, there is no intimal flap or blood flow within the aortic wall. Instead, IMH appears as a crescentic or circumferential thickening of the aortic wall. The presence of thrombus in the aortic wall has higher intensity on CT scanning, and does not enhance with contrast. Aortography can easily miss IMH.

■ **Treatment and prognosis** and similar to classic aortic dissection.

– IMH may convert to classic dissection in ~10 % of cases.
– Surveillance imaging after an acute IMH is similar to classic dissection.

Penetrating Atherosclerotic Ulcer of the Aorta (PAU)

■ **Definition**: An atherosclerotic plaque breaches the internal elastic lamina, allowing blood to penetrate the wall to a varying degree.
■ **Epidemiology**: PAUs are most prevalent in older patients with a history of atherosclerosis, HTN, and smoking.
■ PAUs appear most often in the mid-to-distal descending thoracic aorta (90 %) due to the prevalence of atherosclerosis in this segment.
■ PAU may convert to typical dissection, IMH, a saccular aneurysm, or pseudoaneurysm, which in turn may lead to rupture.
■ **Treatment**: Small PAUs are managed medically with antihypertensives and surveillance imaging. Large or expanding PAUs, or ulcers that have caused pseudoaneurysms, may require intervention, and TEVAR is generally preferred given that this population tends to be older and at high risk from open repair.

Aortic Transsection

■ **Definition**: Through-and-through tear involving all three layers of the aortic wall. It may be partial or complete, in which case the aorta is completely severed. Such injuries may lead to fatal exsanguination, but in some cases the patient survives because the bleeding is contained by a pseudoaneurysm.
■ Traumatic aortic tears result from deceleration injuries, and therefore typically occur near anatomic sites at which the aorta is anchored in the chest, i.e., the ligamentum arteriosum and aortic root.
■ **Diagnosis** is most readily and accurately made by CT angiography.
■ **Treatment**: intervention is required: For tears near the ligamentum arteriosum TEVAR is the treatment of choice; for tears in the aortic root open cardiac surgery is required.

VASCULITIDES INVOLVING THE AORTA [23]

Giant Cell Arteritis (GCA)

Giant cell arteritis (GCA), also known as temporal arteritis, occurs most often in those older than age 50 (especially among those >75 years old). Women outnumber men 2:1, and it is more common among those with northern European ethnicity.

■ It affects elastic arteries, including the aorta and extracranial (but not intracranial) arteries.
■ Polymyalgia rheumatica, an inflammatory condition characterized by constitutional symptoms and shoulder and hip pain and stiffness, is found in about half of patients with GCA.

– Approximately 15 % of patients with polymyalgia rheumatica have GCA.

■ Constitutional symptoms including malaise, anorexia, weight loss, and fevers are common.

■ Aortic aneurysms: More than 10 % can develop thoracic aneurysm as a late manifestation.

■ Therefore surveillance imaging is recommended for up to 10 years after onset.

■ **History and Examination**: mainly due to arterial occlusion:

  – Temporal artery: Ocular symptoms (double or blurry vision may precede permanent blindness), temporal headache, jaw claudication, scalp tenderness.
  – Vertebral artery: Symptoms of vertigo, dizziness, cerebellar signs, stroke.
  – Axillosubclavian arteries: Symptoms of arm claudication, absent pulse.

■ American College of Rheumatology diagnostic criteria include: age >50, new headache, temporal artery tenderness or diminished pulse, erythrocyte sedimentation rate >50 mm/h, necrotizing vasculitis on biopsy.

■ **Treatment**:

  – Corticosteroids are the principal treatment of GCA; therapy over 1–2 years is used to prevent recurrence.
  – Biopsy should not delay initiation of steroids when GCA is suspected; the biopsy will have reasonable yield even within a few days of starting steroids.
  – Other immunomodulators are as efficacious as corticosteroids.

Takayasu Arteritis

■ Takayasu arteritis, sometimes referred to as "pulseless disease," is an idiopathic granulomatous vasculitis affecting large and medium sized muscular arteries (aorta, brachiocephalic arteries, pulmonary artery).

■ Takayasu arteritis is most common in women (Female:Male ~1:10) in the second to third decades. Takayasu arteritis is more common in East Asia and Africa than in Europe or North America.

■ Takayasu arteritis follows an early inflammatory stage (marked by a non-specific systemic inflammatory state with fever, sweats, and weight loss) followed by a later sclerosing phase.

  – The non-specific initial stage results in delayed diagnosis so that 90 % of patients present in the sclerotic phase at diagnosis.
  – Arteritis can manifest by stenosis or aneurysm, and aortic involvement may be patchy.

■ **History and Examination**: vary by affected artery

  – Aorta: AI, myocardial ischemia or infarction due to stenoses of the coronary artery ostia.
    Subclavian: Decreased upper extremity BP (or a BP differential), pain in upper extremities, bruits
  – Carotid: Amaurosis fugax, stroke
  – Renal: Marked HTN

■ **Diagnosis**:

  – Diagnostic criteria from the American College of Rheumatology include intermittent claudication, diminished pulses, subclavian bruits, BP differential, and angiographic evidence of aortic or branch vessel stenoses.
  – Angiography can reveal both stenoses and aneurysms.

■ **Treatment**:

  – High dose corticosteroids are the mainstay of treatment and the treatment course may need to extend 1–2 years. ACC/AHA recommends periodic monitoring of disease activity by exam and/or inflammatory markers.

- Cyclophosphamide, azathioprine, methotrexate, or tumor necrosis factor inhibitors may be used in cases where either systemic inflammatory symptoms recur, vascular disease continues to progress, or inflammatory markers rise.
- Surgical bypass (or reconstruction) and balloon angioplasty are options to treat severe arterial stenoses.

IgG4-Related Disease [24]

■ IgG4-related disease is an autoimmune condition characterized by overproduction of IgG4 with lymphoplasmacytic and eosinophil tissue infiltrate, obliterative phlebitis, and fibrosis.

■ IgG4-related disease affects a number of glandular tissues but a lymphoplasmacytic aortitis has been described that may generate aneurysm and dissection.

■ In a single center experience, IgG4-related disease caused approximately 9 % of non-infectious thoracic aortitis.

QUICK REVIEW (TABLE 11-4)

TABLE 11-4		
QUICK REVIEW	**FINDINGS**	**IMPLICATION**
	Elderly male, abdominal pain, pulsatile mass	AAA rupture
	Ehlers-Danlos syndrome type IV	Risk of ascending aortic aneurysms
	Loeys-Dietz syndrome	Mutations in the TGF-beta receptor; treat with losartan
	↓dP/dt	Principle to reduce wall stress by reducing HR and BP
	Marfan syndrome	High risk for aortic root aneurysms and dissection
	DeBakey classification system	Types I and II involve the ascending aorta
	Stanford classification system	Type A involves the ascending aorta
	Histologic pattern in aneurysm wall	Medial degeneration
	Laplace's Law	Wall tension proportional to product of pressure and radius
	Type A aortic dissection	High risk of rupture, tamponade, and death
	Genetic defect in Marfan syndrome	Mutation in *FBN-1*, the gene for fibrillin-1
	Prevalence of BAV	1–2 % of the general population
	Pseudohypotension	Falsely low BP in due to compromise of branch artery in aortic dissection
	Intramural hematoma	Blood in aortic media that does not communicate with aortic lumen
	Syndrome associated with giant cell arteritis	Polymyalgia rheumatica
	Hoarseness	Recurrent laryngeal nerve compression (Ortner's syndrome) by a large TAA
	Inferior myocardial infarction in aortic dissection	Type A dissection with compromise of the right coronary artery ostium
	Paraplegia after descending thoracic aortic aneurysm repair	Major risk associated with surgery on the descending or thoracoabdominal aorta
	ARB effective in certain TAA syndromes	Pleiotropic effects on TGF-beta pathway
	Aortic injury following a motor vehicle accident	Deceleration injury causing aortic transsection; most often occurs at ligamentum arteriosum
	Circle of Willis aneurysm in aortic dissection patient	Coarctation of the aorta is the likely underlying lesion

REVIEW QUESTIONS

1. **A 41 year old female acquaintance was evaluated for a heart murmur. On exam she had a systolic ejection click and faint systolic ejection murmur. An echocardiogram reported a bicuspid aortic valve with a horizontal commissure and, but the valve functioned well and there was no stenosis and trace aortic insufficiency. Her aortic root diameter was 3.6 cm. Her cardiologist reassured her that there is nothing further to do and she should simply follow-up with her internist annually. She is anxious and has therefore called you for advice. What is the most prudent suggestion to offer?**
   - **(a)** The cardiologist's plan is sound, so she should follow up with her internist.
   - **(b)** She should undergo genetic testing for a mutation in the gene for fibrillin-1.
   - **(c)** Her first degree relative should be screened for thoracic aortic aneurysms.
   - **(d)** She should undergo a CT or MR to determine if her ascending thoracic aorta is dilated.
   - **(e)** She should undergo annual surveillance echocardiograms to monitor her bicuspid aortic valve function.

2. **A 66 year old male new to your practice has a past history of uncontrolled HTN and a descending thoracic aortic aneurysm, and 4 months ago suffered a type B aortic dissection that was managed with TEVAR. Which of the following is not endorsed in ACC/AHA guidelines for this patient?**
   - **(a)** Chronic beta-blocker therapy.
   - **(b)** Surveillance imaging of the thoracic aorta at 1, 3, 6 and 12 months following the aortic dissection.
   - **(c)** D-dimer to assess for degree of thrombosis of false lumen.
   - **(d)** Pan-aortic imaging to exclude e.g. a concurrent AAA.
   - **(e)** Burst precautions.
   - **(f)** All of the above are indicated or recommended.

ANSWERS

1. **(d)** The echocardiogram documented a normal aortic root diameter, but no mention was made of the size of the ascending thoracic aorta. The aortic root and ascending thoracic aorta are distinct anatomically, and one aortic segment may be enlarged while the other is normal in size. Therefore unless both diameters are documented in the report as normal, a dilated aorta cannot be excluded. Half of those with bicuspid aortic valve have a dilated proximal aorta, and the majority of such aneurysms involve the ascending aorta rather than the root, so in any patient diagnosed with a bicuspid aortic valve the ascending thoracic aortic diameter must be evaluated. Since this echocardiogram apparently did not exclude a dilated ascending aorta another imaging study, either a CT or MR, should be obtained. There is no indication to test for the fibrillin-1 mutation in the setting of bicuspid aortic valve, as this is an abnormality associated with Marfan syndrome. The patient has a bicuspid aortic valve but has not yet been found to have a TAA, so there is yet no indication to screen her first-degree relatives for aneurysms. Her bicuspid aortic valve functions well, so there is no indication for annual surveillance echocardiograms to monitor the valve.

2. **(c)** The 2010 ACC/AHA guidelines on thoracic aortic disease highlight beta-blockade as an integral therapy for patients following aortic dissection. Serial imaging is recommended at regular intervals following an acute dissection given the risk of rapid early growth of dissected segments of the aorta. Burst precautions, or avoiding heavy lifting, straining, or pushing that would raise aortic pressure, is prudent. Because of the prevalence of concurrent aneurysms, patients with either TAA or AAA should have the entire aorta imaged on at least one occasion. While degree of thrombosis of a false lumen of a type B dissection correlates with mortality, D-dimer testing is neither helpful nor indicated in this context.

REFERENCES

1. Bengtsson H, Bergquist D, Sternby NH. Increasing prevalence of abdominal aortic aneurysms: a necropsy study. Eur J Surg. 1992;158:19–23.
2. Weintraub NL. Understanding abdominal aortic aneurysm. N Engl J Med. 2009;361:1114–6.
3. Hirsch AT, Haskal ZJ, Hertzner NR, et al. ACC/AHA 2005 Practice Guidelines for the management of patients with peripheral arterial disease (lower extremity, renal, mesenteric, and abdominal aortic). Circulation. 2006;113:e463–654.
4. Lederle FA, Simel DL. Does this patient have abdominal aortic aneurysm? JAMA. 1999;281:77–82.
5. Brown LC, Powell JT. Risk factors for aneurysm rupture in patients kept under ultrasound surveillance. UK Small Aneurysm Trial Participants. Ann Surg. 1999;230:289–96.
6. United Kingdom EVAR Trial Investigators, Greenhalgh RM, Brown LC, et al. Endovascular versus open repair of abdominal aortic aneurysm. N Engl J Med. 2010;362:1863–71.
7. Greenhalgh RM, Powell JT. Endovascular repair of abdominal aortic aneurysm. N Engl J Med. 2008;358:494–501.
8. Rooke TW, Hirsch AT, Misra S, et al. 2011 ACCF/AHA Focused update of the guideline for the management of patients with peripheral artery disease (updating the 2005 guideline): A report

of the American College of Cardiology Foundation/American Heart Association task force on practice guidelines. Circulation. 2011;124:2020–45.

9. Lederle FA, Freischlag JA, Kyriakides TC, Matsumura JS, Padberg FT, Jr., Kohler TR, et al. Long-term comparison of endovascular and open repair of abdominal aortic aneurysm. N Engl J Med. 2012;367(21):1988–97.

10. Jackson RS, Chang DC, Freischlag JA. Comparison of long-term survival after open vs endovascular repair of intact abdominal aortic aneurysm among Medicare beneficiaries. JAMA. 2012; 307:1621–8.

11. Elefteriades JA. Thoracic aortic aneurysm: reading the enemy's playbook. Yale J Biol Med. 2008;81:175–86.

12. Hiratzka LF, Bakris GL, Beckman JA, et al. ACCF/AHA/AATS/ACR/ASA/SCA/SCAI/SIR/STS/SVM guidelines for the diagnosis and management of patients with Thoracic Aortic Disease. Circulation. 2010;121:e266–369.

13. Isselbacher EM. Thoracic and abdominal aortic aneurysms. Circulation. 2005;111:816–28.

14. Siu S, Silversides CK. Bicuspid aortic valve disease. J Am Coll Cardiol. 2010;55:2789–800.

15. Douglas PS, Garcia MJ, Haines DE, Laiw WW, Manning WJ, Patel AR, et al. ACCF/ASE/AHA/ASNC/HFSA/HRS/SCAI/SCCM/SCCT/SCMR 2011 Appropriate Use Criteria for Echocardiography. J Am Coll Cardiol. 2011;57:1126–66.

16. Bonow RO, Carabello BA, Chatterjee K, de Leon Jr AC, Faxon DP, Freed MD, et al. ACC/AHA 2006 guidelines for the management of patients with valvular heart disease. J Am Coll Cardiol. 2006;48:e1–148.

17. Keane MG, Pyeritz RE. Medical management of Marfan syndrome. Circulation. 2008;117:2802–13.

18. Larsson E, Vishevskaya L, Kalin B, et al. High frequency of thoracic aneurysms in patients with abdominal aortic aneurysms. Ann Surg. 2011;253:180–4.

19. Klompas M. Does this patient have an acute thoracic aortic dissection? JAMA. 2002;287(17):2262–72.

20. Hagan PG, Nienaber CA, Isselbacher EM, et al. The International Registry of Acute Aortic Dissection (IRAD) – new insights into an old disease. J Am Med Assoc. 2000;283:897–903.

21. Moore AG, Eagle KA, Bruckman D, et al. Choice of computed tomography, transesophageal echocardiography, magnetic resonance imaging, and aortography in acute aortic dissection: International Registry of Acute Aortic Dissection (IRAD). Am J Cardiol. 2002;89:1235–8.

22. Coady MA, Ikonomidis JS, Cheung AT, et al. Surgical management of descending thoracic aortic disease: open and endovascular approaches. Circulation. 2010;121:2780–804.

23. Evangelista A, Mukherjee D, Mehta RH, et al. Acute intramural hematoma of the aorta: a mystery in evolution. Circulation. 2005;111:1063–70.

24. Weyand CM, Goronzy JJ. Medium- and large-vessel vasculitis. N Engl J Med. 2003;349:160–9.

25. Stone JH, Khosroshahi A, Deshpande V, et al. IgG4-related systemic disease accounts for a significant proportion of thoracic lymphoplasmacytic aortitis cases. Arthritis Care Res. 2010;3: 316–22.

Suggested Reading

Hiratzka LF, Bakris GL, Beckman JA, et al. ACCF/AHA/AATS/ACR/ASA/SCA/SCAI/SIR/STS/SVM guidelines for the diagnosis and management of patients with Thoracic Aortic Disease. Circulation. 2010;121:e266–369.

Hirsch AT, Haskal ZJ, Hertzner NR, et al. ACC/AHA 2005 Practice Guidelines for the management of patients with peripheral arterial disease (lower extremity, renal, mesenteric, and abdominal aortic). Circulation. 2006;113:e463–654.

Isselbacher EM. Thoracic and abdominal aortic aneurysms. Circulation. 2005;111:816–28.

CHAPTER 12

Lauren G. Gilstrap and Malissa J. Wood

Cardiovascular Disease in Women and Pregnancy

CHAPTER OUTLINE

ABBREVIATIONS

AAA	Abdominal aortic aneurysm
ACC	American College of Cardiology
ACE	Angiotensin Converting Enzyme
Afib	Atrial fibrillation
AHA	American Heart Association
AR	Aortic regurgitation
ARB	Angiotensin Receptor Blocker
AS	Aortic stenosis
ASD	Artial septal defect
AVNRT	Atrioventricular nodal reentrant tachycardia
BMI	Body mass index
CAD	Coronary artery disease
CHF	Congestive heart failure
Cigs	Cigarettes
CV	Cardiovascular
CVA	Cerebral vascular accident
DVT	Deep vein thrombosis
EF	Ejection fraction
ESRD	End stage renal disease
GI	Gastrointestinal
HDL	High density lipoprotein
HELLP	Hemolysis elevated liver enzymes, low platelet count
HITT	Heparin induced thrombocytopenia and thrombosis
HOCM	Hypertropic obstructive cardiomyopathy
HR	Hazard ratio
HTN	Hypertension
IMT	Intima media thickness
IUGR	Intra-uterine growth retardation
LDL	Low density lipoprotein
LV	Left ventricle
LVEF	Left ventricular ejection fraction
MI	Myocardial infarction
Mins	Minutes
MR	Mitral regurgitation
MS	Mitral stenosis
PAC	Premature atrial complex
PAD	Peripheral artery disease

PCI   Percutaneous coronary intervention
PDA   Patent ductus arterosis
PE   Pulmonary embolism
PVC   Premature ventricular complexes
RCT   Randomized controlled trial
RR   Relative risk
SERM   Selective estrogen-receptor modulators
TC   Total cholesterol
VSD   Ventricular septal defect
Wk   Week

CARDIOVASCULAR DISEASE IN WOMEN

Worldwide, 8.6 million women will die from cardiovascular (CV) disease each year [1]. Similarly in the US, CV disease is the number one killer of women [2]. In 2007, the Centers for Disease Control reported 1.2 million deaths among US women, 370,000 (30 %) of which were attributable to CV disease (heart disease and stroke). To compare, 293,000 (24 %) were attributable to all forms of cancer combined [2].

Eight million US women are currently living with CV disease and 435,000 will have a heart attack this year [1]. However, while only 24 % of men die within 1 year of their heart attack, 42 % of women do [1]. For women under 50, their first heart attack is twice as likely to be fatal [1]. On average, CV disease presents 10 years later in men than women [3].

RISK FACTORS FOR CARDIOVASCULAR DISEASE IN WOMEN

■ Traditional Framingham risk factors (cholesterol, hypertension (HTN), smoking, diabetes and family history) apply differently to women [4]

  – Elevated Cholesterol

    ■ 14.6 % of Americans >20 years old have elevated total cholesterol [5]
    ■ For men, total cholesterol (TC) and low density lipoprotein (LDL) are the most predictive
    ■ For women, the TC/ high density lipoprotein (HDL) ratio is more accurate (ratio should be ≥4) and for women >65 years of age, HDL and triglycerides (TG) appear are more significant [6]
    ■ Primary Prevention

      – Recent meta-analysis of over 18 randomized controlled trials (RCT) with N=121,235 showed that statins decrease CV events and all-cause mortality in men and women; therefore statin therapy should be used in appropriate patients regardless of gender [7]
      – Benefit to treating low HDL with statin, even with normal LDL, in postmenopausal women

        ■ AFCAPS/TexCAPS Study [8]: In men/postmenopausal women with normal TC and LDL but low HDL, statin decreased incidence of first myocardial infarction (MI) by 46 % in women, 37 % in men

      – No data to support statin use in premenopausal women without history of coronary artery disease (CAD) or multiple risk factors [4]

■ Secondary Prevention

- Benefit from statins with history of MI and normal cholesterol

■ CARE Study [9]: men/women with normal cholesterol but history of MI, statin decreased death/MI 46 % in women, 26 % in men

- Hypertension

■ 30 % of Americans >20 years old have HTN [5]
■ Women with HTN have 3.5 times greater risk of CV disease than women with normal blood pressure (BP) [1]
■ Women are less likely to be aware of HTN, less likely to be treated and less likely to be at goal once on treatment [6]

- Women's Health Initiative: Only 36 % of women with HTN, on meds, achieved goal BP, control is worse with older women [10]

■ Treatment Options

- Thiazides: enhance bone density (decrease urinary excretion of calcium), showed best results as monotherapy in Women's Health Initiative
- Angiotensin Converting Enzyme (ACE) Inhibitors/Angiotensin Receptor Blockers (ARB): some suggest that they may be less effective in women because of low plasma renin activity

■ Meta-Analysis of diuretics and ACE/ARB show no difference in effectiveness when used as monotherapy [11]

- Beta Blockers: less effective BP medication

- Smoking

■ Smoking erases a woman's estrogen protection [1]
■ Heavy Smokers (>20 cigs/day) have two to fourfold increased CV risk [12]
■ Light Smokers (1–4 cigs/day) still have two to threefold increased risk [12]
■ Women who smoke have first MI 19 years earlier, on average, than nonsmokers [1]
■ Mechanism [13]

- Linear relationship between number of cigarettes smoked and cholesterol
- Chronic smokers have higher serum insulin levels but are insulin resistant
- Smoking causes wall damage and accelerated plaque formation
- Smoking + contraceptive use accelerates thrombogenesis

■ Smoking Cessation Decreases Risk

- Nurses Health's Study [14]: 30 % decrease in CAD after 2 years of cessation
- Continued improvement in CV health for 10–15 years, after which risk is equivalent to nonsmoker

- Diabetes

■ Most powerful predictor of CV risk in women
■ Eliminates the 10-year "gender gap"

- Hyperglycemia decreases estradiol-mediated nitric oxide production, causes endothelial dysfunction and promotes platelet aggregation [15]
- Hyperglycemia creates a "hypercoagulable" state by increasing levels of fibrinogen, factor VII and fibrinopeptide A [16]
- Over the age 40, more women than men have diabetes

PRESENTATION OF HEART DISEASE IN WOMEN

- In contrast to men, women do not present with typical angina [6]
- Women are more likely to present with atypical symptoms such as [6]:

  - Shoulder/neck pain
  - Abdominal pain
  - Profound fatigue
  - Dyspnea without pain

- 2/3 of deaths from MI occur in women with no history of chest pain [1]
- 71 % of women do experience early warning symptoms of MI but they are atypical and often involve no chest pain

AMERICAN COLLEGE OF CARDIOLOGY (ACC)/AMERICAN HEART ASSOCIATION (AHA) GUIDELINES FOR RISK FACTOR MANAGEMENT IN WOMEN [4]

- Risk Stratification

  - High Risk (>20 % chance of CV event in the next 10 years)

    - ≥1 of the following: Known CAD, history of cerebral vascular accident (CVA), peripheral artery disease (PAD), abdominal aortic aneurysm (AAA), end stage renal disease (ESRD), diabetes

  - Intermediate Risk (10–20 % chance of CV event in the next 10 years)

    - ≥1 of the following: Smoking, HTN, Hyperlipidemia, obesity, poor diet, physical inactivity, poor exercise capacity, family history in first degree relative, coronary calcification, thick intima media thickness (IMT), autoimmune disease, preeclampsia, gestational diabetes, gestational hypertension

  - Low Risk (<10 % chance of CV event in the next 10 years)

    - All of the following: TC < 200 mg/dL, BP < 120/80 mmHg, Fasting glucose <100 mg/dL, body mass index (BMI) <25 kg/cm², nonsmoker, 150 min/week of moderate exercise or 75 min/week of intense exercise, healthy/DASH-like diet

- Lifestyle Intervention

  - Smoking: Encourage cessation
  - Physical Activity: Minimum 30 min/day on most if not all days
  - Cardiac Rehab: For all women after acute coronary syndrome (ACS)
  - Diet: Encourage fruits/vegetables, grains, low/non fat dairy, lean protein; limit saturated fat <10 % of calories, cholesterol <300 mg/day and trans fatty acid intake

    - In high risk women, limit saturated <7 % of calories, cholesterol <200 mg/day and limit trans fats as much as possible

  - Omega-3-Fatty Acids: Only as adjunct therapy in high risk women
  - Weight: BMI 18.5–24.9
  - Psychosocial: Women with CV disease should be evaluated/treated for depression (Table 12-1)

TABLE 12-1

THERAPEUTIC INTERVENTIONS

	HIGH RISK	INTERMEDIATE RISK	LOW RISK
Blood pressure	Treat all women with BP>140/90 mmHg		
Goal:	Treat all diabetics with BP>130/85 mmHg		
<120/80 mmHg	Use thiazide diuretic in all, unless contraindicated		
Lipids	Statin: Start when LDL>100 mg/dL	Statin: Start when LDL≥130 mg/dL	0–1 risk factor: Consider statin when LDL≥190 mg/dL
Goal: LDL<100 mg/dL HDL >50 mg/dL TG<150 mg/dL	Continue (regardless of LDL) unless contraindicated		>1 risk factor: Consider statin when LDL≥160 mg/dL
	Niacin/fibrate: Start when HDL <40 mg/dL	Niacin/fibrate: Start when HDL is <40 mg/ dL after LDL is at goal	Consider niacin/fibrate if HDL <40 mg/dL once LDL is at goal
Diabetes Goal: HbA1c <7 %	Use all lifestyle and pharmacologic options to maintain HbA1c <7 %		

- Specific Medications

  - Aspirin

    - High Risk: Use 75–162 mg aspirin or clopidogrel, unless contraindicated
    - Intermediate Risk: Consider 75–162 mg aspirin if blood pressure is controlled and risks of gastrointestinal (GI) bleeding do not outweigh risk
    - Low Risk: Routine aspirin use not recommended

  - Beta Blockers

    - Used in all women, indefinitely, with history of MI or chronic ischemic syndrome

  - ACE Inhibitors

    - Used in all high risk women, unless contraindicated

  - ARB

    - Used for high risk women with evidence of heart failure or ejection fraction (EF) <40 % who are intolerant of ACE inhibitors

- Atrial Fibrillation/Stroke Prevention

  - Warfarin: All women with chronic/paroxysmal atrial fibrillation (goal INR 2–3), unless they are low risk (CHADS-2 score 0–1, <1 %/year risk) or are at high risk for bleeding
  - Aspirin: All women with chronic/paroxysmal atrial fibrillation with CHADS-2 score of 0–1 (risk <1 %/year) or women in whom warfarin is contraindicated

- Medications that are Contraindicated for Prevention

  - Hormone therapy and selective estrogen-receptor modulators, selective estrogen-receptor modulators (SERM), (Class III, Level A)
  - Antioxidants, Vitamins E, C and beta carotene, (Class III, Level A)
  - Folic Acid, with or without Vitamin B6/B12 (Class III, Level A)
  - Aspirin for women >65 years old– routine use not recommended to prevent MI (Class III, Level B)

- Stress Testing

  - Exercise ECG's are less accurate in women than men

    - Sensitivity/specificity 61 %/70 % (compared to 72 %/77 % in men)
    - Accuracy improved by adding tests: Duke Treadmill Test, heart rate recovery, maximal exercise capacity

■ Stress Echocardiography

- No effect of gender on test outcome of test
- Mean sensitivity in women 81 %, specificity 86 %
- May be the most cost-effective way to diagnose CAD in women with "indeterminate" likelihood of disease

■ Perfusion Imaging

- Has special features in women such as smaller hearts and breast tissue

    ■ Use of higher count isotope ^{99m}Tc and less attenuation minimizes breast attenuation
- Useful in women who cannot exercise (i.e. stress echocardiography)
- Vasodilator perfusion imaging is more accurate than exercise stress imaging
- SPECT imaging provides gradation of risk (rather than dichotomous presence of disease)

■ CT/MRI

- Data is emerging but at present, there does not appear to be a significant difference in diagnostic accuracy between men and women

■ Observational Data

- Nurses' Health Study [17]: Significant reduction in MI/death

■ RCT Data

- HERS Study [19]: Estrogen + Progesterone vs. Placebo in high risk post menopausal women – showed no difference in rate of nonfatal MI/death but *52 % increase* in CV events during first year of therapy
- ERA Study [20]: Neither Estrogen + Progesterone nor Estrogen only showed angiographic benefit on disease
- WHI Study [21]: 16,000 postmenopausal women – trial stopped early because of hazard ratio (HR) = 1.24 for coronary heart disease among hazard ratio patients. Study concluded that hormone therapy did not provide protective benefit and may cause harm
- WHI (Estrogen Only Arm) [22]: Also stopped early because hormone replace increased risk of CVA and did not decrease risk of heart disease

■ Conclusion

- Based on data from observational/randomized trials, Estrogen + Progesterone or Estrogen only therapy should not be used for primary or secondary prevention

■ Further research into this area is warranted given the somewhat controversial nature of the current literature

TABLE 12-2		
	BENEFITS	**RISKS**
THE CONTROVERSIAL ROLE OF ESTROGEN [17, 18]	Improves lipid profile	Breast cancer (RR=1.35 weeks/>10 years)
	Decreases insulin resistance	Endometrial cancer (RR=8.22 weeks/>8 years)
	May improve body fat distribution	DVT/PE (RR=2)
	Inhibits intimal hyperplasia	Gallbladder disease (RR=2)
	Potentiates endothelium –derived-relaxing factor	
	Increases prostacyclin production	
	Decreases fibrinogen	
	Calcium channel blocking effect	
	Antioxidant effects	

EVALUATION OF CARDIAC DISEASE IN WOMEN

■ Differences from Men

  – Women are more likely to have single-vessel disease
  – Women are more likely to have non-obstructive disease
  – Decreased accuracy of diagnostic testing in women

    ■ Higher rate of false positives

REFERRAL AND TREATMENT OUTCOMES IN WOMEN

■ Referral for Intervention

  – Early data from Gusto IIB [23] suggested women were referred less often for percutaneous coronary intervention (PCI)
  – However, later data suggests that when adjusted for disease burden, there is no difference in the rate of referral between men and women

■ Hospitalization

  – Women have more complications (shock, congestive heart failure [CHF], pain, cardiac rupture, stroke)
  – Mortality is the same, once adjusted for age/baseline risk
  – Reinfarction rates were also similar

■ Primary PCI

  – Referral rates are now the same for women/men
  – Women/men have similar procedural success rates
  – PCI improves survival and decreases hemorrhage risk, compared to thrombolytics
  – Women have higher 30-day mortality and more complications

    ■ This is likely due to differences in baseline risk: later presentation, more challenging initial diagnosis, older age, more comorbidities

■ Thrombolytics

  – Early Study (Gusto I) [24] – similar artery patency, similar early mortality reduction but women's 30-day mortality rates are twice that of men

    ■ No weight based dosing led to higher cerebral hemorrhage rates in women

  – Later Study (TIMI II) [25] – similar mortality benefit for women and men with thrombolytics

HEART FAILURE IN WOMEN

■ Risk Factors in Women

  – HTN and diabetes are most significant for women, compared to CAD for men
  – Diabetic women have higher risk of developing post-MI CHF
  – Gender Specific: Postpartum cardiomyopathy and Takatsubo's
  – Differing structural response of heart tissue may predispose to left ventricular (LV) hypertrophy

■ Gender Specific Cardiomyopathies

  – Postpartum: see section "Cardiovascular Disease in Pregnancy"
  – Takatsubo Cardiomyopathy: stress cardiomyopathy or apical ballooning syndrome

■ Clinical Presentation [26–28]

  – Suggestive of acute MI (chest pain, ST-segment elevation, cardiac biomarker release, and LV dysfunction) and the absence of significant CAD
  – Associated with regional systolic dysfunction of the mid and apical LV and hyperkinesis of the basal segments.
  – More prevalent in post menopausal women following a period of extreme emotional or physical stress.

■ Pathophysiology

  – Catecholamine mediated cardiotoxicity, coronary vasospasm, and coronary microvascular dysfunction
  – In one of the largest prospective cohort studies to date (n = 130), 89 % of cases of stress cardiomyopathy were precipitated by intensely stressful emotional or physical (i.e. non-cardiac illness) events [28]

■ Clinical course

  – Often complicated by CHF
  – Risk factors for CHF include: advanced age, a physical stressor, elevated admission troponin T level, and LVEF < 40 %
  – Majority of cases demonstrate resolution of symptoms, wall motion abnormalities and normalization of LV function

CARDIOVASCULAR DISEASE IN PREGNANCY

Cardiac disease is becoming an important consideration during pregnancy. Risk assessment based on the patient's underlying congenital or acquired disease is the most important predictor of both maternal and fetal outcome. In addition to preexisting cardiac disease, pregnancy itself increases the risk of cardiac disease and postpartum complications.

PHYSIOLOGY OF PREGNANCY [29]

■ Pregnancy: Increased demands on the CV system

  – Plasma volume increases 40–50 %
  – Red cell mass increases 20–30 %
  – Cardiac output increases 20–50 %

    ■ Increased preload due to increased blood volume
    ■ Reduced afterload secondary decreased systemic vascular resistance
    ■ Increased maternal heart rate

  – Stroke volume increases and peaks at 31 weeks

    ■ However, by the third trimester, there is significant caval compression by the uterus which causes stroke volume to fall

  – BP typically falls 10–15 mmHg by the end of the second trimester

■ Labor: Wide hemodynamic/volume swings

  – With each contraction, blood volume increases 300–500 ml – this increases cardiac output by as much as 75 %
  – BP increases during labor
  – Blood loss during delivery is significant: 300–400 mL for vaginal birth/500–800 mL for C-section

	PREGNANCY	LABOR	DELIVERY
Blood volume	↑	↑	↓
Cardiac output	↑	↑	↑ Immediately after delivery, then ↓ to baseline
Heart rate	↑	↑	↓
Stroke volume	↑ (First/second trimester)	↑	↓
	↓ (Third trimester)		
Blood pressure	↓	↑	↓
Systemic vascular resistance	↓	↑	↓

TABLE 12-3

EFFECT OF PREGNANCY/LABOR AND DELIVERY ON CARDIAC PHYSIOLOGY

CRITERIA	EXAMPLE	POINTS
Prior cardiac event	CHF, TIA, CVA	1
Prior arrhythmia	Symptomatic tachy/bradyarrhythmia	1
NYHA III–IV HF	Any cause	1
Severe valvular disease	AS with area <1.5 cm²	1
	MS with area <2 cm²	
	LV outflow obstruction with gradient >30 mmHg	
Myocardial dysfunction	EF<40 % (from any cause)	1
	Cardiomyopathy (restrictive) or HOCM	

TABLE 12-4

CARDIAC RISK STRATIFICATION FOR PREGNANCY

■ Postpartum: Increase in venous return secondary to relief of vena cava compression by uterus

   – Increase in venous return increases both preload and cardiac output
   – It is often accompanied by increased renal perfusion and subsequent diuresis
   – CV system returns to "normal" 3–4 weeks postpartum (Tables 12-3 and 12-4)

■ Score 0 = 3 % risk of maternal cardiac event
■ Score 1 = 30 % risk of maternal cardiac event
■ Score >1 = 66 % risk of maternal cardiac event

CONGENITAL CARDIAC LESIONS [30]

■ Atrial Septal Defect (ASD): Low Risk

   – Most common: ostium secundum
   – Uncorrected ASD → small increased risk of paradoxical embolism
   – As maternal age increases → increased risk of arrhythmia (Atrial fibrillation/flutter)
   – No prophylactic antibiotics at delivery

■ Ventricular Septal Defect (VSD)

   – Isolated VSD → Low Risk
   – VSD + Pulmonary Hypertension/Eisenmenger → High Risk
   – Prophylactic antibiotics at labor/delivery recommended

■ Patent Ductus Arteriosus (PDA): Low Risk

   – Small/Moderate Shunt → Not associated with increased maternal risk (assuming normal pulmonary pressures)
   – No antibiotic prophylaxis

- Mitral Regurgitation (MR): Low Risk

  - Physiology: Generally a balance – the decrease in systemic vascular resistance helps to offset increase in blood volume

    - Development of atrial fibrillation or HTN can disrupt this balance

  - Other causes (same physiologic effect): hypertrophic obstructive cardiomyopathy (HOCM), mitral annual dilatation secondary to dilated cardiomyopathy
  - Treatment: Severe MR may cause CHF, especially during third trimester

    - Medical Management

      - Diuretics, afterload reducers (nitrates, dihydropyradine calcium channel blockers are okay during pregnancy)
      - Hydralazine has been used for pre-eclampsia but it's utility as an afterload reducer during first/second trimester is controversial

    - If known prior to conception → consider surgical correction

- Pulmonic Stenosis: Low Risk

  - If severe → can be treated with percutaneous angioplasty during pregnancy (should be delayed until after first trimester to avoid fetal radiation exposure)
  - Frequently co-exists with more severe congenital defects that can cause cyanosis

- Aortic Stenosis (AS): Moderate Risk

  - Physiology: Stenosis worsens during pregnancy because of increase blood volume
  - Most Common Cause: Bicuspid Valve

    - Bicuspid valves have increased risk of aortic dissection during pregnancy secondary to hormonal effects

  - Less Common Causes: Rheumatic, Calcific, Unicuspid
  - Mild/Moderate AS (with preserved EF) → Low Risk

    - Treatment: Medical management

  - Severe AS (Area < 1 cm², mean gradient > 50 mmHg) → High Risk

    - First/third trimester symptoms include: dyspnea, angina, syncope
    - Treatment

      - If known prior to conception, correct prior to pregnancy

        - Valve replacement superior to percutaneous valvuloplasty
        - Bioprosthetic valves avoid anticoagulation issue during pregnancy – anticoagulation increases risk for maternal/fetal complications

      - If not known until after conception, percutaneous valvuloplasty prior to labor/delivery

        - Subsequent regurgitation (from percutaneous valvuloplasty) is well tolerated during labor/delivery

  - Avoid epidural/spinal anesthesia secondary to vasodilatory effects
  - Prophylactic antibiotics are recommended before delivery
  - Invasive hemodynamic monitoring is recommended for vaginal delivery

- Mitral Stenosis (MS): Moderate Risk

  - Physiology: Worsened during pregnancy secondary to increased volume, women often become symptomatic during end second/third trimester
  - Causes: Rheumatic disease
  - Mild MS

    - Treatment: Conservative medical management

- Severe MS (Area < 1 cm^2) → High Risk

  - Close monitoring required

    - Echocardiography recommended at end of first and second trimester, monthly during third

  - Treatment: Medical management for evidence of pulmonary hypertension (pulmonary artery pressure >50 mmHg) on echo

    - Medications: Beta blockers, diuretics
    - If known prior to conception → surgically correct
    - If not known until after conception and patient is symptomatic → percutaneous valvuloplasty

      - If percutaneous valvuloplasty is not possible, surgical commissurotomy is better than replacement during pregnancy

    - Atrial fibrillation is common with MS secondary to rise in L atrial pressures

      - Rate control with digoxin and beta blockers
      - Decrease left atrial pressures with diuretics
      - If patient decompensates → cardioversion
      - NOT an indication for anticoagulation during pregnancy

    Epidural anesthesia better tolerated than general anesthesia
    - Prophylactic antibiotics are recommended before delivery
    - Invasive hemodynamic monitoring recommended for vaginal delivery and several hours after (given large volume swings)

CARDIOVASCULAR DISEASE IN PREGNANCY

- HTN: affects 12–22 % of pregnancies

  - Chronic

    - Definition: BP > 140/90 mmHg prior to pregnancy or that develops before 20 weeks
    - Risk: Stroke, CV complications
    - Treatment: When diastolic pressure >110 mmHg

  - Gestational

    - Define: BP that develops after 20 weeks with no proteinuria, typically resolves by 12 weeks after delivery
    - Risk: Higher lifetime risk of chronic HTN, stroke, CV complications
    - Treatment: No specific guidelines on when to start treatment

  - Pre-eclampsia: 3–8 % of pregnancies

    - Definition: HTN, proteinuria (>300 mg/24 h) and edema

      - Eclampsia: Grand mal seizures in women w/ pre-eclampsia

    - Risk: Seizures, HTN, HELLP (hemolysis, elevated liver enzymes, low platelets), placental abruption, cerebral hemorrhage, liver/renal failure, pulmonary edema
    - Treatment

      - Start when diastolic pressure >105 mmHg, systolic >160–180 mmHg
      - If any of the aforementioned "risks" develop, delivery is required

- Future Risk of CV Events

  - Women with gestational HTN, gestational diabetes and preeclampsia are at increased risk of developing CV disease

TABLE 12-5

ANTIHYPERTENSIVES IN
PREGNANCY

DRUG	FETAL RISK	RISK CLASS	BREASTFEEDING
First line agents			
Methyldopa	None, longest safety record	C	Safe
	Avoid in depression		
Labetolol	IUGR	C/D	Safe, but observe for bradycardia
	Newborn bradycardia		
Nifedipine	Generally safe	C	Safe
	Avoid sublingual preparation		
Second line agents			
Amlodipine	Generally safe	C	Not known
	Inadequate formal data		
Hydralazine	First trimester: hypospadias	C	Safe
	Third trimester: neonatal thrombocytopenia		
	Maternal/fetal lupus-like syndrome		
	Lower APGAR scores		
Other beta blockers (Atenolol, Metoprolol)	IUGR	First – C	Not safe (bradycardia)
	Newborn bradycardia	Second/ third – D	
Thiazides	Neonatal hypoglycemia, thrombocytopenia and hemolytic anemia	D	Safe, but may decrease lactation
	Maternal electrolyte issues		
Drugs to avoid			
ACE Inhibitors	Second/third trimester: Prematurity, IUGR	D	Not known but should avoid
	Renal damage: Oligohydramnios, anuria, Lung/skull hypoplasia		
	Hypotension		
ARB's	Renal damage: Anuria	D	Not known, but should avoid
	Skull hypoplasia		
	Hypotension		

– Gestational HTN and preeclampsia increase the odds ratio of CV disease by nearly 30 % (odds ratio [OR] 1.27 for gestational HTN, 1.26 for gestational diabetes and 1.31 for preeclampsia) [33]
– Women with pre-eclampsia were at increased risk of developing [34]:

■ HTN: (Relative ratio [RR] 3.70)
■ CAD: (RR 2.16)
■ CVA: (RR 1.81), venous thromboembolism (VTE) (RR 1.79)
■ Absolute risk that a woman with a history of pre-eclampsia would experience an event at age 50–59 years estimated to be 17.8 % compared to 8.3 % in women without preeclampsia

– Women with a history of preeclampsia or early onset IUGR exhibit impaired endothelial function and vasodilatation

■ Possible underlying predisposition for both disorders
■ Preeclampsia results in permanent arterial changes leading to late cardiovascular disease
■ Potential for early metabolic syndrome: insulin resistance, sympathetic overactivity, proinflammatory activity, endothelial dysfunction, and the abnormal lipid profile [35] (Table 12-5)

TABLE 12-6

ANTIARRHYTHMICS IN PREGNANCY

DRUG	FETAL RISK	RISK CLASS	BREASTFEEDING
Adenosine	None	C	Not known
Amiodarone	IUGR Prematurity Neonatal hypothyroidism	C	Not known, but should avoid
Beta blockers	IUGR Neonatal bradycardia	First − C Second/third − D	Safe
Digoxin	IUGR Prematurity	C	Safe
Flecainide	Little data, few reports of fetal death	C/D	Safe
Lidocaine	CNS depression	C/D	Safe
Procainamide	Little data, generally unknown	C	Safe
Sotalol	IUGR, bradycardia	First − B Second/third − D	Safe

Risk Class *A* adequate and well-controlled human studies have failed to demonstrate a risk to the fetus, *B* animal studies failed to demonstrate a risk to the fetus and there are no adequate and well-controlled studies in pregnant women OR Animal studies have shown an adverse effect, but adequate and well-controlled studies in pregnant women failed to demonstrate a risk to the fetus, *C* animal studies showed an adverse effect on the fetus and there are no adequate and well-controlled studies in humans, but potential benefits may warrant use of the drug in pregnant women despite potential risks, *D* positive evidence of human fetal risk based on adverse reaction data from studies in humans, but potential benefits may warrant use of the drug in pregnant women despite potential risks, *X* studies in animals or humans have demonstrated fetal abnormalities and/or there is positive evidence of human fetal risk based on adverse reaction data, and the risks involved in use of the drug in pregnant women clearly outweigh potential benefits

■ Arrhythmias

- Physiology: Commonly premature atrial complexes (PAC)/premature ventricular complexes (PVC), atrial fibrillation/flutter, ventricular tachycardia (rare), bradyarrhythmias (rare)
- Treatment: Medical management

  ■ PAC/PAV's: no treatment required
  ■ Atrial fibrillation /flutter: rate control with beta blockers, digoxin, cardioversion

    - Anticoagulate chronic atrial fibrillation patients

  ■ Atrioventricular nodal reentrant tachycardia (AVNRT): adenosine/beta blocker
  ■ Ventricular Tachycardia: Antiarrhythmic medication
  ■ Bradyarrhythmia: Treat only if symptomatic, hemodynamically significant (Table 12-6)

■ CAD: rare, only 0.01 % of pregnancies

- Physiology: traditional plaque rupture, coronary spasm, coronary thrombosis, coronary dissection
- Treatment: Per traditional advanced cardiovascular life support (ACLS) protocol

  ■ Thrombolytics: increase maternal hemorrhage risk 8 %
  ■ PCI: lead shielding required
  ■ Medical management considered safe

    - 81 mg Aspirin
    - Nitrates
    - Beta blockers
    - Heparin (short term)

- Drug Classes to avoid
  - ACE inhibitors/ARB's
  - Statins
- Diabetes
  - Physiology: Insulin resistance is mediated by pregnancy hormones, typically it is offset by hormonally induced increase in insulin production
  - Gestational Diabetes: Development of diabetes during pregnancy, women who develop diabetes before 24 weeks have 80 % chance of developing diabetes type 2 within in the next 5 years
    - Pregnancy complications: HTN, hyperlipidemia, maternal death
    - Higher glucose levels result in higher birth weights, macrosomia, greater risk of infant mortality
- Anticoagulation
  - Conditions that necessitate anticoagulation during pregnancy: mechanical valves, hypercoagulable disease, history of deep venous thromboembolism (DVT)/pulmonary embolism (PE), Eisenmenger's syndrome
  - Treatment
    - Low Molecular Weight Heparin: preferred treatment
      - Weight adjusted dose, twice a day for first to third trimester
      - Labs: Xa goal 1.0–1.2 U/mL 4 h after injection
      - Risks: Does not cross the placenta – unclear effect on bone mineral density, less risk of heparin induced thrombocytopenia and thrombosis (HITT) than unfractionated heparin
    - Unfractionated Heparin
      - Weight adjusted dose, twice a day, first to third trimester
      - Labs: PTT goal 2–3× baseline 6 h after injection and/or Xa 0.35–0.7 U/mL 4 h after injection
      - Risks: Does not cross the placenta – maternal osteoporosis, hemorrhage, thrombocytopenia, HITT
    - Warfarin
      - Do not use in the first trimester or after week 35 (okay to use week 12–35)
      - Labs: INR goal 2.5–3.5
      - Risks: Freely crosses the placenta, causes abnormal development of fetal bones and cartilage (4–10 % risk), other central nervous system defects (rare)

CARDIOVASCULAR DISEASE RESULTING FROM PREGNANCY

- Peripartum Cardiomyopathy
  - Definition: systolic dysfunction that develops in the last month of pregnancy or up to 5 months after delivery
  - Incidence: 1 in 3–4,000 live births
  - Risk Factors: Age >30 years, multiparity, multiple fetuses, pre-eclampsia/eclampsia, postpartum hypertension, maternal cocaine use or selenium deficiency
  - Treatment
    - During Pregnancy: Digoxin, diuretics, consider beta blockers
      - Consider hydralazine for afterload reduction
      - Consider anticoagulation (no warfarin after 35th week)

■ After Delivery: Traditional management

  – Avoid atenolol/metoprolol during breastfeeding because of infant bradycardia
  – No data on ACE inhibitors/ARB's during breastfeeding
  – Start anticoagulation

    ■ Based on limited data, warfarin does not appear to get into breastmilk and is likely safe [36]

  ■ Prognosis

    – 50–60 % recover completely, usually within 6 months
    – 40–50 % remain stable or continue to deteriorate
    – 30 % ultimately require transplantation
    – 10–50 % overall mortality

  – Women who have had an episode of peripartum cardiomyopathy, even if they recover completely, are at high risk of future pregnancy complications (i.e. severe systolic heart failure and death) and are thus counseled to avoid pregnancy in the future

REVIEW QUESTIONS

1. **A 25 year old female with a history of Marfan syndrome presents for annual cardiology follow up and states that she would like to start a family. She has a history of minimally dilated aortic root and mitral valve prolapse on an echo performed 4 years prior to this visit. Her examination reveals a tall, marfanoid female in no distress. An echocardiogram is performed and reveals normal chamber dimensions and wall thickness, an aortic root dimension of 45 mm, moderate aortic regurgitation (AR) is noted, normal ascending aorta, bileaflet prolapse and moderate to severe mitral regurgitation. Her estimated right ventricular systolic pressure is 24 mmHg. Which of the following would you recommend?**
   (a) The patient should be discouraged from becoming pregnant and referred to a cardiac surgeon for aortic root/valvular repair/mitral valve repair.
   (b) Advising her to undergo genetic counseling by allowing her to proceed with pregnancy, adding an ACE-inhibitor and increasing her dose of beta blocker.
   (c) Repair aortic root but avoid mitral repair as the degree of mitral regurgitation is likely to improve with pregnancy. Tell her to consider genetic counseling.
   (d) Recommend genetic counseling and proceeding with pregnancy but advising her not to curtail strenuous exercise until after the baby is born.

2. **Which of the following physiologic changes are associated with pregnancy?**
   (a) Increased systolic blood pressure
   (b) Decreased systemic vascular resistance
   (c) Decreased cardiac output
   (d) Reduced blood volume
   (e) Increased mitral valvular regurgitation

3. **Takatsubo cardiomyopathy is characterized by which of the following?**
   (a) Diffuse LV hypokinesis
   (b) Hyperdynamic basal LV function
   (c) Diffuse increased LV contractility due to low levels of catecholamines
   (d) Elevated pulmonary artery pressures
   (e) Diffuse thickening of the mitral and tricuspid valves

ANSWERS

1. (a) It is currently recommended that women with Marfan syndrome and aortic root measurement of >45 mm undergo elective root replacement/repair prior to elective pregnancy. The risk of aortic dissection increases substantially in women with aortic root dimensions of >45 mm. The degrees of mitral and aortic regurgitation both suggest that valve repair (if feasibly from surgical standpoint/replacement) should also be performed [37].

2. (b) Physiologic changes associated with pregnancy include decreased systemic vascular resistance, systolic blood pressure, increased cardiac output and blood volume and a reduction in the degree of mitral valvular regurgitation.

3. (b) Takatsubo cardiomyopathy is characterized by regional systolic dysfunction of the mid and apical left ventricle (LV) and hyperkinesis of the basal segments which occurs in the setting of a stressful event and is thought to be in part due to elevated catecholamine levels.

REFERENCES

1. Women's Heart. Women and heart disease facts. 2011. Available from: http://www.womensheart.org/content/HeartDisease/heart_disease_facts.asp. Cited 2012.

2. CDC. Morbidity of heart disease. 2006. Available from: http://www.cdc.gov/nchs/fastats/heart.htm. Cited 2012.

3. Mosca L, Barrett-Connor E, Wenger NK. Sex/gender differences in cardiovascular disease prevention: what a difference a decade makes. Circulation. 2011;124(19):2145–54.

4. Mosca L, Benjamin EJ, Berra K, Bezanson JL, Dolor RJ, Lloyd-Jones DM, et al. Effectiveness-based guidelines for the prevention of cardiovascular disease in women – 2011 update: a guideline from the American Heart Association. J Am Coll Cardiol. 2011;57(12):1404–23.

5. CDC. Heath, United States, 2010. Available from: http://www.cdc.gov/nchs/data/hus/hus10.pdf#066. Cited 2012.

6. Wenger NK. Clinical characteristics of coronary heart disease in women: emphasis on gender differences. Cardiovasc Res. 2002;53(3):558–67.

7. Kostis WJ, Cheng JQ, Dobrzynski JM, Cabrera J, Kostis JB. Meta-analysis of statin effects in women versus men. J Am Coll Cardiol. 2012;59(6):572–82.

8. Brown AS. Primary prevention of coronary heart disease: implications of the Air Force/Texas coronary atherosclerosis prevention study (AFCAPS/TexCAPS). Curr Cardiol Rep. 2000;2(5):439–44.

9. Pfeffer MA, Sacks FM, Moye LA, Brown L, Rouleau JL, Hartley LH, et al. Cholesterol and Recurrent Events: a secondary prevention trial for normolipidemic patients. CARE Investigators. Am J Cardiol. 1995;76(9):98C–106.

10. Wassertheil-Smoller S, Anderson G, Psaty BM, Black HR, Manson J, Wong N, et al. Hypertension and its treatment in postmenopausal women: baseline data from the Women's Health Initiative. Hypertension. 2000;36(5):780–9.

11. Perry IJ, Beevers DG. ACE inhibitors compared with thiazide diuretics as first-step antihypertensive therapy. Cardiovasc Drugs Ther. 1989;3(6):815–9.

12. Wenger NK. Coronary heart disease: the female heart is vulnerable. Prog Cardiovasc Dis. 2003;46(3):199–229.

13. Howard G, Wagenknecht LE, Burke GL, Diez-Roux A, Evans GW, McGovern P, et al. Cigarette smoking and progression of atherosclerosis: The Atherosclerosis Risk in Communities (ARIC) Study. JAMA. 1998;279(2):119–24.

14. Sarna L, Bialous SA, Cooley ME, Jun HJ, Feskanich D. Impact of smoking and smoking cessation on health-related quality of life in women in the Nurses' Health Study. Qual Life Res. 2008;17(10):1217–27.

15. Maggi A, Cignarella A, Brusadelli A, Bolego C, Pinna C, Puglisi L. Diabetes undermines estrogen control of inducible nitric oxide synthase function in rat aortic smooth muscle cells through overexpression of estrogen receptor-beta. Circulation. 2003;108(2):211–7.

16. Lim HS, MacFadyen RJ, Bakris G, Lip GY. The role of hyperglycaemia and the hypercoagulable state in the pathogenesis of cardiovascular events in diabetes mellitus: implications for hypertension management. Curr Pharm Des. 2006;12(13):1567–79.

17. Stampfer MJ, Colditz GA, Willett WC, Manson JE, Rosner B, Speizer FE, et al. Postmenopausal estrogen therapy and cardiovascular disease. Ten-year follow-up from the nurses' health study. N Engl J Med. 1991;325(11):756–62.

18. Grodstein F, Stampfer MJ, Manson JE, Colditz GA, Willett WC, Rosner B, et al. Postmenopausal estrogen and progestin use and the risk of cardiovascular disease. N Engl J Med. 1996;335(7):453–61.

19. Hulley S, Grady D, Bush T, Furberg C, Herrington D, Riggs B, et al. Randomized trial of estrogen plus progestin for secondary prevention of coronary heart disease in postmenopausal women. Heart and Estrogen/progestin Replacement Study (HERS) Research Group. JAMA. 1998;280(7):605–13.

20. Herrington DM, Reboussin DM, Brosnihan KB, Sharp PC, Shumaker SA, Snyder TE, et al. Effects of estrogen replacement on the progression of coronary-artery atherosclerosis. N Engl J Med. 2000;343(8):522–9.

21. Barber CA, Margolis K, Luepker RV, Arnett DK. The impact of the Women's Health Initiative on discontinuation of postmenopausal hormone therapy: the Minnesota Heart Survey (2000–2002). J Womens Health (Larchmt). 2004;13(9):975–85.

22. Hopkins Tanne J. Oestrogen only arm of women's health initiative trial is stopped. BMJ. 2004;328(7440):602 [News].

23. A clinical trial comparing primary coronary angioplasty with tissue plasminogen activator for acute myocardial infarction. The Global Use of Strategies to Open Occluded Coronary Arteries in Acute Coronary Syndromes (GUSTO IIb) Angioplasty Substudy Investigators. N Engl J Med. 1997;336(23):1621–8 [Clinical Trial Comparative Study Multicenter Study Randomized Controlled Trial Research Support, Non-U.S. Gov't].

24. Newby LK, Rutsch WR, Califf RM, Simoons ML, Aylward PE, Armstrong PW, et al. Time from symptom onset to treatment and outcomes after thrombolytic therapy. GUSTO-1 Investigators. J Am Coll Cardiol. 1996;27(7):1646–55 [Clinical Trial Randomized Controlled Trial Research Support, Non-U.S. Gov't].

25. Comparison of invasive and conservative strategies after treatment with intravenous tissue plasminogen activator in acute myocardial infarction. Results of the thrombolysis in myocardial infarction (TIMI) phase II trial. The TIMI Study Group. N Engl J Med. 1989;320(10):618–27 [Clinical Trial Comparative Study Multicenter Study Randomized Controlled Trial Research Support, U.S. Gov't, P.H.S.].

26. Bybee KA, Kara T, Prasad A, Lerman A, Barsness GW, Wright RS, et al. Systematic review: transient left ventricular apical ballooning: a syndrome that mimics ST-segment elevation myocardial infarction. Ann Intern Med. 2004;141(11):858–65 [Review].

27. Tsuchihashi K, Ueshima K, Uchida T, Oh-mura N, Kimura K, Owa M, et al. Transient left ventricular apical ballooning without coronary artery stenosis: a novel heart syndrome mimicking acute myocardial infarction. Angina Pectoris-Myocardial Infarction Investigations in Japan. J Am Coll Cardiol. 2001;38(1):11–8 [Case Reports].

28. Sharkey SW, Lesser JR, Zenovich AG, Maron MS, Lindberg J, Longe TF, et al. Acute and reversible cardiomyopathy provoked by stress in women from the United States. Circulation. 2005; 111(4):472–9.

29. Warnes C, Oakley C, editors. Heart disease in pregnancy. 2nd ed. Oxford: Blackwell Publishing; 2007.

30. Siu SC, Colman JM. Heart disease and pregnancy. Heart. 2001;85(6):710–5 [Review].

31. Hoendermis ES, Drenthen W, Sollie KM, Berger RM. Severe pregnancy-induced deterioration of truncal valve regurgitation in

an adolescent patient with repaired truncus arteriosus. Cardiology. 2008;109(3):177–9 [Case Reports].

32. Stangl V, Bamberg C, Schroder T, Volk T, Borges AC, Baumann G, et al. Pregnancy outcome in patients with complex pulmonary atresia: case report and review of the literature. Eur J Heart Fail. 2010;12(2):202–7 [Case Reports Review].

33. Lawlor DA, Macdonald-Wallis C, Fraser A, Nelson SM, Hingorani A, Davey Smith G, et al. Cardiovascular biomarkers and vascular function during childhood in the offspring of mothers with hypertensive disorders of pregnancy: findings from the Avon Longitudinal Study of Parents and Children. Eur Heart J. 2012;33(3):335–45.

34. Bellamy L, Casas JP, Hingorani AD, Williams DJ. Pre-eclampsia and risk of cardiovascular disease and cancer in later life: systematic review and meta-analysis. BMJ. 2007;335(7627): 974 [Meta-Analysis Research Support, Non-U.S. Gov't Review].

35. Kaaja RJ, Greer IA. Manifestations of chronic disease during pregnancy. JAMA. 2005;294(21):2751–7 [Review].

36. Orme ML, Lewis PJ, de Swiet M, Serlin MJ, Sibeon R, Baty JD, et al. May mothers given warfarin breast-feed their infants? Br Med J. 1977;1(6076):1564–5.

37. Regitz-Zagrosek V, Blomstrom Lundqvist C, Borghi C, Cifkova R, Ferreira R, Foidart JM, et al. ESC Guidelines on the management of cardiovascular diseases during pregnancy: the Task Force on the Management of Cardiovascular Diseases during Pregnancy of the European Society of Cardiology (ESC). Eur Heart J. 2011;32(24):3147–97 [Practice Guideline].

CHAPTER 13

Jackie Szymonifka and Brian C. Healy

Basic Statistics

CHAPTER OUTLINE

ABBREVIATIONS

ACCORD	Action to Control Cardiovascular Risk in Diabetes
AF	Atrial fibrillation
AHA	American Heart Association
ANOVA	Analysis of variance
AUC	Area under the curve
BNP	Brain natriuretic peptide
CABG	Coronary artery bypass graft
CHF	Congestive heart failure
CI	Confidence interval
CVD	Cardiovascular disease
ECG	Electrocardiogram
ER	Emergency room
FN	False negatives
FP	False positives
H_0	Null hypothesis
H_1	Alternative hypothesis
HR	Hazard ratio
IQR	Interquartile range
LR+	Positive likelihood ratio
LR−	Negative likelihood ratio
MI	Myocardial infarction
NPV	Negative predictive value
NT-proBNP	N-terminal prohormone of brain natriuretic peptide
NYHA	New York Heart Association
OR	Odds ratio
PPV	Positive predictive value
PRIDE	Pro-BNP Investigation of Dyspnea in the Emergency Department
ROC	Receiver operating characteristic
SD	Standard deviation
SOC	Standard of care
TN	True negatives
TP	True positives

INTRODUCTION

A general understanding of statistical concepts is necessary for any cardiologist intending to either perform scientific research or understand the results of others' research. The field of statistics is often broken down into two branches: descriptive statistics and inferential statistics. This chapter provides a review of each of these branches and also gives a summary of statistical concepts related to clinical research. Our goal in this chapter is both to prepare readers to successfully answer statistics questions on the cardiology board exams and to provide readers with statistical background knowledge related to clinical trials and medical research. Readers interested in a more thorough discussion of statistical concepts should consult Bernard Rosner's [1] or Rothman et al. [2].

DESCRIPTIVE STATISTICS

Goal of Descriptive Statistics

To describe the characteristics of a sample of data. Example—baseline characteristics of a study sample.

Types of Data

- **Categorical (also known as nominal)**: A variable that can take on two or more values, but there is no ordering of the values. Examples—race, occupation, marital status.
- **Dichotomous (also known as binary)**: A categorical variable that can take on only two values. Examples—normal/abnormal, yes/no, dead/alive.
- **Ordinal (also known as rank)**: A variable that can take on two or more categories with a clear ordering but not necessarily equal magnitude between categories. Examples—NYHA grade, mild/moderate/severe.
- **Continuous**: A variable that can take on an entire range of values with a clear ordering and magnitude of difference. Examples—age, lab values, expression levels.
- **Time-to-event**: A variable that measures the amount of time between two events, typically including censored observations (that is, observations for which only partial information is available). Example—time to death (patients who were alive at the date of last contact are censored since the death/event had not occurred).

Summary Statistics

Dichotomous, Categorical:
- **Frequency**: n, the number of sample members within each category.
- **Proportion**: $p = n/N$, the percent of sample members within each category, where n is the frequency of the category and N is the total sample size.

Continuous:
- **Sample mean**: $\bar{x} = \frac{1}{N}\sum_{i=1}^{N} x_i$, the most commonly used measure of location, but can be affected by outliers or skewed distribution. This is equal to the sum of the observations divided by the number of observations.
- **Sample standard deviation (SD)**: $s = \sqrt{\frac{1}{N-1}\sum_{i=1}^{N}(x_i - \bar{x})^2}$, the most commonly used measure of variability, but can be affected by outliers or skewed distribution.
- **Sample median**: The 50th percentile (i.e. the value that is both >50 % of the sample and <50 % of the sample). This is the most appropriate measure of location for skewed data. For normally distributed data, the median equals the mean.

- **Sample interquartile range (IQR)**: The difference between the 75th percentile and the 25th percentile, typically reported with the median for skewed distribution.

Incidence and Prevalence:
- **Prevalence**: The proportion of the population with a disease or condition of interest.
- **Incidence rate**: The rate of new cases in a given time frame.

$$
\text{– Example––} \quad \frac{\text{\# of new cases}}{\text{total person time at risk}}
$$

INFERENTIAL STATISTICS

Goal of Inferential Statistics

To use a sample (Fig. 13-1) to draw conclusions about a population.

- **Outcome variable**: The dependent variable or the variable to be predicted in an experiment.
- **Explanatory variable(s)**: The independent variable(s) or the variable(s) used to predict the outcome variable.

Estimation

A common goal in medical research is to estimate a quantity of interest.

- **Point estimate**: To estimate a population parameter, we use the sample estimate based upon the type of data (described above). Examples–We can use the sample mean to estimate the population mean, or we can use the sample proportion of success to estimate the population probability of success.
- **Interval estimate/Confidence intervals (CI)**: Gives a range of plausible values for the estimate. In other words, gives a sense of the variability of a sample estimate. Formally, a 95 % CI says if you resample a population 100 times, you expect on average 95 of the CIs to cover the true population parameter and 5 of the CIs to not cover the true population parameter.

  – **Example:** Ho et al. [3] reported that the Framingham age-adjusted hazard ratio (HR) of death (95 % CI) following congestive heart failure for women vs men was 0.64 (0.54, 0.77). This means that our best guess of the true population hazard ratio is 0.64, but any value from 0.54 to 0.77 is considered plausible based on this study.

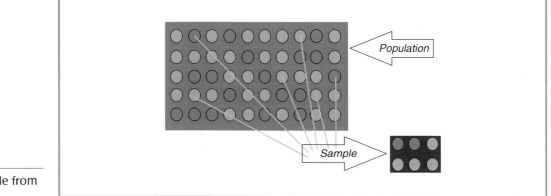

FIGURE 13-1

Selecting a random sample from a population

Hypothesis Testing

A second common goal in medical research is to compare a quantity of interest to a known value or to compare a quantity of interest in two (or more) groups using a hypothesis test.

Reasons for differences between groups:
- **Actual effect**—Observed difference occurred because there truly is a difference between groups.
- **Chance**—Observed difference occurred due to random differences among samples drawn from the population. Statistical tests are designed to determine if observed differences were likely due to chance.
- **Bias**—Observed difference occurred because of intentional or unintentional errors in the study design.
- **Confounding**—Observed difference was caused by another factor that was associated with the groups.

Hypothesis testing:
A formal statistical procedure to assess if the observed result is unlikely due to chance under the null hypothesis.
- **Null hypothesis (H_0)/Alternative hypothesis (H_1)**: Two statements about the relationship between groups that cover all possibilities. Our goal is to make a statement about H_0 (either reject or fail to reject H_0) based on the available data. H_0 is often set up so that there is no difference between groups so that we can reject the null in favor of a difference.
  - **One-sided hypothesis test**: A hypothesis test in which the alternative of interest is in only one direction. Example – H_0: Mean cholesterol in treated patients *is higher than or equal to* the mean cholesterol in placebo treated patients; H_1: Mean cholesterol in treated patients *is lower than* the mean cholesterol in placebo treated patients
  - **Two-sided significance test**: A hypothesis test in which the alternative of interest is in both directions. This is a more conservative test and is more commonly reported in the literature. Example – H_0: Mean cholesterol in males *is equal to* the mean cholesterol in females; H_1: Mean cholesterol in males *is not equal to* the mean cholesterol in females
- **Errors**
  - **Type I error**: Rejecting a null hypothesis when the null hypothesis is actually true (false positive).
  - **Type II error**: Failing to reject the null hypothesis when the null hypothesis is actually not true (false negative).
- **Significance level**: The probability of a type I error, also called the alpha-level, usually set to 0.05. This is how often we allow a type I error if we test the hypothesis at this level.
- **p-value**: The probability of obtaining the observed result or something more extreme assuming that the null hypothesis is true. If the p-value is less than the significance level, we reject the null hypothesis.
- **Parametric vs. non-parametric test**

  Parametric test: A hypothesis test that assumes the data being analyzed come from a specific distribution (e.g., normally distributed). When these assumptions are met, these tests tend to increase statistical power.
  - **Non-parametric test**: A hypothesis test that makes fewer assumptions about the distribution of the data but often has less statistical power.

OUTCOME VARIABLE	EXPLANATORY VARIABLE	STATISTICAL TEST	EFFECT ESTIMATE
Continuous	Dichotomous	t-test, Wilcoxon test, linear regression	Difference in group means
Continuous	Categorical	ANOVA, linear regression	Difference in group means
Continuous	Continuous	Correlation, linear regression	Correlation coefficient
Dichotomous	Dichotomous	Chi-squared test (Fisher's exact test), logistic regression	Odds ratio
Dichotomous	Categorical	Chi-squared test, logistic regression	Odds ratio
Dichotomous	Continuous	Logistic regression	Odds ratio
Time-to-event	Dichotomous	Log-rank, Cox regression	Hazard ratio
Time-to-event	Categorical	Cox regression	Hazard ratio
Time-to-event	Continuous	Cox regression	Hazard ratio

Steps for Hypothesis Testing

1. **Experimental question**
   (a) State your null and alternative hypotheses.
   (b) State the type of data for the outcome and explanatory variable(s).
   (c) Determine the appropriate statistical test.
2. **Computation**
   (a) State the appropriate summary statistic.
   (b) Calculate the p-value.
3. **Interpretation**
   (a) Decide whether to reject or not reject the null hypothesis.
   (b) State your conclusion.

Statistical Tests

Statistical tests to be used for given outcome and explanatory variable types are shown in Table 13-1. For a more complete list, see http://www.ats.ucla.edu/stat/mult_pkg/whatstat/default.htm.

■ **t-test**: A parametric test to assess whether a difference exists between group means. A t-test assumes that data from both samples come from an underlying normal distribution.

  – **Example**: Rivera et al. [4] tested H_0: Mean NT-proBNP levels in obese patients is equal to mean NT-proBNP levels in non-obese patients, against H_1: Mean NT-proBNP levels in obese patients is not equal to mean NT-proBNP levels in non-obese patients.
  – Outcome variable, NT-proBNP level, is continuous, and the explanatory variable, obesity status, is dichotomous.
  – For a continuous outcome and dichotomous explanatory variable, the t-test is appropriate.
  – Mean (SD) NT-proBNP level in obese patients (n=34) was 617 (512) and in non-obese patients (n=77), was 1,683 (2007).
  – For this test, p=0.0029.
  – Since p=0.0029<0.05 (i.e. the significance level), we reject the null hypothesis.
  – Based on this test, we conclude that there is a statistically significant difference in NT-proBNP levels between obese and non-obese patients.

■ **Wilcoxon test**: A non-parametric test to determine whether one group tends to have larger values than the other group. It allows the comparison of a continuous outcome in two groups even if data is not normally distributed or includes outliers. This test also allows group comparisons for ordinal data.

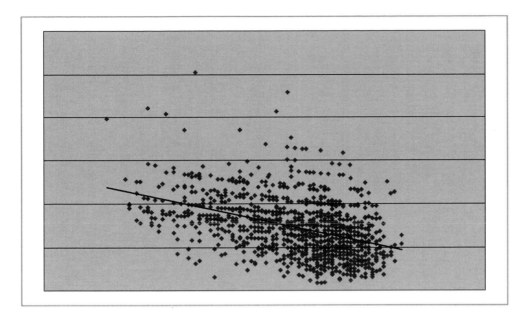

FIGURE 13-2

An example of linear regression modeling: a scatterplot showing the relationship between age and GFR and the estimated linear regression line (Based on data from the PRIDE study [5])

■ **ANOVA**. A parametric test used to compare the means of two or more groups to each other. It assumes data are normally distributed and the null hypothesis is that the means of all groups are equal.

   – If a difference is found, consider looking at specific group comparisons, but be mindful of inflated type I error rates (i.e. false positives) due to multiple comparisons.

■ **Correlation**: The degree to which two continuous variables are linearly related.

   – A negative correlation says that as one variable goes up, the other goes down (negative slope), while a positive correlation says that when one variable goes up, the other goes up as well (positive slope).
   – Correlation ranges from −1 (perfect negative correlation) to +1 (perfect positive correlation), and correlation equal to 0 means there is no linear relationship between the variables.

■ **Linear regression**: An alternative way to assess the relationship between an outcome (y_i) and an explanatory variable (x_i) by using the equation: $y_i = \beta_0 + \beta_1 * x_i + e_i$. An example is shown in Fig. 13-2.

   – This approach estimates the coefficients for this equation by minimizing the residuals (e_i) from the line.
   – The main advantage of linear regression is that it allows any kind of predictor (dichotomous, continuous, etc.) and multiple predictors within the same model.

■ **Chi-squared test/Fisher's exact test**: Both tests are used to assess the relationship between two categorical/dichotomous variables.

   – A contingency table is one way to express data of this type with the outcome and predictor as the row and column, respectively.
   – Each of these approaches tests whether there is an association between the outcome and predictor by looking at the frequency in each entry of the table.
   – A chi-square test should only be applied if all expected table entries are greater than or equal to 5, while Fisher's exact test works with any table entries.

TABLE 13-2	CHF: YES	CHF: NO	TOTAL
A 2×2 CONTINGENCY TABLE SHOWING INCIDENCE OF CHF BY GENDER			
Male	346	1,425	1,771
Female	112	1,587	1,699
Total	458	3,012	3,470

- **Example**:
  - Suppose we conducted a study and we wanted to test H_0: Men and women enrolled in our study were equally likely to experience CHF, H_1: The distribution of CHF was not equally distributed between men and women.
  - The outcome variable is experiencing CHF (dichotomous) and the explanatory variable is gender (dichotomous).
  - A dichotomous outcome variable and dichotomous explanatory variable (with sufficient expected cell counts for each outcome/explanatory pairing) means that the chi-squared test is appropriate.
  - The 2×2 contingency table (Table 13-2) shows the results from the study:
    - The p-value for this test is <0.001.
    - Based on this p-value, reject the null hypothesis stating that men and women in our study were equally likely to experience CHF.
    - This data shows that there was a statistically significant difference in the distribution of CHF between men and women.

- **Logistic regression**: An extension of linear regression that allows a dichotomous outcome.

  - This approach can be used to assess the association between a dichotomous outcome and dichotomous, categorical, and continuous predictors.
  - Logistic regression may be used to compute odds ratios, which for a two group comparison is the odds in one group divided by the odds in the other group

  $$\left(OR = \frac{Odds_1}{Odds_0} = \frac{p_1 / (1 - p_1)}{p_0 / (1 - p_0)} \right)$$

  - Under the null hypothesis of no groups difference, OR = 1.

- **Log-rank test**: A test used to compare time-to-event distributions between two groups. This test is appropriate to use when data contains right censored observations.
  - **Example**: The time-to-death analysis of Framingham patients (matched on age, sex, year) comparing patients w/ and w/o AF, performed by Benjamin, et al. [6], used a log-rank test since AF status is dichotomous and patients who are still alive will have time-to-death censored at date last known to be alive.

- **Cox proportional hazards regression**: An extension of linear regression used for time to event outcomes.

  - This approach can also estimate the hazard ratio (HR). As with the OR, the HR for a two group comparison is the hazard in group 1 divided by the hazard in group 0.
  - Under the null hypothesis of no group difference, the HR = 1.
  - **Example**: D'Agostino et al. [7] used the Framingham Heart Study data to calculate a hazard ratio for developing cardiovascular disease (CVD) of 1.78, comparing male diabetics to non-diabetics. This hazard ratio was reported with a p-value of <0.0001; therefore the group difference is statistically significant, indicating that male diabetics develop CVD at a significantly faster rate than non-diabetic males.

Subgroup Analysis

- Wang et al. [8] explained that subgroup analysis describes the analysis of an outcome in specific subgroups of patients.
- An example is the ICON study [9], comparing NT-proBNP levels of patients with and without acute heart failure. Authors determined the optimal cut-off points for patients with age <50 years, patients with age 50–75 years and patients with age >75 years.
- Subgroup analyses are useful to determine heterogeneity of study results. For example, do we see a difference in NT-proBNP levels for patients >75 years that is not present for patients <75 years? Do we see higher NT-proBNP levels for patients >75 years with heart failure (HF), but lower NT-proBNP levels for patients <75 years with HF?
- A common approach to answering these questions is to run the analysis once in patients >75 years and then repeating the analysis in patients <75 years, but this is not ideal.
- The preferred analysis approach is to look at interaction effects. If an interaction effect is not significant, this doesn't guarantee that there is not a difference between subgroups analyzed because the study may not be powered to detect an interaction effect.
- Multiple comparisons rules do apply to subgroup analyses. For example, if you run 100 subgroup analyses, you'd expect some significant effects by chance alone, so be mindful of test significance levels.

STUDY DESIGN

Types of Studies

- **Cross-sectional study**: A descriptive study which looks at a sample at one specific point in time. This is useful for making statements about disease prevalence, but is limited by being a single look at a population.

  - For example, the prevalence of cardiology procedures scheduled in a surgical unit might be biased if data from the surgical unit is taken the week of the AHA's annual conference.

- **Longitudinal study**: A study that involves measurements of variables over time.

  - For example, the Framingham study collected multiple measurements of cholesterol and blood pressure levels from participants over several decades to determine the effects on CVD.

- **Case–control study**: An observational study in which patients are identified based on the presence or absence of a disease and exposures in patients with a disease (cases) are compared to exposures patients without the disease (controls).

  - Example—Baessler et al. [10] reported on the impact of in-patient cardiac rehabilitation using pairs of siblings with MI and without MI.

- **Cohort study**: An observational study in which patients are identified based on the presence or absence of an exposure, and patients are observed to see if they develop the disease.
- **Randomized clinical trial**: An intervention study which randomizes participants to one of at least two treatment arms (one of which is typically a control arm) and observes differences in outcomes between the study arms.

  - Example—In the CLARITY-TIMI 28 trial [11], ST-elevation myocardial infarction patients receiving fibrinolysis were randomized to receive either aspirin alone or aspirin plus clopidogrel.

Sample Size Calculation

Prior to starting a study, we must determine how many patients will contribute to the study. To complete a sample size calculation, you must identify the outcome variable, explanatory variable and appropriate statistical test using Table 13-1. In addition, we must know:

- Significance level: Usually 0.05.

- Difference between groups: This is the anticipated effect of the explanatory variable on the outcome. For a two group comparison, this is often the difference in the means.
- Variability in the data.
- Power: This is defined as the probability that we will reject the null given the expected difference between groups. This is equal to 1-type II error rate. Desired power is typically 0.8 or 0.9.

Ways to Change Required Sample Size

Each of the four things that we must know for a sample size calculation can be altered to change the sample size requirement:

- If we increase the significance level (i.e. we use 0.1 as our significance level as opposed to 0.05), required sample size goes down.
- If we increase the difference between groups, required sample size goes down.
- If we increase the variability in the data, required sample size goes up.
- If we increase the power (i.e. we want a 90 % chance to reject the null as opposed to an 80 % chance), required sample size goes up.

Example Sample Size Calculation

1. **State the null and alternative hypotheses**. Test H_0: mean cholesterol in patients treated with study drug+standard of care (SOC) is equal to the mean cholesterol in SOC only patients against H_1: mean cholesterol in study drug+SOC patients is not equal to the mean cholesterol in the control (SOC only) group. Randomize patients 1:1 to either study drug+SOC or SOC only. From previous reports, the mean cholesterol level in the SOC only group is 250 mg/dL. We believe the new study drug will lower the mean cholesterol to 225 mg/dL.
2. **State the variability of the outcome**. Assume a standard deviation of 50 and that the standard deviation in the study drug+SOC arm is equal to that of the SOC arm.
3. **State the desired power and significance level**. Use a two-sided 5 % significance level and have 90 % power.
4. **State the statistical test to be used**. We have a continuous outcome variable (mean cholesterol), which is believed to be normally distributed, and a dichotomous explanatory variable (study arm), so a two-sided, two-sample t-test will be used.
5. **Use statistical package to calculate the sample size**. Using statistical software, we see that a total sample size of 170 patients (85 patients per arm) will allow us to achieve the desired alpha and power levels.

DIAGNOSTIC TESTS

- **Gold standard**: A previously established/validated test, necessary for determining whether or not a patient has a disease. For any new diagnostic test, we compare the results of the new test to the gold standard to calculate several measures:
- **True positives (TP)**: The number who test positive and have the disease.
- **False positives (FP)**: The number who test positive and do not have the disease.
- **True negatives (TN)**: The number who test negative and do not have the disease.
- **False negatives (FN)**: The number who test negative and have the disease.
- **Sensitivity**: The proportion of those with the disease who test positive.

$$\text{Sensitivity} = \frac{TP}{TP + FN}$$

- **Specificity**: The proportion of those without the disease who test negative.

$$\text{Specificity} = \frac{TN}{TN + FP}$$

- **Positive likelihood ratio (LR+)**: The number of times more likely that a positive test result comes from a patient with disease than from a patient without disease.

$$LR+ = \frac{\text{Sensitivity}}{1 - \text{Specificity}}$$

	CVD POSITIVE	CVD NEGATIVE	TOTAL
Students' diagnosis: CVD positive	TP=50	FP=31	81
Students' diagnosis: CVD negative	FN=6	TN=225	231
Total	56	256	312

TABLE 13-3

2×2 CONTINGENCY TABLE SHOWING A GROUP OF FIRST YEAR MEDICAL STUDENTS' ER DIAGNOSES COMPARED TO TRUE PATIENT DIAGNOSES

- **Negative likelihood ratio (LR-)**: The number of times more likely that a negative test result comes from a patient with disease than from a patient without disease.

$$LR- = \frac{1-\text{Sensitivity}}{\text{Specificity}}$$

- **Negative predictive value (NPV)**: The proportion of correctly diagnosed negatives among all negative tests. Assuming sample is representative of population of interest:

$$NPV = \frac{TN}{TN+FN}$$

- **Positive predictive value (PPV)**: The proportion of correctly diagnosed positives among all positive tests. Assuming sample is representative of population of interest:

$$PPV = \frac{TP}{TP+FP}$$

- **Accuracy**: The proportion of correctly diagnosed patients among all tested patients. Assuming sample is representative of population of interest:

$$\text{Accuracy} = \frac{TP+TN}{TP+FP+FN+TN}$$

- **Diagnostic Test Example Case 1**

A group of first year medical students' emergency department diagnoses compared to true patient diagnoses (Table 13-3)

$$\text{Sensitivity} = \frac{TP}{TP+FN} = \frac{50}{50+6} = 89.3\%$$

$$\text{Specificity} = \frac{TN}{TN+FP} = \frac{225}{225+31} = 87.9\%$$

$$LR+ = \frac{Sensitivity}{1-Specificity} = \frac{0.893}{1-0.879} = 7.38$$

$$LR- = \frac{1-Sensitivity}{Specificity} = \frac{1-0.893}{0.879} = 0.12$$

$$PPV = \frac{TP}{TP+FP} = \frac{50}{50+31} = 61.7\%$$

$$NPV = \frac{TN}{TN+FN} = \frac{225}{225+6} = 97.4\%$$

$$\text{Accuracy} = \frac{TP+TN}{TP+FP+FN+TN} = \frac{50+225}{50+31+6+225} = 88.1\%$$

Keep in mind:

PPV, NPV and accuracy are affected by the prevalence in the sample. If the prevalence in the sample is different from the prevalence in the group to whom the test is going to be applied, the PPV, NPV and accuracy must be calculated using alternative formulas (see

TABLE 13-4

EXAMPLE OF A 2 × 2 CONTINGENCY TABLE SHOWING A GROUP OF FIRST YEAR RESIDENTS' DIAGNOSES COMPARED TO TRUE PATIENT STATUS AT A CARDIOLOGY CLINIC

	MI POSITIVE	MI NEGATIVE	TOTAL
Residents' diagnosis: MI positive	TP=300	FP=62	362
Residents' diagnosis: MI negative	FN=36	TN=450	486
Total	336	512	848

FIGURE 13-3

Example of 3 ROC Curves from the PRIDE study, reported by Januzzi et al. [9], looking at using NT-proBNP to diagnose acute heart failure in patients with age <50 years, age 50–75 years and age >75 years (Reproduced with permission from Oxford University Press)

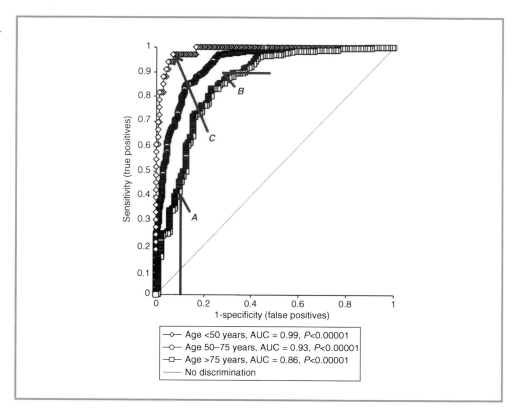

Zhou et al. [12] for more details). In the example above, there was a somewhat low CVD prevalence (17.9 %), which led to a low PPV (61.7 %) and high NPV (97.4 %). High prevalence can have the opposite effect--higher PPV and lower NPV with the same sensitivity and specificity. Consider the next example.

■ **Diagnostic Test Example Case 2**
A group of first year residents' diagnoses compared to true patient diagnoses status at a cardiology clinic (Table 13-4)
  Our sample prevalence in this example is higher (336/848, or 39.6 %), but the sensitivity and specificity are unchanged. Notice that the PPV based on this example is higher: 300/(300+62)=82.9 % and the NPV is lower: 450/(450+36)=92.6 %.

■ For low/high prevalence conditions, negative and positive likelihood ratios may be more informative.

Receiver Operating Characteristic (ROC) Curves

■ **ROC curve**: A graphical plot of sensitivity against 1-specificity, or the true positive rate against the false positive rate, for a varying binary cutpoint (see Fig. 13-3 for 3 ROC curves using NT-proBNP to predict acute heart failure).

– The top left corner (sensitivity = 1.00, specificity = 1.00) indicates perfect classification by a cutoff.

■ **Area under the curve (AUC)**: The AUC of an ROC curve is a measure of a diagnostic test's discriminatory ability [13].

- An AUC of 0.5 indicates that the diagnostic test has no inherent value (this is often labeled "no discrimination"), while an AUC of 1 indicates that the test correctly identifies positives and negatives 100 % of the time.

■ **From these curves, we can draw the following conclusions**:

- NT-proBNP has the most discriminatory value in patients <50 years (AUC=0.99) and the least discriminatory value for patients >75 years (AUC=0.86).
- There's a trade-off between sensitivty and specificity. If we insisted on having at least 90 % specificity for patients >75 years, we could only have sensitivity of approximately 40 % (see point A in Fig. 13-3). Similarly, if we required sensitivity >90 % for patients >75 years, we could not have specificity greater than approximately 70 % (Fig. 13-3, point B).
- In patients <50 years, point C on Fig. 13-3 represents a cutpoint for NT-proBNP close to the top left corner. This point has >90 % specificity (i.e., 1-specificity <0.10, x-axis) and >95 % sensitivity (y-axis).

REVIEW QUESTIONS

1. **A sample of 500 patients selected for the evaluation of a new test is divided, after disease verification, into subpopulations defined in terms of numbers of true positives (TP), true negatives (TN), false positives (FP), and false negatives (FN) as follows:**

   TP: 200, TN: 150, FP: 100, FN: 50.

   Assume that the sample is representative of the population of interest. Which of the following statements is false?
   (a) The disease prevalence in this sample is 50 %.
   (b) The PPV of this test is 67 % and the NPV is 75 %.
   (c) This test has a higher specificity than sensitivity.
   (d) This test's LR + is 2.00 and its LR- is 0.33.

2. **The graph below (Fig. 13-4) shows two ROC curves for new biomarkers, identified as Marker A and Marker B. Which of the following statements is true?**
   (a) There exists a Marker A cutpoint that yields both sensitivity and specificity >80 %.
   (b) The Marker B cutpoint that is closest to the top left corner has 95 % specificity.
   (c) There exists a Marker B cutpoint that yields both sensitivity and specificity >90 %.
   (d) Marker A has lower discrimination value than Marker B based on its AUC.

3. **An investigator is reviewing length of initial hospitalization for 500 patients who have had coronary artery bypass graft (CABG) procedures in the past year. His data does not contain date/time of release for 52 patients, but he does have the last** date/time at which all 52 of these patients were known to be waiting release. Which statistical test would be appropriate for him to use to compare length of initial hospitalizations by patients' age?
   (a) Log-rank test with patient age in years as the explanatory variable
   (b) Cox proportional hazards regression with patient age in years as the explanatory variable
   (c) t-test with patient age dichotomized as >=65 years vs. <65 years as the explanatory variable
   (d) Logistic regression with patient age dichotomized as >=65 years vs. <65 years as the explanatory variable and length of stay treated as a time to event outcome variable

4. An investigator is looking at the results of a logistic regression analysis and sees that within his analysis sample, the odds of an obese patient developing post-operative atrial fibrillation (AF) are 2.06 times the odds of a non-obese patient. His statistical software reports a 95 % confidence interval for this estimate of (1.40, 3.02) and a corresponding (two-sided) p-value of 0.0001. Which of the following statements is true based on this result?
   (a) At the 0.05 significance level, we can conclude that there is a difference between the post-op AF rate of obese patients and of non-obese patients.
   (b) At the 0.01 significance level, we can conclude that there is a difference in the post-op AF rate between obese patients and non-obese patients.
   (c) Both (a) and (b) are true.
   (d) Neither (a) nor (b) are true.

FIGURE 13-4

Two ROC curves for new biomarkers, Marker A and Marker B

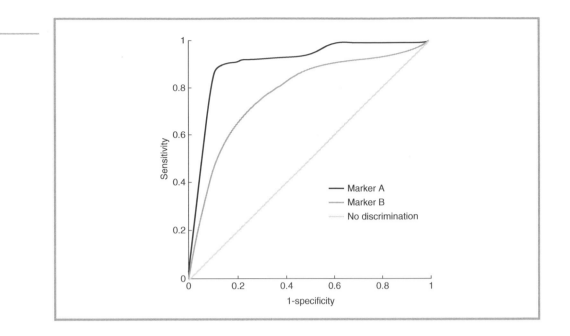

ANSWERS

1. (c) Creating a 2×2 table (Table 13-5), we have:

   Disease prevalence is the proportion of a population with disease, estimated by

   $$\frac{\#\ with\ disease}{sample\ size} = \frac{TP + FN}{TP + FN + FP + TN} = \frac{200 + 50}{500} = 50\,\%$$

   The PPV is the proportion of positive tests which correctly predict disease, or 200 / (200 + 100) = 67 %. The NPV is the proportion of negative tests which correctly predict no disease, or 150/(50 + 150) = 75 %.

   Test sensitivity is the proportion of patients with disease correctly predicted as such by the test, or 200/(200 + 50) = 80 %. Test specificity is the proportion of patients without disease correctly predicted as such, or 150/(150 + 100) = 60 %. Therefore, test sensitivity (80 %) is larger than test specificity (60 %).

   The LR+ is (test sensitivity)/(1−test specificity) = 0.8/(1−0.6) = 2.0. The LR- is (1−test sensitivity)/(test specificity) = (1−0.8)/0.6 = 33 %.

2. (a) The box marked "1" in the Fig. 13-5 indicates values on the Marker A curve which correspond to both sensitivity and specificity >80 %. It is evident that there are multiple points on the Marker A curve within this box, therefore, (a) is true.

   The box marked "2" in the figure above shows all points on the ROC curve for Marker B with specificity >90 %. It is evident that all of the points within this box have sensitivity <45 %. Therefore, there are no Marker B points with both sensitivity and specificity >90 %, so (c) is false.

   Again looking at the box marked "2" showing all points on the ROC curve for Marker B with specificity >90 %, it is clear that none of these Marker B points would be considered closest to the top left corner of the plot. Therefore, the Marker B cutpoint closest to the top left corner must have specificity <90 %, so (b) must also be false.

   Finally, in looking at the curve, it is clear that Marker A curve has the highest AUC value, and thus the highest discrimination value. The Marker B curve is closer to the "no discrimination"

	+ DISEASE	− DISEASE	**TABLE 13-5**
+ Test	200 (TP)	100 (FP)	2 × 2 CONTINGENCY TABLE
− Test	50 (FN)	150 (TN)	

line, and thus has the lower discrimination value and lower AUC. Therefore, (d) is also false.

3. (b) The first step for this investigator to identify an appropriate statistical test is to identify his outcome (dependent) and explanatory (independent) variables. His outcome variable is length of initial hospitalization, and it's important to note that just over 10 % of his patients are missing final date/time of release, which means it will be important for him to choose a statistical test that can handle censored observations.

   Of the choices given, the log-rank test (a) and Cox regression (b) both are intended to handle time-to-event data with censored observations. The key difference between these two tests is that Cox regression models can be used for binary, categorical and continuous explanatory variables, while the log-rank test is unable to handle continuous explanatory variables. Because choice (a) specified age as a continuous variable, the log-rank test is not appropriate. With age as a continuous variable, a Cox regression model, option (b), is most appropriate.

   A t-test is an appropriate test to use for a continuous outcome variable and binary explanatory variable, but this would not be an appropriate test for this investigator because his outcome variable, length of hospitalization, includes censored observations. If he had the dates/times at which all 500 patients were released, a t-test could be applied.

   Finally, logistic regression is an appropriate test when the outcome variable is dichotomous. Because option (d) specified that length of stay was being analyzed as a time to event variable, logistic regression is not appropriate to use. It's worth noting

FIGURE 13-5

Two ROC curves for new biomarkers, Marker A and Marker B. Values that correspond to both sensitivity and specificity >80 % are marked

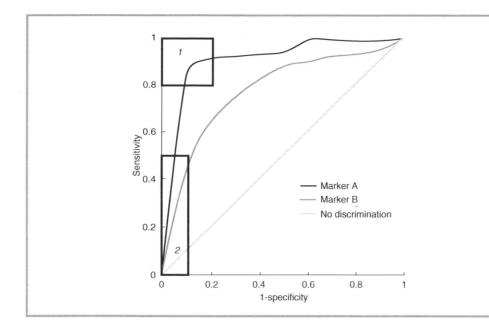

that although this is a less desirable alternative, a logistic regression might be appropriate if the investigator were to dichotomize length of hospitalization (perhaps looking at length of hospitalization, say, <10 days vs. >–10 days) and all of the 52 censored patients were known to have been hospitalized for at least 10 days (or whichever time point is chosen).

4. (c) Using a two-sided p-value in a logistic regression analysis indicates that we are testing the null hypothesis, H_0: the rate of post-op AF in obese patients is equal to the post-op AF rate in non-obese patients, against the alternative hypothesis, H_1: the rate of post-op AF in obese patients is not equal to the post-op AF rate

in non-obese patients. Therefore, if our p-value is lower than our significance level, we should reject the null hypothesis and conclude that the rate of post-op AF in obese and non-obese patients is not equal.

If we had pre-specified either a significance level of 0.05 or 0.01, the observed p-value of 0.0001 would be less than the significance level. Therefore, both (a) and (b) are true, so the correct answer is (c).

REFERENCES

1. Rosner B. Fundamentals of biostatistics. 7th ed. Belmont: Duxbury Press; 2010.
2. Rothman KJ, Greenland S, Lash TL. Modern epidemiology. 3rd ed. Philadelphia: Lippincott Williams & Wilkins; 2008.
3. Ho KK, Anderson KM, Kannel WB, Grossman W, Levy D. Survival after the onset of congestive heart failure in Framingham Heart Study subjects. Circulation. 1993;88:107–15.
4. Rivera M, Cortes R, Salvador A, Bertomeu V, Garcia de Burgos F, Paya R, et al. Obese subjects with heart failure have lower N-terminal pro-brain natriuretic peptide plasma levels irrespective of aetiology. Eur J Heart Fail. 2005;7:1168.
5. Januzzi Jr JL, Camargo CA, Anwaruddin S, Baggish AL, Chen AA, Krauser DG, et al. The N-terminal Pro-BNP investigation of dyspnea in the emergency department (PRIDE) study. Am J Cardiol. 2005;95(8):948–54.
6. Benjamin EJ, Wolf PA, D'Agostino RB, Silbershatz H, Kannel WB, Levy D. Impact of atrial fibrillation on the risk of death: the Framingham Heart Study. Circulation. 1998;98:946.
7. D'Agostino Sr RB, Vasan RS, Pencina MJ, Wolf PA, Cobain M, Massaro JM, et al. General cardiovascular risk profile for use in primary care. Circulation. 2008;117:743.
8. Wang R, Lagakos SW, Ware JH, Hunter DJ, Drazen JM. Statistics in medicine-reporting of subgroup analyses in clinical trials. N Engl J Med. 2007;357:21.
9. Januzzi JL, van Kimmenade R, Lainchbury J, Bayes-Genis A, Ordonez-Llanos J, Santalo-Bel M, et al. NT-proBNP testing for diagnosis and short-term prognosis in acute destabilized heart failure: an international pooled analysis of 1256 patients. Eur Heart J. 2006;27(3):330.
10. Baessler A, Hengstenberg C, Holmer S, Fischer M, Mayer B, Hubauer U, et al. Long-term effects of in-hospital cardiac rehabilitation on the cardiac risk profile, a case–control study in pairs of siblings with myocardial infarction. Eur Heart J. 2001;22(13):1111.
11. Sabatine MS, Cannon CP, Gibson CM, Lopez-Sendon JL, Montalescot G, Theroux P, et al. Addition of clopidogrel to aspirin and fibrinolytic therapy for myocardial infarction with ST-segment elevation. N Engl J Med. 2005;352(12):1179–89.
12. Zhou XH, Obuchowski NA, McClish DK. Statistical methods in diagnostic medicine. 1st ed. New York: John Wiley & Sons; 2009.
13. Pencina MJ, D'Agostino Sr RB, D'Agaostino Jr RB, Vasan RS. Evaluating the added predictive ability of a new marker: from area under the ROC curve to reclassification and beyond. Stat Med. 2008;27:157.

CHAPTER 14

Kimberly A. Parks and James L. Januzzi, Jr.

Diagnosis and Management of Acute Heart Failure

CHAPTER OUTLINE

ABBREVIATIONS

ACC	American college of cardiology
ACE	Angiotensin converting enzyme
ACS	Acute coronary syndromes
ADHF	Acute decompensated heart failure
AHA	American heart association
AR	Aortic regurgitation
ARB	Angiotensin II receptor blocker
BNP	B-type natriuretic peptides
BUN	Blood urea nitrogen
Ca	Calcium
cAMP	Cyclic adenosine monophosphate
CBC	Complete blood count
Cr	Creatinine
CRT	Cardiac resynchronization therapy
CVA	Cerebrovascular accident
CXR	Chest X-ray
HF	Heart failure
HFpEF	Heart failure with preserved ejection fraction
HFrEF	Heart failure with reduced ejection fraction
HFSA	Heart Failure Society of America
ICD	Implantable cardioverter defibrillator
JVP	Jugular venous pressure
K	Potassium
LFT	Liver function tests
LV	Left ventricle
LVEF	Left ventricle ejection fraction
MCS	Mechanical circulatory support
Mg	Magnesium
Na	Sodium
NSAIDS	Nonsteroidal anti-inflammatory drugs
NT-proBNP	N-terminal proBNP
NYHA	New York Heart Association
PAD	Peripheral arterial disease
PCWP	Pulmonary capillary wedge pressure
PVC	Premature ventricular contractions
PVR	Pulmonary vascular resistance
RV	Right ventricular
SVR	Systemic vascular resistance

TIA   Transient ischemic attack
VAD   Ventricular Assist Devices
VT   Ventricular tachycardia

INTRODUCTION

Heart failure (HF) is a complex disorder that consists of a clinical syndrome with symptoms associated with pulmonary or systemic congestion with or without poor cardiac output. Acute heart failure is defined as acute onset of signs and symptoms of HF requiring urgent or emergent intervention. Symptoms may be of new onset or recurrent. Acute HF can be associated with reduced LV systolic dysfunction (HFrEF or Systolic HF) or can occur in patients with preserved LV ejection fraction (LVEF) (HFpEF or diastolic HF); up to 50 % of patients hospitalized with acute HF have preserved LV systolic function [1, 2]. It is important to recognize that acute HF can present without signs and symptoms of congestion and patients may only have manifestations of low cardiac output and cardiogenic shock.

EPIDEMIOLOGY [3]

- 670,000 people are diagnosed with HF annually in the US; more than 290,000 deaths are associated with HF.
- HF is the most common reason for hospitalization in people over age 65.
- Over one million hospitalizations occur annually due to acute HF

    - More than 70 % of admissions are from worsening of chronic HF

        - In-hospital mortality is 4 %, and 1 year mortality is 20 % [4]
        - 30-day readmission rate is high

            - Readmission rates of 26.9 % for HF vs. 19.1 for all comers [5]

- Based on acute HF registries (ADHERE [4], OPTIMIZE-HF [6], EHFS II [7]), most who are admitted with HF are over age 70, have a prior history of admission for HF and 40–52 % have preserved LVEF

PATHOPHYSIOLOGY

Variety of mechanisms, consisting of an underlying substrate, triggering mechanism and perpetuating factors [8]

A. **Substrate: myocardial structure and function**

- Normal myocardial substrate that has suffered an acute injury

    - Ischemia/infarction
    - Inflammation (myocarditis, autoimmune)
    - Could be completely reversible, partially reversible or irreversible

- Abnormal underlying substrate

    - American College of Cardiology (ACC)/American Heart Association (AHA) Stage B with first symptomatic event
    - Those with chronic compensated HF who present with an acute decompensation

        - Most common presentation

B. **Triggering mechanisms**

- Acute coronary syndromes (ACS) /ischemia
- Medication non-compliance, iatrogenic changes in medications, drug interactions.

- ■ Dietary non-compliance
- ■ Worsening renal dysfunction

  – Renal artery stenosis [9] "Pickering syndrome"

- ■ Arrhythmias (Atrial or ventricular)

  – Atrial fibrillation [10]
  – Premature ventricular contractions (PVC) [11]
  – Ventricular tachycardia (VT)

- ■ Pulmonary emboli
- ■ Infection
- ■ Severe hypertension
- ■ Volume administration (e.g. intravenous fluids or blood transfusions)
- ■ Cardiotoxic agents

  – Antineoplastic agents

    ■ Anthracyclines
    ■ Trastuzumab
    ■ Cyclophosphamide
    ■ Imatinib
    ■ Mitoxantrone
    ■ Sunitinib

  – Cocaine
  – ETOH
  – Ephedra

- ■ Medications

  – Nonsteroidal anti-inflammatory drugs (NSAIDS)
  – Corticosteroids
  – Negative inotropes (e.g. verapamil/diltiazem)

- ■ RV pacing [12]
- ■ Hyper/hypothyroidism
- ■ Inflammation
- ■ Sleep apnea

C. **Perpetuating factors lead to chronic HF (see Chap. 15)**

CLASSIFICATION

Two major classification systems have been described for patients with HF [13]
A. New York Heart Association (NYHA) Functional Classification of Heart Failure Symptoms (Table 14-1)
B. ACC/AHA Staging System for HF (Table 14-2)

TABLE 14-1		
NEW YORK HEART ASSOCIATION (NYHA) FUNCTIONAL CLASSIFICATION OF HEART FAILURE SYMPTOMS	Class I	No symptoms with ordinary activity
	Class II	Slight limitation of physical activity; comfortable at rest, but **ordinary physical activity** results in fatigue, dyspnea or angina
	Class III	Marked limitation of physical activity; comfortable at rest, **but less than ordinary physical activity** results in fatigue, dyspnea or angina
	Class IV	Unable to carry out **any physical activity** without symptoms. Symptoms may be present at rest

Stage A	High risk for developing HF	Hypertension CAD Diabetes Mellitus Family history of cardiomyopathy
Stage B	Asymptomatic HF	Previous MI LV Systolic dysfunction Asymptomatic valvular disease
Stage C	Symptomatic HF	Known structural heart disease Shortness of breath and fatigue Reduced exercise tolerance
Stage D	Refractory end-stage HF	Marked symptoms at rest despite maximal medical therapy

TABLE 14-2

AMERICAN COLLEGE OF CARDIOLOGY/AMERICAN HEART ASSOCIATION STAGING SYSTEM FOR HF

INITIAL ASSESSMENT

Presentation

■ Dyspnea on exertion

– most sensitive symptom

■ Paroxysmal nocturnal dyspnea

– most specific symptom [14]

■ Peripheral edema

less common (66 %)

■ Fatigue
■ Cough, particularly nocturnal
■ Chest discomfort

Physical Examination

A rapid initial assessment should be performed to identify (Table 14-3).
■ Evidence of congestion
■ Evidence of low output/ cardiogenic shock
■ Presence of co-morbidities and precipitating factors
NOTE: Clinical evaluation is often inaccurate

Diagnostic Evaluation (Table 14-4)

1. Chest X-ray (CXR)
    ■ Initial radiographs may not show evidence of pulmonary congestion [15]
    ■ >25 % of patients with acute decompensated heart failure (ADHF) present without CXR findings [16]
    ■ CXR findings include:

    – Dilated upper lobe vessels
    – Interstitial edema
    – Enlarged pulmonary arteries
    – Pleural effusion
    – Alveolar edema
    – Prominent superior vena cava
    – Kerley B lines

TABLE 14-3

ESTIMATION OF HEMODYNAMIC PROFILE BASED ON EXAM FINDINGS

CONGESTION	LOW CARDIAC OUTPUT
S3 and/or S4 gallop	Narrow pulse pressure *(Usually less than 25)*
Prominent P2	Cool extremities
Elevated JVP	Lethargy/ altered mentation
JVD > 10 cm corresponds to PCWP > 22 mmHg with 80 % accuracy	
Hepatojugular reflux	Hypotension
Hepatomegaly	Sinus Tachycardia
Edema	Pulsus alternans
Pulsatile liver	
Ascites	
Rales or wheezes (cardiac asthma)	

TABLE 14-4

POSSIBLE ETIOLOGIES OF AHF

Cardiac causes	Progression of underlying cardiomyopathy
	New onset/acute cardiomyopathy
	Postpartum
	Myocarditis
	Tako-tsubo syndrome
	Ischemia
	Arrhythmias
	Pericardial
	Constriction
	Tamponade
	Valvular dysfunction
	Stenosis
	Regurgitation
Pressure overload	Severe hypertension
Volume overload	Renal dysfunction
	Sodium/ volume load
	Medication non-compliance (diuretics)
High output	Thyroid disease
	Shunt
	Intracardiac
	Extracardiac (A-V fistula)
	Anemia
	Septicemia
Miscellaneous causes	Infection
	Pulmonary embolism
	New medications/substances
	NSAIDs
	Corticosteroids
	Cardiotoxic agents

2. Electrocardiogram
   ■ Assess for

   – Acute myocardial ischemia/infarction
   – LV hypertrophy
   – Arrhythmias

   ■ Atrial fibrillation

   – present in 31 % of patients presenting with acute HF

   ■ Heart block
   ■ PVC's

■ Pacemaker malfunction, particularly in those patients with cardiac resynchronization therapy (CRT) devices; assess for adequate biventricular pacing.

3. Laboratory tests
   ■ Electrolytes, including sodium (Na), calcium (Ca), potassium (K) and magnesium (Mg)
   ■ Renal function (blood urea nitrogen (BUN), Creatinine (Cr)) [17]
   ■ Liver function tests (LFT's)
   ■ Thyroid function tests
   ■ Natriuretic Peptides

      – Two forms have been studied:

         ■ B-type natriuretic peptides (BNP), N-terminal proBNP (NT-proBNP)

      – Can be used when the diagnosis of acute HF is uncertain, for prognostication or to guide therapy [18]
      – Levels may be elevated in states other than acute HF, including chronic, compensated HF, acute myocardial infarction, valvular heart disease, and arrhythmias, while non-cardiac causes may include advancing age and renal failure.
      – complete blood count (CBC)

4. Echocardiography
   ■ Assess LV and RV Function
      1. Preserved or reduced
      2. Ventricular structure
      3. Size
      4. Wall thickness
   ■ Other structural abnormalities
      5. Valvular
      6. Pericardial
      7. Right ventricle
      8. Atrial size

INDICATIONS FOR HOSPITALIZATION

A. Per Heart Failure Society of America (HFSA) guidelines [19], hospitalization is recommended for patients with ADHF who present with the following clinical circumstances:
   ■ Hypotension
   ■ Worsening renal function
   ■ Altered mentation
   ■ Rest dyspnea
   ■ Tachypnea
   ■ Hypoxia
   ■ Hemodynamically significant arrhythmias
   ■ New onset rapid atrial fibrillation
   ■ ACS
B. Consideration of hospitalization should be made if:
   ■ Evidence of worsening pulmonary or systemic congestion (even in the absence of dyspnea or weight gain)
   ■ Marked electrolyte disturbances
   ■ Multiple implantable cardioverter defibrillator (ICD) firings
   ■ Co-morbid conditions

      – Pneumonia
      – Diabetic ketoacidosis
      – Pulmonary embolus
      – Transient ischemic attack (TIA)/cerebrovascular accident (CVA)

INITIAL MANAGEMENT OF ACUTE HF SYNDROMES

Goals

- Rapidly relieve symptoms of congestion
- Identify reversible causes, particularly ischemia
- Restore hemodynamics
- Ensure adequate oxygenation
- Prevent end organ damage
- Identify patients with low output states

Management should be based on hemodynamic profile

Rapid assessment and initiation of therapy can be made using the following 2 × 2 diagram demonstrating the various hemodynamic profiles of patients presenting with acute HF (Fig. 14-1) [20]

After Admission

Practice guidelines recommend that the following parameters be monitored in patients hospitalized for acute HF [19]:

- Daily weight
- Daily measurement of fluid intake and output
- Vital signs (more than once daily, as indicated)
- Physical exams signs (at least daily)

    – Increased jugular venous pressure (JVP)
    – Hepatojugular reflux
    – Rales

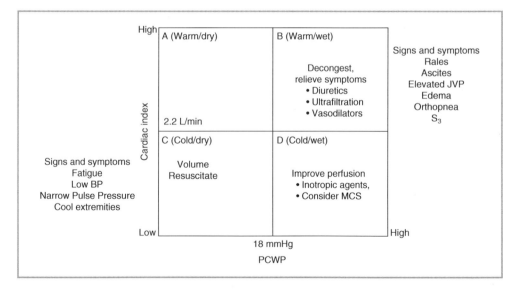

FIGURE 14-1

2 × 2 HF hemodynamic profiles. The above diagram demonstrates the hemodynamic profiles, signs and symptoms and treatment approach of patient's presenting with heart failure. Quadrant *A* represents the patient who is not congested and has adequate perfusion. Quadrant *B* represents the patient who is congested but has adequate perfusion. Quadrant *C* represents the patient who is congested and has poor perfusion. Quadrant *D* represents the patient who has a normal to low volume status and poor perfusion. Treatment approaches overlap in the low output profiles, as those patients who are congested and also poorly perfused may need a separate treatment approaches to both conditions

- Edema
- Hepatomegaly
- Liver tenderness

■ Labs (at least daily)

- Electrolytes
- Renal function

■ Symptoms (at least daily)

- Fatigue
- Dyspnea
- Orthopnea
- Paroxysmal nocturnal dyspnea or cough

Hemodynamic monitoring

■ Studies, such as the ESCAPE study, assessing the use of routine invasive monitoring such as pulmonary artery catheter have been essentially neutral [21]

■ The routine use of invasive hemodynamic monitoring is not recommended, but should be considered under the following circumstances:

- In those patients refractory to initial therapy
- When volume status and cardiac filling pressures are unclear
- When there is clinically significant hypotension, typically:

    ■ SBP <80 mmHg
    ■ worsening renal function during therapy

Management of Congestion

Diuretics are first line therapy in the management of patients with congestion

■ Initial management consists of IV diuresis using loop diuretics [22] at intervals of BID-TID, and in some cases continuous IV infusion.

- Typically 2–2.5 x home daily diuretic dose.

    ■ e.g. in a patient taking 80 mg oral furosemide daily, begin with 200 mg PO equivalent IV dosing, bumex 5 mg IV or Furosemide 100 mg IV. Should see a response within 30 min of administration. Diuretic dose should be escalated until desired effect occurs
    ■ Always watch out for electrolyte depletion (especially K and Mg) with aggressive diuresis.
    ■ Furosemide

        - PO has an onset of 20–30 min, peak of 1–2 h and duration of 6–8 h (50 % bioavailable).
        - IV has an onset of 5 min, peak of 30 min and duration of 2 h (100 % bioavailable).

- Bolus vs. continuous infusion has not been shown to be superior [23]
- Thiazide diuretics can be added when there is sub-optimal response to loop diuretics

    ■ Block reabsorbtion of distal tubule Na
    ■ Antagonize renal adaptation to chronic loop diuretic treatment
    ■ Improve diuretic resistance which occurs with rebound Na retention

- Can augment hypotensive effects of angiotensin converting enzyme (ACE)-I/ angiotensin II receptor blocker (ARB) regardless of volume status

Ultrafiltration

■ Consider in patients who are refractory to IV diuretics [24]

■ Uses a small extracorporeal circuit which is connected to the patient via peripheral or central venous access

- Patients with hypotension may not tolerate ultrafiltration
- The UNLOAD [25] trial compared ultrafiltration to conventional diuretic therapy

  - At 48 h, compared to diuretics, ultrafiltration produced:

    - a greater reduction in weight
    - Greater fluid loss
    - Similar changes in serum creatinine

- More recent data indicate ultrafiltration may not be superior to aggressive diuretic therapy. Choice should be based on response to initial diuretic treatment, therefore.

Non-invasive positive pressure ventilation

- Can be considered in patients with pulmonary edema and severe dyspnea
- Improves dyspnea
- Probably has no impact on mortality or rate of intubation [26]

Vasodilator therapy (nitroglycerin, nitroprusside, nesiritide).

- Recommended for rapid symptom relief in those with pulmonary congestion or hypertension
- Use when symptoms persist despite aggressive diuretic and standard oral regimens
- Do not use if the patient has symptomatic hypotension

Nitroglycerin

- Provides venodilation and thus reduction in preload
- Coronary vasodilation
- At higher doses, provides reduction in systemic afterload
- Tachyphylaxis can occur
- Contraindicated in patients using sildenafil

Nitroprusside

- Indicated when a marked reduction in afterload is desired

  - Hypertensive emergency
  - Severe mitral regurgitation
  - Severe aortic insufficiency
  - Acute ventricular septal rupture

- Potent vasodilation, equal venodilation and arterial dilation
- Accumulation of the metabolites cyanide and thiocyanate may occur and in rare cases can be lethal; drug should only be administered for a limited period of time (24–48 h)
- Use caution if renal or hepatic impairment
- Can get reflex tachycardia
- Rebound vasoconstriction can occur upon discontinuation

Nesiritide

- Recombinant form of human BNP
- Reduces pulmonary capillary wedge pressure (PCWP), systemic vascular resistance (SVR) and pulmonary vascular resistance (PVR), increases cardiac output at higher doses
- Inconsistent effects on urine output, with some studies showing an increase and others with no effect [27].

  - ASCEND-HF trial [28] showed no difference in death or rehospitalization but more hypotension from nesiritide use.

Support of Hemodynamics

Inotropic Therapy (Table 14-5)

Vasodilating inotropes: Milrinone, dobutamine
Vasopressor inotropes: Dopamine, norepinephrine

- Consider in patients who are non-responsive to or intolerant of vasodilators and diuretics
- No evidence that inotropic agents benefit patients without evidence of poor perfusion.

TABLE 14-5

COMPARISON OF VARIOUS VASODILATORS AND INOTROPIC AGENTS USED FOR ACUTE HF

MEDICATION (USUAL DOSE)	MECHANISM OF ACTION	PERIPHERAL VASODILATION	PERIPHERAL VASOCON-STRICTION	INOTROPY	CHRONOTROPY	PULMONARY VASODILATION	ARRHYTHMOGENIC
Nitroglycerin (5–10 µg/min, max 200 µg/min)	Stimulated cGMP production through activation of guanylyl cyclase	+	-	-	-	+	-
Nitroprusside (0.3 µg/kg/min-3 µg/kg/min max 10 µ/kg/min)	Interacts with oxyhemoglobin, forming methemoglobin leading to cyanide ion and nitric oxide (NO) release	++	-	-	-	+	
Nesiritide (0.01–0.03 µg/kg/min)	Recombinant BNP, binds to guanylate cyclase receptor, leading to increased cGMP	+	-	-	-	+	
Milrinone (0.375–0.75 µg/kg/min)	Inhibits phosphodiesterase III	++	-	+	-	+	+
Dobutamine (2.0–20 µg/kg/min, max 40 µg/kg/min)	Stimulates β1 and β2 receptors	+	-	+	+	-	+
Dopamine (2.0–20 µg/kg/min max 50 µg/kg/min)	Dose dependent activation of D1, β1 α1	-	+	+	+	-	+
Norepinephrine (0.01–3 µg/kg/min)	potent α1 agonist, modest β1,β2 agonist	-	+	+	+	-	+
Epinephrine (0.01–0.10 µg/kg/min)	Stimulates β1,β2, and α1 receptors	-	+	+	+	-	+

- Short term therapy using inotropic agents has been associated with significantly higher in hospital mortality than vasodilator therapy [29, 30]
- Should be reserved for patients with hemodynamic instability or evidence of poor cardiac output and end organ hypoperfusion:
  - Systemic hypotension
  - Renal dysfunction

- Use is associated with poor prognosis

Milrinone

- Inhibits phosphodiesterase III, preventing degradation of cyclic adenosine monophosphate (cAMP).

  - Increased cAMP leads to vasodilation

- Reduces RV and LV pre-load and afterload
- Potent pulmonary vasodilator
- Can cause marked hypotension
- Does not act via adrenergic receptors thus may be more desirable in patients on chronic beta blocker therapy
- No improvement in mortality compared to placebo
- Increased incidence of arrhythmias [31]
- Outcomes of a Prospective Trial of Intravenous Milrinone for Exacerbation of Chronic Heart Failure (OPTIME-CHF)

  - Hospitalized patients randomized to a 48-h infusion of intravenous milrinone or placebo.
  - Administration of milrinone was associated with:

    - A higher rate of early treatment failure
    - more sustained hypotension
    - new atrial arrhythmias
    - Had a higher composite rate of death or rehospitalization
    - Patients with an ischemic etiology that were treated with milrinone had a higher 60-day mortality

Dobutamine

- Synthetic catecholamine
- Nonselective beta-1 and beta-2 adrenergic receptor agonist
- Positive inotropy and chronotropy
- Decreases afterload
- Increases heart rate, stroke volume and cardiac output

Dopamine

- Dose dependent activation of D1, Beta 1 and Alpha 1 receptors
- Low dose (2mcg/kg/min), activates vascular D1 receptors (coronary/renal/mesenteric)
- Moderate dose (2–5 mcg/kg/min) binds to beta 1 receptors in the heart leading to inotropy
- High doses (5–15 mcg/kg/min) activates alpha 1 receptors

Mechanical Circulatory Support

In patients who have a persistent low output state despite medical management, immediate consideration should be made for initiation of mechanical circulatory support

- Conditions in which MCS is generally accepted:

  - Fulminant myocarditis with cardiogenic shock

– Acute hemodynamic compromise

  ■ Cardiopulmonary arrest
  ■ Cardiogenic shock

– High risk percutaneous coronary interventions
– In patients who are waiting for transplant

The devices below specifically address acute needs and are for short term support only, and can be used for days to weeks. Long term devices can be used in patients waiting for transplant and are discussed in Chap. 15. A variety of devices are available, the ones most commonly used in clinical practice will be discussed here.

Intraaortic Balloon Counterpulsation

■ Most well studied
■ Increases coronary blood flow, decreases myocardial demand and increases oxygen supply, increases cardiac output
■ Contraindications:

– Aortic dissection
– Severe aortic regurgitation (AR)
– Severe peripheral arterial disease (PAD) (occlusive aortoiliac disease)

Percutaneous Ventricular Assist Devices (VADs)

■ Impella

– Uses a miniature impeller pump that is placed across the aortic valve into the left ventricle; draws blood out of the ventricle and ejects blood through the ascending aorta
– Can pump 2.5 L/min, 4.0 L/min or 5.0 L/min depending on size of pump used
– Requires systemic anticoagulation

■ Tandem heart [32]

– Left atrial-to-femoral artery bypass system using:

  ■ transseptal cannula
  ■ arterial cannula
  ■ centrifugal blood pump

– Provides flow rates up to 4.0 L/min
– Requires systemic anticoagulation

■ Extracorporeal Membrane Oxygenation (ECMO) [33]

– Provides total circulatory support
– Uses a centrifugal pump and membrane oxygenator
– Can be placed percutaneously
– Supports both the left and right ventricle
– Requires systemic anticoagulation
– Two types: venoarterial and venovenous

  ■ Only venoarterial ECMO provides hemodynamic support
  ■ Both venoarterial and venovenous provide respiratory support

Complications of mechanical circulatory support

■ Infection
■ Thrombosis
■ Thrombocytopenia
■ Hemolysis
■ Bleeding
■ CVA

36. Effect of metoprolol CR/XL in chronic heart failure: Metoprolol CR/XL Randomised Intervention Trial in Congestive Heart Failure (MERIT-HF). Lancet. 1999;353(9169):2001–7.

37. Effects of enalapril on mortality in severe congestive heart failure. Results of the Cooperative North Scandinavian Enalapril Survival Study (CONSENSUS). The CONSENSUS Trial Study Group. N Engl J Med. 1987;316(23):1429–35.

38. Cohn JN, Johnson G, Ziesche S, Cobb F, Francis G, Tristani F, et al. A comparison of enalapril with hydralazine-isosorbide dinitrate in the treatment of chronic congestive heart failure. N Engl J Med. 1991;325(5):303–10.

39. Effect of enalapril on survival in patients with reduced left ventricular ejection fractions and congestive heart failure. The SOLVD Investigators. N Engl J Med. 1991;325(5):293–302.

40. Cohn JN, Tognoni G. A randomized trial of the angiotensin-receptor blocker valsartan in chronic heart failure. N Engl J Med. 2001;345(23):1667–75.

41. Pitt B, Zannad F, Remme WJ, Cody R, Castaigne A, Perez A, et al. The effect of spironolactone on morbidity and mortality in patients with severe heart failure. Randomized Aldactone Evaluation Study Investigators. N Engl J Med. 1999;341(10):709–17.

42. Taylor AL, Ziesche S, Yancy C, Carson P, D'Agostino Jr R, Ferdinand K, et al. Combination of isosorbide dinitrate and hydralazine in blacks with heart failure. N Engl J Med. 2004;351(20):2049–57.

43. Moss AJ, Hall WJ, Cannom DS, Daubert JP, Higgins SL, Klein H, et al. Improved survival with an implanted defibrillator in patients with coronary disease at high risk for ventricular arrhythmia. Multicenter Automatic Defibrillator Implantation Trial Investigators. N Engl J Med. 1996;335(26):1933–40.

44. Bristow MR, Saxon LA, Boehmer J, Krueger S, Kass DA, De Marco T, et al. Cardiac-resynchronization therapy with or without an implantable defibrillator in advanced chronic heart failure. N Engl J Med. 2004;350(21):2140–50.

45. Cleland JG, Daubert JC, Erdmann E, Freemantle N, Gras D, Kappenberger L, et al. The effect of cardiac resynchronization on morbidity and mortality in heart failure. N Engl J Med. 2005;352(15):1539–49.

46. McCarthy 3rd RE, Boehmer JP, Hruban RH, Hutchins GM, Kasper EK, Hare JM, et al. Long-term outcome of fulminant myocarditis as compared with acute (nonfulminant) myocarditis. N Engl J Med. 2000;342(10):690–5.

47. Acker MA. Mechanical circulatory support for patients with acute-fulminant myocarditis. Ann Thorac Surg. 2001;71 (3 Suppl):S73–6; discussion S82-5.

48. The effect of digoxin on mortality and morbidity in patients with heart failure. The Digitalis Investigation Group. N Engl J Med. 1997;336(8):525–33.

49. Pelta A, Andersen UB, Just S, Baekgaard N. Flash pulmonary edema in patients with renal artery stenosis–the Pickering Syndrome. Blood Press. 2011;20(1):15–9.

CHAPTER 15

GABRIEL SAYER AND MARC J. SEMIGRAN

Chronic and End-Stage Heart Failure

CHAPTER OUTLINE

ABBREVIATIONS

ACE	Angiotensin-converting enzyme
ACEI	Angiotensin-converting enzyme inhibitor
AF	Atrial fibrillation
AHA	American Heart Association
ARB	Angiotensin-receptor blocker
BB	Beta-blocker
BMI	Body mass index
BNP	B-type natriuretic peptide
BTT	Bridge to transplantation
CAD	Coronary artery disease
cAMP	Cyclic adenosine monophosphate
CO	Cardiac output
CPET	Cardiopulmonary exercise test
Cr	Creatinine
CV	Cardiovascular
DT	Destination Therapy
HCM	Hypertrophic cardiomyopathy
HDZ	Hydralazine
HF	Heart failure
HFpEF	Heart failure with preserved ejection fraction
HFrEF	Heart failure with reduced ejection fraction
HTN	Hypertension
IABP	Intra-aortic balloon pump
ICD	Implantable cardiac defibrillator
ISDN	Isosorbide dinitrate
JVP	Jugular venous pressure
K	Potassium
LV	Left ventricular
LVAD	Left ventricular assist device
LVEF	Left ventricular ejection fraction
LVH	Left ventricular hypertrophy
MCS	Mechanical circulatory support
MI	Myocardial infarction
NIDCM	Nonischemic dilated cardiomyopathy
NYHA	New York Heart Association
PH	Pulmonary hypertension
PVR	Pulmonary vascular resistance

- **Restrictive cardiomyopathy**
  - Idiopathic restrictive cardiomyopathy
  - Infiltrative diseases
    - Sarcoidosis – usually presents with arrhythmias or sudden death
    - Amyloidosis – senile, familial, or associated with abnormal light chain production (AL amyloidosis)
      - Initially normal LV systolic function, with subsequent deterioration of LVEF
  - Storage diseases
    - Fabry's Disease
      - X-linked genetic disorder
      - Deficiency of α-galactosidase A $\rightarrow$ lysosomal storage disease
      - Characterized by marked LVH – may be confused for HCM
      - Can be treated with enzyme replacement
    - Hemochromatosis
      - Inherited genetic order or secondary to large volume of blood transfusions
      - Characterized by myocardial deposition of iron
  - Endomyocardial fibrosis
    - Diffuse fibrosis of ventricular endocardium of unclear etiology
    - Most common worldwide cause of restrictive cardiomyopathy
    - Mostly found in Africa, Asia and South America
  - Radiation Therapy
    - Damages blood vessels $\rightarrow$ inflammation $\rightarrow$ myocardial fibrosis $\rightarrow$ decreased ventricular compliance
- **Right ventricular (RV) failure**
  - Almost always associated with pulmonary hypertension (PH)
  - Final consequence of many congenital heart lesions, particularly in context of Eisenmenger syndrome (irreversible PH)
- **Constrictive Pericarditis**
  - May be caused by:
    - Prior cardiac surgery
    - Radiation
    - Infections (Tuberculosis, bacterial, parasitic)
  - Resolves with surgical pericardiectomy

PATHOPHYSIOLOGY OF CHRONIC HF (FIG. 15-1)

- Acute injury to myocardium causes decreased cardiac output (CO) and end-organ perfusion
- **Neurohormonal activation**
  - Upregulation of **renin-angiotensin-aldosterone system**
    - Increased angiotensin II $\rightarrow$ systemic and renal arterial vasoconstriction
    - Increased aldosterone $\rightarrow$ renal sodium retention
  - **Sympathetic nervous system** activation
    - Release of catecholamines (e.g. norepinephrine)
    - Results in enhanced myocardial contractility and systemic vasoconstriction
    - Decreases distal water delivery in kidney due to reduction in glomerular filtration rate (GFR) $\rightarrow$ decreased excretion of water

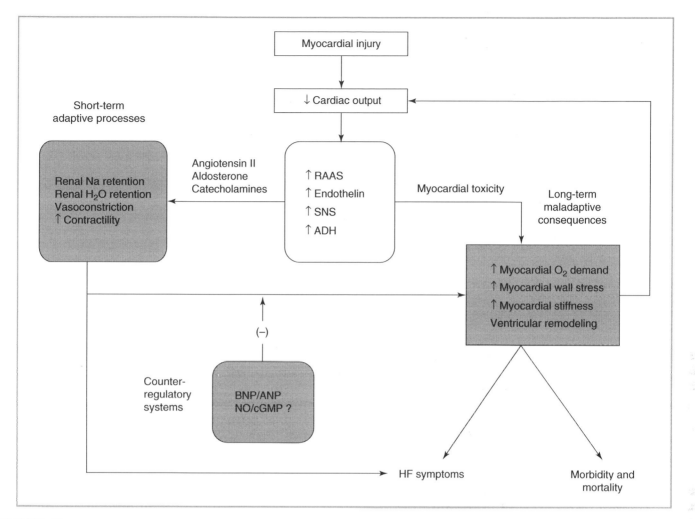

FIGURE 15-1

A schematic representation of the pathophysiology of chronic heart failure due to impaired LV systolic function. The initiating event is an injury that leads to myocardial dysfunction. The body compensates for decreased cardiac output by activating multiple neurohormonal systems. In the acute phase, these mechanisms act to maintain adequate perfusion of systemic organs, but may also result in congestion and HF symptoms. Over time, these compensatory systems have adverse effects on the LV, stimulating further neurohormonal activation, worsening HF symptoms and ultimately leading to HF mortality. Counter-regulatory systems, including the natriuretic peptides, are upregulated to prevent the adverse effects of neurohormonal activation. *Abbreviations*: *RAAS* renin-angiotensin-aldosterone system, *SNS* sympathetic nervous system, *ADH* anti-diuretic hormone, *BNP* B-type natriuretic peptide, *ANP* atrial natriuretic peptide, *NO* nitric oxide, *cGMP* cyclic guanosine monophosphate, *HF* heart failure

- Release of **anti-diuretic hormone**

  ■ Enhances reabsorption of water by renal collecting tubules

- **Ventricular remodeling**

  ■ Type of remodeling depends on type of stress placed on ventricle
  ■ **Pressure overload** (e.g. aortic stenosis)

  – Concentric remodeling → LVH
  – Reduced wall stress via LaPlace's Law (stress inversely proportional to wall thickness)

  ■ **Volume overload** (e.g. mitral regurgitation)

  – Eccentric remodeling → ventricular dilatation
  – Increased preload maintains cardiac output via Frank-Starling mechanism

- **Myocardial injury** (e.g. MI)

  - Stretching of scarred tissue → mixed pressure and volume load on non-infarcted tissue
  - Ventricular dilatation → maintenance of cardiac output

- Acute compensatory responses become deleterious over time

  - Progressive ventricular dilatation → increased wall stress (LaPlace: stress proportional to chamber radius)
  - Ongoing ventricular remodeling causes progressive HF

EVALUATION OF CHRONIC HF

- Comprehensive history with focus on potential etiologies of cardiomyopathy

  - Detailed alcohol, drug, toxin exposure
  - Atherosclerotic risk factors, history of MI
  - Systemic systems indicative of extracardiac disease
  - Family history of HF, CAD or sudden cardiac death

- Symptom assessment

  - Dyspnea most common symptom
  - NYHA Classification
  - Congestion (orthopnea, paroxysmal nocturnal dyspnea)
  - Low CO (fatigue, impaired cognition)

- Physical Examination

  - Signs of congestion

    - Rales and/or pleural effusions on pulmonary exam – can be absent in long-standing HF despite elevated left-sided pressures
    - Elevated jugular venous pressure (JVP)
    - Positive hepatojugular reflex – sustained rise in JVP with compression of right upper quadrant of abdomen
    - Ascites
    - Lower extremity edema

  - Signs of low CO

    - Hypotension
    - Sinus tachycardia
    - Narrow pulse pressure
    - Cool extremities
    - Diminished pulses

  - Other findings

    - Displaced and enlarged point of maximal impulse
    - Third heart sound (S3)
    - RV heave
    - Prominent pulmonic component of second heart sound (P2)
    - Murmurs of functional mitral and tricuspid regurgitation

- Diagnostic testing

  - Laboratory analyses

    - Basic metabolic panel, complete blood count, liver function tests, thyroid-stimulating hormone, urinalysis, hemoglobin A1C or fasting glucose
    - HIV test, iron studies (to screen for hemochromatosis) and sleep study should be considered in most patients
    - Further testing in selected patients depending on risk factors for specific etiologies of HF

  - ECG – arrhythmias, conduction disturbances, voltage (high or low), ectopy
  - Chest X-ray – cardiac chamber enlargement, pleural effusions, interstitial or pulmonary edema
  - Transthoracic echocardiogram (**TTE**)

- ■ LV and RV systolic function
- ■ Presence of scar or wall motion abnormalities – suggestive of CAD
- ■ Diastolic function of LV
- ■ Quantification of chamber dilation and ventricular hypertrophy
- ■ Identification of valvular abnormalities
- ■ Presence of pericardial effusion

- – Assessment for obstructive CAD with **coronary angiography** or **noninvasive imaging** in patients with CAD risk factors
- – **Cardiopulmonary exercise testing (CPET)** – measurement of peak oxygen uptake (VO_2) provides assessment of relative contributions of cardiac disease and pulmonary disease to dyspnea as well as prognostic information
- – Endomyocardial biopsy not helpful in most cases unless specific diagnosis suspected that would alter management
- – Signal-averaged electrocardiogram not recommended in routine assessment

PROGNOSIS OF CHRONIC HF

■ Factors associated with worse prognosis in chronic HF include:

- – LVEF – 39 % increase in mortality for each 10 % drop in LVEF [8]
- – RV ejection fraction (RVEF) <35 % [9]
- – PH [10]
- – QRS length >120 ms [11]
- – VO_2 <14 ml/kg/min [12]
- – Chronic kidney disease – patients with severe renal dysfunction have 2× risk of death at 1 year compared to patients with normal renal function [13]
- – B-type Natriuretic Peptide (BNP)/amino-terminal (NT)-proBNP – one of strongest independent predictors of prognosis [14]
- – Troponin levels [15]

■ Risk scores have been developed for patient stratification

- – Seattle Heart Failure Model

  - ■ Incorporates clinical variables, medications and devices
  - ■ Highly accurate prediction of survival out to 3 years in general HF population [16]

- – Heart Failure Survival Score [17]

  - ■ Incorporates CAD, heart rate, LVEF, blood pressure, intraventricular conduction delay, serum sodium, peak VO_2
  - ■ Used to risk stratify NYHA Class III–IV patients being considered for transplantation

MANAGEMENT OF CHRONIC HF

■ Treatment of comorbid conditions [3]

- – HTN – Maintenance of blood pressure within guideline-recommended limits
- – Identification and treatment of dyslipidemia based on risk level
- – Diabetes – Control of blood glucose within guideline-recommended limits
- – AF

  - ■ Control of ventricular rate
  - ■ Consideration of rhythm control

    - – No survival benefit has been demonstrated but may improve symptoms
    - – Amiodarone and dofetilide only agents with established safety in HF

- – CAD

  - ■ Treatment of angina with nitrates and beta-blockers
  - ■ Consideration of revascularization when indicated

40. Rose EA, Gelijns AC, Moskowitz AJ, Heitjan DF, Stevenson LW, Dembitsky W, et al. Long-term use of a left ventricular assist device for end-stage heart failure. N Engl J Med. 2001;345: 1435–43.

41. Slaughter MS, Rogers JG, Milano CA, Russell SD, Conte JV, Feldman D, et al. Advanced heart failure treated with continuous-flow left ventricular assist device. N Engl J Med. 2009;361: 2241–51.

42. Stehlik J, Edwards LB, Kucheryavaya AY, Aurora P, Christie JD, Kirk R, et al. The registry of the International Society for Heart and Lung Transplantation: twenty-seventh official adult heart transplant report – 2010. J Heart Lung Transplant. 2010;29: 1089–103.

43. Mehra MR, Kobashigawa J, Starling R, Russell S, Uber PA, Parameshwar J, et al. Listing criteria for heart transplantation: International Society for Heart and Lung Transplantation Guidelines for the care of cardiac transplant candidates – 2006. J Heart Lung Transplant. 2006;25:1024–42.

44. Lietz K, John R, Burke EA, Ankersmit JH, McCue JD, Naka Y, et al. Pretransplant cachexia and morbid obesity are predictors of increased mortality after heart transplantation. Transplantation. 2001;72:277–83.

CHAPTER 16

SAMMY ELMARIAH, JAMES L. JANUZZI, JR., AIDAN W. FLYNN, PRAVEEN MEHROTRA, AND IGOR F. PALACIOS

Valvular Heart Disease

CHAPTER OUTLINE

ABBREVIATIONS

AR	Aortic regurgitation
AS	Aortic stenosis
AV	Aortic valve
BAV	Percutaneous balloon aortic valvuloplasty
CSA	Cross sectional area
DFP	Diastolic filling period
DT	Deceleration time
HR	Heart rate
LV	Left ventricular
LVOT	Left ventricular outflow tract
MR	Mitral regurgitation
MS	Mitral stenosis
MVA	Mitral valve area
MVG	Mitral valve gradient
MVR	Mitral valve replacement
NYHA	New York Heart Association
PHT	Pressure half-time
PMV	Percutaneous mitral valvuloplasty
PR	Pulmonic regurgitation
PS	Pulmonic stenosis
RA	Right atrial
RV	Right ventricular
TR	Tricuspid regurgitation
TS	Tricuspid stenosis
VTI	Velocity time integral

INTRODUCTION

Valvular heart disease is a growing public health concern – as our population ages, the prevalence of valvular heart disease will only rise. The expansive topic encompasses numerous disease entities, complex hemodynamics, invasive and noninvasive testing, and involved management decisions. In addition, perhaps more so than any other topic in cardiology, the diagnosis and management of valvular heart disease is dependent on the history and physical examination. Such complexity makes valvular heart disease a prime topic for cardiology board examinations.

AORTIC STENOSIS

Etiology

- The most common cause of aortic stenosis is calcific degeneration [1].
- Calcific aortic stenosis (AS) was historically felt to be due to age-related degeneration; however, it is due to an active process similar to atherosclerosis that includes lipid deposition, inflammation, and active calcification [2–6]. Severe calcific AS most frequently presents in the sixth to seventh decades of life.
- Bicuspid aortic valves are prevalent in 1–2 % of the general population, predominantly men. Severe AS due to a bicuspid aortic valve can occur early in life, but most frequently presents in the fifth and sixth decades of life [7, 8].
- Rheumatic AS rarely occurs in the Western world and is most often associated with concomitant mitral pathology.

Pathophysiology and Hemodynamics

- Aortic stenosis (AS) causes an obstruction to left ventricular outflow tract, resulting in a fixed cardiac output and concentric left ventricular (LV) hypertrophy in compensation for left ventricular pressure overload.

  - Left ventricular hypertrophy occurs in order to maintain normal wall stress (σ) which is proportional to the LV pressure (P) and radius (r) and inversely related to wall thickness (T) as dictated by LaPlace's law:

$$\sigma = (P \times r)/2T$$

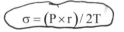

  - Worsening AS leads to progressive LV hypertrophy that in turn leads to diastolic dysfunction and myocardial oxygen supply–demand mismatch.

- Low-flow aortic stenosis

  - In patients with AS and LV systolic dysfunction, AV leaflet opening may be reduced due to a low stroke volume, not severe AS (pseudostenosis).

    - Identification of pseudostenosis is frequently performed by assessing the severity of AS during low-dose dobutamine infusion. An increase in the AVA during dobutamine infusion signifies pseudostenosis; whereas, an increase in AV gradients with a constant AVA suggests true AS [9].

Assessment

- History (See Chap. 1 for important details)

  - AS is typically asymptomatic until valvular stenosis is severe.

    - Symptom development in a patient with moderate AS may suggest the presence of underlying coronary artery disease

	AORTIC SCLEROSIS	MILD	MODERATE	SEVERE
Aortic jet velocity (m/s)	≤2.5 m/s	2.6–2.9	3.0–4.0	>4.0
Mean gradient (mmHg)	–	<20	20–40	>40
AVA (cm²)	–	>1.5	1.0–1.5	<1.0
Indexed AVA (cm²/m²)		>0.85	0.60–0.85	<0.6
Velocity ratio		>0.50	0.25–0.50	<0.25

TABLE 16-1

SEVERITY OF AORTIC VALVE STENOSIS

Adapted from Bonow et al. [10]

- The hallmark of AS is the classical triad of dyspnea on exertion, chest heaviness, and dizziness with exertion.

  - These symptoms do not develop simultaneously, and in many cases, only one of the three is present.

- Physical examination (see Chap. 1 for important details)
  - The physical examination of the patient with AS is very important to remember.
  - Most important hallmarks of severe aortic stenosis on physical examination include:

    - Reduction in the amplitude and velocity of the carotid upstrokes
    - Diminution or entire loss of the second heart sound
    - Mid-to-late peaking nature to the systolic murmur

  - The murmur of AS radiates to the carotids, sometimes associated with a thrill.

    - Radiation may also occur across the precordium

  - The murmur increases with squatting, decreases with standing and handgrip

    - This helps to differentiate it from hypertrophic cardiomyopathy.

  - Other findings include an opening click in patients with a bicuspid valve, as well as the murmur of aortic regurgitation.

- Echocardiography

  - Transthoracic Doppler echocardiography is the standard method for quantifying the degree of aortic stenosis (Table 16-1).
  - The velocity (V) across the stenotic aortic valve on echocardiography can be used to estimate the peak pressure gradient across the valve (ΔP) by use of the Bernoulli equation:

$$\Delta P = 4V^2$$

  - The principle of conservation of mass dictates that flow within the left ventricular outflow tract (LVOT) must be the same as flow through the aortic valve. Hence, the aortic valve area (AVA) can be calculated using the continuity equation:

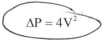

$$AVA \times VTI_{AV} = CSA_{LVOT} \times VTI_{LVOT}$$

  where VTI is the velocity time integral and CSA is cross sectional area.

- Cardiac catheterization

  - Invasive assessment of AS severity is recommended when noninvasive tests are inconclusive or discordant with clinical findings [10].

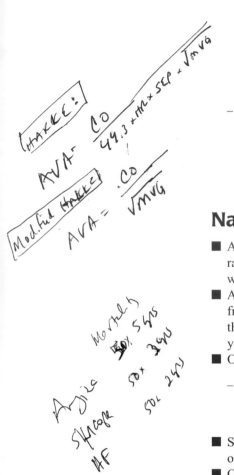

– During cardiac catheterization, the mean gradient across the aortic valve (MVG) is measured and used to calculate the AVA using the Gorlin formula [11]:

$$AVA = CO / \left(44.3 \times HR \times SEP \times \sqrt{MVG}\right)$$

where CO (ml/min) is cardiac output, HR (bpm) is heart rate, SEP (s) is systolic ejection period, and MVG is mean valve gradient.

– The Hakki equation simplified the Gorlin formula for routine use in clinical practice [12]:

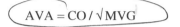

$$AVA = CO / \sqrt{MVG}$$

where CO (L/min) is cardiac output and MVG is mean valve gradient.

Natural History

■ Aortic stenosis typically progresses slowly over decades (latent phase) with an average rate of progression of 0.1–0.2 cm^2/year [13, 14], although more rapid progression is seen with heavily calcified valves [15].

■ Aortic sclerosis progresses to severe AS in some, but not all, individuals. Progression from sclerosis to stenosis over a 5-year interval was observed in approximately 9 % of the Cardiovascular Health Study (CHS) population, all of whom were older than 65 years [16].

■ Once symptoms due to severe AS develop, survival worsens.

– With the development of angina, syncope, or heart failure, only 50 % of patients will survive 5, 3, and 2 years, respectively, if valve replacement is not performed [17] (Fig. 16-1).

■ Sudden death occurs in the setting of severe AS, whether or not symptoms have developed; however, sudden death is rare in asymptomatic AS patients (<1 %/year) [10].

■ Other complications of AS include left ventricular dysfunction, worsening mitral regurgitation from annular dilation, heart failure, and conduction disease from erosion of calcium at the level of the aortic annulus into the upper septum and affecting either the atrioventricular node (first degree block) or the bundles.

■ Concomitant ascending aortic dilation is present in patients with bicuspid aortic valves (independent of the degree of stenosis or regurgitation).

– Dilation of the ascending aorta in a patient with a bicuspid valve is not due to "post-stenotic" turbulence of blood flow; rather it is due to an inherited weakness of the medial smooth muscle integrity.

– Aortic dissection is a dreaded complication in this scenario.

Management of AS

■ Pharmacologic

– Patients with asymptomatic AS have outcomes similar to normal, adult controls.

■ Consequently, with the exception of serial screening for worsening valve stenosis, no further management for asymptomatic AS is needed.

– There is little in the way of medical therapy for slowing progression of AS.

■ While substantial retrospective data suggested that lipid-lowering therapy with statins would slow the progression of AS, randomized clinical trials have not supported this hypothesis [18–20].

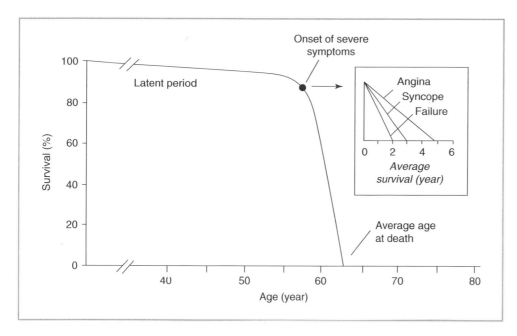

FIGURE 16-1

Survival rate of symptomatic aortic stenosis

- For patients with dilated ascending aorta, use of beta blockers and possibly vasodilators (such as angiotensin receptor blockers) is recommended to retard progression of dilation and reduce risk for dissection.

  ■ Aortic regurgitation should be treated as below

■ Aortic valve replacement

- The current indications for aortic valve replacement (AVR) are listed in Table 16-2.
- Surgical AVR is the standard of care for patients with severe, symptomatic AS and in those with severe AS and LV systolic dysfunction.

  ■ Valve replacement in this setting alleviates symptoms and results in substantial reduction in mortality. Survival after surgical AVR approximates that of age-matched controls [10].

  ■ Surgery should not be considered for asymptomatic patients with severe AS unless there is a need for other cardiac or aortic surgery or if there is a high likelihood of rapid progression [10].

  ■ In patients with low ejection fraction due to the AS, AVR may lead to considerable improvement in ventricular function, in contrast to this situation in aortic regurgitation.

  ■ In patients with a dilated ascending aorta at the time of surgery, replacement of the aneurysm may be indicated, particularly if the size is >40 mm or if there is a family history of aortic dissection.

- In patients at high-risk for surgical AVR, transcatheter aortic valve replacement (TAVR) has recently been introduced and approved by the United States Food and Drug Administration (FDA) based on finding from the PARTNER I trial [21].

■ Percutaneous aortic valvuloplasty

- Percutaneous balloon aortic valvuplasty (BAV) is a procedure in which a balloon is inflated across the stenotic AV in order to increase valve opening [22].
- Aortic valvuloplasty is effective for severe AS in children and adolescents; however, its efficacy is limited in adults with calcific AS due to short-lived and only modest clinical benefits [10].

TABLE 16-2		CLASS
INDICATIONS FOR AORTIC VALVE REPLACEMENT FOR AORTIC STENOSIS	**Aortic stenosis**	
	Symptomatic patients with severe AS	Class I
	Patients with severe AS undergoing cardiac surgery	Class I
	Asymptomatic patients with severe AS and LV systolic dysfunction (LV EF <50 %)	Class I
	Patients with moderate AS undergoing cardiac surgery	Class IIa
	Asymptomatic patients with severe AS and abnormal response to exercise	Class IIb
	Asymptomatic patients with severe AS if there is a high likelihood of rapid progression or surgical delay at the time of symptom development	Class IIb
	Patients with mild AS and evidence that progression may be rapid	Class IIb
	Asymptomatic patients with extremely severe AS (AVA <0.6 cm², mean gradient >60 mmHg, jet velocity >5.0 m/s) if expected operative mortality <1 %	Class IIb

Adapted from Bonow et al. [10]
AS aortic stenosis, *AVA* aortic valve area, *EF* ejection fraction, *LV* left ventricular

- In the current era, BAV is used as a bridge to surgical or transcatheter AVR in unstable patients with severe AS and as a palliative procedure in those in whom other definitive therapies are not feasible.

AORTIC REGURGITATION

Etiology

- Aortic regurgitation (AR) develops due to abnormalities in either the aortic root or the valve leaflets.

  - Acute and chronic AR are distinct clinical entities which will be considered independently.

- There are several causes of chronic AR, the most common of which is dilation of the aortic root and AV annulus. Several other etiologies are also noteworthy (Table 16-3).
- Acute AR is less common and usually due to infective endocarditis, aortic dissection, or trauma [10].

Pathophysiology and Hemodynamics

- In AR, the fundamental insult is LV volume overload. The extent of overload and regurgitation depends on the regurgitant orifice, the diastolic pressure gradient across the AV, and the duration of diastole [23].

  - Chronic aortic regurgitation

    - In response to chronic volume overload, eccentric LV hypertrophy develops in order to increase LV end-diastolic volume. Thus, the compliant LV can accommodate the increased volume load without an increase in end-diastolic pressures [10].
    - Eccentric hypertrophy also results in a larger stroke volume in the setting of preserved LV function; thereby, maintaining effective forward stroke volume.
    - With progressive chronic AR, LV systolic dysfunction ultimately ensues. This further increases LV end-diastolic volume and pressure, resulting in marked LV dilation and dysfunction.

  - Acute aortic regurgitation

    - With acute AR, forward cardiac output drops substantially as the LV does not have the opportunity to adapt to the volume load of AR [24].
    - In severe cases, hemodynamic instability and cardiogenic shock ensue. Mean left atrial pressure rises, resulting in pulmonary edema as well.

TABLE 16-3

CAUSES OF AORTIC REGURGITATION

Leaflet abnormalites

Chronic regurgitation

  Bicuspid aortic valve

  Calcific valve disease

  Rheumatic valve disease

  Myxomatous valve disease

  Rheumatoid arthritis

  Nonbacterial thrombotic endocarditis

  Systemic lupus erythematosus

  Pharmacologic agents

Acute regurgitation

  Endocarditis

  Iatrogenic leaflet damage

  Ruptured leaflet fenestration

  Blunt chest trauma

Abnormalities of the aorta

Chronic regurgitation

  Marfan syndrome

  Bicuspid aortic valve disease

  Hypertensive aortic dilation

  Familial aortic aneurysm

  Cardiovascular syphilis

  Ankylosing spondylitis

  Other systemic inflammatory disorders

Acute regurgitation

  Aortic dissection

- The pre-existence of pressure-overload in which the LV is small and non-compliant results in more dramatic decompensation as these patients possess a steeper diastolic pressure volume relationship [10, 24].
- Myocardial perfusion pressure may also diminish as LV end-diastolic pressure approaches the diastolic aortic pressure, resulting in subendocardial ischemia.

Assessment

- History

  - Until left ventricular end diastolic pressure begins to rise, patients with AR are frequently asymptomatic.
  - Symptoms may relate to exaggerated cardiac output with increased stroke volume, including a sense of pounding in the chest.
  - Dyspnea is an ominous sign, implying a rise in left ventricular end diastolic pressure with the onset of heart failure.

- Physical examination (see Chap. 1 for important details)

  - The exam of the patient with AR is important to understand.
  - Vital sign hallmarks of significant AR include a pulse indicative of both elevated cardiac output and diastolic "run off".
    - The 'Waterhammer' pulse is an exaggerated upstroke most notable in the carotid pulse.
    - The pulse pressure in chronic AR is usually wide.
    - The pulse pressure may re-narrow in the context of a high left ventricular end diastolic pressure, such as in heart failure.

PARAMETER	MILD	MODERATE	SEVERE
Jet width/LVOT (%)	<25	25–65	>65
Vena contracta (cm)	<0.3	0.3–0.6	>0.6
Pressure half-time (ms)	>500	200–500	<200
Regurgitant volume (mL/beat)	<30	30–60	>60
Regurgitant fraction (%)	<30	30–50	>50
Regurgitant orifice area (cm²)	<0.10	0.1–0.3	>0.30

Adapted from Refs. [10, 24]
LVOT left ventricular outflow tract

– The point of maximal impulse is usually displaced in severe chronic AR but may be normally located in acute AR.
– The diastolic murmur of AR.

  ■ Most often musical ("blowing"), but may be harsh when due to aortic leaflet eversion, tearing, or perforation.
  ■ The murmur of AR typically radiates along the left sternal border and is best heard with the patient sitting up and leaning forward with a full expiration.
  ■ If the murmur radiates along the right sternal border, it is suggestive of an ectatic aortic root, such as which occurs in syphilis.
  ■ With worsening aortic regurgitation and onset of ventricular failure, the murmur may shorten.
  ■ Very significant AR is frequently accompanied by a mitral diastolic rumble (the "Austin-Flint" murmur) due to impingement on the mitral valve by the regurgitant volume.

– Other stigmata of AR are discussed in Chap. 1 but the classical findings of chronic AR (such as head bobbing, to-and-fro murmurs over the vascular structures, or higher leg blood pressures compared to arm) are less evident or absent in acute AR.

■ Echocardiography

– Echocardiography can be invaluable in identifying the etiology and severity of AR and allows assessment of the ascending aorta.

  ■ Doppler and color flow echocardiography is used to grade the severity of AR using several parameters (Table 16-4) [10, 25].
  ■ The ratio of AR jet width/area to LVOT diameter/area correlate with angiographic AR severity.
  ■ The time required for the AV pressure gradient in diastole to fall by half ("pressure half-time") also correlates with AR severity; however, the ability of this measure to distinguish between grades of AR is limited. Shorter pressure half-times are associated with more severe AR.
  ■ Quantification of the volume and fraction of regurgitant flow is performed by echocardiography as follows [25, 26]:

$$SV_{LVOT} = \left(LVOT\ diameter\right)^2 \times 0.785 \times VTI_{LVOT}$$

$$SV_{MV} = \left(MV\ annulus\ diameter\right)^2 \times 0.785 \times VTI_{MV\ inflow}$$

$$RV = SV_{LVOT} - SV_{MV}$$

$$RF = \left(RV\ /\ SV_{LVOT}\right) \times 100\ \%$$

GRADE OF REGURGITATION	
1	Small amount contrast enters LV in diastole and is cleared with each beat
2	More contrast fills LV with faint opacification of the entire LV
3	LV is well opacified with contrast density equal to the ascending aorta
4	Complete and dense opacification of the LV on the first beat with contrast density greater than the ascending aorta

Adapted from Maroo et al. [26]
LV left ventricle

TABLE 16-5

SELLER'S CRITERIA FOR GRADING AORTIC REGURGITATION BY ANGIOGRAPHY

where MV is mitral valve, RF is regurgitant fraction, RV is regurgitant volume, and SV is stroke volume.

– Regurgitant orifice area (ROA) is a robust measure of AR severity that is calculated by dividing the regurgitant volume by regurgitant flow (VTI$_{AR}$) [23]:

$$ROA = RV / VTI_{AR}$$

– Other findings consistent with severe AR include premature closure of the mitral valve, mitral valve fluttering, reversed doming of the anterior mitral valve leaflet, and holodiastolic flow reversal in the descending aorta.

■ Cardiac catheterization

– Invasive assessment of AS severity is recommended when noninvasive tests are inconclusive or discordant with clinical findings [10].
– Invasive hemodynamic measurements can be helpful in evaluating patients with mixed aortic valve stenosis and regurgitation.
  Supravalvular aortography can be used to grade AR severity based on the degree of contrast regurgitation into the LV (Table 16-5) [27].

Natural History

■ Acute AR is often a medical emergency that requires immediate intervention.
■ Asymptomatic patients with preserved LV function and without severe LV dilatation possess a good prognosis.

– The rate of progression to LV dysfunction and/or symptom development is only 4.3 %/year and the rate of sudden death only 0.2 %/year [10].
– The guidelines for valve replacement surgery in the asymptomatic patient are listed in Table 16-6.

Management

■ Pharmacologic

– Chronic aortic regurgitation

  ■ Vasodilators are the primary therapy for asymptomatic patients with chronic severe AR.
  ■ Vasodilators such as hydralazine, nifedipine and felodipine increase cardiac output and reduce the regurgitant fraction [28, 29].
  ■ Therapy with angiotensin-converting enzyme inhibitors (ACE-I) reduces end-diastolic volume if doses sufficient to reduce systemic blood pressure are administered [10, 30].
  ■ Long-term therapy with vasodilators is only indicated for those without an indication for valve replacement or in those who cannot undergo surgery [10].

TABLE 16-6		CLASS
INDICATIONS FOR AORTIC VALVE REPLACEMENT FOR AORTIC REGURGITATION	Symptomatic patients with severe AR	Class I
	Asymptomatic patients with severe AR and LV systolic dysfunction (LV EF ≤50 %)	Class I
	Asymptomatic patients with severe AR undergoing cardiac surgery	Class I
	Asymptomatic patients with severe AR with severe LV dilatation (EDD >75 mm or ESD >55 mm)	Class IIa
	Patients with moderate AR undergoing cardiac surgery	Class IIb
	Asymptomatic patients with severe AR with LV dilatation (EDD >70 mm or ESD >50 mm) when there is evidence for progressive LV dilatation, declining exercise tolerance, or abnormal hemodynamic response to exercise	Class IIb

Adapted from Bonow et al. [10]

AR aortic regurgitation, *EDD* end diastolic dimension, *EF* ejection fraction, *ESD* end systolic dimension, *LV* left ventricular

- Short-term therapy can be instituted for hemodynamic optimization prior to surgical AVR [10].

  – Acute aortic regurgitation

  ■ Medical therapy for acute severe AR should be used solely to maintain hemodynamic stability prior to surgical AVR.
  ■ Intravenous vasodilators, such as nitroprusside, should be used to reduce afterload and LV end-diastolic pressure and to augment cardiac output.
  ■ Inotropic agents can also be used to further increase cardiac output if needed, but are generally not useful.
  ■ β-blockers should be avoided, although these agents can be used cautiously in the setting of acute AR due to aortic dissection in order to reduce dP/dT [10, 26].

■ Surgical management of AR (Table 16-6)

  – Surgical AVR is a class I indication for symptomatic patients with severe AR regardless of LV dimensions and function [10].
  – Surgery is a class I indication for asymptomatic patients with LV dysfunction (ejection fraction ≤50 %) and those asymptomatic patients with severe AR undergoing concomitant cardiac surgery.
  – AVR may be considered (Class II) in asymptomatic patients with severe LV dilatation.
  – Despite high operative risk, clinical outcomes with AVR in patients with NYHA class IV symptoms and/or severe LV dysfunction (LV ejection fraction ≤25 %) are better than with medical therapy alone [31].
  – Surgical aortic valve repair (rather than replacement) for AR is feasible, especially in those with bicuspid aortic valves or those with AR due to cusp prolapse.

MITRAL STENOSIS

Etiology

■ Most common cause of mitral stenosis (MS) is rheumatic heart disease due to previous rheumatic fever.

  – Rheumatic MS involves mitral valve leaflet thickening and calcification, commissural fusion, chordal fusion, and ultimate obstruction [32].
  – There is a variable interval between the occurrence of rheumatic fever and the development of hemodynamically significant MS (up to in excess of 20 years).
  – Early phase inflammatory and edematous changes progress to fibrosis and calcification over time, leading to the characteristic thickened leaflet tips, and commissural fusion.

■ Other causes of MS are less common, and include calcific encroachment on the mitral orifice (not uncommonly seen in patients with advanced renal failure).

  – Other rare causes include congenital MS, malignant carcinoid disease, systemic lupus erythematosis, and rheumatoid arthritis.

■ Left atrial outflow obstruction (simulating MS) may be caused by cor triatriatum (persistent atrial membrane which isolates pulmonary venous flow from the left atrial body) or left atrial myxoma.

Pathophysiology and Hemodynamics

■ MS obstructs left ventricular inflow, a lesion that is overcome by an increase in left atrial pressure.

  – Elevated left atrial pressure is transmitted through the pulmonary vasculature leading to dyspnea, orthopnea, and paroxysmal nocturnal dyspnea.

    ■ Tachycardia shortens the time for left ventricular filling (diastolic filling period) and increases the trans-mitral flow rate (and thus the transmitral pressure gradient), thereby perpetuating symptoms and the hemodynamic consequences of MS.
    ■ Because of the importance of heart rate in MS, patients are frequently asymptomatic at rest with the development of symptoms with exertion or with the onset of atrial fibrillation.

  – Elevated left atrial pressure increases left atrial volume, which can lead to stasis of blood and an increased risk of thromboembolic events.

Assessment

■ History

  – The symptoms of MS typically relate to degree of obstruction and elevation of left atrial pressure.

    ■ Dyspnea
    ■ Orthopnea
    ■ Paroxysmal nocturnal dyspnea
    ■ Palpitations (if atrial fibrillation develops)
    ■ Chest discomfort
    ■ Hemoptysis
    ■ Peripheral or cerebral embolization
    ■ Fatigue
    ■ Right heart failure symptoms (including ascites, edema, and hepatomegaly)
    ■ Wasting
    ■ Importantly, all of these symptoms may acutely worsen during pregnancy, to the point of cardiogenic shock.

■ Physical examination (see Chap. 1 for important details)

  – On palpation, the apex of the heart is typically non-displaced but if there is pulmonary hypertension, a right ventricular heave may be detected.
  – Auscultation of the heart in MS is best achieved with the patient in the left lateral decubitus position, and has several important hallmarks:

    ■ Loud S1
    ■ Opening snap
    ■ Mid-diastolic rumbling murmur, which may have pre-systolic accentuation if the patient is in sinus rhythm

  In advanced cases, signs and symptoms of pulmonary congestion, pulmonary hypertension, and right heart failure may be present.

  – Atrial fibrillation is commonly present.

- ■ Echocardiography

  - – In rheumatic MS, echocardiography characteristically reveals a "hockey-stick" deformity of the anterior mitral leaflet (also described as a "doming" pattern), due to restriction of the tip of the leaflets with free motion of the body.

    - ■ The posterior leaflet is typically fixed in an apical configuration, and may be thickened with the appearance of an "onlay" lesion.
    - ■ Fusion of the commisures is best appreciated in the parasternal short-axis view on echocardiography. This view also allows for direct planimetry of the mitral valve orifice area.
    - ■ Subvalvular involvement (chordal apparatus) can be evaluated using echocardiography.
    - ■ The Wilkins scoring system, incorporating leaflet thickening, leaflet mobility, leaflet calcification and sub-valvular involvement (with each component given a score of 1–4, based on increasing severity) allows identification of patients suitable for percutaneous intervention rather than surgical intervention [33] (Table 16-7) [34].
    - ■ In calcific MS, encroachment of calcium may lead to narrowing of the orifice of the mitral valve, with relatively normal leaflet appearance.

  - – Transthoracic Doppler echocardiography is the standard method for quantifying the degree of MS (Table 16-8) [10].

    - ■ Mitral valve area is calculated from the empiric formula:

    $$MVA = 220 / PHT$$

    where MVA is mitral valve area (cm^2) and PHT is pressure half-time (s).
    - ■ Pressure Half-Time is the time for the peak pressure gradient to half and is equal to:

    $$PHT = V_{max} / 1.4$$

    where V_{max} is the peak inflow velocity (m/s).
    - ■ PHT is also directly related to the deceleration time (DT) in milliseconds and can be calculated using the equation:

    $$PHT = 0.29 \times DT$$

    - ■ Mitral valve area may be calculated using the continuity equation as well:

    $$MVA = LVOT_{VTI} \times LVOT_{CSA} / MV_{VTI}$$

    where LVOT is left ventricular outflow tract, VTI is velocity time integral, CSA is cross-sectional area.

  - – Exercise echocardiography allows evaluation of symptoms and assessment of right ventricular systolic pressure with exercise.

    - ■ An increase to >60 mmHg has been associated with adverse clinical outcomes.
    - ■ Exercise echocardiography is particularly useful in patients with MS with confusing symptoms in the context of either equivocal resting gradients or relatively normal resting pulmonary pressures.

- ■ Cardiac catheterization

  - – Catheter-based measurement of the left atrial and ventricular pressures allows calculation of the mean transmitral gradient.

    - ■ While pulmonary capillary wedge pressure can be used to estimate left atrial pressure, direct left atrial pressure measurement using transseptal puncture should be utilized to avoid incorrect gradient quantification.

TABLE 16-7

WILKINS SCORE FOR ASSESSING
APPROPRIATENESS OF
PERCUTANEOUS BALLOON MITRAL
VALVULOPLASTY

Leaflet mobility

1. Highly mobile valve leaflets with restriction at the leaflet tips
2. Mid portion and base of leaflets have reduced mobility
3. Valve leaflets move forward in diastole primarily at the base
4. No or minimal forward movement of the leaflets in diastole

Valve thickening

1. Near normal leaflets (4–5 mm)
2. Mid leaflet thickening and/or pronounced thickening of the margins
3. Thickening of the entire leaflets (5–8 mm)
4. Pronounced thickening of all leaflet tissue (> 8–10 mm)

Subvalvar disease

1. Minimal thickening of chordal structures immediately below the valve
2. Thickening of up to one third of the chordal length
3. Thickening to the distal third of the chordae
4. Extensive thickening and shortening of all chordae extending to the papillary muscle

Valve calcification

1. A single, focal area of increased echo brightness
2. Scattered areas of brightness at the leaflet margins
3. Brightness extending into the mid portion of leaflets
4. Extensive brightness throughout most of the leaflet tissue

Adapted from Wilkins et al. [33]

TABLE 16-8

SEVERITY OF MITRAL VALVE
STENOSIS

	MILD	MODERATE	SEVERE
Mean gradient (mmHg)	<5	5–10	>15
MVA (cm²)	>1.5	1.0–1.5	<1.0
Pulmonary artery systolic pressure (mmHg)	<30	30–50	>50

Adapted from Bonow et al. [10]

■ The MVA can be calculated using the Gorlin formula [11]:

$$MVA = CO / 38 \times HR \times DFP \times \sqrt{MVG}$$

where CO is cardiac output (ml/min), HR is heart rate (bpm), DFP is diastolic filling period (s), and MVG is mean valve gradient (mmHg).

■ The Hakki equation simplified the Gorlin formula for routine use in clinical practice [12]:

$$MVA = CO / \sqrt{MVG}$$

where CO (L/min) is cardiac output and MVG is mean mitral valve gradient.

Natural History

■ The progression of MS is variable, with a longer duration between rheumatic fever and symptomatic MS in temperate climates (United States and Western Europe) and a shorter duration in developing countries [32].

– In the United States, there is an asymptomatic interval of 15–20 years between rheumatic fever and the development of symptoms.

– In developed countries, symptom progression from mild to severe disability occurs over approximately 5–10 years. The hemodynamic rate of progression results in a decrease in mitral valve area of approximately 0.1 cm²/year.
– In developing countries, the intervals are considerably shorter, possibly because of the relative prevalence of rheumatic fever (leading to recurrent episodes in places of higher prevalence) and the relative lack of primary and secondary preventative measures.

■ In symptomatic patients who decline intervention (valvotomy), the 5-year survival rate is approximately 44 %. Surgical or percutaneous intervention significantly improves survival.

Management

■ Pharmacologic

– Medical treatment includes diuretics for heart failure symptoms (noting that such symptoms are an indication for gradient relief), beta-blockers to slow the heart rate (both in sinus rhythm and atrial fibrillation), digoxin for atrial fibrillation and warfarin for thromboembolic prophylaxis.
– Systemic anticoagulation

■ Indicated for thromboembolic prophylaxis in all patients with mitral stenosis and atrial fibrillation and patients in sinus rhythm with left atrial thrombus or prior thromboembolic event.
■ Beyond these indications, anticoagulation can be considered in those patients with a significantly dilated left atrium (≥55 mm) or spontaneous contrast on echocardiography [10].

■ Percutaneous mitral valvuloplasty (PMV)

– PMV is the procedure of choice for severe or symptomatic MS, provided the valve morphology is favorable [10, 35, 36].

■ In asymptomatic patients, the onset of atrial fibrillation may be a relative indication for gradient relief.
■ Reactive pulmonary hypertension during exercise is also a relative indication.
■ Short-term and long-term results of PMV are outstanding in well-selected patients [37].
■ Complications of PMV include worsened mitral regurgitation, due to leaflet tearing during balloon inflation. Thus, patients with significant degrees of regurgitation are poor candidates for the procedure and should probably be referred for surgical replacement.

■ Mitral Valve Replacement

– Surgical mitral valve replacement (MVR) is indicated when PMV is not available or is contraindicated due to thrombus in left atrium or moderate or severe mitral regurgitation.
– Surgical MVR is also indicated in those with calcific mitral stenosis and in rheumatic mitral stenosis with an unfavorable Wilkins score [33, 34].
– Surgical open commissurotomy is less commonly employed due to the improvements in PMV [35, 36, 38].

MITRAL REGURGITATION

Etiology

■ The most common causes of mitral regurgitation (MR) are organic causes, such as mitral valve prolapse (MVP) and functional causes, such as ischemic MR due to coronary artery disease [23, 32].

– MVP is the most common structural cause of MR, affecting 1–3 % of the population.

- More common in women
- More common in patients with connective tissue disorders such as Marfan syndrome, and Ehlers-Danlos syndrome.
- Most often due to myxomatous degeneration of the mitral valve leaflets and weakening/elongation of the chordae tendineae with or without rupture.
- The most common leaflet affected by MVP is the posterior, with most cases involving the middle portion of the leaflet. However, both leaflets may be affected, leading to so-called "Barlow's Syndrome".

   – MR due to ischemic heart disease is the second most common cause, and is typically due to left ventricular and/or mitral annular dilation.

- Displacement of the papillary muscles with apical tethering and incomplete mitral leaflet coaptation occurs.
- An important cause of MR from ischemic heart disease is partial or complete transection of a papillary muscle head following acute MI. This most often affects the posteromedial papillary muscle head due to the fact this zone is subtended by only one vessel (the right coronary artery).

   – Other notable causes include mitral annular calcification, rheumatic heart disease, infective endocarditis, hypertrophic cardiomyopathy (with or without systolic anterior motion of the valve), trauma, and congenital disorders.

Pathophysiology and Hemodynamics

- Three distinct phases of MR are recognized: acute MR, chronic compensated MR, and chronic decompensated MR [23, 32].

   – Acute severe MR

- Important causes of acute severe MR include transection of a papillary muscle head, rupture of a chordae tendinea (such as following isotonic exercise), or due to endocarditis.
- In acute MR, the total stroke volume is maintained (and indeed increased) by compensatory mechanisms including reduced end-systolic volume and increased preload (Frank Starling principle)
- Increased preload, decreased afterload and increased myocardial contractility (reduced left ventricular late-systolic pressure allows enhanced myocardial fiber shortening) all contribute to an increase in the measured ejection fraction.
- Although total stroke volume increases, a percentage of the stroke volume is transmitted to the left atrium, resulting in a decrease in forward stroke volume. The increase in left atrial pressure results in acute, often severe, dyspnea.

   – Chronic compensated MR

- In chronic, compensated MR, the end-diastolic volume increases due to chronic volume overload.
- Eccentric LV hypertrophy is frequently present.
- The increased end-diastolic volume and normal muscle function allows further elevation in total stroke volume, and a return to normal of forward stroke volume.
- Left atrial enlargement allows accommodation of regurgitant volume at a lower pressure, with a reduction in symptoms.

   – Chronic decompensated MR

- As myocardial dysfunction develops, the LV ejection fraction declines from a "supranormal" level to within previously normal levels.
- Consequently, an ejection fraction of <60 % should be considered abnormal.
- Symptoms may or may not be present at this point, thus vigilance regarding ventricular function is important.

Assessment

- History

  - The symptoms associated with MR depend on the phase of disease

    - In acute severe MR, the patient typically has hallmark symptoms of acutely decompensated heart failure
    - In chronic compensated MR, symptoms may be entirely absent
    - In chronic decompensated MR, symptoms may be very subtle and relate to decreased exercise tolerance and volume sensitivity.

- Physical examination (see Chap. 1 for more details)

  - Findings on physical examination associated with MR depend on the phase of the disease

    - In acute severe MR, the apical impulse is usually normal in location and hyperdynamic.
    - The murmur or acute severe MR may be quite subtle if "wide open" regurgitation is present (such as due to transection of a papillary muscle head), but when due to rupture of a chordae, the murmur is typically quite harsh.
    - In chronic forms of MR, the apical impulse may be displaced. Auscultation reveals a relatively soft first heart sound, followed by a holosystolic blowing murmur.
    - In patients with chronic MR due to MVP, a mid-systolic click may be appreciated, but as the degree of MR progresses, this may be lost.
    - Radiation of the MR murmur is dependent on the vector of regurgitation.

      - For central MR, the murmur is typically heard to radiate to the back or clavicular area.
      - For eccentric MR (such as which occurs in those with asymmetric leaflet pathology, including MVP), the murmur radiates differentially: anterior leaflet pathology results in radiation to the axilla, while posterior leaflet pathology results in radiation to the base, sometimes masquerading as AS.

    - An S3 gallop is typically present in advanced MR
    - Echocardiography [25]

      - Doppler echocardiography is useful to reveal the etiology and severity of MR.

    - In some cases trans-esophageal echocardiography is necessary to assist in identifying mechanism and severity of MR, such as papillary muscle head transection, or chordal rupture.
    - In addition, transesophageal echocardiography is sometimes necessary to accurately visualize and grade very eccentric jets of MR.
    - Transesophageal echocardiography is also useful to "map" the mitral valve prior to proposed repair (see below).

  - The severity of MR is assessed on Doppler and 2-D echocardiography using integration of multiple parameters (Table 16-9).
  - Quantification of the volume and fraction of regurgitant flow is performed by echocardiography as follows [25, 26]:

    - The proximal isovelocity surface area (PISA), also known as the flow convergence method, allows for quantification of MR as follows:

$$Q_{MR} = 2\pi r^2 \times V_a$$

$$ROA = Q_{MR} \times V_{MR}$$

where Q_{MR} is mitral regurgitant flow, r is the PISA radius, V_a is the aliasing velocity, ROA is regurgitant orifice area, and V_{MR} is the peak velocity of the regurgitant jet.

TABLE 16-9

PARAMETER	MILD	MODERATE	SEVERE
Color Doppler jet area	<4 cm² or <20 % LA area		>40 % of LA area or swirling in LA
Vena contracta (cm)	<0.3	0.3–0.7	>0.7
Regurgitant volume (mL/beat)	<30	30–60	>60
Regurgitant fraction (%)	<30	30–60	>60
Regurgitant orifice area (cm²)	<0.20	0.2–0.4	>0.40

MEASURES OF MITRAL REGURGITATION SEVERITY

Adapted from Refs. [10, 24]
LA left atrium

- Regurgitant volume is can then be calculated as:

$$RV = ROA \times VTI_{MR}$$

  where RV is regurgitant volume and VTI_{MR} the velocity time integral of the regurgitant jet.
- Systolic flow reversal in the pulmonary veins is consistent with severe MR.
- Exercise echocardiography allows assessment of pulmonary artery systolic pressure with exertion and allows evaluation of functional capacity

- Cardiac catheterization

  - Invasive assessment of the severity of MR is indicated when non-invasive data provide inadequately diagnostic information.

    - Seller's criteria, a semi-quantitative angiographic measure of MR, assesses the severity of MR based on the density of contrast in the left atrium, following injection into the left ventricle (Table 16-10) [27].

Natural History

- Natural history of MR is dependent on its cause and severity.
- Asymptomatic patients with mild MR may remain stable for many years.
- Acute severe MR has a poor short-term prognosis without intervention, regardless of the etiology.
- Following an initial compensated phase, symptomatic chronic severe MR is associated with a poor short-term prognosis without intervention [23, 32].

  - Indications for surgical intervention in chronic MR are discussed below.

Management

- Pharmacologic

  - Acute severe MR

    - Afterload reduction with intravenous vasodilators such as nitroprusside with or without intra-aortic balloon counterpulsation.
    - Intravenous inotropes are often utilized in order to increase cardiac output.

  - Chronic MR

    - Afterload reduction with ACE inhibitors and diuretic therapy for symptomatic patients.
    - Control of coronary ischemia with beta blockers.

TABLE 16-10	GRADE OF REGURGITATION	
SELLER'S CRITERIA FOR GRADING MITRAL REGURGITATION BY ANGIOGRAPHY	1	Small amount contrast enters LA in diastole and is cleared with each beat
	2	More contrast fills LA with faint opacification of the entire LA; contrast does not clear with each beat
	3	LA is well opacified with contrast density equal to the LV within 2–3 beats
	4	Complete and dense opacification of the LA on the first beat; contrast refluxes into pulmonary veins

Adapted from Maroo et al. [26]
LA left atrium, *LV* left ventricle

- There is insufficient evidence to support the use of ACE inhibitors or other vasodilators in chronic asymptomatic MR in the absence of other indications for these therapies.

- Surgical

  – Indications for surgical intervention for MR are listed in Table 16-11
  – Acute severe MR is a surgical urgency/emergency.
  – Other primary indications for surgery are the presence of symptoms, and/or the development of reduced ejection fraction.
  – Mitral valve repair is preferred to mitral valve replacement and ideally, should be performed for the majority of patients with MR.

    - Repair is preferred due to its favorable effects on LV function, the durability of the repair, and the ability to avoid long-term anticoagulation [10, 39, 40].
    - Mitral valve surgery is reasonable in asymptomatic patients with severe MR and preserved LV function if the likelihood of valve repair is >90 % [10].
    - In asymptomatic patients with severe MR due to MVP, it is reasonable to consider surgery for those with new onset atrial fibrillation or elevated pulmonary artery systolic pressure (>50 mmHg at rest or >60 mmHg during exercise), particularly if the valve is repairable.

  – In patients with MR due to ischemia undergoing surgery for other reasons (e.g. bypass surgery), the decision to repair or replace the valve should be made prior to the procedure, as the degree of MR decreases by a full grade under anesthesia.
  – Mitral valve repair for MVP typically involves resection of the prolapsed section of the valve ("quadrangular resection"), with the insertion of an annuloplasty ring to reduce the orifice size.
  – Mitral valve replacement is typically achieved with implantation of either a bioprosthesis or mechanical tilting disc valve, the latter of which has a longer life span.

TRICUSPID STENOSIS (TS)

Etiology

- Rheumatic heart disease is the most common (>90 %) cause of TS.

  – Rheumatic TS is characterized by fusion and thickening of the leaflets and shortening of the chordae tendinae.
  – Isolated TS is very rare and coexisting mitral stenosis is almost always present [41].

	CLASS
Symptomatic patients with acute severe MR	Class I
Symptomatic patients with chronic severe MR in the absence of severe LV dysfunction (LV EF <30 %) and/or ESD >55 mm	Class I
Asymptomatic patients with chronic severe MR and LV systolic dysfunction (LV EF ≤50 %)	Class I
Asymptomatic patients with chronic severe MR and mild to moderate LV dysfunction (LV EF 30–60 %) and/or ESD ≥40 mm	Class I
MV repair is recommended over MV replacement in the majority of patients	Class I
Asymptomatic patients with chronic severe MR with preserved LV function (LV EF >60 % and ESD <40 mm) if likelihood of MV repair is >90 %	Class IIa
Asymptomatic patients with chronic severe MR with preserved LV function and new onset atrial fibrillation or pulmonary hypertension (PASP >50 mmHg at rest or >60 mmHg with exercise)	Class IIa
Severely symptomatic patients (NYHA class III or IV) with chronic severe MR due to primary valve dysfunction and severe LV dysfunction (LV EF <30 %) and/or ESD >55 mm if MV repair is likely	Class IIa
Patients with chronic severe secondary MR and severe LV dysfunction (LV EF <30 %) and/or ESD >55 mm with severe symptoms (NYHA class III or IV) despite optimal therapy and cardiac resynchronization	Class IIb

TABLE 16-11

INDICATIONS FOR MITRAL VALVE SURGERY FOR MITRAL REGURGITATION

Adapted from Bonow et al. [10]
EF ejection fraction, *ESD* end-systolic dimension, *LV* left ventricular, *MR* mitral regurgitation, *MV* mitral valve, *NYHA* New York Heart Association, *PASP* pulmonary artery systolic pressure

- Carcinoid syndrome, the second most common cause of TS, exposes the right heart to serotonin and other vasoactive substances leading to endocardial and valvular damage by means of myofibroblast proliferation, collagen deposition, and inflammation [42, 43].

  - Concomitant left sided disease is rare but occurs in patients with a patent foramen ovale or lung metastases [44]

- Other causes of TS include infective endocarditis, congenital tricuspid atresia, right atrial tumors, endomyocardial fibrosis, extracardiac tumors, pacemaker leads, and drug induced.

Pathophysiology and Hemodynamics

- Structural changes in the tricuspid valve apparatus prevent proper opening of the valve during diastole and subsequent RV inflow leading to elevated RA pressure and a diastolic pressure gradient between the RA and RV.
- Resting cardiac output is markedly reduced and passive venous congestion ensues.
- A gradient of at least 2 mmHg is sufficient to establish a diagnosis of TS, while a gradient of ≥5 mmHg is enough to cause systemic venous congestion.

Assessment

- History

  - Symptoms of TS are very nonspecific and include those of congestion of the right heart.

    - Neck fluttering or fullness
    - Fatigue
    - Abdominal fullness, particularly in the right upper quadrant
    - Protein losing enteropathy is more common in TS

- Physical examination (see Chap. 1 for more details)

  - Physical findings in TS include marked elevation of neck veins, cannon A waves, as well as a mid-diastolic rumbling murmur that increases with inspiration.

- Echocardiography [44]

  - Transthoracic echocardiography demonstrates a thickened, calcified tricuspid valve with restricted mobility and diastolic doming.
  - In carcinoid syndrome, tricuspid valve leaflets are retracted and have a "frozen appearance".
  - Right atrial and IVC enlargement are common.
  - Hemodynamically significant TS is identified by:

    - Mean gradient >5 mmHg
    - Peak velocity approaching 2 m/s
    - Valve area by continuity equation ≤1.0 cm2
    - Pressure half time ≥190 ms

  - Color Doppler will often demonstrate concomitant tricuspid regurgitation (TR).

- Cardiac Catheterization

  - Simultaneous RA and RV pressure tracings demonstrate significant diastolic gradient between the two chambers which increases with inspiration and decreases with expiration.
  - Other common findings include elevated RA pressure with very tall *a* wave and low cardiac output.
  - With concomitant MS, the left atrial, pulmonary artery, and right ventricular pressures may be significantly elevated.

Management

- Pharmacologic

  - Medical therapy for tricuspid stenosis is limited to diuretics and sodium restriction in order to minimize peripheral edema.

- Surgical

  - Timing of surgery for severe, rheumatic TS is usually dictated by severity of left-sided lesions.
  - Surgical options include:

    - Open valvotomy: The stenotic tricuspid valve is converted into a functionally bicuspid valve (commissure between anterior and posterior leaflet is not opened for fear of developing severe TR) [32].
    - Valve replacement is the procedure of choice in select patients with carcinoid-related TS and when valvuloplasty or open valvotomy is not feasible or unsuccessful.

- Percutaneous

  - Percutaneous balloon valvuloplasty is feasible and safe, but experience with the procedure is limited [45].
  - Hemodynamic and symptomatic improvement is often attained, but there are high rates of TR after balloon valvuloplasty.

TRICUSPID REGURGITATION

■ Mild TR is common and found in up to 70 % of adults [46].

Etiology

■ Functional (secondary) TR is most common cause of acquired TR and may occur due to left-sided heart disease (particularly mitral valve disease), pulmonary hypertension, or right ventricular infarction [47].
■ Organic (primary) TR can be caused by rheumatic heart disease, carcinoid syndrome, infective endocarditis, myxomatous disease/prolapse, pacemaker leads, repeated endomyocardial biopsies after cardiac transplant, trauma, connective-tissue disorders, drug-induced, and endomyocardial fibrosis.
■ In carcinoid syndrome and rheumatic disease, mixed TS and TR are common.
■ Congenital causes of TR include Ebstein's anomaly, pulmonic stenosis (functional), Eisenmenger's syndrome (functional due to pulmonary hypertension), perimembranous VSD (due to formation of septal aneurysm with tricuspid valve tissue), and cleft tricuspid valve with AV canal defects (discussed in Chap. 20)

Pathophysiology and Hemodynamics

■ Tricuspid annular and right ventricular dilatation leads to functional TR, while in organic TR, structural changes in the tricuspid valve apparatus prevent proper coaptation at end-diastole and lead to subsequent incompetence [47].
■ TR results in RV volume overload and when severe will lead to poor cardiac output and passive systemic venous congestion.
■ TR is dynamic and the degree of TR can change with the respiratory cycle [48].
■ RA and RV pressure are also usually elevated with significant TR even if pulmonary hypertension is not present.

Assessment

■ History

  – Symptoms from TR are rare unless severe regurgitation is present.
  – If symptomatic, complaints related to right heart failure predominate, as with TS.

■ Physical examination (see Chap. 1 for more details)

  – The jugular venous pressure is usually elevated, with a prominent 'v' wave

    ■ This may lead to overestimation of filling pressures if TR is not recognized.

  – A low frequency holosystolic murmur along the left sternal border is typically present.

    ■ This murmur increases with inspiration.

  – Parasternal heave and a right-sided S3 gallop (increasing with inspiration) may also be present.
  – A pulsatile liver is frequently palpable in severe TR
  – Lower extremity edema

■ Echocardiography [25]

  – Transthoracic echocardiography can help to identify valve morphology and grade severity of TR.
    ■ The valve may appear structurally normal in functional TR but coaptation may be poor when TR is severe.
    ■ Pulmonary artery systolic pressure may be elevated and should be estimated by applying the modified Bernoulli equation to the peak TR velocity:

$$P = 4V_{TR}^2 + RA \text{ pressure}$$

    where P is the pulmonary artery systolic pressure gradient across the tricuspid valve, V_{TR} is velocity of the TR jet (m/s) and RA is right atrial.
    ■ Color Doppler is useful to grade TR

      – Severe TR is characterized by regurgitant jet area >10 cm^2, vena contracta width >0.7 cm, and systolic flow reversal in the hepatic vein.

    ■ Dilated right heart chambers and inferior vena cava, paradoxical septal motion, and septal flattening in diastole are also present with significant TR and indicative of right ventricular (RV) volume overload.

■ Cardiac Catheterization

  – The right atrial (RA) waveform demonstrates a large right atrial c-*v* wave ("ventricularization" of RA pressure), absence of x descent, and rapid and prominent *y* descent.
  – A RV or pulmonary arterial pressure >55 mmHg suggests that the TR is secondary, while a RV pressure <40 mmHg suggests a primary cause of TR [32].

Management

■ Pharmacologic

  – Diuretic therapy and sodium restriction are the primary therapies for TR.
  – For functional TR, treatment of the primary left-sided lesion is also appropriate.
  – Vasodilators are beneficial in the setting of LV dysfunction.

■ Surgical

  – Tricuspid valve repair (annuloplasty ring) is indicated for severe TR in patients with mitral valve disease undergoing mitral valve surgery [10].
  – Functional TR in the absence of pulmonary hypertension and annular dilatation generally does not require surgery [32].
  – Tricuspid valve repair is preferred over replacement; however, patients with organic TR with abnormal leaflets will need valve replacement.
  – Valvectomy with delayed valve replacement (6–9 months after initial surgery) is a reasonable option for TR without pulmonary hypertension due to endocarditis in IV drug users [32].

PULMONIC STENOSIS

Etiology

■ Congenital pulmonic stenosis (PS), the most common etiology, is discussed in Chap. 20 and may be sub-valvular, valvular, or supra-valvular.
■ The most common acquired cause of PS is carcinoid disease. PS due to carcinoid often occurs in conjunction with tricuspid valve disease [25, 44].

■ Rheumatic heart disease rarely can lead to fusion of pulmonary valve cusps.
■ Functional PS can be due to extrinsic compression of the right ventricular outflow tract by tumor.

Pathophysiology

■ PS is characterized by RV pressure load that leads to RV hypertrophy.

– RV dysfunction presents in late stages of the disease.

Assessment

■ History

– Typically asymptomatic
– May lead to fatigue and right heart congestive symptoms if severe

■ Physical examination (see Chap. 1 for more details)

– Palpation may reveal an RV heave or a thrill, but both are rare
– Auscultation findings include a harsh systolic murmur that increases with inspiration.
– Associated congenital lesions may be present, including right to left shunting with cyanosis.

■ Echocardiography

– Leaflet fusion (rheumatic)
– Retraction (carcinoid)
– Thickening with systolic doming (congenital)
– Subvalvular/infundibular stenosis (congenital)
– Continuous wave Doppler helps with assessing severity of lesion (peak gradient: mild <36 mmHg, moderate 36–64 mmHg, and severe >64 mmHg) [44].

■ Cardiac catheterization

– Simultaneous pulmonary artery and RV pressure measurements can confirm pulmonic valve gradient when echocardiography is inconclusive regarding the severity of PS.

Management

■ Therapy for congenital PS is balloon valvuloplasty (discussed in Chap. 20).
■ PS due to carcinoid syndrome may necessitate valve replacement.
■ Management of pregnant patients with PS is discussed in Chap. 20.

PULMONIC REGURGITATION

■ Mild pulmonic regurgitation (PR) is observed in nearly 80 % of healthy adults [25].

Etiology

■ Pulmonary arterial hypertension is the most common cause of PR, followed by infective endocarditis.
■ Marfan syndrome can cause pulmonary arterial dilation and concomitant PR.
■ Other rare causes of PR include rheumatic heart disease, carcinoid disease, congenital heart disease, and trauma.

Pathophysiology

- PR is characterized by RV volume overload.
- Early stages of disease are well tolerated unless occurring with significant pulmonary hypertension.
- Late stages of disease are manifested by RV enlargement and dysfunction.

Assessment

- History

  - Almost always asymptomatic
  - If severe, PR may result in right sided congestive symptoms.

- Physical examination (see Chap. 1 for more details)

  - Decrescendo murmur heard best over the lower left sternal border

- Echocardiography is the primary means of imaging and grading PR [25].

  - 2D imaging can identify valve morphology and motion (doming or prolapse), RV enlargement/hypertrophy, RV function, and pulmonary arterial dilatation.

Management

- Surgical correction of PR is rarely necessary.
- PR secondary to pulmonary arterial hypertension and infective endocarditis usually improve with treatment of the underlying condition.
- In cases of severe PR following tetralogy of Fallot repair with intractable right heart failure, valve replacement with a bioprosthesis or allograft is usually recommended.

REVIEW QUESTIONS

1. A 64-year-old male with no known cardiovascular history is referred for cardiac consultation for a heart murmur. The patient has remained active without cardiovascular symptoms. Physical examination reveals a blood pressure of 105/40 mmHg and an exaggerated carotid upstroke. In addition, a II/VI, blowing, diastolic murmur is heard along the right sternal border and a II/VI diastolic rumble is noted at the apex. An echocardiogram is obtained demonstrating severe aortic regurgitation, a left ventricular ejection fraction of 55 %, and left ventricular end systolic dimension of 57 mm.

   What is the best next step in the management of this patient?

   (a) Initiation of an angiotensin-converting enzyme inhibitor
   (b) Percutaneous mitral balloon valvuloplasty
   (c) Surgical aortic valve replacement
   (d) Exercise echocardiography
   (e) Hospital admission for nitroprusside infusion

2. A 58-year-old lady with no known medical history presents to her primary care physician for routine evaluation. She is asymptomatic without exertional dyspnea, heart failure symptoms, or palpitations. Physical examination reveals a loud first heart sound and a mid-diastolic rumble. A transthoracic echocardiogram was performed and shows rheumatic mitral stenosis with a mean gradient of 7 mmHg. The pulmonary artery systolic pressure is 40 mmHg. She is in normal sinus rhythm. She has a valve morphology that is suitable for percutaneous balloon valvuloplasty.

   Which of the following is the next best step?

   (a) Percutaneous balloon valvuloplasty
   (b) Mitral valve replacement
   (c) Transesophageal echocardiogram
   (d) Exercise echocardiography
   (e) Right and left heart catheterization with coronary angiography

3. A previously asymptomatic 73-year-old man with a history of mitral valve prolapse and mild mitral regurgitation presents to his primary care physician with a 4-month history of dyspnea on moderate exertion. Physical examination reveals a Grade III/VI holosystolic murmur, loudest at the apex, and radiating to the axilla. Transthoracic echocardiography reveals severe mitral regurgitation and evidence of rupture of a chordae tendineae to the posterior leaflet. Left ventricular function and dimensions are normal (ejection fraction 65 %).

   Which of the following is the next best step?

(a) Immediate transfer to the Emergency Department for management of acute severe MR.

(b) Exercise echocardiography, 24 h Holter and transesophageal echocardiography.

(c) Elective mitral valve repair.

(d) Elective mitral valve replacement.

(e) Continue with optimal medical therapy, and annual echocardiographic assessment of left ventricular function.

4. A 43-year-old male with a history of hypertension and IV drug abuse presents with a 1-week history of fever and productive cough. Physical exam reveals jugular venous distension, an early systolic mumur at the left sternal border which increases with inspiration, and lower extremity edema. Chest x-ray reveals bilateral infiltrates. Laboratory data is as follows:

Sodium 132 mEq/L

Potassium 3.6 mEq/L

Chloride 100 mEq/L

Bicarbonate 24 mEq/L

Urea Nitrogen 35 mg/dL

Creatinine 1.2 mg/dL

WBC Count: 15.3×10^3/mL

Hematocrit: 34.8 %

Hemoglobin 11.6 g/dL

Platelets 332×10^3/mL

What is the most likely diagnosis?

(a) Community acquired pneumonia

(b) Tricuspid valve endocarditis

(c) Acute mitral regurgitation due to ruptured chordae tendinae

(d) Flow murmur related to iron-deficiency anemia and fever

(e) Pulmonic regurgitation

ANSWERS

1. (c) Surgical aortic valve replacement. Asymptomatic severe aortic regurgitation is an indication for surgical aortic valve replacement in the presence of left ventricular dysfunction (ejection fraction ≤50 %; Class I) or severe dilatation (end diastolic dimension >75 mm or end systolic dimension >55 mm). Vasodilators are the mainstay of therapy for asymptomatic severe aortic regurgitation if surgery is not yet indicated. They may be used for hemodynamic optimization prior to surgery, but the patient presented here has no evidence of heart failure and has a relatively low blood pressure. While the patient has a diastolic murmur in the mitral position ("Austin-Flint" murmur), indicative of severe AR, the mitral valve is morphologically normal without mitral stenosis on echocardiography. Exercise testing is reasonable in patients with severe AR for assessment of functional status and symptoms, although the role of observed changes in left ventricular function with exercise are unclear. Poor exercise tolerance in an "asymptomatic" patient with normal left ventricular size and function may be used to justify aortic valve replacement in the absence of other clear reason. Nitroprusside infusion is useful for afterload reduction in patients with severe acute aortic regurgitation.

2. (d) Exercise echocardiography. Asymptomatic moderate mitral stenosis in the absence of elevated pulmonary artery systolic pressure (>50 mmHg at rest; >60 mmHg with exercise) is not an indication for percutaneous balloon valvuloplasty or mitral valve surgery. In addition, when suitable, percutaneous balloon valvuloplasty is preferred to mitral valve surgery for rheumatic mitral stenosis. Exercise echocardiography would be useful to evaluate the pulmonary artery systolic pressure with exercise, and to observe the exercise capacity, which may reveal previously unidentified symptoms. Transesophageal echocardiography is necessary prior to percutaneous balloon valvuloplasty to assess for left atrial thrombus and moderate to severe mitral regurgitation, both of which are Class III indications (contraindications) for the procedure. There is no indication for right and left heart catheterization and coronary angiography based on the information supplied. A 24 h Holter Monitor may be useful in assessing for atrial fibrillation, which, if present, would be a Class IIb indication for percutaneous balloon valvuloplasty in the setting of moderate asymptomatic mitral stenosis.

3. (c) Elective mitral valve repair. Mitral valve prolapse is one of the most prevalent cardiac valvular abnormalities, and spontaneous rupture of the chordae tendineae is the most common cause of intensification of the MR. The patient described above presents with symptomatic chronic severe MR. Surgical intervention for symptomatic chronic severe MR is recommended. Exercise echocardiography and 24 h Holter monitor recording will not aid in the decision making process for this patient. Transesophageal echocardiography may be necessary to define the valvular abnormality and assess the suitability for repair in some cases. Mitral valve repair is preferable to replacement, as preservation of the mitral apparatus leads to better post-operative LV function and survival. In addition, the risks of chronic anticoagulation are avoided. Continuing with medical therapy alone is inappropriate in patients with symptomatic severe MR who are candidates for surgical intervention.

4. (b) Tricuspid valve endocarditis. Individuals with intravenous drug abuse have a high incidence of staphylococcal infection including endocarditis. This patient presents with an early systolic murmur which increases with inspiration and jugular venous distension – findings which are consistent with a murmur of tricuspid regurgitation. The jugular venous pulse characteristically demonstrates an elevated v wave and prominent y descent. Septic emboli due to tricuspid valve endocarditis typically travel to the lung and present with cough and pulmonic infiltrates on chest x-ray. Community acquired pneumonia can present with a productive cough and can occur in a patient with IV drug abuse, but this answer does not explain the murmur and jugular venous distension. Acute mitral regurgitation may present with an early systolic murmur, but the murmur is heard best at the apex and should not vary in intensity with the respiratory cycle. Flow murmurs are usually mid-systolic and are best heard at the base. The murmur of pulmonic regurgitation is typically diastolic.

REFERENCES

1. Selzer A. Changing aspects of the natural history of valvular aortic stenosis. N Engl J Med. 1987;317:91–8.
2. Mohler 3rd ER, Gannon F, Reynolds C, et al. Bone formation and inflammation in cardiac valves. Circulation. 2001;103:1522–8.
3. O'Brien KD, Shavelle DM, Caulfield MT, et al. Association of angiotensin-converting enzyme with low-density lipoprotein in aortic valvular lesions and in human plasma. Circulation. 2002;106:2224–30.
4. Otto CM, Kuusisto J, Reichenbach DD, et al. Characterization of the early lesion of 'degenerative' valvular aortic stenosis. Histological and immunohistochemical studies. Circulation. 1994;90:844–53.
5. Rajamannan NM, Subramaniam M, Rickard D, et al. Human aortic valve calcification is associated with an osteoblast phenotype. Circulation. 2003;107:2181–4.
6. Goldbarg SH, Elmariah S, Miller MA, et al. Insights into degenerative aortic valve disease. J Am Coll Cardiol. 2007;50:1205–13.
7. Michelena HI, Desjardins VA, Avierinos JF, et al. Natural history of asymptomatic patients with normally functioning or minimally dysfunctional bicuspid aortic valve in the community. Circulation. 2008;117:2776–84.
8. Roberts WC, Janning KG, Ko JM, et al. Frequency of congenitally bicuspid aortic valves in patients >/=80 years of age undergoing aortic valve replacement for aortic stenosis (with or without aortic regurgitation) and implications for transcatheter aortic valve implantation. Am J Cardiol. 2012;109:1632–6.
9. Blais C, Burwash IG, Mundigler G, et al. Projected valve area at normal flow rate improves the assessment of stenosis severity in patients with low-flow, low-gradient aortic stenosis: the multicenter TOPAS (Truly or Pseudo-Severe Aortic Stenosis) study. Circulation. 2006;113:711–21.
10. Bonow RO, Carabello BA, Chatterjee K, et al. 2008 Focused update incorporated into the ACC/AHA 2006 guidelines for the management of patients with valvular heart disease: a report of the American College of Cardiology/American Heart Association Task Force on Practice Guidelines (Writing Committee to Revise the 1998 Guidelines for the Management of Patients With Valvular Heart Disease): endorsed by the Society of Cardiovascular Anesthesiologists, Society for Cardiovascular Angiography and Interventions, and Society of Thoracic Surgeons. J Am Coll Cardiol. 2008;52:e1–142.
11. Gorlin R, Gorlin SG. Hydraulic formula for calculation of the area of the stenotic mitral valve, other cardiac valves, and central circulatory shunts. I. Am Heart J. 1951;41:1–29.
12. Hakki AH, Iskandrian AS, Bemis CE, et al. A simplified valve formula for the calculation of stenotic cardiac valve areas. Circulation. 1981;63:1050–5.
13. Otto CM, Pearlman AS, Gardner CL. Hemodynamic progression of aortic stenosis in adults assessed by Doppler echocardiography. J Am Coll Cardiol. 1989;13:545–50.
14. Cheitlin MD, Gertz EW, Brundage BH, et al. Rate of progression of severity of valvular aortic stenosis in the adult. Am Heart J. 1979;98:689–700.
15. Rosenhek R, Binder T, Porenta G, et al. Predictors of outcome in severe, asymptomatic aortic stenosis. N Engl J Med. 2000;343:611–7.
16. Novaro GM, Katz R, Aviles RJ, et al. Clinical factors, but not C-reactive protein, predict progression of calcific aortic-valve disease: the Cardiovascular Health Study. J Am Coll Cardiol. 2007;50:1992–8.
17. Ross Jr J, Braunwald E. Aortic stenosis. Circulation. 1968;38:61–7.
18. Cowell SJ, Newby DE, Prescott RJ, et al. A randomized trial of intensive lipid-lowering therapy in calcific aortic stenosis. N Engl J Med. 2005;352:2389–97.
19. Rossebo AB, Pedersen TR, Boman K, et al. Intensive lipid lowering with simvastatin and ezetimibe in aortic stenosis. N Engl J Med. 2008;359:1343–56.
20. Chan KL, Teo K, Dumesnil JG, et al. Effect of Lipid lowering with rosuvastatin on progression of aortic stenosis: results of the aortic stenosis progression observation: measuring effects of rosuvastatin (ASTRONOMER) trial. Circulation. 2010;121:306–14.
21. Leon MB, Smith CR, Mack M, et al. Transcatheter aortic-valve implantation for aortic stenosis in patients who cannot undergo surgery. N Engl J Med. 2010;363:1597–607.
22. Cribier A, Savin T, Saoudi N, et al. Percutaneous transluminal valvuloplasty of acquired aortic stenosis in elderly patients: an alternative to valve replacement? Lancet. 1986;1:63–7.
23. Freeman RV, Otto CM. Aortic valve disease. In: Fuster V, Walsh R, Harrington R, editors. Hurst's the heart. 13th ed. New York, NY: McGraw-Hill; 2010.
24. Stout KK, Verrier ED. Acute valvular regurgitation. Circulation. 2009;119:3232–41.
25. Zoghbi WA, Enriquez-Sarano M, Foster E, et al. Recommendations for evaluation of the severity of native valvular regurgitation with two-dimensional and Doppler echocardiography. J Am Soc Echocardiogr. 2003;16:777–802.
26. Maroo A, Deedy M, Griffin BP. Aortic valve disease. In: Griffen BP, Topol EJ, editors. Manual of cardiovascular medicine. 2nd ed. Philadelphia, PA: Lippincott Williams & Wilkins; 2004.
27. Sellers RD, Levy MJ, Amplatz K, et al. Left retrograde cardioangiography in acquired cardiac disease: technic, indications and interpretations in 700 cases. Am J Cardiol. 1964;14:437–47.
28. Bolen JL, Alderman EL. Hemodynamic consequences of afterload reduction in patients with chronic aortic regurgitation. Circulation. 1976;53:879–83.
29. Greenberg BH, DeMots H, Murphy E, et al. Beneficial effects of hydralazine on rest and exercise hemodynamics in patients with chronic severe aortic insufficiency. Circulation. 1980;62:49–55.
30. Lin M, Chiang HT, Lin SL, et al. Vasodilator therapy in chronic asymptomatic aortic regurgitation: enalapril versus hydralazine therapy. J Am Coll Cardiol. 1994;24:1046–53.
31. Bonow RO, Nikas D, Elefteriades JA. Valve replacement for regurgitant lesions of the aortic or mitral valve in advanced left ventricular dysfunction. Cardiol Clin. 1995;13:73–83, 5.
32. Otto CM, Bonow RO. Valvular heart disease. In: Libby P, Bonow RO, Mann DL, Zipes EP, editors. Braunwald's heart disease: a textbook of cardiovascular medicine. 8th ed. St. Louis, MO: W.B. Saunders; 2007.
33. Wilkins GT, Weyman AE, Abascal VM, et al. Percutaneous balloon dilatation of the mitral valve: an analysis of echocardiographic

variables related to outcome and the mechanism of dilatation. Br Heart J. 1988;60:299–308.

34. Abascal VM, Wilkins GT, O'Shea JP, et al. Prediction of successful outcome in 130 patients undergoing percutaneous balloon mitral valvotomy. Circulation. 1990;82:448–56.

35. Palacios IF. Farewell to surgical mitral commissurotomy for many patients. Circulation. 1998;97:223–6.

36. Reyes VP, Raju BS, Wynne J, et al. Percutaneous balloon valvuloplasty compared with open surgical commissurotomy for mitral stenosis. N Engl J Med. 1994;331:961–7.

37. Palacios IF, Sanchez PL, Harrell LC, et al. Which patients benefit from percutaneous mitral balloon valvuloplasty? Prevalvuloplasty and postvalvuloplasty variables that predict long-term outcome. Circulation. 2002;105:1465–71.

38. Ben Farhat M, Ayari M, Maatouk F, et al. Percutaneous balloon versus surgical closed and open mitral commissurotomy: seven-year follow-up results of a randomized trial. Circulation. 1998;97:245–50.

39. Enriquez-Sarano M, Schaff HV, Orszulak TA, et al. Valve repair improves the outcome of surgery for mitral regurgitation. A multivariate analysis. Circulation. 1995;91:1022–8.

40. Gillinov AM, Cosgrove DM, Blackstone EH, et al. Durability of mitral valve repair for degenerative disease. J Thorac Cardiovasc Surg. 1998;116:734–43.

41. Hauck AJ, Freeman DP, Ackermann DM, et al. Surgical pathology of the tricuspid valve: a study of 363 cases spanning 25 years. Mayo Clin Proc. 1988;63:851–63.

42. Moller JE, Connolly HM, Rubin J, et al. Factors associated with progression of carcinoid heart disease. N Engl J Med. 2003;348:1005–15.

43. Simula DV, Edwards WD, Tazelaar HD, et al. Surgical pathology of carcinoid heart disease: a study of 139 valves from 75 patients spanning 20 years. Mayo Clin Proc. 2002;77:139–47.

44. Baumgartner H, Hung J, Bermejo J, et al. Echocardiographic assessment of valve stenosis: EAE/ASE recommendations for clinical practice. J Am Soc Echocardiogr. 2009;22:1–23.

45. Al Zaibag M, Ribeiro P, Al Kasab S. Percutaneous balloon valvotomy in tricuspid stenosis. Br Heart J. 1987;57:51–3.

46. Singh JP, Evans JC, Levy D, et al. Prevalence and clinical determinants of mitral, tricuspid, and aortic regurgitation (the Framingham Heart Study). Am J Cardiol. 1999;83:897–902.

47. Taramasso M, Vancrmen H, Maisano F, et al. The growing clinical importance of secondary tricuspid regurgitation. J Am Coll Cardiol. 2012;59:703–10.

48. Topilsky Y, Tribouilloy C, Michelena HI, et al. Pathophysiology of tricuspid regurgitation: quantitative Doppler echocardiographic assessment of respiratory dependence. Circulation. 2010;122:1505–13.

CHAPTER 17

RORY B. WEINER AND AARON L. BAGGISH

Dilated, Restrictive/Infiltrative, and Hypertrophic Cardiomyopathies

CHAPTER OUTLINE

ABBREVIATIONS

ACE	Angiotensin converting enzyme
AF	Atrial fibrillation
ANA	Anti-nuclear antibody
AR	Aortic regurgitation
ARB	Angiotensin receptor blocker
ARVC	Arrhythmogenic right ventricular cardiomyopathy
BNP	B-type natriuretic peptide
CAD	Coronary artery disease
CMV	Cytomegalovirus
CRT	Cardiac resynchronization therapy
CT	Computed tomography
CXR	Chest x-ray
DCM	Dilated cardiomyopathy
E'	Early peak diastolic tissue velocity
ECG	Electrocardiogram
HCM	Hypertrophic cardiomyopathy
HIV	Human immunodeficiency virus
HOCM	Hypertrophic obstructive cardiomyopathy
ICD	Implantable cardioverter defibrillator
LV	Left ventricle or left ventricular
LVEF	Left ventricular ejection fraction
LVH	Left ventricular hypertrophy
LVOT	Left ventricular outflow tract
MR	Mitral regurgitation
MRI	Magnetic resonance imaging
NTproBNP	N-terminal pro B-type natriuretic peptide
RV	Right ventricle or right ventricular
SAM	Systolic anterior motion
SCD	Sudden cardiac death
SPEP	Serum protein electrophoresis

Electronic supplementary material
The online version of this chapter (doi:10.1007/978-1-4471-4483-0_17)
contains supplementary material, which is available to authorized users.

TABLE 17-1

TYPICAL FEATURES OF THE VARIOUS FORMS OF CARDIOMYOPATHY

PARAMETER	DCM	RESTRICTIVE/ INFILTRATIVE	HCM
Definition	Ventricular dilation/ impaired contractility	Impaired ventricular filling due to decreased compliance	Marked LVH in the absence of a pressure load
Common causes	CAD	Myocardial infiltration (amyloid, sarcoid, hemochromatosis)	Familial
	Valve disease	Endomycardial (Löeffler's endocarditis)	Sporadic
	Idiopathic		
	Familial		
	Infectious		
	Toxin		
Classic echocardiographic findings	Ventricular dilation ± thrombus	↑ wall thickness	LVH (asymmetric)
	↓ LVEF	Biatrial enlargement	SAM
	MR		LVOT gradient

INTRODUCTION

Cardiomyopathies represent a heterogeneous group of heart muscle diseases that are a major cause of morbidity and mortality [1, 2]. Classification schemes for cardiomyopathy have been complex, and efforts have been made to classify the disease states based on myocardial characteristics and etiologies [3]. The etiology, diagnosis, and management of dilated cardiomyopathy (DCM), restrictive/infiltrative cardiomyopathy, and hypertrophic cardiomyopathy (HCM) are the subject of this chapter and several features of each form of cardiomyopathy are highlighted in Table 17-1.

DCM

Definition

■ Ventricular dilation and impaired contractility (left ventricle [LV] and/or right ventricle [RV]); typically normal LV wall thickness
■ Prevalence 1.2,500

Etiology [4]

■ Cardiac causes: Ischemia/coronary artery disease (CAD); valvular heart disease (i.e. chronic volume overload from aortic regurgitation [AR] or mitral regurgitation [MR])
■ Idiopathic (possibly undiagnosed genetic mutations [titin] or infectious causes)
■ Familial (20–35 % of DCM): mutations in contractile sarcomeric, nuclear envelop, and transcriptional coactivator proteins

– Defined as DCM of unknown cause in two or more closely related family members

■ Infectious

– Viral (i.e. Coxsackie, Adenovirus, cytomegalovirus [CMV], human immunodeficiency virus [HIV])
– Bacterial (i.e. Lyme), Fungal, Parasitic (Chagas disease, typically LV apical aneurysm)

■ Toxic

– Alcohol, cocaine
– Chemotherapeutic agents: anthracyclines (increased risk with dose >550 mg/m^2), cyclophosphamide, trastuzumab

FIGURE 17-1

Transthoracic echocardiogram from a patient with DCM (parasternal long-axis view) demonstrating LV dilation (*red line* shows the increased LV inner dimension at end-diastole)

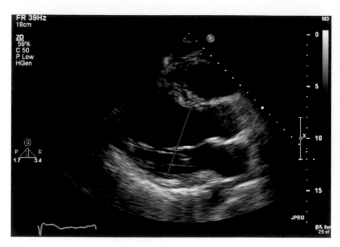

- Tachycardia-mediated: proportional to heart rate and duration of tachycardia
- Stress-induced (Takotsubo): classically apical ballooning (other variants possible); post menopausal women in response to psychological or physiological stressor
- LV noncompaction: prominent trabeculations, particularly in LV apex
- Infiltrative cardiomyopathy: can present as a mix of DCM and restrictive cardiomyopathy; LV systolic dysfunction more common in late-stage disease.
- Arrhythmogenic right ventricular cardiomyopathy (ARVC): fibrofatty tissue replacement, can also involve the LV
- Metabolic: hypothyroidism, pheochromocytoma, acromegaly, thiamine deficiency
- Peripartum: final month of pregnancy to first 5 months after delivery
- Autoimmune

  - Collagen vascular disease (i.e. systemic lupus erythematosus, scleroderma, polymyositis, rheumatoid arthritis, polyarteritis nodosa)
  - Idiopathic giant cell myocarditis: can be fulminant in presentation
  - Eosinophilic: hypersensitivity (mild) or acute necrotizing (severe)

History/Physical Examination and Diagnostic Evaluation

- Chest pain with certain etiologies (coronary artery disease, myocarditis)
- Elicit history of alcohol or drug use, current or past exposure to chemotherapy, and the ability of the patient to perform daily activities.
- Careful family history for ≥3 generations
- Symptoms and signs of left and/or right sided heart failure (dyspnea, orthopnea, jugular venous distention, lower extremity edema)
- Diffuse and laterally displaced point of maximal impulse, S3 gallop, murmur (i.e. MR)
- *Initial diagnostic evaluation*

  - 12-lead electrocardiogram (ECG): Evaluate for poor R wave progression, Q waves, left atrial enlargement, bundle branch block, atrial fibrillation (AF)
  - Chest x-ray (CXR): Increased cardiac silhouette, pleural effusions, Kerley B lines
  - Transthoracic echocardiogram (Fig. 17-1 and Video 17-1): LV dilation, decreased LV ejection fraction (LVEF), global or regional LV hypokinesis, MR (papillary muscle displacement and incomplete mitral valve closure), RV dilation and hypokinesis, LV thrombus
  - Laboratory studies: complete blood count, serum electrolytes, blood urea nitrogen and serum creatinine, fasting blood glucose or hemoglobin A1C, urinalysis, lipid profile, liver function tests, and thyroid-stimulating hormone.
  - Measurement of natriuretic peptides (BNP and NT-proBNP) can be useful in the urgent care setting in patients in whom the diagnosis of heart failure is uncertain.

■ *Disease-specific evaluation*

  – Ischemic (CAD):

    ■ Stress test: useful if negative, but can have high false positive rate, even with imaging
    ■ Coronary computed tomography (CT) angiogram: most useful when low pre-test probability
    ■ Coronary angiography [5]

      – Should be performed in patients with angina or ischemia unless the patient is not eligible for revascularization of any kind (Class I, Level of Evidence B)
      – Reasonable for patients who have chest pain that may or may not be cardiac in origin who have not had evaluation of their coronary anatomy and who have no contraindication to revascularization (Class IIa, Level of Evidence C)
      – Reasonable in patients who have known or suspected CAD but who do not have angina, unless the patient is not eligible for revascularization of any kind (Class IIa, Level of Evidence C)

  – Cardiac magnetic resonance imaging (MRI): useful in evaluation of myocarditis or infiltrative disease
  – Iron studies, anti-nuclear antibody (ANA), serum protein electrophoresis (SPEP), HIV, selenium, thiamine, etc. based on clinical suspicion for specific causes

■ Endomyocardial biopsy [6]

  – New-onset heart failure of <2 weeks' duration with hemodynamic compromise (Class I, Level of Evidence B)
  – New-onset heart failure of 2 weeks' to 3 months' duration and new ventricular arrhythmias, second- or third-degree heart block, or failure to respond to usual care within 1–2 weeks (Class I, Level of Evidence B)
  – Should not be performed as a part of routine evaluation (Class III, Level of Evidence C) [5]

Treatment and Prognosis

■ Identification and treatment of underlying cause if possible
■ See Chaps. 14 and 15 for detailed treatment including medical therapy (β-blocker, angiotensin converting enzyme [ACE] inhibitor or angiotensin receptor blocker [ARB], aldosterone antagonist), device therapy (implantable cardioverter defibrillator [ICD], cardiac resynchronization therapy [CRT])
■ Consideration of reversibility is needed before implantation of device therapy
■ Immunosuppression for giant cell myocarditis, eosinophilic disease, collagen vascular disease and peripartum cardiomyopathy
■ Prognosis depends on etiology, worst for ischemic cardiomyopathy [4]; overall, DCM most frequent cause of heart transplantation
■ Screening of family members for familial DCM (after other more common causes, i.e. CAD, cardiotoxic agents, etc.) have been excluded [7]

  – Genetic testing should be considered for the 1 most clearly affected person in a family to facilitate family screening and management
  – Clinical screening (history, physical exam, ECG, echocardiogram) for DCM in asymptomatic 1st degree relatives is recommended; interval of screening depends on genotype status
  – Genetic and family counseling is recommended for all patients and families with familial DCM

RESTRICTIVE AND INFILTRATIVE CARDIOMYOPATHY

Definition

- Impaired ventricular filling (restrictive filling) due to decreased compliance in the absence of pericardial disease
- Normal or decreased volume of both ventricles associated with biatrial enlargement; normal or increased LV wall thickness

Etiology [8]

Myocardial

- Infiltrative

    - Amyloidosis [9]: primary (AL), familial (transthyretin), senile; more common in males, average age of presentation approximately 60 years

        - evaluate for systemic signs and symptoms (nephrotic syndrome, peripheral neuropathy, macroglossia, etc.).

    - Sarcoidosis: conduction abnormalities, arrhythmia (i.e. ventricular tachycardia); clinical evidence of myocardial involvement in ~5 % of patients with sarcoidosis (20–30 % show cardiac involvement at autopsy) [10]
    - Hemochromatosis: liver function abnormalities, diabetes, skin hyperpigmentation

- Storage diseases: Gaucher's, Fabry's (neuropathic pain, impaired sweating, skin rashes; can mimic HCM), Hurler's, glycogen storage disease
- Autoimmune (scleroderma, polymyositis-dermatomyositis)
- Diabetes mellitus
- Friedrich's ataxia (gait abnormalities)
- Idiopathic

Endomyocardial

- Löeffler's endocarditis (hypereosinophilic syndrome): temperate climates, mural thrombi that have embolic potential
- Endomyocardial fibrosis: tropical regions (Africa), variable eosinophil levels

    - Bimodal incidence peak at ages 10 and 30
    - Echocardiography shows apical fibrosis of LV and/or RV, giant atria, restrictive Doppler filling pattern on mitral inflow (similar findings can be seen in Loeffler's, which may also have localized thickening of the posterobasal LV wall)

- Radiation
- Serotonin: carcinoid, ergot alkaloids, serotonin agonists

History/Physical Examination and Diagnostic Evaluation

- Right > left-sided heart failure
- Peripheral edema refractory to diuretics
- Tachyarrhythmias (i.e. ventricular tachycardia)
- Thromboembolic complications
- Increased jugular venous pressure with hepatojugular reflux; S4 ± S3
- Edema: sacral, ascites, lower extremity edema

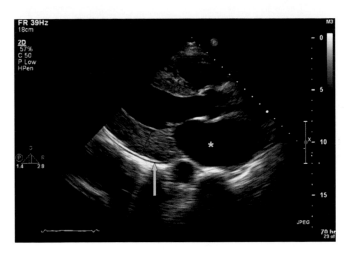

FIGURE 17-2

Transthoracic echocardiogram from a patient with amyloidosis (parasternal long-axis view) demonstrating increased wall thickness (*red lines*), left atrial enlargement (*yellow asterisk*), and a trace pericardial effusion (*blue arrow*)

■ 12-lead ECG: low-voltage in amyloidosis, pseudoinfarct pattern (Q waves), arrhythmia (atrial or ventricular), conduction abnormalities

■ CXR: Normal size cardiac silhouette, atrial enlargement

■ Transthoracic echocardiogram

- Increased wall thickness
- Biatrial enlargement
- Short deceleration time (<160 ms)
- Mitral and tricuspid regurgitation
- Reduced early peak diastolic tissue (E') Doppler velocity (<10 cm/s)

■ Echocardiographic features of specific disease states:

- Amyloid (Fig. 17-2 and Video 17-2): granular myocardial texture, biventricular wall thickening, valve thickening, small pericardial effusion
  Sarcoid: basal septal wall motion abnormality

■ Cardiac MRI: late gadolinium enhancement pattern

- Amyloidosis: diffuse throughout both ventricles, particularly the subendocardium
  Sarcoidosis: patchy, basal and lateral LV walls

■ Cardiac catheterization for hemodynamic evaluation

  Dip and plateau (*square root sign*) in the ventricular pressure tracing (Fig. 17-3a): deep and rapid early decline in ventricular pressure at the onset of diastole, with a rapid rise to a plateau in early diastole

- The dip and plateau manifests in the atrial pressure tracing as a prominent y descent followed by a rapid rise and plateau. The x descent may also be rapid. The combination results in the M or W characteristic waveform in the atrial pressure tracing (Fig. 17-3b)
- Square root sign and M or W pattern are typical for restriction, but are also characteristic of pericardial constriction. Differentiating features of restrictive cardiomyopathy and constrictive pericarditis are highlighted in Table 17-2.

■ Endomyocardial biopsy: heart failure with unexplained restrictive cardiomyopathy (Class IIa, Level of Evidence C) [6]

- Specific for ruling out certain diseases (i.e. amyloidosis)

Treatment and Prognosis

■ Identification and treatment of underlying cause if possible

- There is no specific treatment for idiopathic restrictive cardiomyopathy

FIGURE 17-3

Hemodynamic pressure tracings obtained at cardiac catheterization in a patient with restrictive cardiomyopathy. (**a**) The characteristic hemodynamic feature of restrictive cardiomyopathy (as well as constrictive pericarditis) is a deep and rapid decline in ventricular pressure at the onset of diastole (*red arrow*), with a rapid rise to a plateau in early diastole (*blue arrow*). This dip and plateau is referred to as the *square root sign*. (**b**) Right atrial pressure tracing showing a prominent y descent (*red arrow*) followed by a rapid rise and plateau. The x descent is also rapid (*green arrow*). The combination results in the M or W waveform

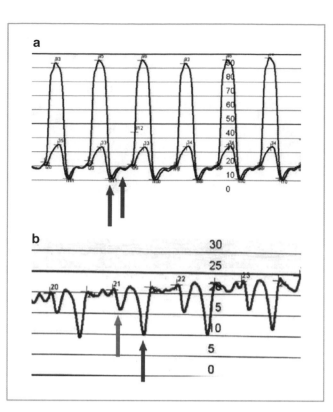

TABLE 17-2		

FEATURES OF RESTRICTIVE CARDIOMYOPATHY COMPARED WITH CONSTRICTIVE PERICARDITIS

FEATURE	RESTRICTION	CONSTRICTION
Physical exam	± Kussmaul's sign Powerful PMI Murmurs of MR or TR	+ Kussmaul's sign Absent PMI + Pericardial knock
Echocardiogram	Increased wall thickness Biatrial enlargement Reduced E′ MR / TR frequent *Normal* respiratory variation of mitral E velocity	Normal wall thickness Septal "bounce" Increased E′ MR / TR infrequent *Exaggerated* respiratory variation of mitral E velocity
CT/MRI	Normal pericardium	Thick pericardium
Cardiac catheterization	LVEDP>RVEDP RVSP>55 mmHg RVEDP < 1/3 RVSP *Concordance* of LV and RV pressure peaks with respiration	LVEDP=RVEDP RVSP<55 mmHg RVEDP > 1/3 RVSP *Discordance* of LV an RV pressure peaks during respiration
Endomyocardial biopsy	± Specific etiology	Typically normal

LVEDP LV end-diastolic pressure, *PMI* point of maximal impulse, *RVEDP* RV end-diastolic pressure, *RVSP* RV systolic pressure, *TR* tricuspid regurgitation

- ■ Heart rate control and maintenance of sinus rhythm to improve diastolic filling
- ■ In clinical syndrome of heart failure, use of medical therapy including ACE inhibitor and β-blocker
- ■ Diuretics as tolerated to reduce pulmonary and systemic congestion
- ■ Digoxin is proarrhythmic in amyloidosis
- ■ Poor prognosis in symptomatic restrictive cardiomyopathy

  – 37 % survival at 10 years in symptomatic idiopathic restrictive cardiomyopathy [11]

- ■ Refractory cases may require cardiac transplantation

HCM

Definition

- Marked LV hypertrophy (LVH), typically ≥15 mm (and/or RV hypertrophy) in the absence of a hemodynamic pressure load to produce the hypertrophy
- LV morphology is variable. Common geometric variants include:

    - Concentric/non-obstructive
    - Septal predominant ± obstruction (≥1.3:1 septal to posterior wall thickness ratio)
    - Apical
    - Apical predominant

- Prevalence 0.2 % (1 in 500) [12]
- Pathology characterized by myocyte fiber disarray and hypertrophy
- LV outflow tract [LVOT] obstruction can result from several factors: hypertrophied interventricular septum, systolic anterior motion (SAM) of the anterior mitral valve leaflet, and abnormal papillary muscle location

    - LVOT obstruction increased with decreased preload (volume depletion) or increased contractility

Etiology

- Differentiate HCM from other causes of LVH: hypertension, aortic stenosis, athlete's heart, Fabry's disease, sarcoidosis, LV noncompaction

    - HCM vs. athlete's heart

        - Most difficult to distinguish in cases of concentric LVH induced by isometric (pressure) training; less overlap with eccentric LVH induced by isotonic (volume) training
        - "Gray zone" LV wall thickness of 13–15 mm
        - Adjunctive features that favor athlete's heart: dilated LV cavity, symmetric LVH, regression of LVH with detraining, no family history of sudden cardiac death (SCD) [13]

- HCM is 50 % sporadic/gene mutation negative; 50 % familial with clearly identifiable gene mutation

    - Familial: autosomal dominant mutations in cardiac sarcomere genes (i.e. β-myosin heavy chain, cardiac troponin, etc.)

History/Physical Examination and Diagnostic Evaluation

- Majority are asymptomatic
- Dyspnea: can be the result of diastolic dysfunction or MR due to SAM
- Angina: can result from microvascular dysfunction in the absence of epicardial coronary artery disease or from concomitant CAD
- Palpitations or syncope: arrhythmia (atrial or ventricular)
- SCD: ≤1 % annually [14]

    - Risk factors for SCD (Table 17-3)

Risk factors	TABLE 17-3
Personal history of unexplained syncope	
Family history of SCD	RISK FACTORS FOR SCD IN HCM
LV wall thickness ≥30 mm	
Systolic blood pressure increase <20 mmHg with exercise	
Ventricular arrhythmia on Holter monitor	
Possible: delayed gadolinium enhancement on cardiac MRI	

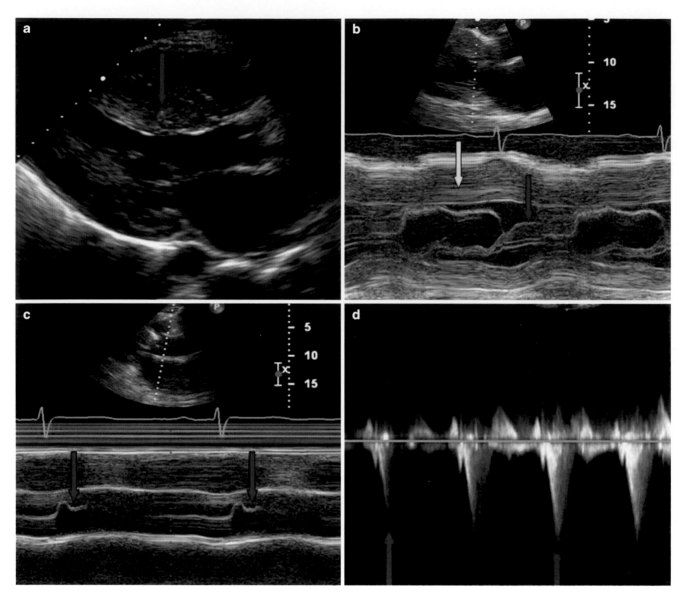

FIGURE 17-4

(**a**) Transthoracic echocardiogram from a patient with septal predominant HOCM (parasternal long-axis view) demonstrating asymmetric LVH (markedly thickened interventricular septum; *red arrow*). (**b**) M-mode of a parasternal long-axis view demonstrating SAM of the mitral valve (*red arrow*). Note the markedly thickened interventricular septum (*yellow arrow*). (**c**) M-mode of a parasternal long-axis view demonstrating mid-systolic closure (*red arrows*) of the aortic valve. (**d**) Continuous wave Doppler demonstrating a late-peaking systolic gradient in the LVOT at rest (*red arrow*), which is dynamic and increases with the Valsalva maneuver (*blue arrow*)

- Bisferiens carotid pulse (double peak)
- Sustained point of maximal impulse
- Systolic crescendo-decrescendo murmur at the left-lower sternal border: increased with Valsalva maneuver and standing (decreased preload)
- Apical holosystolic murmur (MR) may be present
- 12-lead ECG: voltage criteria LVH ± ST-segment and T wave abnormalities

    - Prominent T wave inversions in leads V5–V6 suggestive of apical variant

- Transthoracic echocardiogram (Fig. 17-4 and Video 17-3)

    - Typical wall thickness ≥15 mm or septum to posterior wall thickness ratio ≥1.3:1
    - SAM and posteriorly directed MR in hypertrophic obstructive cardiomyopathy (HOCM)

- – Mid-systolic closure of the aortic valve in HOCM
- – Dynamic, late-peaking LVOT gradient (i.e. dagger shaped) in HOCM

- ■ Stress testing: assess blood pressure response to exercise, and ischemia if symptoms of chest pain or angina equivalent
- ■ Holter monitoring: assess for subclinical ventricular arrhythmia
- ■ Cardiac MRI: Assess for LVH and delayed hyperenhancement

    - – Useful in cases of suspected HCM with equivocal echocardiograms
    - – Subsets with LV apical aneurysm or myocardial crypts

- ■ Cardiac catheterization

    - – Coronary angiography to exclude concomitant CAD in symptomatic patients with an intermediate to high likelihood of CAD (Class I, Level of Evidence C) [15]
    - – Measure LVOT pressure gradient
    - – Brockenbrough sign: post-extrasystolic beat demonstrates decreased pulse pressure (due to increased contractility and obstruction resulting in decreased systolic pressure)

Treatment and Prognosis [15]

- ■ Medical therapy to treat symptoms (negative inotropy/chronotropy): β-blocker, verapamil and/or disopyramide
- ■ Attempt to avoid vasodilators and diuretics
- ■ Avoid digoxin
- ■ Consider anticoagulation with warfarin in the setting of AF regardless of $CHADS_2$ score
- ■ Competitive sport restriction [16]

    - – Participate in Class IA sports only (golf, billiards, bowling, cricket, curling, riflery)

- ■ If obstructive physiology and symptoms refractory to medical therapy, consider septal reduction therapy with surgical myectomy, or alcohol septal ablation in patients with prohibitive surgical risk

    In a nonrandomized retrospective evaluation of HOCM patients <65 years old, survival free from recurrent symptoms favored myectomy over ablation (89 % vs. 71 %, p=0.01) [17]
    - – Procedural success is associated with very low mortality (<1 % for myectomy; 0–4 % for ablation)
    - – High-grade atrioventricular block requiring permanent pacemaker can occur in 10–20 % of patients undergoing septal ablation [18]

- ■ Dual chamber pacemaker with shortened AV delay (useful if pacemaker indicated for other reasons; not a first-line therapy)
- ■ ICD for SCD prevention typically considered if at least one risk factor (Table 17-3) is present
- ■ Family Screening [15]

    - – Evaluation of familial inheritance and genetic counseling is recommended as part of the assessment of patients with HCM (Class I, Level of Evidence B)
    - – Screening (clinical, with or without genetic testing) is recommended in 1st degree relatives of patients with HCM (Class I, Level of Evidence B)
    - – Genetic testing is reasonable in the index patient to facilitate the identification of 1st degree family members at risk of developing HCM (Class IIa, Level of Evidence B)
    - – Genetic testing is not indicated in relatives when the index patient does not have a definitive pathogenic mutation (Class III, Level of Evidence B)
    - – Clinical screening: transthoracic echocardiography and ECG

        - ■ Age <12 years: optional, unless symptoms, patient is a competitive athlete, or high risk features in the family
        - ■ Age 12 to 18–21 years: every 12–18 months
        - ■ Age >18–21 years: every 5 years or at onset of symptoms (can be more frequent in families with high risk features)

REVIEW QUESTIONS

1. A 34-year-old man who previously immigrated from South America presents with difficulty swallowing. He also reports palpitations and ambulatory monitoring reveals non-sustained ventricular tachycardia. He therefore has a transthoracic echocardiogram (TTE). Figure 17-5 shows the TTE apical four-chamber view with contrast administration to better delineate the borders of the left ventricular apex. Which of the following is true regarding this diagnosis?
   (a) It is caused by a previous viral infection
   (b) It is part of an inherited familial syndrome
   (c) It is caused by infection with *Tyrpanosoma cruzi*
   (d) It is the result of iron overload

2. A 62-year-old man presents with several months of increasing dyspnea and lower extremity edema. He also reports numbness in his extremities and lightheadedness with standing. A transthoracic echocardiogram parasternal long-axis view is shown in Fig. 17-6. Which of the following is true of the diagnosis?
   (a) QRS voltage is increased on 12-lead ECG
   (b) Renal disease is uncommon in this disease

   (c) An abdominal fat pad aspirate is a useful diagnostic procedure
   (d) Cardiac involvement portends a favorable prognosis

3. Differentiation of pericardial constriction and restrictive cardiomyopathy has important treatment implications. The following are all typical features of restrictive cardiomyopathy, except:
   (a) Discordance of LV and RV pressure peaks with respiration
   (b) Increased wall thickness on echocardiography
   (c) Pulmonary hypertension
   (d) Normal pericardium on CT or MRI

4. A 19-year-old male basketball player has syncope during a basketball game. A transthoracic echocardiogram is consistent with the diagnosis of hypertrophic obstructive cardiomyopathy (HOCM). All of the following are accepted risk factors for sudden cardiac death (SCD) in this condition, except:
   (a) Personal history of unexplained syncope
   (b) Family history of SCD
   (c) Systolic blood pressure increase <20 mmHg with exercise
   (d) Maximum left ventricular wall thickness ≥20 mm

FIGURE 17-5

TTE apical four-chamber view with contrast administration to better delineate the borders of the left ventricular apex

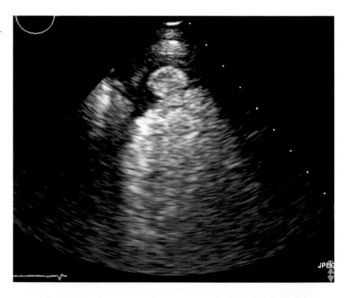

FIGURE 17-6

TTE parasternal long-axis view showing classic features of cardiac amyloidosis in primary (AL) amyloidosis

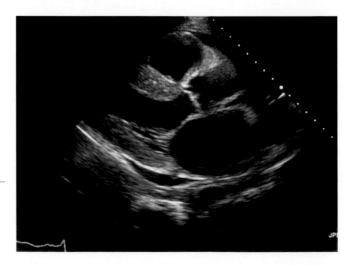

ANSWERS

1. (c) A left ventricular (LV) apical aneurysm, as seen in the TTE image, is a manifestation of Chagas cardiomyopathy. Chagas disease is caused by infection with the protozoan Trypanosoma cruzi. The disease is prevalent in Central and South America. The major cardiovascular manifestation is an extensive myocarditis that typically becomes evident years after the initial infection. Ten to 15 % of asymptomatic patients have evidence of apical aneurysm on echocardiography. The echocardiographic findings in advanced disease included dilated cardiomyopathy with reduced ejection fraction and increased end-diastolic and end-systolic volumes. The right ventricle can also be involved.
   Viral cardiomyopathy as a result of infection with viruses such as Coxsackie virus can result in dilated cardiomyopathy but do not classically cause an LV apical aneurysm. Familial dilated cardiomyopathy is another cause of cardiomyopathy, but does not classically cause LV apical aneurysm. Iron overload, secondary to hemochromatosis, can cause a dilated or restrictive cardiomyopathy, and is classically associated with bronze skin and diabetes mellitus.

2. (c) The TTE shows classic features of cardiac amyloidosis in primary (AL) amyloidosis. Renal, cardiac, gastrointestinal, and neurologic manifestations are typical of this disease. Orthostatic hypotension occurs in approximately 10 % of cases. The classic ECG finding is low QRS voltage despite the increased wall thickness on echocardiography. The classic echocardiographic features in addition to increased wall thickness are small ventricular chambers

and dilated atria. A small pericardial effusion and thickened valve leaflets (with regurgitation) can also be seen. Abdominal fat aspirate is a very useful diagnostic procedure, as it is safe, easy to perform and sensitive. Biopsy of the rectum, gingiva, and other tissues, including endomyocardial biopsy, can be useful if the abdominal fat aspirate is negative. The prognosis of cardiac amyloidosis is poor, with a median survival of 6 months if there is cardiac involvement.

3. (a) At cardiac catheterization, restrictive cardiomyopathy shows concordance of LV and RV pressure peaks with respiration. In contrast, pericardial constriction shows discordance of LV and RV pressure peaks during respiration. The discordance in pericardial constriction results from a dissociation of intrathoracic and intracardiac pressures and is a sign of ventricular interdependence. Distinguishing features of restriction vs. constriction are shown in Table 17-2.

4. (d) Hypertrophic cardiomyopathy is the leading cause of death in young athletes in the United States. Risk factors for sudden cardiac death (SCD) in HCM have been identified and include a personal history of unexplained syncope, family history of SCD, LV wall thickness ≥30 mm, systolic blood pressure increase <20 mmHg of exercise, and ventricular arrhythmia on Holter monitor. These features are used to determine the need for implantable cardioverter defibrillator (ICD) implantation, and an ICD is typically considered if at least one of these risk factors is present.

REFERENCES

1. Watkins H, Ashrafian H, Redwood C. Inherited cardiomyopathies. N Engl J Med. 2011;364(17).1643 56.
2. McMurray JJ. Systolic heart failure. N Engl J Med. 2010;362(3): 228–38.
3. Maron BJ, Towbin JA, Gaetano T, Antzelevitch C, Corrado D, Arnett D, et al. Contemporary definitions and classification of cardiomyopathies. Circulation. 2006;113:1807–16.
4. Felker GM, Thompson RE, Hare JM, Hruban RH, Clemetson DE, Howard DL, et al. Underlying causes and long-term survival in patients with initially unexplained cardiomyopathy. N Engl J Med. 2000;342(15):1077–84.
5. Hunt SA, Abraham WT, Chin MH, Feldman AM, Francis GS, Ganiats TG, et al. 2009 focused update incorporated into the ACC/AHA 2005 guidelines for the diagnosis and management of heart failure in adults. Circulation. 2009;119(14):e391–479.
6. Cooper LT, Baughman KL, Feldman AM, Frustaci A, Jessup M, Kuhl U, et al. The role of endomyocardial biopsy in the management of cardiovascular disease: a scientific statement from the American Heart Association, the American College of Cardiology, and the European Society of Cardiology. Circulation. 2007;116(19):2216–33.
7. Hershberger RE, Lindenfeld J, Mestroni L, Seidman CE, Taylor MRG, Towbin JA. Genetic evaluation of cardiomyopathy – a Heart Failure Society of America practice guideline. J Card Fail. 2009;15:83–97.
8. Seward JB, Casaclang-Verzosa G. Infiltrative cardiovascular diseases: cardiomyopathies that look alike. J Am Coll Cardiol. 2010;55(17):1769–79.
9. Selvanayagam JB, Hawkins PN, Paul B, Myerson SG, Neubauer S. Evaluation and management of the cardiac amyloidosis. J Am Coll Cardiol. 2007;50(22):2101–10.
10. Kim JS, Judson MA, Donnino R, Gold M, Cooper Jr LT, Prystowsky FN, et al. Cardiac sarcoidosis. Am Heart J. 2009; 157(1):9–21.
11. Ammash NM, Seward JB, Bailey KR, Edwards WD, Tajik AJ. Clinical profile and outcome of idiopathic restrictive cardiomyopathy. Circulation. 2000;101(21):2490–6.
12. Maron BJ. Hypertrophic cardiomyopathy: a systematic review. JAMA. 2002;287:1308–20.
13. Maron BJ. Distinguishing hypertrophic cardiomyopathy from athlete's heart physiological remodelling: clinical significance, diagnostic strategies and implications for preparticipation screening. Br J Sports Med. 2009;43(9).649–56.
14. Maron BJ. Contemporary insights and strategies for risk stratification and prevention of sudden death in hypertrophic cardiomyopathy. Circulation. 2010;121(3):445–56.
15. Gersh BJ, Maron BJ, Bonow RO, Dearani JA, Fifer MA, Link MS, et al. 2011 ACCF/AHA guideline for the diagnosis and treatment of hypertrophic cardiomyopathy. Circulation. 2011; 124(24):2761–96.
16. Mitchell JH, Haskell W, Snell P, Van Camp SP. Task force 8: classification of sports. J Am Coll Cardiol. 2005;45(8):1364–7.
17. Sorajja P, Valeti U, Nishimura RA, Ommen SR, Rihal CS, Gersh BJ, et al. Outcome of alcohol septal ablation for obstructive hypertrophic cardiomyopathy. Circulation. 2008;118(2):131–9.
18. Chang SM, Nagueh SF, Spencer 3rd WH, Lakkis NM. Complete heart block: determinants and clinical impact in patients with hypertrophic obstructive cardiomyopathy undergoing nonsurgical septal reduction therapy. J Am Coll Cardiol. 2003;42(2): 296–300.

CHAPTER 18

Ravi V. Shah, Ron Blankstein, and Gregory D. Lewis

Pericardial Diseases and Hemodynamics

CHAPTER OUTLINE

ABBREVIATIONS

ADA	Adenosine deaminase
ANA	Antinuclear antibody
CAD	Coronary artery disease
COPD	Chronic obstructive pulmonary disease
CRP	C-reactive protein
CT	Computed tomography
EBV	Epstein-Barr virus
ECG	Electrocardiogram
EP	Electrophysiology
ESR	Erythrocyte sedimentation rate
HBV	Hepatitis B virus
HCV	Hepatitis C virus
IPP	Intra-pericardial pressure
IVC	Inferior vena cava
LV	Left ventricular
LVEDP	Left ventricular end diastolic pressure
MRI	Magnetic resonance imaging
NSVT	Nonsustained ventricular tachycardia
PE	Pulmonary embolism
PEEP	Positive end expiratory pressure
RA	Rheumatoid arthritis
RV	Right ventricular
RVEDP	Right ventricular end diastolic pressure
RVSP	Right ventricular systolic pressure
SLE	Systemic lupus erythematosus
TB	Tuberculosis
TEE	Transesophageal echocardiography
TMP-SMX	Trimethoprim–sulfamethoxazole

Electronic supplementary material
The online version of this chapter (doi:10.1007/978-1-4471-4483-0_18)
contains supplementary material, which is available to authorized users.

INTRODUCTION

Pericardial diseases and associated hemodynamic findings represent an important but difficult area in cardiovascular physiology and disease. In this chapter, we will discuss several different key aspects of pericardial physiology and pathology, including acute and chronic inflammatory states of the pericardium, cardiac tamponade, and chronic constrictive pericarditis. The outline of each section will include a discussion of the etiology of the specific pericardial pathology, a description of salient diagnostic features (by physical examination, echocardiography, hemodynamic measurements, and/or advanced imaging techniques, where applicable), and a discussion of management and follow-up.

NORMAL PHYSIOLOGY OF THE PERICARDIUM

■ Anatomy:

– Two layers: the outermost fibrous pericardium and the inner 2-component serous pericardium (*visceral* and *parietal*); approximately 2 mm thick in non-pathologic conditions
– *Pericardial sac* between the visceral and parietal contains 35–50 ml of serous fluid
– Pericardium is by *pericardial reflections*, with the <u>left atrium and pulmonary veins mostly outside the pericardium</u>
    Phrenic nerves run adjacent to the parietal pericardium (accounting for referred phrenic nerve irritation during pericardial inflammation)
– Pericardial arteries supply blood to the dorsal portion of the pericardium

■ Physiology: Normal pericardium serves several key roles:

– "Pericardial restraint": the compliance of the pericardium varies with the volume in the heart; initially, the pericardium is supple, and can expand with minimal increases in intrapericardial pressure with cardiac filling; at higher volumes, the intrapericardial pressure rises, and impedes systemic and pulmonary venous return (Fig. 18-1). This explains why acute increases in pericardial fluid volume lead to very high intrapericardial pressures and impedance to cardiac filling and ejection (e.g., **cardiac tamponade**) whereas slowly growing effusions are more well tolerated
– Barrier to infection
– Respiratory-cardiac coupling (pericardium transmits intrathoracic pressure to the heart; for example, during inspiration, intrapleural pressure falls; normal pericardial function will transmit a negative intrapleural pressure to the heart, to decrease intracardiac pressures and provide an impetus for systemic venous return)

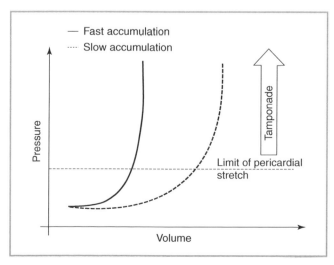

FIGURE 18-1

Pericardial restraint. Slow accumulation of pericardial fluid leads to a "give" in the pericardium, gradual increase in pericardial compliance, and a less exuberant rise in intrapericardial pressure (a higher threshold for tamponade). In rapid accumulation, the gradual increased pericardial compliance is not permitted, and tamponade ensues at a lower pericardial fluid volume (Courtesy of Dr. Hanna Gaggin)

TABLE 18-1

ETIOLOGIES AND THERAPIES
OF ACUTE PERICARDITIS

ETIOLOGY	EVALUATION	TREATMENT
Idiopathic	Standard	NSAIDs
Infectious (e.g., viral, bacterial, fungal, TB)	Viral titers/cultures, HIV, pericardial fluid analysis (ADA and PCR for TB), pericardial biopsy (rare)	Anti-infective therapy, drainage of fluid (for bacterial)
Post-MI	Standard	Aspirin (no NSAIDs due to infarct remodeling), avoid anticoagulation if possible
Aortic dissection	Urgent echocardiography or cardiac CT/MRI	Surgical (do not drain percutaneously)
Traumatic	Urgent echocardiography or cardiac CT/MRI	NSAIDs, avoid anticoagulation, close monitoring
Cancer	Standard, pericardial fluid cytology or flow cytometry/tumor markers	NSAIDs or intra-pericardial steroids, pericardial window for refractory cases
Renal failure	Standard	Intensify dialysis
Autoimmune disease	ANA, ESR, CRP, complement, anti-dsDNA	Rheumatologic evaluation, NSAIDs or steroid therapy (anti-inflammatory therapy)
Post-cardiotomy	Standard	NSAIDs, avoid anticoagulation
Drug reaction	Can be linked to autoimmune markers (see above)	Discontinue offending agents; NSAID or steroid therapy

Adapted from Lange and Hillis [4]

ACUTE PERICARDITIS

Acute pericarditis is an acute inflammatory process of the pericardium affecting both layers of the pericardium. Here, we review the clinical profile, evaluation, management, and follow-up of patients with acute pericarditis

■ Etiology (Table 18-1) – etiology often not known and ~80 % are considered idiopathic [1]

- Infections in immunocompetent hosts

  ■ Viral (e.g., HIV, coxsackievirus, adenovirus, parvovirus B19, HCV/HBV)
  ■ Bacterial (e.g., via extension from lung infection, endocarditis; Lyme disease, tuberculosis)

- Infections in immunocompromised hosts

  ■ Same as above, plus a variety of fungal or mycobacterial infections

- Autoimmune (e.g., SLE/RA, dermatomyositis, vasculitis)

  ■ Post-myocardial infarction (Dressler) syndrome (weeks after large, transmural infarction; associated with markers of systemic inflammation, e.g., elevated ESR, fever)
  ■ Drugs (e.g., procainamide, hydralazine)

- Cancer (e.g., via direct anatomic extension, pericardial metastases, or cardiac invasion; e.g., EBV-associated non-Hodgkin's lymphoma, melanoma, sarcoma, pulmonary)
- Radiation (acutely after radiation)
- Post-pericardiotomy syndrome (e.g., after cardiac surgery; usually more prominent effusions present after aortic or mitral valve surgery)
- Hemopericardium (e.g., from aortic dissection into the pericardium, traumatic, iatrogenic – EP ablation procedures, or anticoagulation-associated spontaneous bleed)

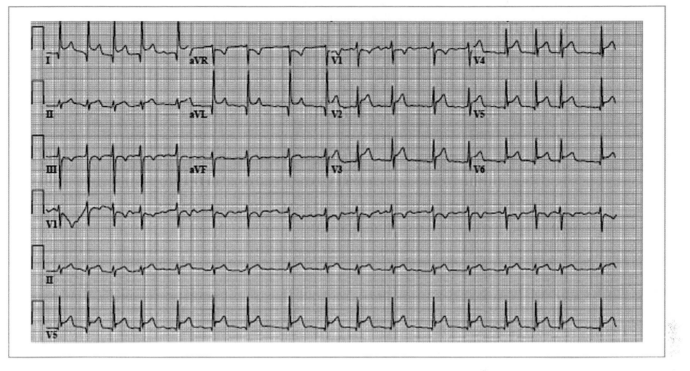

FIGURE 18-2

12-lead electrocardiogram of an 80 year old male with an aortic dissection complicated by severe aortic insufficiency and rupture of aorta into pericardium, resulting in acute pericarditis. Note rapid atrial fibrillation with associated PR depression and diffuse ST elevation

- – Endocrine disorders (e.g., thyroid disorder)
- – Uremia (e.g., patients with stage V chronic kidney disease)

■ Clinical presentation—History and Physical Examination.

- – Acute onset chest pain (sharp, pleuritic, radiation to the ipsilateral shoulder, neck and trapezius, better with sitting forward, worse while lying back)
- – Can be associated with subjective dyspnea, palpitations/supraventricular arrhythmias (e.g., new onset atrial fibrillation), or hiccups (e.g., phrenic nerve irritation)
- – **Nearly 85 % have a pericardial friction rub** on auscultation heard best at left lower sternal border; rub = movement of pericardial surfaces against each other during cardiac motion (up to 3 components: 1—ventricular systole; 2—early ventricular filling; 3—atrial contraction); variable during acute pericarditis [2]
- – Assessment should include signs of heart failure or ventricular irritability (e.g., NSVT; indicating concurrent *myocarditis*) or tamponade (see below)
- – History should focus on etiology of pericarditis (e.g., concurrent malignancy, rheumatologic disorders, recent viral infections, etc.)

■ Clinical presentation—Electrocardiography:

- – Classically described as **diffuse ST segment elevation** with **reciprocal PR depression** (most prominent in leads II and V_5–V_6; Fig. 18-2). However, opposite pattern in lead aVR where PR segment elevation may be seen and is a specific marker for pericarditis
- – Note: ECG changes can be localized to one territory, and PR changes can occur independent of ST elevations
- – Acute pericarditis can be differentiated from acute MI by (1) absence of reciprocal ST depression, (2) convexity of ST segment (vs. concave down with MI), (3) rapid evolution of ST segments to biphasic T waves and T wave inversion; (4) appearance of Q waves and (5) loss of R wave height

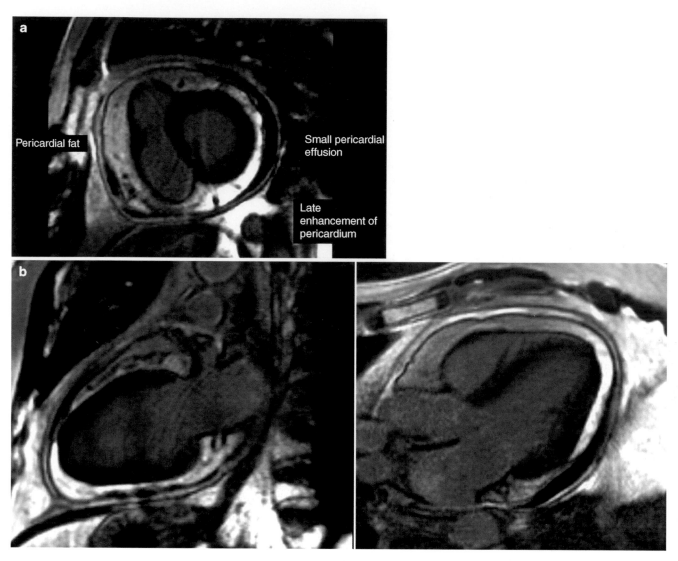

FIGURE 18-3

Late gadolinium enhancement imaging, indicating enhancement of the visceral and parietal pericardium and an associated pericardial effusion in a short-axis view (**a**), two-chamber view (**b**-left), and three-chamber view (**b**-right)

- Acute pericarditis can be differentiated from normal variant repolarization by ST to T wave height ratio in lead $V_6 > 0.25$ [3]
- ECG in acute pericarditis can progress through 4 phases: (1) ST segment elevation; (2) normal; (3) T wave inversions in same leads; (4) normal. These changes occur over a variable time period (e.g., weeks to months); nearly 80 % patients with acute pericarditis have ST-elevations at the time of initial presentation [4]

■ Clinical presentation—Laboratory and imaging findings

- Non-specific
- Elevation in ESR or CRP
- Troponin elevated in nearly 50 % of patients in one series with pericarditis, specifically in those with ST elevation [5]; no real prognostic importance [6]
- ANA often positive (~40 %) although titer usually 1:40–1:80. If higher → suspect rheumatologic disease [7]
- Chest x-ray, echocardiography usually unremarkable; used to exclude pulmonary disease, heart failure, and/or cardiac tamponade

- Cardiac MRI: pericardial inflammation/increased T2 signal of pericardium (Fig. 18-3a, b). MRI can differentiate myopericarditis (sub-epicardial enhancement) from infarction (sub-endocardial enhancement) with high accuracy.

■ Acute pericarditis: Clinical evaluation & examination

- Standard evaluation should include *complete blood count* (rule-out infection), *renal function* (rule-out uremia), *chest x-ray* (concomitant disease), *echocardiography* (underlying ventricular disease, effusion), *cardiac troponin* (serially, to exclude significant myocardial injury/acute MI), *thyroid stimulating hormone level, HIV testing, age-appropriate cancer screening,* and *ESR* (to assess for disease activity)
- Additional testing can be conducted on the basis of focused physical examination and history, including viral panels, blood investigations for infectious causes, serum rheumatologic studies (e.g., ANA panel), additional imaging studies to search for malignancy
- Cardiac MRI (for assessment of pericardial enhancement) may be used to confirm diagnosis; identify/exclude concomitant myocarditis or myocardial infarction. Coronary angiography may be considered in cases where clinical presentation is unclear with regard to acute MI vs. pericarditis, particularly if MRI not available and high suspicion for obstructive CAD
- Coronary CT angiography may be useful for excluding obstructive CAD in selected cases when suspicion for obstructive CAD lower; pericardial contrast enhancement may be visualized on CT to support presence of pericardial inflammation.

■ Acute pericarditis: Management (idiopathic only)

- Limited randomized evidence in the management of acute pericarditis
- Does the patient have to be hospitalized? Indicators of adverse clinical profile [8, 9]:

  ■ Fever
  ■ Subacute onset of symptoms (e.g., weeks-months; indicating more insidious underlying disorder)
  ■ Failure of aspirin or NSAID therapy (after at least 7 days)
  ■ Trauma
  ■ Oral anticoagulation
  ■ Evidence of myocarditis
  ■ Large effusion or tamponade

- It is important to recognize that these recommendations are for patients with idiopathic (or viral) pericarditis only; pericarditis associated with other specific underlying diseases (e.g., malignancy, trauma, aortic dissection) are treated differently
- First-line therapy: non-steroidal anti-inflammatory agents (e.g., ibuprofen 800 mg TID, indomethacin 80 mg TID) or high dose aspirin (650 mg QID) in patients with pericarditis associated with MI (as NSAIDs can impair infarct healing)

  ■ Usual duration: 14 days
  ■ Relieve chest pain in up to 90 %, generally within days of initiation [4]
  ■ Adjunct colchicine has been advocated as an *initial adjunctive therapy* with NSAIDs to prevent recurrent pericarditis (has been studied in small trials; dose 1–2 mg loading, 0.5–1.0 mg daily for 3 months) [10]

- Second-line therapy: If initial therapy is unsuccessful at relief of chest pain, add colchicine therapy and/or switch to a different NSAID [4]
- Third-line therapy: If these efforts fail, initiation of steroid therapy (prednisone 1–1.5 mg/kg/day) may prove useful, with very slow taper over the course of months

  ■ If higher dose steroids are employed, concomitant clinical prophylaxis should be implemented (e.g., TMP-SMX for P. jiroveci pneumonia; proton pump inhibitors, and osteroporosis protection)
  ■ Steroids may increase risk of recurrent pericarditis and constriction

■ Reserved for refractory pericarditis

■ Patients unable to taper steroids without recurrence of pericardial symptoms should be considered for steroid-sparing therapies (e.g., immunomodulatory agents, such as azathioprine, methotrexate) [11] or intrapericardial steroid therapy [4]

■ Acute pericarditis—Follow-up:

– Patients should be advised to refrain from vigorous exercise given the risk of ventricular and supraventricular arrhythmias until completion of NSAID therapy and resolution of symptoms

– Follow-up echocardiography is warranted if initial echocardiography demonstrated effusion (of any size) or other abnormalities; note that "constrictive physiology" by echo (see below) during initial evaluation of pericarditis should be re-assessed after a period of treatment (e.g., acute pericardial inflammation can mimic chronic constrictive pericarditis; the diagnosis of constriction should be made after recovery of acute pericardial inflammation, if possible)

– Up to 30 % patients with acute pericarditis will have recurrent pericarditis [4]

CARDIAC TAMPONADE

Major issues involving pericardial effusions revolve around (1) assessment of clinical significance (e.g., progression to tamponade) by clinical, imaging, and hemodynamic parameters and (2) therapy. Given the overlap in etiology between acute pericarditis and pericardial effusions, we will focus here on clinical evaluation and therapy of cardiac tamponade, with specific emphasis on physical examination, imaging, and hemodynamics

■ Cardiac tamponade—hemodynamics:

– Cardiac tamponade refers to impedance to cardiac filling secondary to increased intrapericardial pressures (IPP): accumulation of fluid in the pericardial sac increases IPP; when IPP exceeds central venous pressure (CVP), systemic venous return (preload) is reduced, and right ventricular (and left ventricular) stroke volume falls by a Frank-Starling mechanism. Although compensatory tachycardia may assist in initially maintaining cardiac output, hemodynamic collapse, hypotension, and cardiogenic shock will eventually occur

– It is important to recognize that tamponade can occur <u>without significant pericardial effusion</u> (though rare) if the rate of accumulation of fluid is very rapid (e.g., postoperative or trauma)

– The key hemodynamic concept is the presence of **ventricular interdependence** (an exaggerated reciprocal relationship between RV and LV filling and cardiac output with respiration due to pericardial effusion)

– Right heart hemodynamics (Fig. 18-4):

■ **Elevation in right atrial pressure** (generally >10 mmHg; *low-pressure* tamponade can occur in states of hypovolemia, and can be unmasked with a 1 l fluid challenge during catheterization, if clinically feasible)

■ **"Blunting" or loss of the *y* descent of the right atrial pressure tracing**: The *y*-descent occurs at the time of early RV filling; "pericardial restraint" impedes ventricular filling throughout the cardiac cycle (early and late diastole), leading to a very short period of initial flow from the RA into the RV in early diastole, with subsequent rise and equalization in RA and RV pressures, and restriction of further RA to RV flow (e.g., "blunted" *y* descent; this is in contradistinction to hemodynamic measurements in constriction, see below)

■ **Equalization of right and left ventricular** end-diastolic **and mean right and left atrial pressures** (equal to the IPP; this is an expression of "pericardial restraint")

■ **Pulsus paradoxus** (a > 10 mmHg inspiratory fall in systolic blood pressure is characteristic of tamponade): Explained by an inspiratory increase in venous return to the right heart, which shifts the interventricular septum to the LV side, decreasing LV filling and LV output, leading to paradoxical pulse.

- CAUTION: Other causes of paradoxical pulse exist, including severe COPD/asthma/airway obstruction, massive pulmonary embolism, RV infarction, auto-PEEP on ventilator support; therefore, the diagnosis of tamponade does not rest on demonstration of a paradoxical pulse alone.
- CAUTION: Pulsus paradoxus also may not occur in states of poor LV function or heart failure, interatrial or interventricular septal defect, or severe aortic insufficiency, even when tamponade is present, due to high venous pressures and inability to alter cardiac output with inspiration

■ **These hemodynamic features may not be seen in cases of localized tamponade** (e.g. post-cardiac surgery with pericardial hematoma posterior to the LV). **In these cases, a high index of suspicion and** direct visualization **of the pericardial collection** (e.g., via transesophageal echocardiography or cardiac MRI, or direct surgical visualization) is required

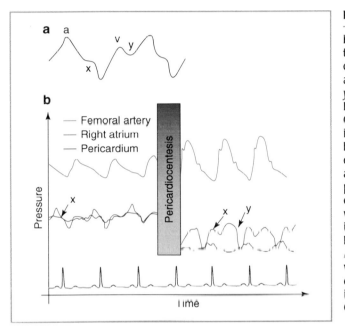

FIGURE 18-4

Hemodynamics of tamponade via right heart catheterization. (**a**) Right atrial pressure with blunted *y* descent (Courtesy of Dr. Hanna Gaggin). (**b**) Concomitant right atrial and intrapericardial pressure before and after pericardiocentesis. Note the decreased aortic pulse pressure before pericardiocentesis and the characteristic RA waveform with equalization of RA and intrapericardial pressure before relief of tamponade. After tamponade is relieved with pericardial fluid drainage, pressures normalize (Courtesy of Dr. Hanna Gaggin)

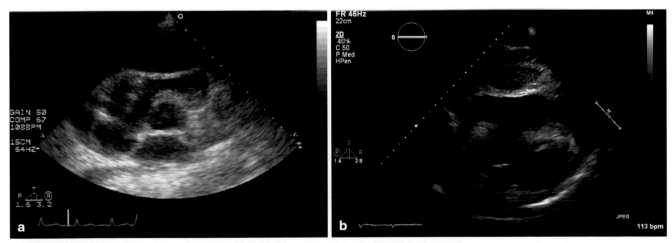

FIGURE 18-5

Echocardiography of pericardial disease (Courtesy of Dr. John Groarke, BWH). (**a**) Right ventricular collapse in two views in cardiac tamponade. (**b**) Exaggerated variation in peak E transmitral velocities with tamponade. (**c**) Cardiac tamponade by M-mode through right ventricular outflow tract. Notice M-mode evidence of diastolic inversion of the RV free wall, indicating elevated intrapericardial pressures and tamponade physiology. (**d**) M-mode echocardiogram through the RV outflow tract in the parasternal long-axis view, demonstrating diastolic collapse

FIGURE 18-5

(continued)

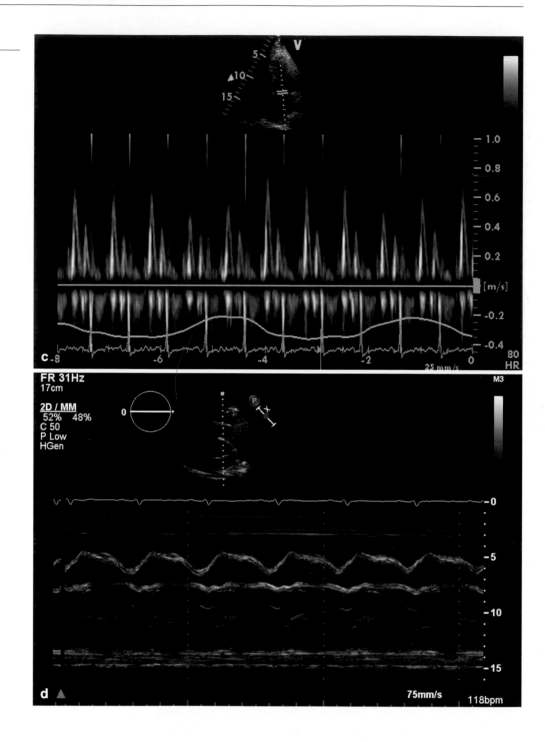

– Echocardiography in cardiac tamponade (Fig. 18-5 and Chap. 34):

■ Although transthoracic imaging is the mainstay of evaluation, transesophageal echocardiography may be required to visualize inaccessible areas prone to loculated pericardial effusion/hematoma (e.g., posterior LV). **A high index of suspicion is required (based on hemodynamics) to proceed to early TEE to make this potentially life-saving diagnosis**

■ **Large pericardial effusion (>20 mm)**: usually large, circumferential effusions are required for tamponade; however, smaller or loculated effusions (e.g., posterior to the left atrium; more difficult to visualize on transthoracic echocardiography) are possible etiologies as well

■ **Intrapericardial echoes** (strands or echogenic material): can indicate pericardial hematoma or metastatic disease

- **Right atrial systolic collapse** (inversion for >1/3 of systole, 94 % sensitivity, 100 % specificity for tamponade in presence of effusion [12]): increased IPP impairs filling of right atrium during <u>ventricular</u> systole, leading to collapse. The more severe the collapse (e.g., longer duration in systole), the higher the probability of tamponade
- **Right ventricular diastolic collapse** (60–90 % sensitive, 85–100 % specific [12]): indenting or compression of RV free wall (best seen in subcostal or parasternal long-axis view or via M-mode imaging; Videos 18-3 and 18-4) during diastole indicates high IPP impeding diastolic filling; again, the longer this occurs in diastole, the more significant the hemodynamic effect of the effusion
- **Septal shift** (during respiration; explained above in pulsus paradoxus)
- **Exaggerated respirophasic changes in mitral and tricuspid flow**: With inspiration, systemic venous return increases, leading to higher trans-<u>tricuspid</u> peak E wave velocities; pulmonary venous return decreases (due to larger lung vessels and more capacitance for pulmonary blood volume), leading to less pulmonary venous return to the left atrium and lower trans-<u>mitral</u> peak E wave velocity. These features are exaggerated during tamponade, such that a>25 % decrease in peak E wave velocity of transmitral flow is consistent with tamponade physiology
- **Dilated IVC** (>18 mm, subcostal view, with <50 % respirophasic change in diameter): Suggestive of high right atrial pressures, and supports the diagnosis of tamponade (97 % sensitive, but only 40 % specific [12])

- Cardiac tamponade—History and physical examination:

  - Clinical signs/symptoms include dyspnea (sensitivity 87–89 %), tachycardia (sensitivity 77 %), elevated jugular venous pressure (sensitivity 76 %), pulsus paradoxus (sensitivity 82 %), cardiomegaly on chest x-ray (sensitivity 89 %) [13]
  - Exam: Narrow pulse pressure ; Presence of pulsus paradoxus >10 mmHg with a large pericardial effusion yields a 3.3-fold increased likelihood of tamponade [13]
  - *Beck's triad*: elevated jugular venous pressure, hypotension, distant heart sounds
  - Clear lungs (but can be present in other conditions, e.g., massive PE, RV infarction, or severe airway obstruction/auto-PEEP)
  - Historical features should focus on similar features as acute pericarditis (aimed at etiology of pericardial disease)
    In large effusions, electrocardiogram can show evidence of **electrical alternans** (a beat to beat variation in P wave or QRS amplitude owing to "swinging" motion of the heart in the thoracic cavity) or **low QRS voltage** (<5 mm in all limb leads, and <10 mm in all precordial leads; due to insulating effect of pericardial fluid on cardiac electrical activity)
  - Initial management should carry a high index of suspicion, and should focus on bedside echocardiography to delineate hemodynamic impact of effusion on ventricular hemodynamics

- Cardiac tamponade—Management:

  - Little randomized evidence to guide therapeutic decisions
  - **Diagnosis of tamponade is clinical**; echocardiographic and right heart hemodynamics may support the clinical evaluation
  - Urgency of management (e.g., drainage vs. observation/anti-inflammatory therapy) depends on degree of hemodynamic significance and symptoms (e.g., severe dyspnea or breathlessness due to a large, but non-tamponade, effusion)
  - Surgical vs. percutaneous drainage? (surgical preferred if failed prior percutaneous drainage, loculated, or biopsy is required)
  - **Pericardial effusions without tamponade**: generally small to moderate in size (<20 mm), but patients can present with large, slowly accumulating effusions without tamponade

    - Initial management focused on pinpointing etiology (see Acute pericarditis above)

- Pericardiocentesis in small/moderate effusions has very low diagnostic yield, and is not routinely indicated (higher risk) unless specific diagnosis (e.g., infection, malignancy) is highly suspected
- For large effusions <u>without</u> tamponade, pericardiocentesis can be considered, but an initial approach of NSAID therapy is also reasonable
- Serial echocardiography and close follow-up of patients with large effusions who are not drained is required

■ **Pericardial effusion with tamponade**: hemodynamic stability governs management

- In general, percutaneous drainage (via pericardiocentesis) is indicated to prevent decompensation. **(CAUTION: in patients with suspected aortic dissection with pericardial effusion, surgical drainage only should be performed**, as percutaneous drainage could improve cardiac contractility and extend dissection)
- Right heart catheterization can be performed during pericardiocentesis to evaluate for concomitant constriction (*effusive-constrictive pericarditis*, see below under Constriction) and to assess for resolution of tamponade physiology (Fig. 18-5)
- Surgical drainage can be considered for patients with loculated effusions or where pericardial biopsy is being considered
- Generally, a pericardial drain is left in place with attendant anti-inflammatory therapy (e.g., colchicine, steroids, or NSAIDs) and discontinued only when drain output falls below a prescribed level (e.g., 25 cc/24 h)
- Serial echocardiography within 48 h of pericardiocentesis (generally before drain is discontinued) and within 48 h after drain discontinuation is critical to assess for reaccumulation
- Recurrent effusions (e.g., malignancy-related or chronic idiopathic recurrent pericarditis) can be treated with **surgical pericardiotomy** or **balloon pericardiotomy** (in the catheterization laboratory) for suitable candidates
- Pericardial fluid should be evaluated for leukocytes, hematocrit, protein content, cultures and gram stain (ADA level and additional PCR-based methods for TB), and cytology/flow cytometry (if lymphoma or malignancy is suspected)

■ Cardiac tamponade—Additional considerations:

- **Diagnostic pericardiocentesis without tamponade**

  ■ Unclear role; given higher risk of complications with smaller effusions, **can be performed only if high suspicion of specific diagnosis that has been cryptic by other methods** (e.g., malignancy, TB, or bacterial infection)
  ■ This is especially true for **purulent pericariditis** (which should be treated as a pericardial abscess and drained emergently)
  ■ Also can be performed if **large effusion unresponsive to NSAID/steroid therapy with unclear diagnosis** (e.g., behaving differently from a chronic idiopathic pericardial effusion)

- **Pericardial biopsy?**

  ■ Unclear role
  ■ Should be performed during **every** surgical drainage
  ■ Considered in patients with unclear diagnosis with persistent symptoms (>3 weeks in duration) and if diagnosis would change management (e.g., malignancy, TB, bacterial infection)

CONSTRICTIVE PERICARDITIS

Constrictive pericarditis is the end result of chronic pericardial inflammation and scarring, the physiologic outcome of both pericardial surfaces adherent to the heart. The most common etiologies of constriction are post-infectious/idiopathic (e.g., viral), post-cardiac surgical, or radiation-mediated, with others caused by autoimmune disorders, TB, or other etiologies of acute pericarditis. Of note, bacterial, TB, and malignancy-associated pericarditis carry the highest cumulative risk for subsequent constriction. Pathologically, thickened, calcified, adherent pericardium restrict diastolic cardiac filling, resulting in elevated biventricular filling pressures, right heart and systemic venous congestion (in the early stages), and decreased cardiac output (in the later stages). In this review, we will detail the clinical and hemodynamic presentation of constriction, its treatment, and differentiation from other pericardial and myocardial disease (e.g., restrictive cardiomyopathy)

■ Constrictive pericarditis—Hemodynamics (Fig. 18-6):

– The key hemodynamic manifestations of constriction rely on three major pathophysiologic observations:

■ Intrathoracic pressures are not clearly transmitted to the heart with constriction (**as opposed to tamponade**, where the pericardium itself is generally fairly normal)
■ Pericardial restraint creates ventricular interdependence (**similar to tamponade**)

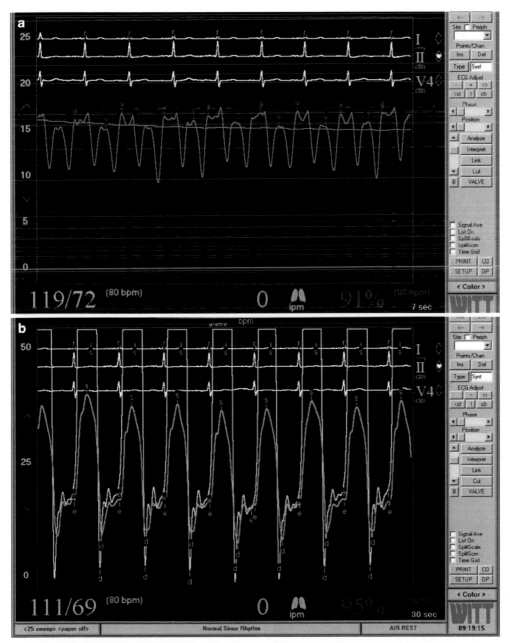

FIGURE 18-6

Hemodynamics of constrictive pericarditis by right and left heart catheterization. (Courtesy of Dr. Michael Fifer, MGH). (**a**) Right atrial pressure. Notice rapid x and y descents in this pressure tracing (in a characteristic "W" pattern, without any significant variation in mean right atrial pressure with respiration; a Kussmaul sign). (**b**) Dip and plateau in RV diastolic pressures ("square root sign"). (**c**) Concomitant RV and LV pressure tracing: Notice the end-diastolic equalization of pressures (no more than 5 mmHg difference between LVEDP and RVEDP), suggesting pericardial restraint. (**d**) An example of discordant LV and RV pressure, suggestive of restrictive cardiomyopathy (see discussion in text)

FIGURE 18-6

(continued)

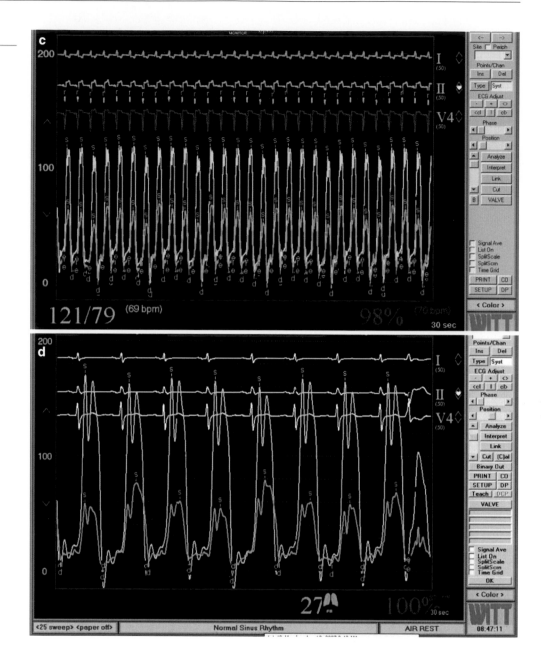

■ Early diastolic filling is usually rapid, whereas later diastolic filling is limited by the presence of a stiff, fibrotic pericardium

– During inspiration, the negative intrapleural pressure (which are transmitted to the pulmonary veins) cannot be transmitted to the heart; subsequently, the pulmonary pressures fall and capacitance increases, leading to reduced pressure gradient for left heart filling, and a lower left heart output. The septum shifts toward the left heart, and this promotes increased RV filling, leading to **ventricular interdependence** (and even a pulsus paradoxus in <20 % of patients with constriction!)

– Right heart hemodynamics: None of these features is 100 % sensitive or specific for the diagnosis of constriction. <u>The diagnosis of constriction requires the integration of clinical, hemodynamic, and imaging findings</u>.

- **Elevated right atrial pressure** (generally >10 mmHg; similar to tamponade; can be provoked by fluid challenge in patients with overdiuresis or volume depletion)
- **Failure of right atrial pressure to fall on inspiration** (hemodynamic Kussmaul sign): lack of transmission of intrapleural pressures to the RV leads to lack of increased RV filling on inspiration, and the blood cannot empty from right atrium and jugular veins into RV; this is also seen in other conditions (e.g., massive PE, RV infarction or RV failure, pulmonary hypertension)
- **Rapid x and *y* descents in the right atrial pressure tracing**: initial diastolic filling rapid in constriction, but once pericardial restraint is reached (e.g., the heart "bangs" the stiff pericardium as it tries to relax), the atrial pressure abruptly rises
- **Pulsus paradoxus** (explained above)
- **Equalization of RV and LV end-diastolic pressures with mean right and left atrial pressures** (due to pericardial restraint)
- **"Square root sign" (or "dip and plateau") in RV and LV diastolic pressures**: initial RV relaxation during diastolic is unimpeded (leading to a rapid **dip**), but once heart "bangs" into the stiff pericardium in mid-diastole, RV and LV pressures rapidly rise (leading to a **rapid rise to a plateau**)
- **Discordance of RV and LV pressure tracings**: This is the hallmark feature of constriction that distinguishes this from restrictive cardiomyopathy.

    CONSTRICTION: There is ventricular interdependence, such that the RV filling occurs at the expense of LV filling, and vice versa. Therefore, on inspiration, the peak systolic RV pressure progressively *rise* as venous return increases, while the peak LV systolic pressure *falls* (**discordance**)
    – **RESTRICTION**: In restrictive cardiomyopathy, the myocardium itself is stiff; therefore, the septum shifts and influences of respiration (e.g., ventricular interdependence) <u>does not exist</u>. As a result, the peak systolic pressures in the RV and LV track with each other during respiration (**concordance**)

- **Normal pulmonary arterial systolic pressure** (considered <55 mmHg)
- **Lack of significant difference in LVEDP and RVEDP** (no significant LV myocardial disease; defined as LVEDP-RVEDP <5 mmHg)
- **Lack of high RVEDP** (lack of significant RV myocardial disease; defined as **RVEDP/RVSP ratio <1/3**)

– Echocardiography: The hemodynamic diagnosis of constriction with echocardiography is extensive, and a full discussion of these characteristics is outside the scope of this discussion.

- **Thickened, hyper-reflective pericardium** (parasternal long-axis view)
- **Exaggerated respirophasic changes in mitral and tricuspid flow** (as in tamponade, with >25 % decrease in transmitral peak E wave velocity; >40 % increase in trans-tricuspid peak E wave velocity) Note: higher yield if fluids given
- **Diastolic septal bounce** (abnormal septal motion during diastole reflecting motion of septum during opening of mitral and tricuspid valves)
- **Decreased systolic phase and increased atrial phase** in pulmonary venous Doppler (corresponding to elevated left atrial pressures and impedance to LV filling)
- **Increased *y* descent in hepatic venous Doppler** (analogous to the right atrial waveform)
- **Hepatic venous flow reversal on inspiration** (equivalent of a Kussmaul sign)
- **Smaller ventricular volumes**
- **Preserved tissue Doppler myocardial function** (e.g., E' velocities >8 cm/s) indicating normal tricuspid and mitral annular motion. (e.g. vs. reduced motion in restrictive cardiomyopathies)

TABLE 18-2

RESTRICTIVE CARDIOMYOPATHY VERSUS CONSTRICTIVE PERICARDITIS

CHARACTERISTICS	RESTRICTIVE CM	CONSTRICTIVE PERICARDITIS
Physical examination	AV regurgitation murmurs	Pericardial knock
	S_3 and S_4 can be present	Kussmaul sign present
	Kussmaul sign present	Pulsus paradoxus can be present
	Evidence of systemic disease (e.g., amyloidosis, hemochromatosis)	Right-sided heart failure signs predominantly (e.g., ascites, edema)
	Evidence of pulmonary edema (left heart failure)	
Electrocardiogram	Low voltage can be present	Generally normal ECG
	AV block	
	Atrial or ventricular arrhythmias	
Hemodynamics	Concordance of LV/RV systolic pressure	Discordance of LV/RV systolic pressure
	LVEDP-RVEDP >5 mmHg	LVEDP-RVEDP <5 mmHg
	RVEDP/RVSP >1/3	RVEDP/RVSP <1/3
	Pulmonary hypertension	Ventricular interdependence
		No pulmonary hypertension
Therapy	Supportive care, cardiac transplantation	Diuretics, CHF management Pericardiectomy

■ **Restriction or constriction?** (Table 18-2)

   – Common clinical scenario (and likely to be represented on the Boards)
   – Your approach to distinguishing these two entities should rely on a examination of some general features
   – Features of restriction

      ■ **No ventricular interdependence** (e.g., discordance of RV/LV filling; lack of respiratory septal shift, paradoxical pulse)
      ■ **Evidence of abnormal myocardium** (e.g., decreased tissue Doppler E' velocities, valvular regurgitation and pulmonary hypertension, myocardial scar by cardiac MRI)
      ■ **Left heart symptoms predominate**

   – Table shows some salient features that differentiate these two entities.

■ Constrictive pericarditis—Management

   – Early post-operative "constriction" is likely to recover within weeks-months of initial diagnosis (e.g., with NSAID therapy), and **constriction should not be diagnosed in the acute or immediate post-operative setting**
   – The mainstay of initial management of constrictive pericarditis is **relief of congestive symptoms** with judicious diuretic therapy
   – With diuretic-refractory symptoms or low-output symptoms, pericardiectomy should be considered
   – Mortality rate for pericardiectomy is proportional to functional status at the time of surgery (in general a high peri-operative mortality between 5–15 %)
   – Careful selection for and timing of surgery critical; early pericardiectomy in medically refractory patients preferred; patients with advanced end-organ dysfunction (e.g., renal failure, malabsorption syndromes, poor nutrition, compromised perfusion) or overlying restrictive cardiomyopathy (e.g., with radiation or other myocardial diseases) fare poorly post-operatively
   – Symptoms generally improve gradually; consideration should be given to **complete** (not partial) pericardiectomy at the time of surgery given the potential for recurrent pericarditis and constriction in remaining pericardium

REVIEW QUESTIONS

1. A 32 year old female with a history of joint pain and stiffness presented with pleuritic chest pain and dyspnea. ECG demonstrates diffuse ST elevation. Physical examination demonstrates a blood pressure of 110/50 mmHg with 15 mmHg of inspiratory paradox, and a holosystolic murmur at the cardiac apex. There is no friction rub. Jugular venous pressure is 12 cm of water. The pulmonary and abdominal examinations are normal. Initial troponin T concentration was 0.25 ng/ml (reference normal <0.03 ng/ml). Chest radiograph demonstrates an enlarged cardiac silhouette. What is the next step in management?

    (a) Transthoracic echocardiography
    (b) Transesophageal echocardiography
    (c) NSAID therapy
    (d) IV fluid administration
    (e) Emergent pericardiocentesis

2. A 55-year-old male is post-operative day 2 after a mechanical aortic valve replacement for severe aortic stenosis. His medical history is significant for prior GI bleed, critical bicuspid aortic stenosis, and smoking. His current vital signs are significant for a blood pressure of 70/40 mmHg, on vasopressor support. He is intubated and not hypoxemic. Jugular venous pressure is elevated. Physical examination discloses clear lungs, and an S4 heart sound, but is otherwise normal. Hemodynamics demonstrate a central venous pressure of 12 mmHg, a pulmonary arterial diastolic pressure of 22 mmHg, a pulmonary capillary wedge pressure of 30 mmHg, and a depressed cardiac index. Emergent limited transthoracic echocardiography demonstrates normal left ventricular function with a small LV, and normal right ventricular function. Transvalvular gradients are normal. Chest tube output is normal. He is on therapeutic anticoagulation therapy for his mechanical aortic valve. What is the next step in management?

    (a) Administration of thrombolytic therapy for prosthetic valve thrombosis
    (b) Dobutamine administration for cardiogenic shock
    (c) Observation
    (d) Emergent transesophageal echocardiography
    (e) Reversal of anticoagulation

3. The patient in question (2) recovers well post-operatively. He is dismissed on post-operative day 10, and on follow-up echocardiography at 1 month, diastolic septal bounce and signs of interventricular dependence are observed on TTE (Video 18-5). The valvular gradients are normal, and there is no evidence of patient-prosthetic mismatch. There is no pericardial effusion. He has no evidence of elevated central venous pressure or peripheral edema and feels well. What is the appropriate next step in management?

    (a) Observation
    (b) Cardiac MRI or CT to evaluate for evidence of constrictive pericarditis
    (c) Steroid therapy
    (d) Pericardiectomy

4. Right heart catheterization in a dyspneic 78-year-old patient with prior mantle radiation shows:

Central venous pressure	15 mmHg
Right ventricular pressure	55/20 mmHg
Pulmonary arterial pressure	55/22 mmHg
Pulmonary capillary wedge pressure	20 mmHg
Left ventricular pressure	120/30 mmHg

Echocardiography shows normal LV function without any significant wall motion abnormalities or left ventricular hypertrophy. LV and RV pressures were not simultaneously recorded. What finding on cardiac imaging would be consistent with the primary suggested etiology of these hemodynamics?

    (a) Transmural late gadolinium enhancement of the anterior wall on cardiac MRI
    (b) A septal tissue Doppler myocardial velocity >10 cm/s
    (c) Large cardiac silhouette on chest x-ray
    (d) Lack of septal shift and transmitral peak E wave velocity on respiration

ANSWERS

1. (a) This patient shows signs of cardiac tamponade with overlying pericarditis. A TEE is not indicated as the initial evaluation, and given her clinical stability, immediate or emergent pericardiocentesis is not warranted before establishing an echocardiographic diagnosis.

2. (d) In the setting of a mechanical aortic valve and therapeutic anticoagulation, cardiac tamponade is a suspected diagnosis, especially given the absence of valvular abnormalities and normal LV function. In cases of localized left atrial tamponade, right heart hemodynamics may not always reflect diastolic equalization of pressure. An emergent TEE would visualize the oblique sinus and left atrium to identify a localized pericardial hematoma, and would interrogate the prosthetic valve. If TEE is not available or is delayed, a reasonable management would be reoperation for refractory hypotension.

3. (a) Early (within 6–8 weeks of pericardiotomy) echocardiographic "evidence" of constriction is not confirmatory evidence of constrictive pericarditis. These changes usually resolve by 1–2 months post-operatively, and should be followed, especially in the absence of symptoms. If the patient had symptoms of "volume overload," after excluding other causes of heart failure, a course of NSAID therapy with diuretic management would be appropriate, with follow-up imaging (via echocardiography or cardiac MRI) in 3 months for resolution of constrictive physiology.

4. (d) The hemodynamic profile presented above is consistent with elevated biventricular filling pressures, pulmonary hypertension, and lack of diastolic equalization of filling pressure. While this could be consistent with valvular heart disease or systolic dysfunction, these etiologies are unlikely given the normal echocardiogram. These findings could be consistent with restrictive cardiomyopathy (elevated CVP >10 mmHg; RVEDP/RVSP >1/3 with PA pressure >50 mmHg). Choice (a) represents a large anterior infarct, which is not likely given the absence of wall motion on the echocardiogram, (b) represents normal (or even supranormal) myocardial function, which is unlikely in RCM, (c) represents either a dilated cardiomyopathy or pericardial effusion, both excluded by echocardiography, and (d) represents characteristic findings on TTE for RCM.

REFERENCES

1. Imazio M, Brucato A, et al. Diagnosis and management of pericardial diseases. Nat Rev Cardiol. 2009;6(12):743–51.
2. Zayas R, Anguita M, et al. Incidence of specific etiology and role of methods for specific etiologic diagnosis of primary acute pericarditis. Am J Cardiol. 1995;75(5):378–82.
3. Ginzton LE, Laks MM. The differential diagnosis of acute pericarditis from the normal variant: new electrocardiographic criteria. Circulation. 1982;65(5):1004–9.
4. Lange RA, Hillis LD. Clinical practice. Acute pericarditis. N Engl J Med. 2004;351(21):2195–202.
5. Bonnefoy E, Godon P, et al. Serum cardiac troponin I and St-segment elevation in patients with acute pericarditis. Eur Heart J. 2000;21(10):832–6.
6. Imazio M, Demichelis B, et al. Cardiac troponin I in acute pericarditis. J Am Coll Cardiol. 2003;42(12):2144–8.
7. Imazio M, Brucato A, et al. Antinuclear antibodies in recurrent idiopathic pericarditis: prevalence and clinical significance. Int J Cardiol. 2009;136(3):289–93.
8. Imazio M, Demichelis B, et al. Day-hospital treatment of acute pericarditis: a management program for outpatient therapy. J Am Coll Cardiol. 2004;43(6):1042–6.
9. Imazio M, Cecchi E, et al. Indicators of poor prognosis of acute pericarditis. Circulation. 2007;115(21):2739–44.
10. Imazio M, Bobbio M, et al. Colchicine in addition to conventional therapy for acute pericarditis: results of the COlchicine for acute PEricarditis (COPE) trial. Circulation. 2005;112(13):2012–6.
11. Maisch B, Seferovic PM, et al. Guidelines on the diagnosis and management of pericardial diseases executive summary; the task force on the diagnosis and management of pericardial diseases of the European society of cardiology. Eur Heart J. 2004;25(7):587–610.
12. Otto CM. Pericardial disease. In: Textbook of clinical echocardiography, 2004; W.B. Saunders Company, Philadelphia, PA.
13. Roy CL, Minor MA, et al. Does this patient with a pericardial effusion have cardiac tamponade? JAMA. 2007;297(16):1810–8.
14. Sagrista-Sauleda J, Angel J, et al. Effusive-constrictive pericarditis. N Engl J Med. 2004;350(5):469–75.

CHAPTER 19

TIMOTHY C. TAN AND JUDY W. HUNG

Tumors of the Heart

CHAPTER OUTLINE

ABBREVIATIONS

AV	Atrioventricular
CCT	Cardiac Computed Tomography
EKG	Electrocardiogram
RA	Right atrium
ESR	Erythrocyte Sedimentation Rate
HCM	Hypertrophic cardiomyopathy
IAS	Inter atrial septum
IL-6	Interleukin-6
IVC	Inferior vena cava
LA	Left atrium
LV	Left ventricle
MRI	Magnetic Resonance Imaging
MR	Mitral valve regurgitation
MS	Mitral valve stenosis
PET	Positron Emission Tomography
PR	Pulmonic valve regurgitation
PS	Pulmonic valve stenosis
PND	Paroxysmal nocturnal dyspnea
RV	Right ventricle
SOB	Shortness of breath
SVC	Superior vena cava
TEE	Transesophageal echocardiogram
TIA	Transient Ischemic Attack
TR	Tricuspid valve regurgitation
TS	Tricuspid valve stenosis
TTE	Transthoracic echocardiogram
VEGF	Vascular endothelial growth factor
WBC	White Blood Cell Count

FIGURE 20-1

Lymphocyte rich infiltrate associated with myocardial necrosis in patient with acute myocarditis (Adapted from Sagar et al. [12])

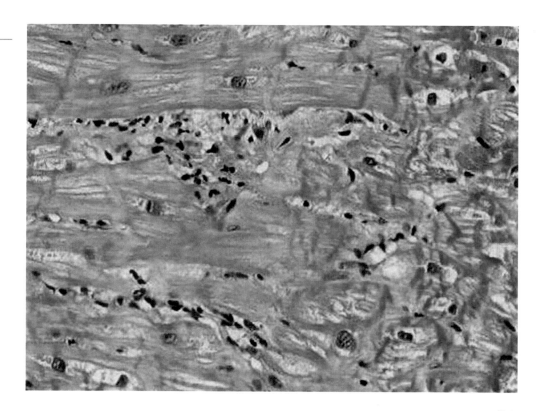

PATHOGENESIS/ETIOLOGY

■ Three stages of pathogenesis in viral myocarditis
1. Acute myocarditis with viremia and a high fatality rate.
2. Subacute myocarditis with lymphocytic infiltrates in the myocardium, increasing antibody titers and inflammatory cytokines such as interleukin (IL)-2, tumor necrosis factor (TNF)- α and interferon (IFN)-γ.
3. Chronic myocarditis with fibrosis and progressive ventricular dilatation leading to a chronic dilated cardiomyopathy
■ Myocyte damage can also occur via interaction of viral genome with the host protein or directly via apoptosis in the absence of active inflammation (Fig. 20-1).

CLINICAL PRESENTATION AND DIAGNOSIS

A. **Clinical Presentation:** There is a wide spectrum of clinical presentation in myocarditis.
   ■ Non-specific symptoms of dyspnea, chest pain (CP), or palpitations.
   ■ Can vary from non-specific electrocardiogram (ECG) findings to cardiogenic shock or even sudden cardiac death
   ■ Patients may report viral prodrome with fevers, myalgias, respiratory or gastrointestinal symptoms

B. **Diagnosis:**
   ■ Diagnosis of acute myocarditis remains a largely clinical one, although there is an increasing use of non-invasive imaging techniques:

   ■ <u>Symptoms and Biomarkers</u>

   – Cardiac enzyme elevations occur in a minority of patients, troponin I has more specificity (89 %) than CK-MB subunits but overall limited sensitivity (34 %) in the diagnosis of myocarditis [4].
   – ECG with ST segment, non-specific ST-T wave abnormalities, occasionally ST elevations in two or more contiguous leads, mimicking an ST-elevation myocardial infarction (STEMI).

- May also present with heart block or non-sustained VT but this is more common in Giant Cell Myocarditis or cardiac sarcoidosis

- ■ **Non-invasive Imaging**

  - **Echocardiogram** findings are varied and non-specific but useful for excluding other known causes of acute HF and cardiomyopathy [5]
  - Left ventricular (LV) dysfunction is frequently observed but LV dilatation is minimal or absent
  - Segmental wall motion abnormalities on echocardiogram can simulate myocardial infarction (MI).
  - **Cardiac MRI (CMR)** is becoming a routine non-invasive test for the diagnosis of myocarditis.
  - **Three CMR techniques have been applied in myocarditis** [6]

    1. Late gadolinium enhancement (for detection of myocardial necrosis/fibrosis)
    2. T2-weighted images for assessment of myocardial edema
    3. T1-weighted sequences before and after contrast imaging for detection of myocardial hyperemia

       ■ Per "Lake Louise Criteria", CMR findings are consistent with myocarditis if 2 of 3 of the above findings are positive/pathologic.

- Sensitivity and specificity vary depending on sequence used. Combination of T2-weighted imaging and post-gadolinium early and late T1 –enhanced imaging provides the best sensitivity (61 %) and specificity (91 %) for the diagnosis of acute myocarditis [7]
- In combination with endomyocardial biopsy, diagnostic yield of over 95 % in the diagnosis of acute myocarditis

- ■ **Histopathology**

  - **Endomyocardial Biopsy**: Gold standard of diagnosis with histopathologic classification according to the Dallas Criteria [8]
  - Not routinely indicated in the evaluation of suspected myocarditis, however per American College of Cardiology (ACC)/American Heart Association (AHA)/European Society of Cardiology (ESC) guidelines, endomyocardial biopsy may provide clinically meaningful information in the setting of:

    ■ Unexplained, new-onset HF of <2 weeks duration associated with a normal-sized or dilated LV in addition to hemodynamic compromise.
    ■ Dilated ventricle with 2 weeks to 3 months of symptoms, new ventricular arrhythmias or heart block who fail to respond to usual care within 1–2 weeks [9]

  - **Limitations**: significant sampling error due to patchy nature of inflammation, intraobserver variability and risks of cardiac perforation and death with native heart biopsy. Sensitivity of biopsy using Dallas Criteria for the diagnosis of suspected myocarditis is about 10 % from several case series.
  - Diagnostic yield of endomyocardial biopsies can be improved by

    ■ Immunohistological evaluation to enable specific detection and quantification of infiltrates
    ■ Molecular analysis with DNA-RNA extraction and amplification of the viral genome with polymerase chain reaction (PCR)
    ■ Biopsies guided with MRI where available

MANAGEMENT

In general, treatment of viral myocarditis is largely supportive, based on conventional HF management except in specific subtypes of myocarditis as discussed below.

■ Treatment should follow current ACC/AHA guidelines for the management of left ventricular dysfunction.

- Primum defects typically have left axis deviation, sinus venosus and secundum generally have a rightward axis.
- Sinus venosus may have a low ectopic atrial rhythm (negative p waves in leads II, III, aVF).

- **Chest X Ray (CXR)**: may reveal the curvilinear shadow of an anomalous pulmonary vein (with inferior sinus venosus defects, Scimitar sign Fig. 21-1b)
- **Echo findings**:

  - Right heart enlargement.
  - Atrial septal drop out (Fig. 21-1c).
  - Main pulmonary artery (PA) enlargement and increased transpulmonic flow.
  - In primum ASD, evaluation for mitral valve (MV) anterior leaflet cleft (Fig. 21-1d) and MR is important, rule out caval type ventricular septal defect (VSD).
  - In secundum ASD, a transesophageal echocardiogram (TEE) defines location and anatomy to determine candidacy for device closure.
  - Diagnosis of sinus venosus defect difficult with 2D echo and usually requires TEE.

- **CT/MR**: May be used for sinus venosus defect and partial vein imaging if not seen on echocardiogram.
- **Cardiac catheterization**: hemodynamic assessment of pulmonary vascular resistance (PVR) and reversibility (response to pulmonary vasodilator therapy: 100 % O_2, nitric oxide [NO]), and shunt calculation is essential to determine closure candidacy. In some, test balloon occlusion in the catheterization lab may facilitate decision process.
- **Management**:

  - ACC/AHA Class I recommendation: closure of an ASD either percutaneously or surgically is indicated for RA or RV enlargement with or without symptoms in predominantly left-to-right shunts, or bidirectional shunting through a larger ASD with low or responsive PVR [2].
  - ACC/AHA Class III recommendation: closure not indicated if severe irreversible pulmonary hypertension (Eisenmenger physiology) [2].
  - Percutaneous closure: uncomplicated secundum defects with appropriate anatomy [3]
  - Surgical closure: large secundum ASDs, unusual anatomy, and all sinus venosus, primum ASDs and coronary sinus defects; Pre-operative imaging will define anomalous pulmonary venous drainage and MV abnormalities that may also require repair. For sinus venosus defects with anomalous pulmonary venous drainage, a Warden technique is sometimes used.
  - Post-operative complications: residual shunt, MR and atrioventricular (AV) conduction abnormality (rare, and all more likely with primum ASD repair). Sinus venosus surgical complications include sinus node dysfunction/supraventricular tachycardia (SVT), pulmonary venous obstruction at anastomosis site, and rarely superior vena cava (SVC) obstruction. Typically, RV size and function improve post operatively even in advanced age.

- **Pregnancy and delivery**: well tolerated in most patients. Ideal to discuss and repair if needed preconception. With large bidirectional shunts, IV filters are recommended.

Ventricular septal defects (VSD)

- **Epidemiology**: among most common congenital heart entities in early childhood, 2/3 close by early school age; larger VSDs present volume burden to the left atrium (LA) and LV and in some, the RV
- **Types** (Fig. 21-2a):

  - Perimembranous: 60–70 %
  - Muscular: singular or multiple (10 %), in adults generally small and restrictive
  - Supracristal: (5 %) more common in Asian populations, usually small defects located beneath the aortic annulus, may lead to progressive aortic leaflet prolapse and insufficiency (right and noncoronary cusp); typically asymptomatic until aortic regurgitation (AR) is severe.

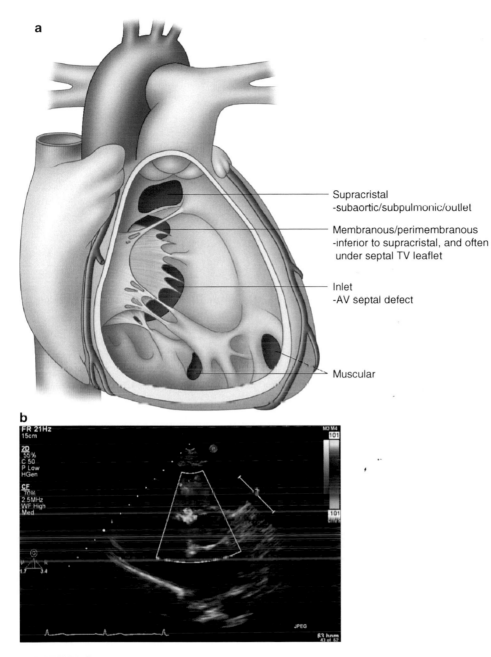

a

Supracristal
-subaortic/subpulmonic/outlet

Membranous/perimembranous
-inferior to supracristal, and often
under septal TV leaflet

Inlet
-AV septal defect

Muscular

b

FIGURE 21-2

Ventricular septal defects. (**a**) Depiction of types of VSDs. (**b**) Parasternal short axis view of perimembraneous VSD, systolic flow noted around 10'o clock

- AV canal defect: common in Down's syndrome, typically involves anterior mitral cleft and occasionally cleft tricuspid septal leaflet; primum ASD may coexist

■ **Clinical presentation**: varies depending on prior management

- If small isolated restrictive defect, typically asymptomatic with a murmur
- If well repaired earlier, typically asymptomatic. Residual VSD is usually small, heart block may occur, and residual or recurrent AR (in a supracristal VSD) or MR (in AV canal VSD)

  If large defect uncorrected in childhood → Eisenmenger syndrome

- **ECG**: typically RBBB (pre or post repair); marked left axis deviation (and sometimes AV block) with AV canal VSDs, right axis deviation/right ventricular hypertrophy (RVH) if significant pulmonary hypertension and in rare patients with progressive RV infundibular hypertrophy.
- **Physical exam**:

  - Classic small restrictive VSD murmur is holosystolic, loud and harsh, augments with isometrics.
  - Associated diastolic murmur of AR if aortic cusp prolapse is present
  - In AV Canal patients, an MR or tricuspid regurgitation (TR) murmur from a cleft valve may also be appreciated
  - If prior pulmonary banding (previously done in infancy to avoid pulmonary volume overload until corrective repair could be undertaken), a loud systolic ejection murmur of supravalvular pulmonic stenosis can be appreciated, and if RVH, there may be a jugular venous *a* wave on exam
  - Eisenmenger exam-see below

- **Echocardiography**:

  - Define detailed VSD anatomy (Fig. 21-2b), estimate RV pressure and gradient across the defect(s), and identify associated lesions
  - If corrected, evaluate for residual shunt and assess RV pressure and rule out associated lesions

- **Catheterization**: performed pre-operatively for pulmonary vascular assessment, coronary screening in older patients, and define associated lesions.
- **Management**:

  - Small, restrictive lesions rarely require specific management
  - ACC/AHA Class I recommendation: closure of a VSD is indicated when there is a Qp/Qs (pulmonary-to-systemic blood flow ratio) of 2.0 or more and clinical evidence of LV volume overload, OR if a patients has had a history of endocarditis [2]
  - ACC/AHA Class III recommendation: closure of a VSD is not recommended in patients with severe irreversible pulmonary hypertension [2]
  - Role for percutaneous approach is evolving for VSDs remote from the tricuspid valve (TV) and aorta

- **Complications**:

  - Endocarditis
  - Potential right-to-left thrombotic complication avoid intracardiac RV pacer or implantable cardioverter defibrillator (ICD) wires
  - Progressive aortic cusp prolapse and insufficiency, and rarely sinus of Valsalva aneurysm or fistula (fistula will result in continuous murmur)
  - Large VSDs left untreated may lead to increased PVR from long term increased pulmonary flow, and reversal of the shunt (Eisenmenger syndrome).
  - Heart block is an occasional early or late post operative complication

Patent ductus arteriosus (PDA)

- **General**: PDA is essential for prenatal survival. It typically closes early in infancy, with a higher incidence of PDA in premature infants and those living at high altitudes. Commonly associated with Congenital Rubella Syndrome as is branch pulmonic stenosis.
- **Clinical Presentation**: varies according to size, from asymptomatic (incidentally noted), to LA and LV volume overload or Eisenmenger syndrome when large and unrepaired

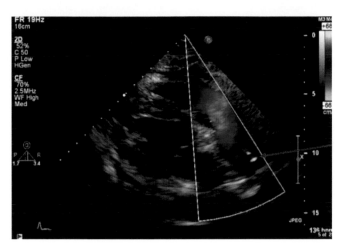

FIGURE 21-3

Patent ductus arteriosus: modified parasternal view with laminar flow across the pulmonic valve leaflets and main PA, and PDA flow from the aorta into the LPA (*red arrow*)

■ **Physical Exam**:

- Small PDA: soft continuous infraclavicular, left sternal border or left upper back murmur, enhanced with isometrics (Fig. 21-3)
- Moderate PDA: ventricular enlargement and a displaced point of maximal impulse on palpation
  Large PDA: LA and LV enlargement; If pulmonary hypertension, there will be a prominent pulmonic component to the second heart sound and RV heave with cyanosis and clubbing [Eisenmenger individual: may have differential cyanosis. cyanosis of feet (clubbing of toes) and perhaps left hand with normal right hand pulse oximetry]
- Differential for continuous murmur includes: PDA, coronary AV fistula, aortopulmonary window, pulmonary AV malformation (Peutz Jaeger syndrome) or the systolic/diastolic murmur of aortic stenosis (AS)/AR

■ **Complications**: endarteritis, left heart failure, pulmonary vascular disease if large and unrepaired; in older adults calcification, aneurysm and dissection risk which may complicate repair

■ **Management**:

ACC/AHA Class I recommendation: closure of PDA either percutaneously or surgically is indicated if there is LA and or LV enlargement, if pulmonary hypertension is present in the presence of net left-to-right shunting OR prior endarteritis. Surgical closure is most appropriate when PDA is too large for percutaneous closure device, or if PDA is aneurysmal, or there is endarteritis [2]

- ACC/AHA Class III recommendations: closure is not indicated if pulmonary hypertension with net right-to-left shunt [2]

Sinus of Valsalva fistula:

■ **Description**: Typically arise from the right or noncoronary sinus of Valsalva and enter the right heart. May be associated with a VSD high in the basal septum; Commonly associated with connective tissue abnormality

■ **Clinical presentation**: new onset prominent diastolic or continuous murmur, occasionally precipitated by strenuous isometric exertion

■ **Management**:

- Endocarditis and AR risks exist
- Surgical repair; transcatheter occlusion for selected patients
- Recurrence may occur

OBSTRUCTIVE LESIONS

Left Ventricular Outflow Tract (LVOT) Obstruction

<u>Congenital Aortic Valvular Stenosis:</u>
- **Bicuspid Aortic Valve (BAV):**

  - **Epidemiology**: most common congenital heart lesion, male predominance, estimated 1–2 % of population, may be familial, multiple morphologic variants, may be undiagnosed for many years
  - Can be associated with aortic coarctation, should be ruled out in Turner's Syndrome
  - Important association with medial connective tissue abnormalities of the ascending aorta

    - Abnormalities of smooth muscle, extracellular matrix, elastin and collagen of the ascending aorta sometimes result in progressive dilation and increase dissection risk with age
    - Ascending aortic dilation does not correlate with valve stenosis severity

  - **Clinical presentation and physical exam**: varies with severity of stenosis or regurgitation

    - Asymptomatic evident by only soft systolic flow murmur and early systolic ejection sound (uncommon after age 40 years)
    - Severe LV outflow obstruction, syncope, chest pain, heart failure and endocarditis
    - Stenosis may be progressive in mid life as well as with advanced age and renal dysfunction
    - Regurgitation is less common than stenosis

  - **Echocardiography**:

    - Mean Doppler gradients correlate well with transcatheter pull back gradients
    - Important to assess ascending aortic dimensions serially (frequency of imaging varies with size of aorta at initial assessment: if <40 mm → every 2 years, if ≥40 mm → annually or more frequently if rapid change or new symptoms) even in previously operated aortic valve patients who have not had prior ascending aortic intervention. CT angiography (CTA) is preferable as aortic size approaches surgical dimensions (see below).

  - **Intervention**: transcatheter balloon dilation may be appropriate in younger adults with severe stenosis without significant AR, otherwise, surgical valvuloplasty or valve replacement per valve guidelines.

    - ACC/AHA Class I recommendation: aortic surgical intervention is indicated in a patient with a BAV and ascending aorta is 5.0 cm or more, or if there is progressive dilatation at a rate greater than 5 mm per year [2]

- **Unicuspid aortic valve**: rare, may present with stenosis or regurgitation. It may be associated with ascending aortic dilation. Transcatheter balloon dilation may cause AR, therefore surgical intervention for severe obstruction or insufficiency is recommended.
- **Quadricuspid aortic valve**: very rare. Presents typically late in life with AR requiring aortic valve replacement, stenosis is rare.

<u>Discrete subaortic membrane:</u>
- **General**:

  - Congenital or acquired, (occasionally associated with primum ASD, double chamber RV, or tetralogy of Fallot [TOF])
  - Prevalence among patients with ACHD is approximately 6.5 %.

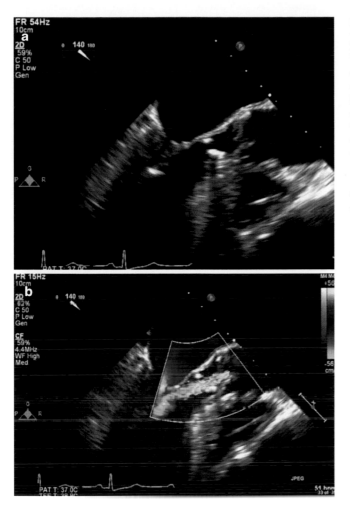

FIGURE 21-4

Subaortic membrane: (**a**) Transespophageal echocardiogram, membrane noted approximately 1.2 cm below the aortic valve along the anterior surface of the ventricular septum, as well as the anterior aspect of the mitral valve. Note the aortic valve leaflets appears thickened and degenerated. (**b**) Associated aortic insufficiency

- Membranes vary in thickness, morphology and distance below the aortic valve (Fig. 21-4), AR is common due to high velocity flow jet causing aortic valve sclerosis
- Familial occurrence approaches 15 % among primary relatives (who should be screened)
- Bacterial endocarditis occurs
- Infrequent ascending aortic dilation

■ **Physical exam**:

- Systolic crescendo decrescendo murmur and absence of ejection sound
- AR murmur (more than 50 %)

■ **Management**:

- Percutaneous balloon dilation is rarely successful
- Surgical resection for significant obstruction or insufficiency, aortic valve should be evaluated at the time of surgery as well.

  ■ ACC/AHA Class I recommendation: Surgical intervention indicated with peak gradient of 50 mmHg or mean gradient of 30 mmHg by echocardiography OR for lesser gradients if progressive aortic regurgitation and LV dilation (end diastolic diameter of 50 mm or more or LV ejection fraction less than 55 %) [2] – however each case should be considered independently as significant heterogeneity exists.

FIGURE 21-5

Supravalvular aortic stenosis (*green arrow*) in a patient with William syndrome, CT angiography, *red arrow* depicts collateral vessels (Sidhu MS et al. MGH cardiovascular imaging 2011)

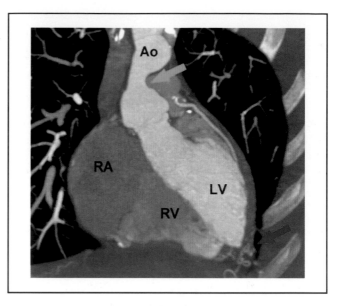

■ **Post operative issues**:

– Residual hypertrophic LVOT obstruction, AR, left bundle branch block (LBBB) or surgical VSD can occur
– Membranes may recur post operatively (15 %)

Supravalvular Aortic Stenosis: Ascending aortic narrowing (Fig. 21-5) commonly associated with Williams Syndrome. Obstruction may be discrete or diffuse, may extend variably cephalad in the ascending aorta and arch. Generally spares the coronary arteries and aortic valve. Surgical revision when obstruction is significant. Differential diagnosis includes: Takayasu and rarely homozygous hypercholesterolemia with secondary lipomatous deposition in the proximal ascending aorta.

Coarctation of the aorta:
■ **Definition/anatomy**:

– Typically focal narrowing in the region of the ligamentum arteriosum adjacent to the origin of the left subclavian artery (Fig. 21-6a)
– May be discrete obstruction or more diffuse narrowing extending proximally towards the arch, may involve associated stenosis of the left subclavian artery
– Distal origin of the right subclavian below the coarctation site occurs in a small percentage and masks the hypertension seen by the coronary arteries and cerebral vasculature as both arm blood pressures may be reflective of post-coarctation pressure.
– Presence of large collaterals may reduce the gradient across the coarctation site
– Shone's complex: coarctation associated with left heart obstructions (subaortic stenosis, BAV, parachute MV, or supramitral ring)

■ **General**:

– Male predominance
– Associated with BAV (50–60 %)
– Associated circle of Willis aneurysm (ACC/AHA Class I recommendation: Intracranial vessels should be screened with MR or CT in all patients with coarctation [2])

■ **Physical exam**:

– Pulse and blood pressure evaluation in all four extremities
– BAV findings (when present): systolic ejection sound, precordial outflow murmur, AR murmur

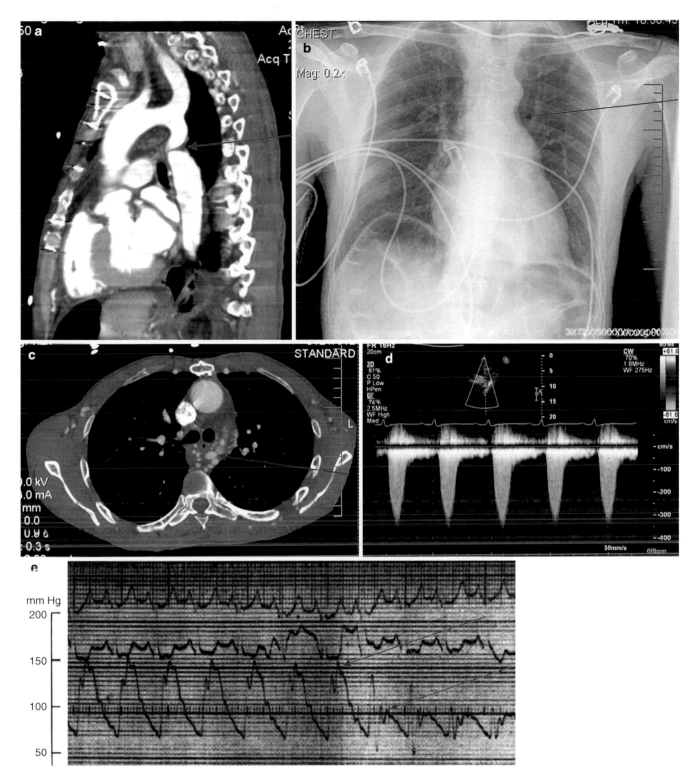

FIGURE 21-6

Coarctation of the aorta. (**a**) Depiction of discrete coarctation (*arrow*) anatomy by CT angiography, sagittal section. (**b**) Classical CXR with the 3 sign (*red arrow*) and subtle rib notching. (**c**) Chest CTA, axial section, demonstrating prominent collateral flow axial imaging, small proximal descending aorta (*arrow*). (**d**) 2D Echocardiogram, Doppler profile of anterograde diastolic flow in the abdominal aorta. (**e**) Invasive hemodynamics with catheter pullback across the coarctation site demonstrating significant drop in pressure (approximately 50 mmHg) distal to the area of coarctation (*arrow*)

- Coarctation findings:
  - ■ Systolic bruit over the upper left back
  - ■ Radial-femoral delay

■ **CXR findings**:

- Aortic indentation at the coarctation site "3 sign" (Fig. 21-6b)
- Notching on the underside of the ribs from collateral vessels

■ **Echocardiography**:

- Best viewed from suprasternal notch
- May see collateral vessel flow (also well defined by MRI and CTA Fig. 21-6c)
- Abdominal aorta demonstrates anterograde diastolic flow (Fig. 21-6d)

■ **Indications for surgical or percutaneous intervention**:

- ACC/AHA Class I recommendation: peak to peak catheterization gradient of 20 mmHg or greater (Fig. 21-6e) regardless or presence or absence of hypertension OR lesser gradient in the presence of imaging evidence of significant coarctation with significant collateral flow [2]
- Percutaneous approach may be considered in experienced hands if narrowed site is amenable
- Surgical intervention for complex anatomy, long segment tubular lesions, prior aneurysm, calcification or poorly compliant arterial system.
- Advanced imaging, whether MRI or CT, may add to delineation and management

■ **Long term follow up**:

- Lifelong adult congenital cardiology follow up is advised with interval assessment for development of resting or exercise-induced hypertension
- Repair or re-repair is appropriate regardless of advanced age
- For complex coarctation, bypass grafting from left subclavian artery to descending aorta or ascending to descending aorta is often advisable.
- ACC/AHA Class I recommendation: evaluation of coarctation repair site by MRI/CT should be performed at intervals of 5 years or less (depending on anatomy of repair) to assess for coarctation site aneurysm or residual obstruction [2]

■ **Pregnancy**:

- With unrepaired or postoperative recurrent coarctation, as well as with aneurysms, there is an increased risk of 3rd trimester or peripartum dissection, which may be fatal
- Hypertension and pre-eclampsia may also occur in select individuals
- Pre-pregnancy counseling is critical, maternal and fetal risks can exist and vary based on prior repair and anatomy
- Pre-pregnancy coarctation imaging is essential to inform risk discussion
- Genetic transmission should be discussed and fetal echocardiography is recommended

Right Ventricular Outflow Tract (RVOT) Obstruction/ Pulmonic Stenosis (PS)

■ <u>Valvular PS</u>: Congenital PS most often occurs at valve level, whether bi or tricommissural. Varies significantly in severity and clinical presentation.

- Noonan syndrome may be associated with myxomatous valvular PS (may also have associated LV hypertrophic cardiomyopathy)

- **Physical exam**:

  - Systolic ejection murmur (intensity, time to peak and duration, vary with severity)
  - Presence of early systolic ejection sound; closer the ejection sound to S1, the more severe stenosis—of note the pulmonic valve ejection click is the **only** right heart finding which **decreases** in intensity with inspiration
  - Pulmonic closure intensity decreases and delay of P2 from A2 increases with severity of stenosis.
  - Jugular venous *a* waves and RVH are present in significant stenosis
  - Low pitched diastolic murmur of PR may coexist

- **Echocardiography**: defines and quantifies PS anatomy and severity
- **CXR**:

  - Prominent main and left pulmonary branch dilation (even if stenosis is not severe)

- **Management**:

  - Surgically managed since the mid 1950s with excellent survival
  - Since early 1980s, transcatheter balloon dilation has supplanted surgery for a majority
  - Balloon valvotomy ACC/AHA Class I recommendations [2]:

    - If asymptomatic with favorable valve anatomy: peak instantaneous Doppler gradient is 60 mmHg or greater, or mean Doppler gradient of 40 mmHg or greater
    - If symptomatic: peak instantaneous gradient of 50 mmHg and mean of 30 mmHg
    - Moderate or greater PR is a relative contraindication.

- **Supravalvular PS:** (or Branch PS) is uncommon but noteworthy and occurs in Congenital Rubella syndrome, Williams syndrome and Takayasu arteritis. Balloon dilation is favored if the lesion in amenable. May occur iatrogenically in the branches from previous systemic to pulmonary palliative shunts, or at the main PA from prior pulmonary artery banding.
- **Subpulmonic stenosis:** rare but does occur in patients with valvular PS, tetralogy of Fallot and some transposition patients.
- **Double chambered RV:** Anomalous muscle bundles that divide the RV into a higher pressure proximal chamber and a lower pressure distal chamber. Associated lesions are VSD, valvular PS, subaortic membranes. In the elderly, double chambered RV may be complicated by ventricular tachyarrhythmia.

COMPLEX LESIONS

Tetralogy of Fallot (TOF):
- **General:**

  - Most common cyanotic congenital heart lesion after infancy
  - Spectrum of morphology and severity, with pulmonary atresia and VSD the most severe form

- **Anatomy**: RV outflow obstruction (valvular and subvalvular/infundibular with generally small pulmonary arteries), large VSD with an overriding aorta and RV hypertrophy (Fig. 21-7a). Right aortic arch is associated in 25 % of cases. Suspect TOF as a diagnosis in cyanotic patients with a right aortic arch.

  - ~ 5 % of TOF patients have aberrant course of the left anterior descending (LAD) or left main arising from the proximal right coronary artery (RCA) or right sinus of Valsalva, traversing the RVOT (coronary anatomy should be assessed pre-operatively)

– Approximately 15 % patients have ascending aortic dilation, most notably those with AR, right aortic arch, and severe degrees of pulmonary stenosis, particularly pulmonary atresia

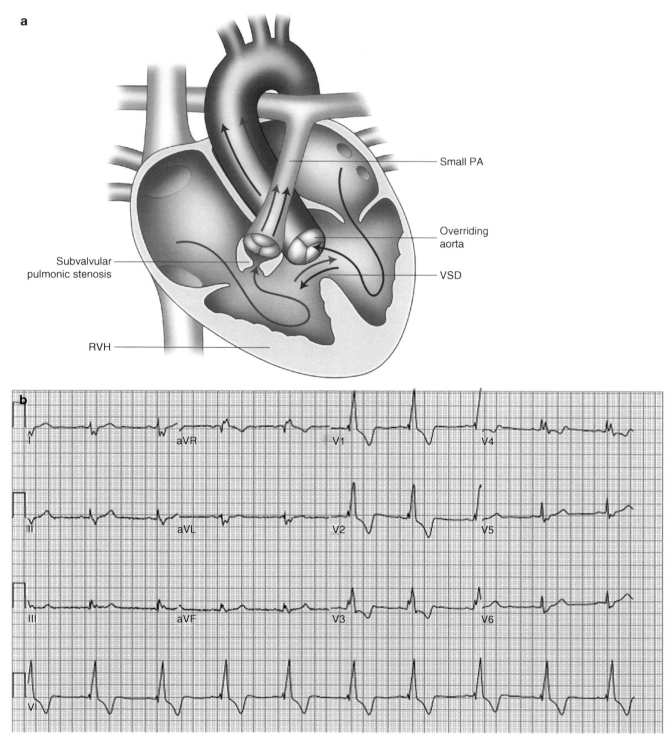

FIGURE 21-7

Tetralogy of Fallot. (**a**) Depiction of TOF. (**b**) Classical ECG with RBBB, right ventricular hypertrophy (patient status post PVR for severe PR). (**c**) Palliative shunts. (**d**) 2D echocardiogram of continuous wave Doppler profile across the RVOT consistent with severe pulmonic regurgitation. Note: steep deceleration of pulmonic regurgitant jet, correlates with short decrescendo diastolic murmur

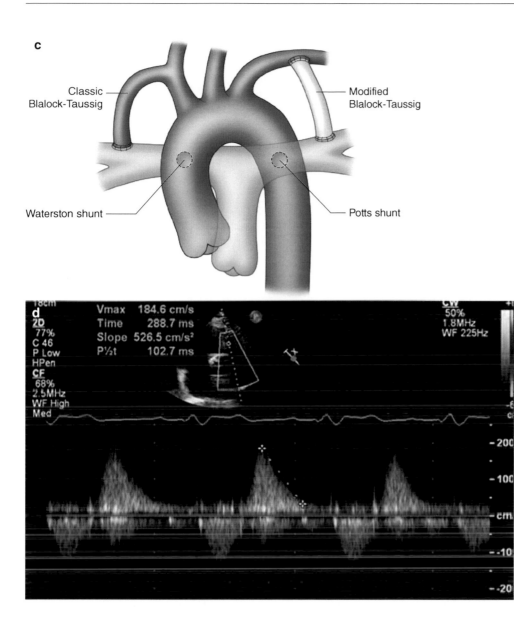

FIGURE 21-7

(continued)

- **Clinical presentation in adults:**

  - Patients present s/p remote palliative procedures (see below), but most present s/p remote complete repair. It is rare to present as an adult with no prior interventions, though teenagers in immigrant populations may present with native disease.
  - Post complete repair: asymptomatic or may have significant late complications including significant pulmonary insufficiency and RV dilation and dysfunction, and ventricular tachycardia (VT), sudden cardiac death.

- **Physical exam:**

  - Evidence of residual RVOT obstruction with systolic murmur over the pulmonic area
  - Harsh holosystolic murmur of a residual VSD
  - Pulmonary incompetence: low-pitched diastolic decrescendo murmur; shorter murmurs generally more severe

- **ECG:**

  - RBBB, RVH, RA enlargement (Fig. 21-7b)
  - T wave inversions over anterior precordium
  - PR prolongation and complete heart block rarely
  - SVT or VT

- **Palliative interventions** (Fig. 21-7c and Table 21-1): do not correct the pulmonary stenosis or the right-to-left shunt

  - Blalock-Taussig shunt is most common. Waterston and Potts are rarely used today.
  - Blalock-Taussig shunt (subclavian artery to branch PA): allowed survival to complete repair; ligated at time of complete repair
  - Potts shunt (descending aorta to left PA window): may be complicated by pulmonary vascular obstruction of the left lung or left PA hypoplasia (challenging surgical revision)
  - Waterston shunt (ascending aorta to right PA window): complications include right PA stenosis and hypoplasia. Transcatheter right PA dilation may be helpful

- Rastelli procedure: (See Table 21-1, Figure 21-18) used in patients who have degrees of transposition of the great arteries associated with their VSD and pulmonary stenosis where traditional complete TOF repair is not possible

  - Baffle from the LV to the ascending aorta (occasionally complicated by AV block) and valved conduit placement from the RV to the main PA
  - Late stenosis of the RV to PA conduit is common and requires with either percutaneous dilation or surgical replacement. Experience with percutaneous valve placement in the Rastelli conduit is growing at select institutions.
  - Stenosis occurs at the take off or touch down conduit site or at the level of the valve within the conduit (transcatheter techniques for pulmonary valve dilation or replacement are rapidly evolving)

- **Complete repair** (VSD closure, RVOT augmentation): now mostly performed in infancy or early childhood
- **Late post repair complications:**

  - PR may be progressive over several decades (Fig. 21-7d). ACC/AHA Class I recommendation: Pulmonic valve replacement is indicated for severe PR with any of the following: (1) symptoms of decreased exercise tolerance, (2) moderate to severe RV dysfunction or enlargement (3) sustained atrial or ventricular arrhythmias or (4) moderate to severe TR [2]
  - Significant residual VSD is increasingly less common as is significant residual PS.
  - SVT is increasingly common beyond the fifth decade
  - Ventricular tachycardia (VT) /fibrillation (sudden cardiac death):

    - High risk features: LV dysfunction, palliation for many years prior to complete repair/older age at time of repair, significant RV dilation and dysfunction, high RV mass to volume ratio, inducible VT on electrophysiology testing, and QRS duration >180ms
    - Aggressive antiarrhythmic management and assessment and implantable defibrillator should be considered in high risk patients. It is important to address repair of significant hemodynamic lesions in patients with an arrhythmia burden as well.

- **Pregnancy:**

  - Well repaired stable TOF adults manage well through pregnancy and delivery, but always advisable to involve high risk obstetrics and congenital heart specialist
  - Risk of right heart failure and arrhythmia is increased with significant RV dysfunction

Ebstein Anomaly

- **General**: approximately 1 % of all CHD, wide spectrum of severity of anatomic and functional abnormalities of the TV and RV

- **Anatomy:** "Apical displacement" of the TV caused by failure of delamination of the tricuspid leaflets from the RV muscle, compromise in size of the portion of the RV below the TV and enlargement of the RA by portion of the RV above the TV ('atrialized' RV)

- **Major clinical issues:**

  - Degree of tricuspid regurgitation
  - RV cardiomyopathy/ RV function
  - Presence of an associated interatrial communication (ASD or stretched patent foramen ovale [PFO])
  - Atrial arrhythmias

- **Clinical presentation is highly variable:**

  - From asymptomatic with a nearly silent clinical exam to marked right heart failure, cyanosis, and early death
  - Wolff-Parkinson-White syndrome (WPW) is present in 25 % of patients and presents with palpitations or SVT. Ventricular arrhythmias may occur.
  - Progressive exercise intolerance and fatigue from TR and RV dysfunction may occur
  - Acute systemic desaturation from right-to-left shunt through an ASD or PFO is poorly tolerated. Paradoxical embolus can rarely occur.

- **Clinical exam**

  - Tricuspid holosystolic murmur and multiple systolic clicks exist but can be subtle
  - Both first and second heart sounds are widely split
  - "Sail sound" of a loud systolic sound created by the large anterior leaflet may be heard
  - Rocking motion of the heart with an easily palpable RV in more severe disease
  - Right heart failure: elevated jugular venous pressure, hepatojugular reflux, lower extremity edema, hepatic congestion, cyanosis

- **ECG:** wide and splintered QRS complex (right precordial leads), RA enlargement, first degree AV block and when present, Type B WPW pattern (Fig. 21-8a)
- **CXR:** varies with severity and shows RA enlargement, pulmonary vasculature usually normal unless marked cyanosis, and cardiac silhouette can be massive with enlargement progressing with age (Fig. 21-8b).
- **Echocardiography** is the diagnostic gold standard and defines anatomy and severity of TR, RV size and function, RA size, interatrial communication and associated LV abnormalities (Fig. 21-8c).

- **Management:**

  - IV filters when ASD or PFO present
  - SVT and accessory pathway management can be challenging secondary to multiple bypass tracts, variation in atrialized RV and tricuspid annular anatomy, thickened atrialized RA tissue and thin RV walls.
  - Anticoagulation is recommended if history of paradoxical embolism or atrial fibrillation

- **Surgical timing:** cannot be generalized and differs with each individual

  - Surgery is best performed in experienced centers
  - Options include TV repair vs. replacement, inter-atrial communication closure, simultaneous Maze procedure, and in some, cardiac transplant
  - Post operatively: management includes avoidance of right ventricular afterload and positive pressure, and arrhythmia and AV block surveillance.

- **Pregnancy:** pre-pregnancy counseling is important; successful delivery is often accomplished without difficulty in uncomplicated patients; but with significant RV failure, TR, and cyanosis, pregnancy should be discouraged.

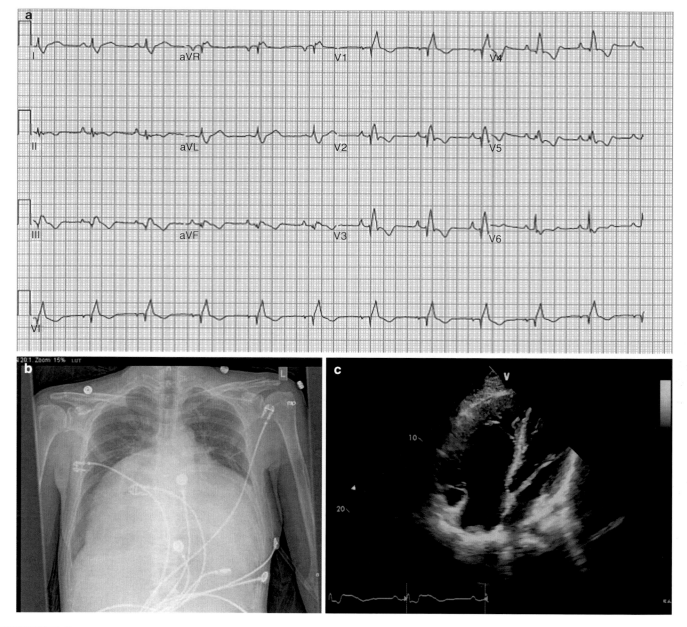

FIGURE 21-8

Ebstein's anomaly. (**a**) ECG with right axis deviation, first degree AV block and complete right bundle branch block with marked splintering of the R' deflection. (**b**) CXR of marked cardiomegaly. (**c**) 2D echocardiogram, four chamber view demonstrating marked apical displacement of the septal leaflet of the tricuspid valve, large atrialized portion of the RV

Transposition of the Great Arteries (TGA)

■ **D-TGA:**

– **Anatomy**: great vessels arise from the incorrect ventricle (i.e., ventriculoarterial discordance: aorta arises from the morphologic RV and PA arises from the morphologic LV) resulting in parallel circulations (Fig. 21-9a)

– **General**: most common cause of cyanotic CHD in neonates

– **Surgery**: adults with D-TGA have had some form of intervention in infancy including:

■ Rashkind balloon atrial septostomy to allow sufficient mixing of deoxygenated and oxygenated blood and enable survival for the early post delivery months

■ Blalock Hanlon surgical atrial septectomy
■ **Atrial switch: Senning and Mustard procedures (until 1980s)** – (Fig. 21-9b):

– re-routes systemic venous return to the MV and LV and lungs, and allows pulmonary venous flow to the TV and RV and aorta.
– **Clinical exam**:

■ RVH with loud (single sounding) second heart sound from the anteriorly placed aorta, often no murmur
■ outflow murmur if there is associated sub pulmonic stenosis
■ holosystolic murmur if there is (systemic) TV regurgitation

– **ECG**: marked right axis deviation and RVH (Fig. 21-9c)
– **Echocardiography:** defines the status of the atrial baffle (rule out baffle leak or obstruction), rule out AV valvular regurgitation, presence of subpulmonic obstruction, and evaluate biventricular dysfunction.
– **CT/MRI**: useful in diagnosing baffle leak or obstruction, and assessing ventricular volumes and function (Fig. 21-9d)
– **Long term complications**:

■ Sinus node dysfunction, sudden death, atrial arrhythmias, ventricular arrhythmias
■ Atrial baffle leak allowing an atrial level shunt
■ Atrial baffle obstruction resulting in inhibition of systemic or pulmonary venous return
■ Systemic atrioventricular valve regurgitation and systemic RV dysfunction

– **Management**:

■ Medications/ablation for atrial arrhythmias, pacemaker for significant sinus node dysfunction
■ Percutaneous intervention for both baffle leaks and obstruction
■ Systemic right ventricle failure with progressive TR should be managed with aggressive systemic afterload reduction but may require cardiac transplantation

■ **Arterial switch: Jatene Procedure** (Fig. 21-9e)

– Has largely supplanted the atrial switch procedure since the 1980s
– Normal exam (healed incision) and generally normal ECG
Potential complications:

■ Aortic dilation and AR
■ Supra- aortic and supra- pulmonic anastomotic site stenosis
■ Coronary ostial obstruction (rare)

■ **Congenitally corrected Transposition of the Great Arteries (CC-TGA, L-TGA, ventricular inversion):**

– Anatomy: systemic venous flow (vena cavae) enter the RA, traverse a MV to a subpulmonary LV and exit the PA to the lungs. The pulmonary veins enter the LA and traverse the TV to the RV to the aorta (making the TV the "systemic" ventricle).
– Associated anomalies include VSD, pulmonic stenosis, or systemic AV valve (tricuspid) insufficiency (occasionally Ebstein-like valve) and complete heart block.

– **Clinical exam:**

■ Consider L-TGA in any young adult with unexplained heart block
■ Loud second heart sound (from the anteriorly placed aorta)
■ Systemic AV valve insufficiency murmur (if tricuspid valve is abnormal or RV annulus is dilated)
■ If VSD and PS are present, there may be cyanosis and clubbing

– **ECG**: (Fig. 21-10a)

■ Classic ECG is diagnostic: Q wave in right precordial leads (septal depolarization direction is altered) with varying degrees of heart block

– **CXR**: (Fig. 21-10b)

■ Flat or convex upper left-sided cardiac silhouette, reflecting the abnormal ascending aorta position and take off

– **Echocardiogram**: (Fig. 21-10c)

■ Gold standard for diagnosis and detection of associated lesions.
■ Apically placed TV which enters the RV receives LA inflow and communicates with the aorta. Apical 4 chamber best demonstrates the "inverted ventricles".

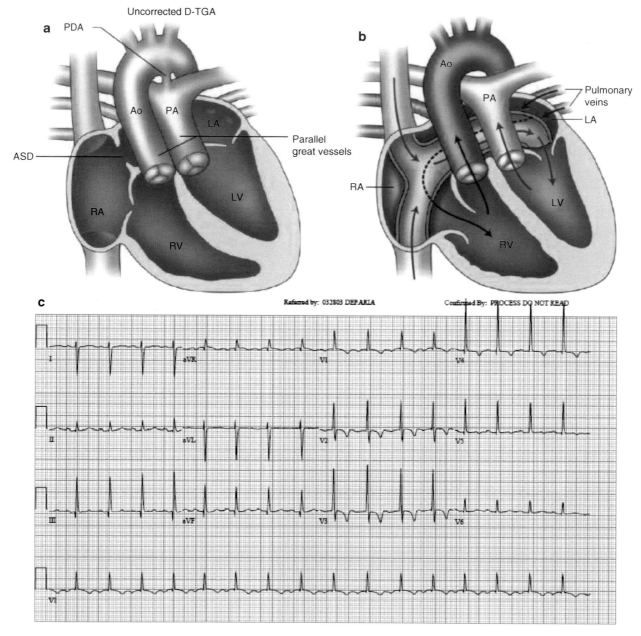

FIGURE 21-9

D Transposition of the Great Arteries. (**a**) Depiction of D TGA anatomy. (**b**) Schematic of Mustard anatomy with baffle directing SVC and IVC flow across the intraatrial septum to the morphologic right ventricle. (**c**) ECG of patient status post Mustard atrial switch with RVH and right axis deviation. (**d**) CTA and MRI of patient with D TGA demonstrating intraatrial baffle directing flow from the pulmonary veins to the LA across the tricuspid valve to hypertrophied systemic RV. (**e**) Schematic of Jatene arterial switch procedure

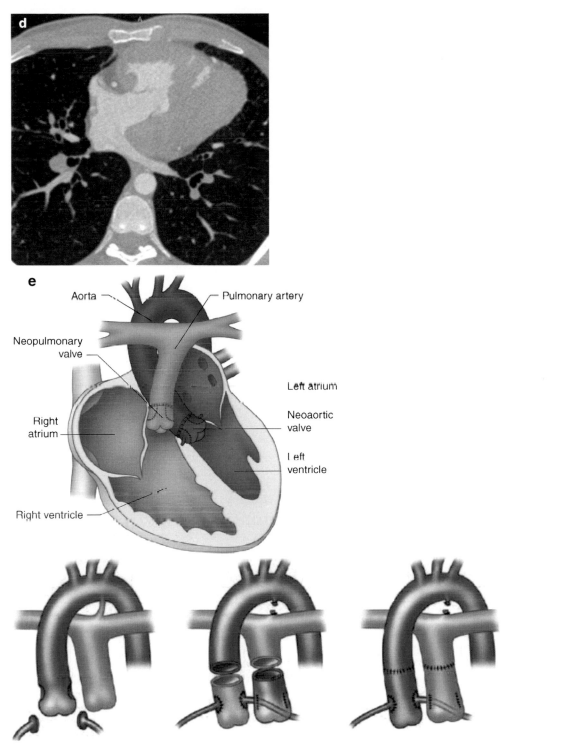

FIGURE 21-9

(continued)

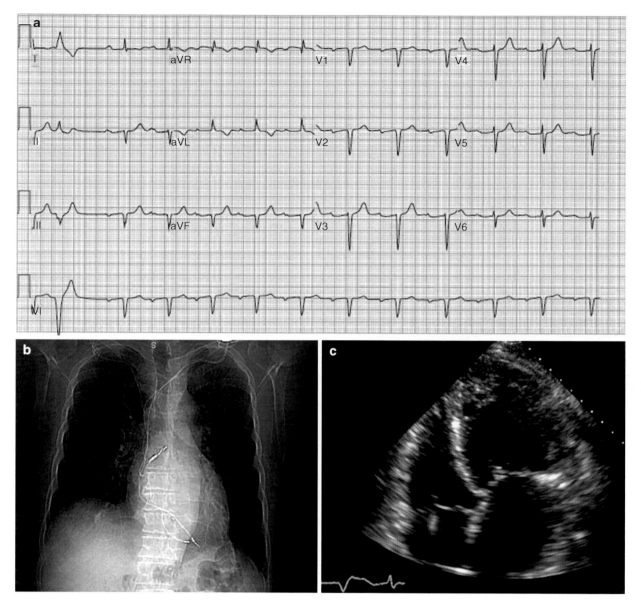

FIGURE 21-10

L Transposition of the Great Arteries. (**a**) ECG with first degree AV block, Q waves in II, III, F, absence of septal Q waves in V5-V6 due to inversion of the right and left bundle branches causing septal activation to occur from right to left axis deviation and PVC not necessarily seen in L-TGA. (**b**) CXR of patient with L- TGA and dual chamber pacer. (**c**) 4-chamber view demonstrating apical displacement of the systemic AV valve indicating this is a tricuspid valve and systemic right ventricle, pacer lead also noted in the morphologic (subpulmonary) LV

- **Outcomes:**

  - May survive well into older age with essentially normal lifestyle including pregnancy and delivery.
  - Complete heart block may require pacemaker placement (active fixation leads may be needed for the smooth LV septal surface).
  - Can present with progressive systemic (tricuspid) AV valve regurgitation and progressive systemic RV dilation, dysfunction and failure

- **Management:**

  - Afterload reduction and maintaining lower blood pressure is helpful
  - Pacemakers for complete heart block, small studies reveal cardiac resynchronization may have a role in some patients with systemic RV failure.

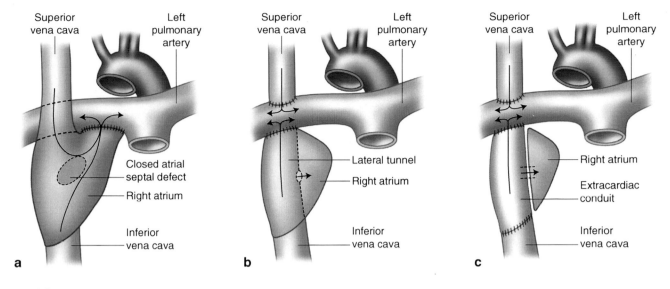

FIGURE 21-11

Fontan circulation

- TV replacement (less often repair) for significant TR if systemic ventricular function is not severely compromised may help preserve systemic ventricular function.
- Clinical management of L-TGA patients can be challenging and expert ACHD input is strongly recommended.
- Cardiac transplantation may be needed for medically refractory heart failure

Univentricular Heart and Fontan revision (Fig. 21-10)
(Tricuspid or Mitral atresia, hypoplastic left or right heart syndrome)
- **Early Interventions Include:**

  - Pulmonary artery banding: protect the lungs from overcirculation for patients with no natural pulmonary flow obstruction
  - Modified Blalock-Taussig shunt (subclavian artery to PA prosthetic conduit): often used for infants with severe pulmonic stenosis or pulmonary atresia and cyanosis, and staged prior to the Fontan procedure
  - Glenn procedure: direct connection of SVC to right PA (may cause late right pulmonary arteriovenous malformations - secondary to absence of inferior venous cava flow to the right lung which may carry "liver factors" which prevent pulmonary arteriovenous malformation)

- **Fontan procedure**: allows systemic venous flow to be directed to the lungs without the aid of a ventricular pump (Fig. 21-11).

  - **Complications**:

    - RA to PA Fontan: RA enlargement, thrombus formation, atrial arrhythmias, hepatic congestion and eventual cirrhosis
    - Lateral tunnel Fontan: Atrial arrhythmias, hepatic congestion
    - Extracardiac conduit: Hepatic congestion may still occur
    - Fistulous communications from the systemic to the pulmonary circulation may present as new onset progressive desaturation, often amenable to transcatheter occlusion

- Univentricular dysfunction as well as AV incompetence may be progressive in adult life, hence early and continued management with afterload reduction and avoidance of systemic hypertension is an essential feature for these patients.

  - When Fontan patients require intubation avoidance of positive pressure is essential

- **Pregnancy:** can be very challenging, contraindicated in severe cyanosis, may not do well with depressed single ventricle ejection fraction

Eisenmenger Syndrome

■ **General:** seen in patients with large left-to-right shunt lesions who were not appropriately intervened upon in childhood (generally because of limited access to health care); defined as progressive increase in PVR which leads to reversal of shunting (right-to-left) and ultimately subpulmonary ventricular failure and death; overall, increasingly uncommon

■ **Clinical Exam:**

- Cyanosis, clubbing, jugular venous a wave
- Prominent RV heave, loud P2
- Often no murmur, but occasionally the holosystolic murmur of TR or diastolic murmur of functional PR from elevated PVR
- Hepatosplenomegaly from chronic congestion

■ **CXR:** Large main PA and central PA with oligemic periphery (pruning) (Fig. 21-12a, b)

■ **Complications:**

- Systemic emboli or abscess from right-to-left shunting
- Erythrocytosis as a response to chronic hypoxemia, thrombocytopenia from splenic sequestration; neurologic events may occur due to hyperviscosity syndrome
- Hemoptysis may occur
- Arrhythmia and sudden cardiac death

■ **Management:** Medical therapy with pulmonary arterial vasodilators is an option and may prolong survival [4] and the only surgical option is heart-lung transplant. ACC/AHA Class I recommendations:

- Avoidance of dehydration, moderate to severe strenuous activity, isometric exercise, excessive heat, chronic high altitude exposure and iron deficiency [2]
- Annual monitoring of hemoglobin, platelet count, iron stores, creatinine, and uric acid annually; assess oximetry with and without oxygen annually [2]
- Right-to-left shunt precautions are essential with all IVs [2]

Other recommendations: Endocarditis prophylaxis, phlebotomy when appropriate (neurologic symptoms from hyperviscocity), anticoagulation may be considered, avoidance of unessential surgery or anesthesia is important. With appropriate and experienced clinically guided care, Eisenmenger patients can survive to midlife and on occasion beyond

■ **Pregnancy:** strictly contraindicated

Dextrocardia and cardiac malposition

■ **Mirror Image Dextrocardia:** (Fig. 21-13a)

- Total situs inversus: heart chambers and body viscera are all in mirror image position
- Many have no associated congenital cardiac anomaly
- ECG, Echo, CXR: when present, can trigger identification (Fig. 21-13b)

■ **Kartagener's syndrome:**

- Bronchiectasis, sinusitis, ciliary dysmotility, infertility
- Limited to those with mirror image dextrocardia and not seen in dextroversion (heart is dextrorotated but visceral abdominal organs are in normal position)

Congenital Coronary anomalies

■ **ALCAPA:** anomalous left coronary artery origin from the PA (rare)

- In the absence of surgical intervention, most infants die in early infancy. Rare natural survivors may have acute myocardial infarction (MI), MR and LV failure and survive to childhood.

- **Management in Infancy involves:**

  ■ Creation of a tunnel in the posterior PA to redirect the anomalously arising left coronary artery blood flow to a neo left coronary ostium and the left coronary artery.

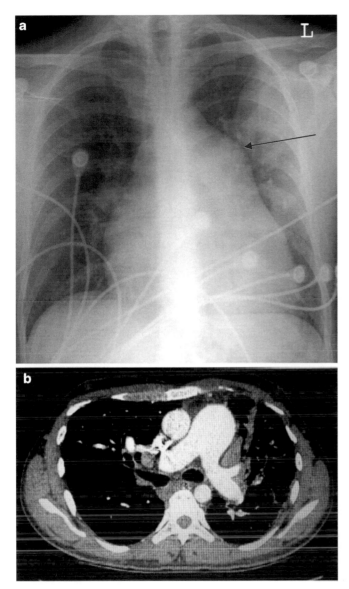

FIGURE 21-12

Eisenmenger physiology. (**a**) CXR of patient with Eisenmenger with markedly enlarged pulmonary artery (*arrow*). (**b**) Chest CT angiography demonstrating PA is significantly larger than aorta, PA branches are dilated

- ■ Long term results of this procedures are still evolving but are encouraging with near normal LV function.
- ■ Even in patients who had significant LV damage with their presentation as infants, LV recovery often seems very favorable.
- ■ Exercise treadmill testing with imaging, arrhythmic monitoring and in many beta blockade or angiotensin converting enzyme (ACE) inhibition for less than normal LV function is likely prudent.

- **Adult presentation**:

  - ■ Infants can grow to adulthood with minimal complications and no significant heart failure post repair
  - ■ Approximately 5 % of ALCAPA patients are unrepaired and survive by natural intercoronary collateral flow and may present in adult life with a palpable left ventricular aneurysm, MR, ventricular tachyarrhythmia and a continuous flow bruit over the anterior wall from the right to the left coronary circulation
  - ■ ECG: may demonstrate LV aneurysm or remote anterior myocardial infarction pattern (Q waves and ST changes with loss of R waves in the anterior precordial leads).

– **Diagnosis:**

  ■ Targeted ultrasound of coronary artery origins can be diagnostic (parasternal short axis above the level of the aortic valve)
  ■ MRI and CTA can be confirmatory (define the course of the vessel, assess for dominance of the artery and caliber of the proximal lumen and of the ostium. CT can assess for atherosclerosis which can change a previously benign clinical presentation)

– **High risk features:**

  ■ Age at presentation < 50 years
  ■ Proximal hypoplasia and stenosis of the ectopic artery, or proximal oblique (or 'slit-like') orifice
  ■ Interarterial course: anterior to the aorta and posterior to the RVOT alone may not be the strongest risk factor, however the presence of a dominant ectopic vessel with proximal anatomic or functional obstruction suggests high risk and surgical intervention should be considered. Individuals with an interarterial course alone and age >50 years have anecdotally survived well with no intervention.
  ■ Presentation with ventricular arrhythmia in adolescence or young adulthood especially with exertion.
  ■ Presence of detectable ischemia on stress testing in the distribution perfused by the ectopic artery

– **Management:**

  ■ Without high risk features: beta blockade (data are limited) and lifestyle modification
  ■ With high risk features: beta blockade and consider surgical revascularization
  ■ Anomalous coronary artery assessment and management can be challenging and expert ACHD consultation (with multidisciplinary evaluation) is often prudent.
  ■ ACC/AHA Class I recommendations (Level of Evidence B): surgical revascularization if:

    – anomalous left main courses between the aorta and PA/RVOT
    – documented ischemia due to coronary compression
    – anomalous origin of the right coronary between the aorta and PA/RVOT with evidence of ischemia [2]

■ **Congenital coronary AV fistula:**

– **Clinical exam:** (in larger congenital coronary AV fistula)

  ■ Precordial continuous murmur (see differential above under PDA, physical exam)

– **Presentation:**

  ■ Subclinical, incidental findings by ultrasound or at the time of coronary angiography (particularly small left main to PA congenital coronary AV fistula – Fig. 21-14c)
  ■ Heart failure, cardiomegaly (when large, usually from RCA or left circumflex, entering right heart)
  ■ Thrombosis
  ■ Ischemia secondary to steal phenomenon, where the fistula redirects flow away from the coronary distal to the fistula takeoff

– **Management:**

  ■ Observation for small fistulas
  ■ If amenable, transcatheter coils are the treatment of choice
  ■ Surgical approach is also an option in select cases, and preferable with large aneurysms.

REVIEW QUESTIONS

1. A 31 year old man with a history of testicular cancer, received a chest, abdomen, and pelvic CT which revealed right ventricular and pulmonary arterial enlargement. An echocardiogram was recommended, but was read as only right heart enlargement. Images are below (Fig. 21-15). What anomaly can be seen in association with this diagnosis?
    (a) tetralogy of Fallot
    (b) ciliary dysmotility syndrome
    (c) partial anomalous pulmonary venous connection
    (d) absent radius

2. A 26 year old woman presents with hypertension and lower extremity claudication. Echocardiogram and CT (Fig. 21-16a, b). Which of the following statements are true?
    (a) This lesion is associated with bicuspid aortic valve in 60 % of cases
    (b) There is a high risk for mother and fetus if a gradient >30 mmHg is present
    (c) She should be offered a brain MRI or CT to evaluate for Berry aneurysm
    (d) Surgical and percutaneous approach have both been validated in this lesion
    (e) All of the above

3. A young man from Cape Verde with right aortic arch, infundibular and valvar pulmonic stenosis presented for surgical correction. Post operatively, after infundibular resection and PVR, he developed florid heart failure. Which of the following was the most likely etiology?
    (a) peri-operative myocardial infarction
    (b) sudden pulmonary embolism
    (c) left to right shunt through an associated VSD once RV pressure declined
    (d) over-aggressive fluid resuscitation intra-operatively

4. A 21 year old woman presents to you to establish primary care. She states she has a history of D transposition of the great vessels and had a surgical procedure when she was a young child. She currently denies any symptoms. Her exam is notable for normal vital signs, a median sternotomy scar, jugular venous pressure of 5cmH$_2$0, normal S$_1$ with prominent A$_2$ and no murmurs or heaves, liver is normal in size without pulsatility and she has no peripheral edema. Her ECG is below (Fig. 21-17). Which of the following below statements are true.
    (a) Her systemic ventricle is her morphologic right ventricle
    (b) She is at high risk for atrial arrhythmias
    (c) A potential complication of her surgery is ostial coronary stenosis and aortic regurgitation
    (d) Her PA diameter should be intermittently monitored with serial echos to screen for dilation
    (e) She may have significant tricuspid regurgitation that cannot be heard on exam due to abnormal cardiac anatomy

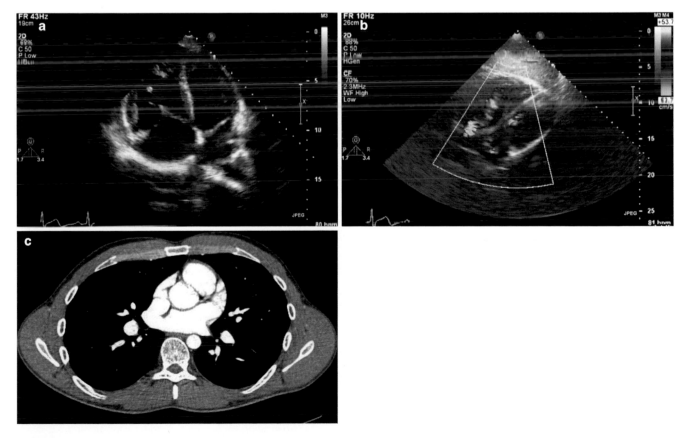

FIGURE 21-15

Question 1 (Echo and CT)

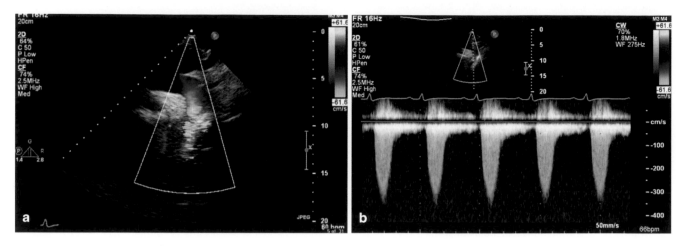

FIGURE 21-16

Question 2 (Echo)

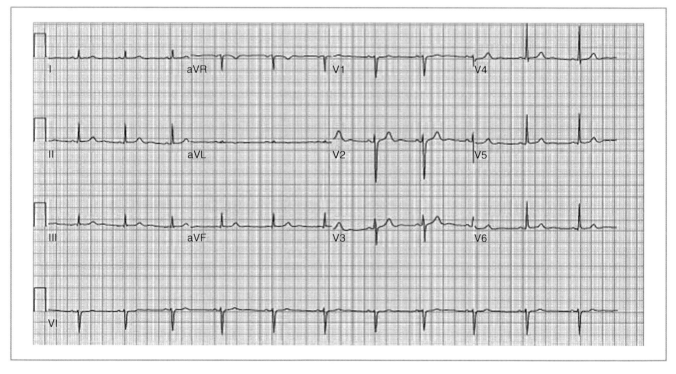

FIGURE 21-17

Question 4

ANSWERS

1. (c) Sinus venosus septal defect, pictured above, is commonly seen in association with anomalous pulmonary venous return. In cases of right heart enlargement where a secundum ASD is not readily visualized, TEE and MRI can be used to assess for sinus venosus or coronary sinus septal defects, as well as anomalous pulmonary venous return. Remember that while atrial level shunts cause right heart enlargement, large VSDs are more likely to cause left heart enlargement with some effect on the RV size, and PDA will create only left heart enlargement. Surgical correction of SV septal defect with PAPVR can be performed with a patch repair or a Warden procedure, where the SVC is transected cranial to the anomalous vein entrance and reattached to the RA appendage, while the SVC stump serves as a reservoir for the pulmonary vein which is directed into the left atrium via the sinus venosus defect. Superior sinus venosus with right upper pulmonary vein anomaly is more common than inferior sinus venosus defects or return of pulmonary venous drainage to the IVC (known as Scimitar Syndrome when accompanied by additional findings).

2. (e) Coarctation of the aorta should always be in the differential diagnosis of hypertension in the young individual. Symptoms may include headaches from hypertension, claudication, fatigue. The diagnosis may also be incidental in the setting of evaluation for a BAV click or murmur. On physical exam, with a significant

coarctation, there will be a radial-femoral (or brachial femoral) pulse delay which is palpable. Intervention is recommended at a peak to peak gradient of 20 mmHg. At 30 mmHg for any LV outflow lesion, the risk in pregnancy rises significantly. Patients should be informed of the risks of long term hypertension even with excellent and lasting repair, premature coronary artery disease, presence of an intracerebral aneurysm, and risk of recoarctation or aortic dilation. Intervention can be surgical (most commonly end to end anastomosis; however some individuals may have had a left subclavian flap repair, and therefore will have a poor pulse and blood pressure in that arm). Guidelines recommend imaging of the aorta with CT/MRI once every 5 years.

3. (c) The presence of RVOT obstruction and right arch should raise suspicion for TOF, as 25 % of TOF patients will have right aortic arch. TOF consists of overriding aorta, VSD, RVH, and RVOT obstruction. The VSD, both in TOF and as an isolated lesion, can be unrecognized due to overlying tricuspid apparatus which can effectively "close" the defect. In this case, with relief of RVOT obstruction and placement of a pulmonic valve prosthesis, the RV

pressure dropped and acute left to right shunting across the VSD ensued as the LV to RV pressure differential overpowered the thin septal leaflet which was covering the VSD. This acute shunt development can result in clinical heart failure.

4. (c) D TGA occurs with atrioventricular concordance (blood flows from RA through TV to RV) and ventriculoarterial discordance (RV to aorta), similarly LA through MV to LV to the PA. Options for correction in infants and children include atrial switch procedures (Mustard or Senning) where systemic venous flow is baffled through the intra-atrial septum to the morphologic LV out the PA. Complications of atrial switch procedures include atrial arrhythmias, baffle leaks, and systemic RV dysfunction. The arterial switch operation (or Jatene procedure) requires aortic and PA root excision and reimplantation to the appropriate ventricular chamber, and coronary buttons are reimplanted to the neo aortic root. Patients who have undergone arterial switch operations have nearly normal exam and ECG, and potential long term complications include aortic regurgitation or issues with ostial coronary stenosis (Table 21-2).

SURGICAL PALLIATION OR CORRECTION	DESCRIPTION	COMPLICATIONS
TABLE 21-1 SURGICAL PALLIATION OR CORRECTIVE PROCEDURES		
Blalock Taussig Shunt (Fig. 21-7c)	Subclavian artery to branch PA connection	(Note: Reduced BP and pulse in affected arm)
Waterston Shunt (Fig. 21-7c)	Ascending aorta to right PA shunt	Right PA stenosis and kinking, pulmonary overcirculation if left open for too long
Potts Shunt (Fig. 21-7c)	Descending aorta to left PA shunt	Pulmonary overcirculation, left PA kinking and challenging late surgical revision
Mustard/Senning (Fig. 21-9b)	Atrial switch for D TGA-redirects venous inflow (Mustard: pericardial or Gore-Tex patch, Senning: native atrial tissue)	Atrial arrhythmias, baffle obstruction, baffle leak, systemic right ventricle failure, systemic TR, ventricular arrhythmias, subpulmonary stenosis
Jatene arterial switch (Fig. 21-9e)	Arterial switch for D TGA (began in 1980s)	Aortic dilation, coronary reimplantation concerns, suprapulmonic or supraaortic anastomotic site stenosis
Glenn Shunt	SVC to right PA shunt	Right pulmonary AVMs if no IVC flow is presented to right lung
Fontan (total cavopulmonary anastomosis) (Fig. 21-11)	Redirecting systemic venous return to the lungs without a ventricular pump (RA to PA, lateral tunnel, extracardiac)	Atrial arrhythmias, baffle leak (cyanosis), RA thrombus, thromboembolism (deep venous thrombosis, pulmonary embolus, stroke), liver dysfunction/ascites, systemic to pulmonary venous collaterals (causing cyanosis), ventricular dysfunction, Failing Fontan (protein losing enteropathy, plastic bronchitis)
Rastelli (right ventricle to PA conduit) (Fig. 21-18)	Used in Double outlet right ventricle and D-TGA morphology most commonly. LV patch directed to aorta: RV conduit to PA	RV to PA conduit stenosis and insufficiency (may require multiple reinterventions). RVH. Right heart failure symptoms, occasionally heart block and subaortic obstruction
PA banding	Surgically created stenosis of the main PA; palliative procedure to protect the lungs against high pulmonary blood flow when definitive repair is not immediately feasible	Band site PA stenosis; RV hypertension
Warden procedure	Baffle technique in SV ASD with PAPVD in the SVC	Sinus node dysfunction, atrial tachycardia and SVC obstruction

FIGURE 21-18

Depiction of Rastelli procedure
(RV to PA conduit)

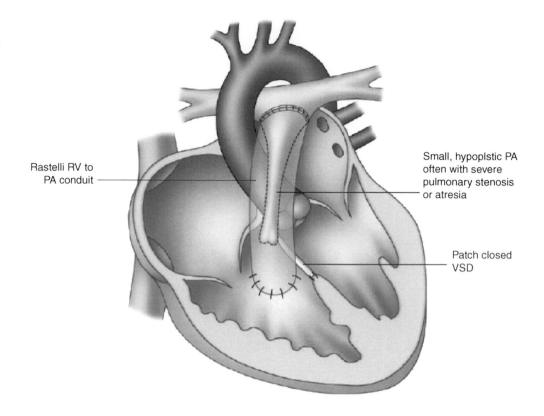

Rastelli RV to
PA conduit

Small, hypoplstic PA
often with severe
pulmonary stenosis
or atresia

Patch closed
VSD

TABLE 21-2

SYNDROMES ASSOCIATED WITH
CONGENITAL HEART DISEASE

SYNDROME	DESCRIPTION	ASSOCIATED CONGENITAL LESIONS
Holt Oram	Congenital abnormality of the hand and radius; autosomal dominant	Atrial septal defect
Williams Syndrome	Deletion of elastin gene (7q11.23)	Supravalvular aortic stenosis
Noonan Syndrome	Facial dysmorphism, short stature; autosomal dominant	Pulmonic stenosis/dysplasia, hypertrophic cardiomyopathy, pectus excavatum
Down Syndrome	Trisomy 13, intellectual disability	Primum ASD and AV canal type VSD, PDA, TOF
Turners Syndrome	45X karyotype; Females; gonadal dysgenesis; short stature, primary amenorrhea	Aortic valvular disease (20–30 %) and aortic coarctation (3–10 %)
Congenital Rubella Syndrome	Hearing impairment, cataracts/congenital glaucoma, retinopathy	PDA, branch pulmonary stenosis

REFERENCES

1. Liberthson RR. Congenital heart disease: diagnosis and management in children and adults. Boston: Little, Brown; 1989.
2. Warnes CA, Williams RG, Bashore TM, Child JS, Connolly HM, Dearani JA, et al. ACC/AHA 2008 guidelines for the management of adults with congenital heart disease. Circulation. 2008;118:e714–833.
3. Du ZD, Hijazi ZM, Kleinman CS, Silverman NH, Larntz K. Comparison between transcatheter and surgical closure of secundum atrial septal defect in children and adults: results of a multicenter nonrandomized trial. J Am Coll Cardiol. 2002;39: 1836–44.
4. Dimopoulos K, Inuzuka R, Goletto S, Giannakoulas G, Swan L, Wort SJ, et al. Improved survival among patients with Eisenmenger syndrome receiving advanced therapy for pulmonary arterial hypertension. Circulation. 2010;121(1):20.

SUGGESTED READINGS

Rhodes JF, Hijazi ZM, Sommer RJ. Obstructive lesions pathophysiology of congenital heart disease in the adult. Part II: simple. Circulation. 2008;117:1228–37.
Sommer RJ, Hijazi ZM, Rhodes Jr JF. Pathophysiology of congenital heart disease in the adult: part I: shunt lesions. Circulation. 2008a;117:1090–9.
Sommer RJ, Hijazi ZM, Rhodes JF. Pathophysiology of congenital heart disease in the adult: part III: complex. Circulation. 2008b;117:1228–37.

CHAPTER 22

JONATHAN CLARKE AND GREGORY D. LEWIS

Pulmonary Hypertension

CHAPTER OUTLINE

ABBREVIATIONS

6 MW	6 Minute Walk
APAH	Associated with Pulmonary Arterial Hypertension
BMP	Bone Morphogenic Protein
CCB	Calcium Channel Blockers
COPD	Chronic Obstruction Lung Disease
CTEPH	Chronic Thromboembolic Pulmonary Hypertension
DVT	Deep Venous Throbosis
FPAH	Familial Pulmonary Arterial Hypertension
HFpEF	Heart Failure with preserved Ejection Fraction
IPAH	Idiopathic Pulmonary Arterial Hypertension
JVP	Jugular Venous Pressure
LFT	Liver Function Test
LVEF	Left Ventricular Ejection Fraction
mPAP	Mean Pulmonary Artery Pressure
NO	Nitric Oxide
NYHA	New York Heart Association
PA	Pulmonary Artery
PAH	Pulmonary Arterial Hypertension
PAP	Pulmonary Artery Pressure
PCH	Pulmonary Capillary Hemangiomatosis
PCWP	Pulmonary Capillary Wedge Pressure
PDE-5	Phosphodiesterase-5
PE	Pulmonary Embolism
PH	Pulmonary Hypertension
PVOD	Pulmonary Veno-Occlusive Disease
PVR	Pulmonary Vascular Resitance
RV	Right Ventricle
RVEF	Right Ventricular Ejection Fraction
TAPSE	Tricuspid Annular Plane Systolic Excursion
TTE	Transthoracic echocardiogram
WHO	World Health Organization

INTRODUCTION

The right ventricular-pulmonary vascular unit is a low resistance, high compliance system that is normally capable of accommodating large increases in blood flow with a minimal increment in pressure. The development of elevated pulmonary arterial pressures, either in unselected populations or in individuals with a variety of cardiopulmonary diseases, is increasingly recognized to be associated with a markedly increased risk of mortality. Regardless of the etiology, pulmonary hypertension leads to right ventricular dysfunction that is closely associated with impaired exercise capacity, renal and hepatic dysfunction. This chapter will briefly review the epidemiology and pathophysiology of pulmonary hypertension (PH) in addition to current diagnostic and treatment approaches with particular emphasis on PH arising in the setting of other cardiovascular diseases.

1. Overview of pulmonary hypertension
2. Diagnostic work up
3. WHO Group Classification with particular attention to:
   (a) Idiopathic Arterial Pulmonary Hypertension
   (b) Pulmonary Venous Hypertension
   (c) Hypoxia Associated Pulmonary Hypertension
   (d) Chronic Thromboembolic Pulmonary Hypertension

DEFINITIONS

A. **Pulmonary Hypertension (PH)**

 ■ Definition: An abnormally high blood pressure within the arteries of the lungs
 ■ Hemodynamic diagnostic criteria

   – Mean pulmonary artery pressure > 25 mmHg.

B. **Pulmonary arterial hypertension (PAH)**

 ■ Definition: A syndrome caused from restricted blood flow through the pulmonary circulation leading to elevation in pulmonary resistance and subsequent right heart failure. Hemodynamic characteristics include

   – Mean pulmonary artery pressure (PAP) >25 mmHg and
   – Pulmonary capillary wedge pressure (PCWP) or left ventricular end diastolic pressure ≤15 mmHg and
   – Pulmonary vascular resistance (PVR) >3 Woods units

C. **Pathology**

 ■ Elevated PVR due to
 ■ loss of vascular luminal cross sectional area due to vascular remodeling from excessive cell proliferation and decreased rates of apoptosis
 ■ impaired endothelial function with excessive vasoconstriction (low nitric oxide and prostaglandin bioavailability, increased thromboxane A2) thrombosis in situ (platelets depleted of serotonin)
 ■ smooth muscle cell proliferation
 ■ 2 hit hypothesis

   – Permissive genotype (i.e. Bone Morphogenic Protein [BMP] 2 mutation)
   – Second insult (i.e. thromboembolism, toxin, infection)

 ■ Histology

   – Predominantly small pulmonary arteries
   – Intimal hyperplasia, medial hypertrophy, adventitial proliferation, thrombosis in situ, inflammation

■ Genetics

- 10 % of cases are familial
- 2 known genetic mutations: BMP-2 and activin-like kinase 1

D. World Health Organization (WHO) Group Classifications

1. Pulmonary arterial hypertension (PAH3)
    1.1. Idiopathic (IPAH)
    1.2. Familial (FPAH)
    1.3. Associated with (APAH):
        1.3.1. Collagen vascular disease
        1.3.2. Congenital systemic-to-pulmonary shunts
        1.3.3. Portal hypertension
        1.3.4. HIV infection
        1.3.5. Drugs and toxins
        1.3.6. Other (thyroid disorders, glycogen storage disease, Gaucher disease, hereditary hemorrhagic telangiectasia, hemoglobinopathies, myeloproliferative disorders, splenectomy)
    1.4. Associated with significant venous or capillary involvement
        1.4.1. Pulmonary veno-occlusive disease (PVOD)
        1.4.2. Pulmonary capillary hemangiomatosis (PCH)
    1.5. Persistent pulmonary hypertension of the newborn
2. Pulmonary hypertension with left heart disease
    2.1. Left-sided atrial or ventricular heart disease
    2.2. Left-sided valvular heart disease
3. Pulmonary hypertension associated with lung diseases and/or hypoxemia
    3.1. Chronic obstructive pulmonary disease
    3.2. Interstitial lung disease
    3.3. Sleep-disordered breathing
    3.4. Alveolar hypoventilation disorders
    3.5. Chronic exposure to high altitude
    3.6. Developmental abnormalities
4. Pulmonary hypertension due to chronic thrombotic and/or embolic disease (CTEPH)
    4.1. Thromboembolic obstruction of proximal pulmonary arteries
    4.2. Thromboembolic obstruction of distal pulmonary arteries
    4.3. Non-thrombotic pulmonary embolism (tumor, parasites, foreign material)
5. Miscellaneous
    5.1. Sarcoidosis,
    5.2. Histiocytosis X
    5.3. Lymphangiomatosis
    5.4. Compression of pulmonary vessels

DIAGNOSTIC WORK UP

A. History

■ Symptoms: Dyspnea on exertion, fatigue, chest pain, syncope, palpitations, lower extremity edema (Table 22-1)

B. Physical Exam (Table 22-2 [1]**)**

C. Diagnostic Studies

■ CXR

- Right ventricular (RV) enlargement, peripheral hypovascularity, hilar enlargement

TABLE 22-1

MEDICAL HISTORY ASSOCIATED WITH PULMONARY HYPERTENSION

GROUP I–PULMONARY ARTERIAL HYPERTENSION	GROUP II–PH WITH LEFT HEART INVOLVEMENT	GROUP III–PH ASSOCIATED WITH LUNG DISEASE AND/OR HYPOXIA	GROUP IV–PH ASSOCIATED WITH TO CHRONIC THROMBOTIC AND/OR EMBOLIC DISEASE	GROUP V–MISCELLANEOUS
Hemoglobinopathies	Atrial or ventricular disease	COPD	Pulmonary embolism	Sarcoidosis
Sickle cell	Systolic heart failure	Interstitial lung disease		Histiocytosis X
β-thalessemia+/+	Heart failure with preserved EF	Obstructive sleep apnea		Lymphangiomatosis
Hereditary spherocytosis	Constrictive or restrictive disease			Compression of pulmonary vessels
Family history of PAH (BMPR2 mutation)	Dilated cardiomyopathy			Adenopathy
Connective tissue disease	Valvular disease			Tumor
Limited cutaneous form of systemic sclerosis	Mitral regurgitation			Fibrosing mediastinitis
SLE	Mitral stenosis			
MCTD				
RA				
Liver disease/cirrhosis				
HIV				
Congenital heart disease with systemic shunt				
Drugs/toxin				
Fenfluramine				
Rapeseed oil				
Methamphetamine				
Cocaine				
Other				
Hereditary hemorrhagic telangiectasia				
Glycogen storage disease				
Gaucher disease				
Thyroid disorders				
Splenectomy				

+/+Standard nomenclature for homozygous gene

TABLE 22-2

SIGNS OF PULMONARY
HYPERTENSION [1]

EARLY PH	MODERATE TO SEVERE PH	ADVANCED PH WITH RV FAILURE
Accentuated S2 (best heard at apex)	Holosystolic murmur that increases with inspiration	Right ventricular S3
Early systolic click	Increased jugular 'v' waves	Distension of jugular veins
Mid systolic ejection murmur	Pulsatile liver	Heptomegaly
Left parasternal lift	Diastolic murmur	Peripheral edema
Right ventricular S4	Hepatojugular reflux	Ascites
Increased jugular 'a' wave		Hypotension, decreased pulse pressure, cool extremities

FIGURE 22-1

Echocardiographic differentiation
of elevated RV systolic pressure

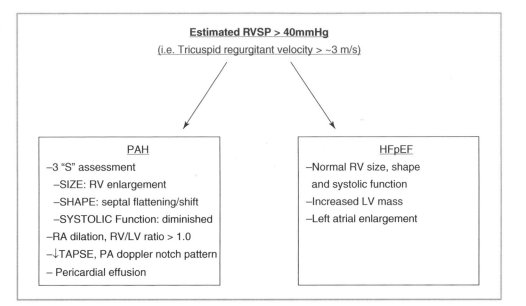

ECG

- Right ventricular hypertrophy, right atrial enlargement, right axis deviation

Trans-thoracic echocardiography (Fig. 22-1)

Further testing for diseases associated with pulmonary hypertension

- ANA & other connective tissue disease serologies
- Sleep study
- Liver function tests
- Pulmonary function tests
- V/Q scan
- HIV

D. Right heart catheterization

- Assess pulmonary vascular resistance to isolate pre-capillary and post-capillary contributions to pulmonary artery pressure
- **Pulmonary arterial hypertension** is characterized by elevations in both mean pulmonary artery pressure (mPAP) and transpulmonary gradient (pre-capillary pulmonary hypertension) (Fig. 22-2) [35]

    - mPAP>25 mmHg
    - PCWP <15 mmHg
    - PVR>3 Woods units

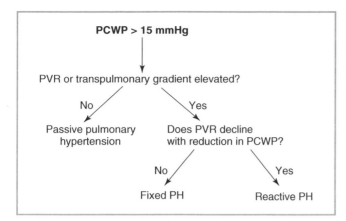

FIGURE 22-2

Diagnosing pulmonary venous/passive/post-capillary hypertension vs pulmonary arterial/pre-capillary hypertension (Adapted from Chatterjeee and Lewis [35])

	NITRIC OXIDE	**ADENOSINE**	**EPOPROSTENOL**
Route of administration	Inhaled	IV infusion	IV infusion
Dose titration	Nne	50 mcg/kg/min every 2 min	2 ng/kg/min every 10–15 min
Dose range	20–40 ppm for 5 min	50–250 mcg/kg/min	2–10 ng/kg/min
Side effects	↑ Left heart filling pressures	Dyspnea, chest pain, AV block	Headache, nausea, lightheadedness

TABLE 22-3

AGENTS FOR ACUTE VASODILATOR TESTING [1]

■ **Passive pulmonary hypertension** (post-capillary pulmonary hypertension)

- mPAP >25 mmHg
  PCWP >15 mmHg
- PVR <3 Woods Units

■ **Mixed (or "Out of Proportion") pulmonary hypertension**

- mPAP >25 mmHg
- PCWP >15 mmHg
- PVR >3 Woods Units

■ Pulmonary hypertension can be due to high pulmonary flow in the setting of high cardiac output
■ Assess for significant intra-cardiac shunt (O_2 saturations from the superior vena cava, right ventricle, pulmonary artery, and femoral artery)
■ Assess for low cardiac output (<2.1 L/min/m^2)
■ Assess for vasoreactivity to pulmonary vasodilators (Table 22-3)
■ Criteria for positive response

- ↓mPAP by ≥10 mmHg and absolute value <40 mmHg without fall in cardiac output
- >20 % reduction in PAP and PVR with no reduction in cardiac output
- 26.6 % of 64 IPAH patients responded with 94 % survival at 5 years compared to 55 % survival of non-responders [3]
- 12.6 % of 557 IPAH patients responded to vasodilator [4]

  ■ 95 % survival at 5 years (responders) vs 48 % (non-responders)

FIGURE 22-3

Treatment algorithm for
Group 1 PAH (Adapted from
McLaughlin et al. [1])

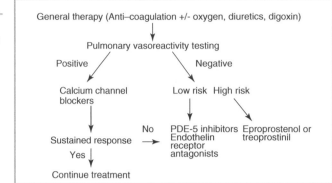

GROUP 1–PULMONARY HYPERTENSION

A. **Epidemiology**, **Natural Survival**, **and Prognosis**

■ ~15 cases/1,000,000 people [5]

– Idiopathic PAH: ~5 cases/1,000,000 people
– Familial PAH: ~1–2 cases/1,000,000 people
– Associated with PAH: 8–9 cases/1,000,000 people
– Historical 1, 3, 5 year survival → 68, 48, and 34 %, Median survival 2.8 years [6]
– Congenital heart disease-> IPAH->Connective tissue disease->HIV (Best outcome → worse)

B. **Treatment** (Fig. 22-3)

■ General recommendations

– Low level graded aerobic exercise
– Avoid heavy physical exertion or isometric exercise as this may cause syncope
– High altitudes may not be tolerated (If O_2 sat <92 %, then supplemental O_2 on airplanes)
– Avoid pregnancy (30–50 % mortality rate)

■ Tables 22-4a, 22-4b, and 22-4c shows therapies for Group 1 Pulmonary Arterial Hypertension

■ Warfarin therapy with INR 1.5–2.5 for all Group 1 patients

– Recommendations only for IPAH, not other forms of PH

■ No randomized control trials – data are only from 3 non-controlled observational studies
■ Mortality benefit seen in only calcium channel blockers (CCB) non-responders

– 1, 3, and 5 year survival: 91, 62, and 47 % (anti-coagulated) vs 52, 31, and 31 % (not anti-coagulated) [3]

■ Oxygen therapy to maintain O_2 sat >90 %
■ Diuretics for RV volume overload
■ Calcium channel blockers for pulmonary vasodilator- responders. (long acting nifedipine, diltiazem, or amlodipine. Verapamil not used due to negative inotropy)

– If no improvement to NYHA Class I or II, then not a chronic responder and alternative therapy should be started.

TABLE 22-4a

PROSTACYCLINS–VASODILATION WITH ANTI-PROLIFERATIVE EFFECTS

NAME	MODE OF DELIVERY	POPULATION	ADVANTAGES	DISADVANTAGES
Epoprostenol (Flolan)	IV or inhaled	Studied in IPAH and with PAH associated with scleroderma spectrum of disease patients with Class III and IV symptoms	Improved survival at 1 year 85–88 % and 3 years 63 % vs historic baseline survival of 59 % at 1 year and 35 % at 3 years [2] Improved 6 min walk test at 12 weeks [34]	Approved in only class III-IV unlike treprostinol Short half life–6 min Side effects–headache, jaw pain, flushing, nausea, diarrhea, skin rash, and muscle cramping Chronic use can result in high output heart failure
Treprostinil (Remodulin, Tyvaso)	Remodulin: IV or sc Tyvaso: inh	Studied in IPAH, connective tissue, and CHD related patients with Class II-IV symptoms	Half life: 4–5 h Improved 6 min walk test [29] Head to head trial vs epoprostenol, improved 6 MW test at 12 weeks, but with increased PA pressures and slightly decreased cardiac index–though dose of iv treprostinil at end of study was more than twice the dose of epoprostenol [16] Approved for class II symptoms	85 % of patients get pain and erythema at site of subcutaneous infusion Increased risk of gram negative bacteremia with intravenous treoprostinil due to soluent [15]
Iloprost (Ventavis)	inh	Studied in IPAH, PAD associated with the scleroderma spectrum of diseases or appetite suppressants, PH related to inoperable chronic thromboembolic disease with Class III and IV symptoms	Half life 20–30 min Combined clinical end point of improved 6 MW and improvement of one functional class at 12 weeks and 1 year [14, 19]	

TABLE 22-4b

ENDOTHELIN RECEPTOR ANTAGONISTS—PROMOTES VASODILATION AND DECREASES SMOOTH MUSCLE PROLIFERATION

NAME	MODE OF DELIVERY	POPULATION	ADVANTAGES	DISADVANTAGES
Bosentan (Tracleer)	Oral	Studied in IPAH and scleroderma spectrum with Class III or IV symptoms and IPAH, FPAH, PAH associated with connective tissue disease, HIV, and CHD with mild Class II symptoms Half life 5 h	Improved 6 MW, cardiac index and functional class, lower mPAP and PVR Prolonged time to clinical worsening defined by death, lung transplantation, hospitalization for PH, lack of clinical improvement or worsening leading to discontinuation of therapy, need for epoprostenol therapy, or atrial septostomy [8] Survival of 85–97 % at 1 year and 70–91 % at 2 years, however 44 % required epoprostenol at follow up [30, 31] Open label compared to historical survival rates—97 % and 91 % at 1 and 2 years respectively vs 91 % and 84 % for epoprostenol cohort, but baseline statistics suggest that epoprostenol cohort had more severe disease [10]	Black Box Warning: Dose dependent abnormal hepatic function—check LFTS every 3 months Teratogenic: barrier techniques recommended as hormonal methods may be less effective May cause testicular cancer and male infertility Syncope, flushing, anemia, and erythema
Ambrisentan (Letairis)	Oral	Studied in IPAH, PAH associated with connective tissue disease, anorexigen use, HIV infection in Class II and III patients	Increased 6 MW and prolonged time to clinical worsening [36]	LFT abnormalities Teratogenic Anemia May cause testicular atrophy Lower extremity edema in patients >65 years

TABLE 22-4c

PHOSPHODIESTERASE 5
INHIBITORS—REDUCES CGMP
DEGREDATION AND POTENTIATES
VASODILATORY EFFECTS OF NO

NAME	MODE OF DELIVERY	POPULATION	ADVANTAGES	DISADVANTAGES
Sildenafil (Revatio)	Oral	Studied in IPAH or PAD associated with connective tissue disease, or repaired congenital systemic-to-pulmonary shunts	Improved 6 MW test, functional class [20] Long term at 1 year showed sustained improvement in 6 MW test	Did not prolong time to clinical worsening Headaches, flushing, dyspepsia, epistaxis
Tadalafi (Adcirca)	Oral	Studied in idiopathic/heritable or related to anorexigen use, connective tissue disease, HIV infection, or congenital systemic-to-pulmonary shunts in Class II–IV patients	Improved 6 MW test and prolonged time to clinical worsening [32]	Headaches, myalgias, flushing

- ⊥ Digoxin
- Prostacyclin (Table 22-4a)
- Endothelin Receptor Antagonists (Table 22-4b)
- Phosphodiesterase Type 5 Inhibitors (Table 22-4c)
- Surgical interventions [1]

  - Atrial septostomy: 15 % mortality, improvement in 6 MW, NYHA functional class, and 30–40 % bridge to transplant. Consider only for severe PAH and intractable RV failure despite maximal therapy. Goals are palliation and bridge to transplant.
  - Heart/Lung or Lung transplant: increased operative mortality, but 3, 5, and 10 year outcomes similar for other indications. Reserved for those with intractable RV failure on inotropic support in the absence of other end organ disease.
  - Pulmonary thromboendarterectomy: for CTEPH patients with accessible disease and are suitable surgical candidates
  - Right Ventricular Assist Device: Experimental in patients with PAH

- Combination therapy

  - Inhaled treprostonil vs placebo + sildenafil or bosentan for 12 weeks [9]

    - Study population: idiopathic or familial PAH or PAH associated with collagen vascular disease, human immunodeficiency virus infection, or anorexigen use. Class III with 6 minute walk (6 MW) test of 200–450 m.
    - Improved 6 MW test, quality of life, and decreased pro-BNP levels.

  - Sildenafil vs placebo + intravenous epoprostenol for 16 weeks [26]

    - Study population: idiopathic, familial, associated with anorexigen use or connective tissue disease, or occurring after surgical repair of congenital systemic-to-pulmonary shunts with class II-III symptoms.
    - Improvements in mPAP, cardiac output, and time to clinical worsening

- Limitations of therapy studies

  - Small trials: most were not powered to detect differences in survival
  - Limited duration 8–16 weeks
  - 6 MW test affected by co-morbidities

    - Annual cost of therapy (approximately) [1, 12]
    - Sildenafil $13,000

TABLE 22-5

RISK STRATIFICATION OF WHO
GROUP 1 PULMONARY
HYPERTENSION [1]

DETERMINANTS OF RISK	LOWER RISK	HIGHER RISK
6 MW distance (m)	>400	<400
Peak VO$_2$ (ml/kg/min)	>10.2	<10.2
Echo variables	Preserved RV function	RA, RV enlargement, RV dysfunction, pericardial effusion
Hemodynamics	RAP<10, CI>2.5	RAP>20, CI<2.0
Biomarkers	Normal BNP, troponin	BNP, troponin elevation

- Tadalafil $13,000
- Bosentan $56,000
- Ambrisentan $57,000
- Iloprost $92,000
- Epoprostenol $32,000 (lower dose for 70 kg)
- Treprostinil $97,000

■ Risk Stratification of WHO Group 1 Pulmonary Hypertension is shown in Table 22-5 [1].

GROUP II–PULMONARY VENOUS HYPERTENSION (DUE TO LEFT HEART DYSFUNCTION)

A. **Overview**

■ Incidence greatly outnumbers the population with Group 1 pulmonary hypertension (Fig. 22-4).

■ Even with optimization of underlying etiology of elevated PA pressures, there will be a population who have PA pressures "out of proportion" to the expected pulmonary vascular response (Fig. 22-5).

■ Often initially presents at passive congestion with pulmonary venous hypertension with subsequent remodeling of pulmonary arteries leading to an increase in pulmonary artery resistance as a possible mechanism for preventing pulmonary edema.

■ RV Dysfunction and pulmonary hypertension determines survival in patients with moderate systolic and diastolic heart failure

- 20 % survival at 5 years with RV Ejection Fraction (RVEF) <35 % and high PA pressures vs 80 % survival with normal RVEF and PA pressures [33].

■ Pulmonary hypertension (PASP>35 mmHg) is common in HFpEF prevalence >80 %
■ Elevated PASP is a prognostic factor in HFpEF [11]

- Estimated 50 % survival of patients with HFpEF at 3 years if PASP >48 mmHg
- Better predictor of mortality than E/e' ratio, left atrial volume index, relative wall thickness, left ventricular mass index

B. **Treatment**

■ Optimizing neurohormonal medications for systolic heart failure
■ Epoprostenol is contraindicated in Group II pulmonary hypertension as the FIRST study showed an increased mortality, even in the face of improved hemodynamic measurements [7]
■ Endothelin antagonist studies failed to show an improvement in outcomes and some had an increased risk of heart failure exacerbations [17]

■ Phosphodiesterase-5 (PDE-5) inhibitors have shown consistent short-term improvements in 6 MW distance, hemodynamics, and peak VO$_2$. A long term outcomes trial (PITCH-HF) has been initiated (Table 22-6).

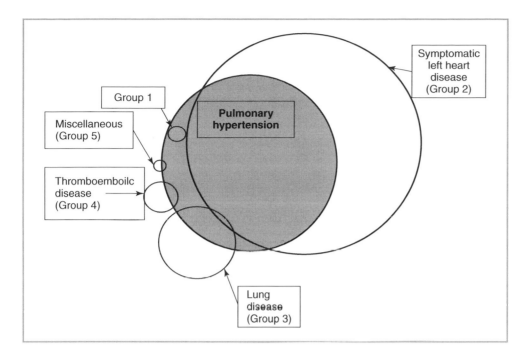

FIGURE 22-4

Pulmonary hypertension epidemiology synopsis

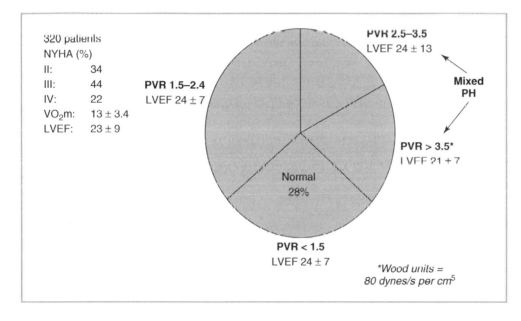

FIGURE 22-5

Pulmonary hypertension out of proportion to PCWP is common in Heart Failure with a preserved Ejection Fraction (HFpEF) [24]

GROUP III–HYPOXIA ASSOCIATED PULMONARY HYPERTENSION

A. Chronic Obstructive Pulmonary Disease (COPD)

- Retrospective series showed 3 % of patients with COPD had severe PH (>40 mmHg) and most had another possible cause of PH including anorexigen exposure, connective tissue disease, thromboembolic disease, or left ventricular disease [18]

- Only 1 % had COPD as the only potential etiology and this group had an unusual pattern of cardiopulmonary hemodynamics: mild-moderate obstruction, severe hypoxia, hypocapnea, and very low diffusing capacity.

- Most patients (50.2 %) have mildly elevated mean PA pressures (25–35 mmHg), 35 % had normal pressures and 15 % had moderate or worse (>35 mmHg) pressures [21].

- Treatment should be directed towards the underlying COPD, but if mean PA pressures >35 mmHg a work up for other causes of pulmonary hypertension should ensue

TABLE 22-6

SUMMARY OF PDE5 INHIBITOR STUDIES IN GROUP II PULMONARY HYPERTENSION.

DRUG	AUTHORS/JOURNAL	STUDY POPULATION	N	DURATION (WEEKS)	DOSE (MG TID)	1° ENDPOINT	2° ENDPOINT(S)	FINDINGS
Sildenafil	Lewis G, *Circulation* 2007;116: 1555–62 [22]	NYHA 2–4, LVEF<0.35, mPAP>25	30	12	25–75	Δ peak VO_2	Hemodynamics ΔLVEF, RVEF, ΔMLHF, Δ6MWT	pVO_2 +15 % ↑ RVEF ↑ 6MWT
Sildenafil	Guazzi M, *JACC* 2007;50: 2136–44 [23]	NYHA 2–3 LVEF<0.45 Age<65	46	24	50	Δ peak VO_2 ΔVE/VCO_2	Δ Ergoreflex Δ FMD	pVO_2 +26 % ↑FMD ↓VE/VCO_2
Sildenafil	Behling A, *J Card Fail* 2008;14:189–97 [13]	NYHA 1–3 LVEF<0.4	19	4	50	Δ peak VO_2 Δ echo PASP	Δ VE/VCO_2	pVO_2 +21 % ↓VE/VCO_2
Sildenafil	Tedford RJ, *Circulation* 2008;1:213–9 [37]	Post-LVAD PVR>3WU	26	15	25–75	Δ PVR, CO	ΔRV contractility, Δ TAPSE	PVR−50 % ↑dP/dt 50 %
Sildenafil	Guazzi M, *Circulation* 2011;124: 164–74 [38]	HFpEF	44	52	50	Δ PAP	Δ PVR, Δ RV function, Δ TAPSE	
Sildenafil	NIH HF Network RELAX	HFpEF	215	24	20–60	Δ peak VO_2	Clinical score 6MWT	

B. **Interstitial lung disease**

■ Similar to COPD, the magnitude is often modest, but a small population has severe disease

■ Treatment is directed toward underlying disease with oxygen and immunomodulators and workup for other potential causes of pulmonary hypertension should be performed

C. **Sleep disordered breathing**

■ Generally modest elevations, if severe and out of proportion look for other causes

GROUP IV—THROMBOEMBOLIC PULMONARY HYPERTENSION

A. **Risk after PE**

■ 4 % risk at 2 years after an acute pulmonary embolism [25]

B. **Pathophysiology**

■ Gradual formation of organized thromboemboli after deep venous thrombosis (DVT) or pulmonary embolism (PE) with distal pulmonary microvascular changes due to

– Obstruction of small, subsegmental elastic pulmonary arteries
– Vasculopathy of the small muscular arteries with pathology similar to IPAH [39]

C. **Diagnosis**

■ V/Q scan more sensitive than CT scan for initial characterization of CTEPH
■ Angiogram is the gold standard

D. **Treatment**

■ Diuretics
■ Oxygen
■ Lifelong anticoagulation
■ Epoprostenol can be considered in

High-risk patients with poor hemodynamics as a bridge to embolectomy
– Post-surgery patients with persistent pulmonary hypertension
– Patients for whom surgery is contraindicated

■ Thromboendarterectomy can be highly effective in carefully selected patients with proximal disease

PULMONARY HYPERTENSION IN THE CARDIAC SURGERY PATIENT

■ Post-operatively, PAH specific therapy may be considered when left sided filling pressures are normal or near normal, but PA pressures remain elevated
■ Persistent PH often is present post-mitral and aortic valve repair
■ Inhaled NO and prostacyclin are effective short term strategies and more effective and tolerable when compared to nitroprusside [27]
■ Inhaled iloprost has been used successfully in patients with RV failure during and following heart transplant [28]
■ Chronic oral therapy for persistent PH following surgery for valvular heart disease has not been adequately studied to make formal recommendations

Pathophysiology of AF

■ Two mechanisms account for the majority of cases of atrial fibrillation

- Foci in the pulmonary veins with very rapid rates initiate and maintain atrial fibrillation in many patients with paroxysmal AF
- Multiple unstable and varying "wavelet" depolarization circuits, reentrant circuits, or rotors in both atria, resulting in fibrillatory conduction contribute to arrhythmia perpetuation, particularly in patients with persistent AF

■ AF results in hemodynamic changes resulting from the lack of an appropriately-timed atrial contraction leading to less-efficient left ventricular filling and ejection

■ Clinical effects

- AF is often not perceived by normal subjects at rest, since the cardiac output can be maintained by increased contractility
- Exercise tolerance and maximum cardiac output are compromised, leading to the dyspnea experienced by some patients
- This becomes clinically important in cases of impaired LV diastolic function (aortic stenosis, left ventricular hypertrophy, hypertrophic cardiomyopathy), where atrial transport is important, as well as in patients with systolic HF and low reserve, where AF may cause decompensation and hospitalization
- AF with fast ventricular rates may precipitate angina in patients with CHD and is particularly dangerous in patients with accessory atrioventricular pathways with short refractory periods where it may degenerate to VF
- Fast rates may cause mechanical remodeling of the ventricles leading to LV systolic dysfunction and HF (tachycardia-induced cardiomyopathy)

■ Structural and electrical remodeling of the atria resulting from prolonged AF promotes persistence of the arrhythmia

Treatment Considerations for AF

Cardioversion

■ New onset AF may be an indication for urgent cardioversion, deferred cardioversion after 3 weeks of antithrombotic therapy, or rhythm control without cardioversion (see Electrical Cardioversion)

- Cardioversion should be considered for all patients with new-onset AF in the absence of spontaneous conversion

■ Major issues in the long-term treatment of atrial fibrillation are the choice of rhythm versus rate control strategies and antithrombotic therapy

Rate vs. Rhythm Control

■ Rate control

- Rate control is initial treatment for patients who do not require urgent cardioversion
- Agents used for rate control include BB, non-dihydropyridine CCB (e.g. diltiazem and verapamil), and digoxin to control the ventricular rate to below 100 bpm at rest
- Amiodarone can be used for rate control if other agents fail and is also useful to maintain sinus rhythm
- BB (e.g. metoprolol, or esmolol for intravenous administration in the acute setting) are preferred in patients with CHD, especially in the presence of angina or acute coronary syndromes
- CCB are used preferentially in patients with intolerance to BB
- Digoxin is a preferred agent in patients with HF, but should only be used as chronic therapy together with BB

■ Rhythm Control

   – In patients with symptomatic AF and no structural heart disease, class IC agents are generally employed as first-line therapy

   – Amiodarone is more effective in maintaining sinus rhythm than Class IC antiarrhythmic agents (e.g. propafenone, flecainide) or sotalol (Class III) but is considerably more toxic than other agents and is generally reserved for elderly patients or as a last line agent in younger individuals

   – Dronedarone (an amiodarone analog with short half-life and no iodine moiety) is less effective than amiodarone, is contraindicated in patients with HF, and requires monitoring of liver function tests due to risk for hepatic necrosis

   – Dofetilide (Class III) is less frequently used because of restricted access, proarrhythmia, and the requirement for continuous monitoring

   – Class IA antiarrhythmic agents (e.g. procainamide, disopyramide) are not commonly used, except occasionally in in patients with hypertrophic cardiomyopathy or vagally-mediated atrial fibrillation

   – BB are indicated for prevention of exercise-induced atrial fibrillation and are sometimes used before rhythm control therapy to control the ventricular rate

   – Class I antiarrhythmic drugs should always be used in conjunction with a BB (or a CCB if BB are not tolerated) to prevent the occurrence of class IC-induced atrial flutter with 1:1 AV conduction

   – Catheter ablation is an option as second line therapy for rhythm control in symptomatic patients who have failed at least one antiarrhythmic drug and in whom additional trials of antiarrhythmic drugs are not preferred by the patient (see Catheter Ablation) [5]

■ There is no evidence that survival is significantly different between rhythm and rate control strategies

Antithrombotic Therapy

■ The $CHADS_2$ score may be used to estimate the risk of stroke in patients with non-rheumatic AF [6]

   – The letters stand for **C**ongestive HF (1 point), **H**ypertension, **A**ge 75 and above, **D**iabetes, (each 1 point) and **S**troke or TIA history (2 points)

   – $CHADS_2$ stratifies patients with a tenfold range of annual risk of stroke ranging from 1.9 to 18.2 % and has found wide application in estimating the advisability of antithrombotic therapy

   – Patients with a $CHADS_2$ score of 0 have a low risk of stroke, and thus the risk/benefit ratio dictates use of aspirin (ASA) alone; those with score of 1 may be given either ASA or warfarin and those with 2 or higher are at high risk for future stroke and should be treated with oral anticoagulants such as warfarin, dabigatran, or rivaroxaban

   – The CHA_2DS_2-VASc score [7] adds: '**A2**: age 75 and above' (2 points), **A**ge 65–74 (1 point), **V**ascular disease, and **Sc** (sex category; female gender) (1 point each), and **S2** (history of peripheral embolism, stroke, or TIA) (2 points)

      ■ Patients with a CHA_2DS_2-VASc score of 0 may be given ASA, those with a score of 1 may be given ASA or oral anticoagulation and those with a score of 2 should be given oral anticoagulation

■ ASA is prescribed in doses of 75–325 mg

■ Warfarin (goal INR 2–3) remains the mainstay of antithrombotic therapy in the majority of patients

   – New antithrombotic agents have been approved for AF and are now supplanting warfarin

   – In addition to comparable or better efficacy, these agents:

- Have predictable pharmacodynamics and do not require monitoring
- All appear to be associated with a lower risk of intracranial hemorrhage compared with warfarin
- Unlike warfarin, there are no clinically available antidotes to reverse the effects of newer agents in the event of major bleeding

  - Dabigatran (a direct thrombin inhibitor), administered 150 mg twice daily for those age <75 years or with preseSSSrved renal function

    - For older patients or those with chronic kidney disease, a dose of 75 mg twice daily is recommended
    - Concern has been raised regarding excessive bleeding, and a higher rate of myocardial infarctions

  - Rivaroxaban (an orally-active direct factor Xa inhibitor), administered 20 mg once daily with the evening meal

    - Lower doses (15 mg daily) are recommended for those with renal failure (CrCl 15–50 mL/min)

  - Apixaban (an orally-active direct factor Xa inhibitor), administered 5 mg twice daily

    - administered 2.5 mg twice daily if serum creatinine >1.5 or age >80 or weight < 60kg

Atrial Flutter (AFL)

- AFL is a reentrant arrhythmia similar to AF

  - As in AF, the SAN and AVN are not required for the initiation or maintenance of the arrhythmia
  - The difference between AF and AFL lies in the regularity of the atrial cycle length (F-F interval) in AFL, with a rate usually in the range of 250–320 bpm
  - Lower flutter rates are observed in the presence of antiarrhythmic agents (Class I, III) and in some patients with diseased atria

- The commonest form of AFL (Type I or typical AFL) is due to a single reentrant circuit circulating around the tricuspid annulus in the RA
- This circuit is most often counterclockwise in direction but may be clockwise in some individuals

  - AFL usually results in a ventricular rate of about 150 bpm, with an atrial rate of about 300 bpm and 2:1 AV nodal conduction

    - Other even AV conduction ratios (e.g. 4:1, 6:1) may also occur
    - Odd AV conduction ratios (e.g. 3:1, 5:1) are less common
    - Irregular ventricular response (usually with Wenckebach periodicity) may be seen in the presence of medications affecting the AV node (e.g. digoxin, beta blockers, calcium channel blockers) or in the presence of AV nodal disease

  - AFL with 1:1 AV conduction will result in very high ventricular rates

    - May be associated with wide QRS duration due to ventricular aberration
    - May cause hemodynamic instability

- The classical ECG has a saw tooth appearance (most visible in V1-2 or in the inferior leads)

  - This may not be present in patients with atypical (Type II) AFL, which has a different locations and reentrant circuits than typical AFL

- Transition between AFL and AF is commonly observed in patients with all types of AFL
- Vagal maneuvers, adenosine, or esmolol may be used to slow AV conduction and reveal the sawtooth F-wave pattern in cases of AFL with 2:1 conduction where the diagnosis may be in doubt
- Unlike AVNRT or AVRT that may break after these maneuvers or medications, AFL does not typically break in response to AV nodal blocking agents, as the AV node does not participate in the reentrant circuit

Typical (Type I) Atrial Flutter

- Typical (Type I) AFL results in a negative F wave in lead II and positive F wave in aVL and aVR
- The reentrant circuit in Type I AFL includes the cavotricuspid isthmus (located between the IVC, the ostium of the coronary sinus, and the tricuspid valve annulus)

  - Referred to as "isthmus dependent" and can be entrained (since there is an excitable time gap in the reentry loop) and ablated at the isthmus
  - Type I AFL may proceed in a counterclockwise (90 % of the cases, positive F waves in V1) or clockwise (negative F waves in V1) fashion

- Example: Chap. 33, ECG #37

Atypical (Type II) Atrial Flutter

- Atypical (Type II) AFL results in faster atrial rates (340–440 bpm), and often cannot be entrained unless the stimulating catheter is in close proximity to the reentrant circuit
- Positive F waves may observed in the inferior leads
- Activation of the atria at the fast rates may result in fibrillatory conduction (described in the AF section)
- The reentrant pathway may be located in either the RA or LA
- Type II AFL may be distinguished from coarse AF by the regularity of F waves
- While the majority of type I (typical/right-sided) flutters are isthmus-dependent, this occurs only in a minority of type II (atypical) cases

Atrioventricular Nodal Reentrant Tachycardia (AVNRT)

- AVNRT is a common supraventricular arrhythmia
- Usually manifested at a young age
- Most patients do not have structural heart disease
- Characterized by regular narrow QRS tachycardia at rates between 120 and 220 bpm with abrupt onset and offset

  - The AV node may be divided functionally into two pathways with different refractory periods and conduction velocities (fast and slow) which creates the substrate for AV node reentry

- AVNRT may be classified into typical, atypical, and intermediate subtypes

Typical (Slow-Fast) AVNRT

- Accounts for 90 % of cases
- Antegrade conduction (toward the ventricles) proceeds through the slow pathway and retrograde activation through the fast pathway (Fig. 23-1a)

  - This causes rapid retrograde activation of the atria (P negative in II, III and aVF, positive in aVR) that is simultaneous with antegrade ventricular activation and, as a result, the P wave occurs at the within or at end of QRS complex (pseudo R prime)
  - The RP interval is shorter than half of the RR interval of the AVNRT (Short RP tachycardia)

- Example: Chap. 34, ECG #40

FIGURE 23-1

Schematic diagrams illustrating mechanisms of atrioventricular nodal reentrant tachycardias. (**a**) Typical (slow-fast) AVNRT. (**b**) Atypical (fast-slow) AVNRT (Modified from Braunwald [8])

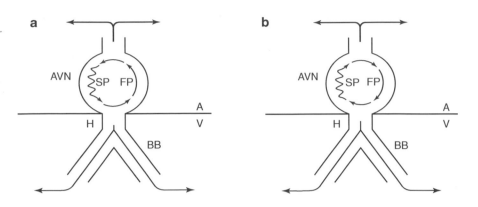

Atypical (Fast-Slow) AVNRT

■ Activation occurs in the opposite direction to that of typical AVNRT
■ Antegrade conduction is via the fast pathway and there is late activation of the atria from retrograde conduction via the slow pathway (Fig. 23-1b)

– The P wave occurs late and within the ST segment in this long RP tachycardia

■ AVNRT is usually precipitated by a premature beat (either atrial or ventricular) that is blocked in either the slow or fast pathway as a result of different refractory periods between the two pathways, creating the substrate for reentry

– Usually APC in typical AVNRT
– Either PVC or APC in atypical AVNRT

Atrioventricular Reentrant Tachycardia (AVRT)

■ Atrioventricular reentrant tachycardias (AVRTs) are associated with the presence of accessory pathways that function as part of the tachycardia reentrant circuit
■ A classical example is the Wolff-Parkinson-White (WPW) syndrome

– The baseline electrocardiogram in classical WPW shows a short PR and wide QRS with a delta wave at the onset of the QRS and secondary T-wave changes (in the opposite direction to the QRS)
– Atrial pacing at increasing rates results in widening of the QRS complex and magnifies the delta wave by prolonging the conduction time through the AV node and increasing the degree of manifest preexcitation (conduction via the accessory pathway)

■ The macro-reentrant circuit between the atria and the ventricles involves conduction via an accessory pathway between the atria and ventricles (e.g. bundle of Kent), as well as the AV node

– Orthodromic AVRT – conduction occurs antegrade through the AV node and retrograde via the accessory pathway, resulting in a narrow-complex tachycardia with retrograde P waves occurring after the QRS complex typically within the ST segment (Fig. 23-2a), Example: Chap. 33, ECG #41
– Antidromic AVRT (less common) – conduction occurs antegrade through the accessory pathway and retrograde via the AV node, resulting in a wide-complex, short RP tachycardia (Fig. 23-2b and Chap. 33 ECG #42)

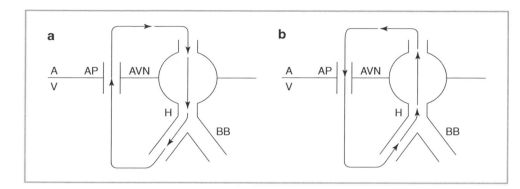

FIGURE 23-2

Schematic diagrams illustrating mechanisms of atrioventricular reentrant tachycardias. (**a**) Orthodromic AVRT. (**b**) Antidromic AVRT (Modified from Braunwald [8])

- In both orthodromic and antidromic AVRTs, the RP interval remains constant if the SVT rate changes, ST-T changes may be present, and the arrhythmia is initiated by an APC or PVC
- Arrhythmias related to a concealed accessory pathway (no delta wave on baseline ECG) conducting only in the retrograde direction manifest on the surface ECG as narrow QRS tachycardias with heart rates between 120 and 200 BPM
- In addition to the bundle of Kent, accessory pathways include

  - James fibers – intranodal or paranodal fibers that bypass all or part of the AV node to enter the bundle of His before the bifurcation, resulting in an electrocardiogram with a short PR with normal duration QRS (enhanced AV conduction may also result in the same electrocardiographic configuration)
  - Lown-Ganong-Levine (LGL) syndrome is the occurrence an ECG with a short PR and normal duration QRS together with tachyarrhythmias
  - Mahaim fibers are atriofascicular pathways that are typically associated with left bundle branch block (LBBB) tachycardias in which the atriofascicular fiber (typically RA to right bundle branch (RBB) connection) is used as the antegrade limb and the AV node as the retrograde limb of the reentrant circuit
    More rarely, nodoventricular and fasiculoventricular connections may be present
  - In a small percentage of patients, multiple accessory pathways may coexist and other congenital anomalies may be present in association with preexcitation (e.g. hypertrophic cardiomyopathy, Ebstein's anomaly)

- The development of atrial fibrillation in patients with accessory pathways (pre-excitation syndromes) is a serious event, since it can lead to very high ventricular rates and may degenerate to ventricular fibrillation (VF) and death in patients in whom one or more accessory pathways is associated with a short antegrade refractory period
- Pre-excitation predisposes to atrial fibrillation (occurring in 10–20 % of cases)

  - The ECG demonstrates irregularly irregular RR intervals with wide QRS configuration (which may vary from beat to beat due variation in the degree of preexcitation)
  - The ability of the accessory pathway to rapidly conduct during AF is an independent predictor of death in this context

    - Usually due to hemodynamic collapse and/or VF
- Patients with preexcitation syndromes should be risk stratified with respect to the risk of sudden cardiac death (SCD)

  - The incidence of SCD overall is rather low (1–2 per 1,000 per years) [9]
  - The majority of patients who suffer SCD experience recurrent AVRT before SCD, underscoring the importance of risk stratification and appropriate treatment in all patients with symptomatic arrhythmias associated with preexcitation
  - Patients with symptomatic AVRT or AF, syncope, presyncope, and those with multiple accessory pathways should undergo catheter ablation (rare exceptions include patients

who prefer pharmacological therapy with antiarrhythmic drugs to curative catheter ablation and those in whom catheter ablation is considered high risk because of proximity of the accessory pathway to the bundle of His)

- Electrophysiologic study (EPS) to evaluate prognosis in asymptomatic patients is generally not necessary unless there is family history of sudden death or the patients are engaged in high-risk professions (e.g. airline pilots) or competitive athletics
- Class IA antiarrhythmic agents (e.g. IV procainamide), amiodarone or cardioversion may be used to terminate the arrhythmia
- Verapamil and adenosine are contraindicated for termination of preexcited AF and digoxin is contraindicated in patients with preexcitation (may increase conduction via the accessory pathway and result in higher ventricular rates due to shortening of the accessory pathway refractory period)

Non-paroxysmal Junctional Tachycardia (NPJT)

- Uncommon tachycardia
- Due to enhanced automaticity of a focus in the bundle of His
- May develop following myocardial infarction, digoxin toxicity, myocarditis, or cardiac surgery
- Retrograde P waves may be present
- Permanent junctional reciprocating tachycardia (PJRT), typically found in the pediatric population, is rarely encountered in adults

DIFFERENTIAL DIAGNOSIS OF TACHYARRHYTHMIAS

Narrow Complex Tachycardias (NCT) (Table 23-1)

- Table 23-1 provides a diagnostic approach to the evaluation of narrow complex tachycardias (NCT).

TABLE 23-1	

APPROACH TO THE NARROW COMPLEX TACHYCARDIA	Evaluate regularity of the ventricular response
	  Irregularly irregular ventricular rate suggests AF or MAT.
	    In MAT there are distinct P waves of at least 3 configurations (and at least 3 each of PP, PR, and RR intervals)

	What is the atrial rate?
	  100–150 bpm suggests ST, IST, MAT, NPJT
	  150–250 bpm suggests AT, AVNRT, AVRT, PJRT
	  250–350 bpm suggests AFL
	  >350 bpm suggests AF

	What is the P wave configuration?
	  In ST, IST and AT (when the focus is near the SA node) similar to sinus rhythm
	  Inverted in the inferior leads in AVNRT, AVRT with septal pathway, and typical flutter

	What is the RP interval?
	  Short (less than half of the RR interval) in orthodromic AVRT and the typical (slow-fast) AVNRT where the P wave has a retrograde configuration (e.g. negative in lead II, positive in aVR)
	    Less commonly, a short RP tachycardia may be JT or AT with first-degree AV block
	  Long in cases of antidromic AVRT and atypical (fast-slow) AVNRT; may be long in AT with first degree AV block

	Response to vagal maneuvers or pharmacologic AV nodal blockade?
	  The atrial activity of AF and AFL may become apparent
	  AVNRT and AVRT may be terminated
	  Administration of adenosine, non-dihydropyridine CCB (diltiazem, verapamil) or beta blockers (esmolol, metoprolol) may have similar effects
	    These techniques should not be performed in patients with AF and a history of preexcitation

Wide Complex Tachycardias
(WCT; See Also Chap. 24)

■ Although the great majority of NCT are supraventricular (VT may rarely be associated with a narrow QRS), wide QRS tachycardias may be either ventricular or supraventricular

- Although several have been proposed, there is no criterion or combination of criteria that can correctly identify the arrhythmia in all cases [10, 11]
- Many patients with WCT are hemodynamically unstable and require urgent therapy, possibly cardioversion
- On the other hand, hemodynamic stability does not exclude VT as a cause of the arrhythmia

■ See Chap. 24 for variables predicting VT and clinical assessment
■ When the diagnosis remains unclear, it is prudent to treat the arrhythmia as ventricular rather than supraventricular

ELECTRICAL CARDIOVERSION

■ Electrical cardioversion is useful in patients with sustained symptomatic atrial tachyarrhythmias
■ Table 23-2 summarizes recommended uses of cardioversion in this context
■ The risks of direct current cardioversion are mainly related to thromboembolism and arrhythmias such (bradycardia and ventricular tachyarrhythmias) as well as hypotension and other anesthesia-related complications

- Patients with AF of unknown duration or lasting 48 h or longer should receive oral anticoagulation (warfarin INR 2.0–3.0, dabigatran, or rivaroxaban) for at least 3 weeks prior to and 4 weeks after cardioversion

    ■ It is important to continue anticoagulation after cardioversion due to stunning of the left atrium and atrial appendage by cardioversion, which may increase the risk of thrombus formation and systemic embolism

■ Transesophageal echocardiography (TEE) may be performed immediately prior to cardioversion to assure the absence of left atrial thrombus in patients who are not therapeutically anticoagulated prior to the procedure and in whom immediate cardioversion is deemed appropriate

    Spontaneous echo contrast, or "smoke," is a marker of stasis and propensity to develop thrombi and may be related to fibrinogen-mediated erythrocyte aggregation

■ Atrial arrhythmias that are reentrant in mechanism may be terminated by pacing and capturing the atria at a rate faster than that of the underlying arrhythmia
■ Continuous atrial overdrive pacing (continuous electronic adjustment to pace the atrium at a rate slightly higher than the patient's intrinsic sinus rhythm, as a means of potentially preventing the initiation of atrial fibrillation) does not prevent the occurrence of atrial fibrillation (ASSERT trial)

CATHETER ABLATION

■ Catheter ablation is commonly employed to treat patients with supraventricular tachyarrhythmias

- Common SVTs subjected to catheter ablation are AFL, AT, AVRT and AVNRT
- More recently, catheter ablation has been widely applied to the treatment of both paroxysmal and persistent AF

(a) Sinus tachycardia
(b) Atypical AVNRT
(c) Typical AVNRT
(d) Antidromic AVRT
(e) Atrial flutter

2. **What is the best initial treatment for the patient described in Question 1?**
(a) IV amiodarone
(b) IV digoxin
(c) IV adenosine
(d) IV procainamide
(e) DC cardioversion

3. **A 78-year-old man with hypertension on amlodipine and irbesartan, DM on metformin, and hypercholesterolemia on atorvastatin, presents with a 1–2 week history of exertional dyspnea. He has no chest pain or fever. His blood pressure is 160/70 and his heart rate is 110 bpm, with an irregularly irregular pulse. Cardiac auscultation reveals no murmurs or extra heart sounds. Physical examination is otherwise normal. What diagnostic tests would be appropriate?**

(a) Transthoracic echocardiogram
(b) Pulmonary function tests
(c) 12-lead electrocardiogram
(d) Thyroid function tests
(e) (a) and (b)
(f) (a) and (c)
(g) (a), (b), (c)
(h) (a), (c), (d)
(i) (a), (b), (c), (d)

4. **What are the important therapeutic considerations for the patient described in Question 3?**
(a) Immediate DC cardioversion
(b) DC cardioversion after 3–4 weeks of therapeutic anticoagulation
(c) Radiofrequency ablation
(d) Long-term therapeutic anticoagulation
(e) (a) and (d)
(f) (b) and (d)

ANSWERS

1. (c) The sudden onset of the arrhythmia and the absence of physical findings related to increased sympathetic tone (e.g. fever) argue against sinus tachycardia. Atrial flutter would demonstrate regular F waves (at this rate, likely with 2:1 conduction). Among the remaining choices, typical AVNRT is the most common. Atypical AVNRT would have a long RP interval and P waves would likely be seen. Typical AVNRT will usually have P waves that are either hidden within the QRS complex (i.e. not visible) or attached to the terminal portion of the QRS complex. AVRT always exhibits P waves that occur after the QRS complex, usually in the ST segment.

2. (c) Reentrant supraventricular tachyarrhythmias that include the AV node in the reentrant pathway are almost always interrupted with AV nodal-blocking agents, particularly adenosine. These include adenosine, beta-blockers (e.g. IV esmolol and metoprolol), non-dihydropyridine calcium channel blockers (e.g. IV diltiazem), and digoxin. Although digoxin may terminate this arrhythmia, it has a far slower onset of action and lower efficacy than the other agents listed. In addition, digoxin alone is not indicated for prevention of this arrhythmia (without concomitant use of beta blockers). Amiodarone is a multichannel antiarrhythmic and may terminate this arrhythmia, but it would take far longer than adenosine. Procainamide is a class IA antiarrhythmic that is typically used to terminate wide-complex tachycardias involving an accessory pathway or ventricular tachycardias that are hemodynamically well tolerated. DC cardioversion would likely terminate this arrhythmia, but there is no indication for its use, given that the patient is hemodynamically stable.

3. (h) The first appropriate test would be a 12-lead electrocardiogram to confirm the diagnosis of atrial fibrillation and to exclude an acute myocardial infarction or ongoing ischemia. Thyroid function testing should be performed for newly-diagnosed atrial fibrillation unless there is a clear alternative etiology (e.g. mitral stenosis, systemic infection, alcohol use). In this patient, a transthoracic echocardiogram would also be useful to ascertain whether there is left ventricular systolic or, more likely, diastolic dysfunction, or any significant valvular disease. In these situations, effective left atrial contraction is necessary for optimal left ventricular filling and, in the presence of atrial fibrillation, may cause early heart failure. Furthermore, the safety and selection of antiarrhythmic drugs is determined largely by the presence or absence of underlying structural heart disease.

4. (f) The patient is hemodynamically stable and is in no acute distress, therefore immediate DC cardioversion is not indicated. After effective rate control therapy is initiated with either a BB or CCB, DC cardioversion following at least 3 weeks of therapeutic anticoagulation is appropriate. Following cardioversion, anticoagulation should be continued for at least 4 weeks in all patients, to reduce the risk of thromboembolic events. In this patient, given the patient's age, hypertension, and diabetes, his CHADS2 score is at least 3, suggesting that long-term therapeutic anticoagulation would be indicated.

REFERENCES

1. Josephson ME. Clinical cardiac electrophysiology: techniques and interpretations. 4th ed. Philadelphia: Lippincott Williams & Wilkins; 2008.

2. Shine KI, Kastor JA, Yurchak PM. Multifocal atrial tachycardia. Clinical and electrocardiographic features in 32 patients. N Engl J Med. 1968;279(7):344–9.

3. Healey JS, Connolly SJ, Gold MR, Israel CW, Van Gelder IC, Capucci A, et al. ASSERT Investigators. Subclinical atrial fibrillation and the risk of stroke. N Engl J Med. 2012;366(2):120–9.

4. Fuster V, Rydén LE, Cannom DS, et al. ACCF/AHA/HRS focused updates incorporated into the ACC/AHA/ESC 2006 Guidelines for the management of patients with atrial fibrillation. J Am Coll Cardiol. 2011;57(11):101–98.

5. Calkins H, Kuck KH, Cappato R, et al. HRS/EHRA/ECAS expert consensus statement on catheter and surgical ablation of atrial fibrillation: recommendations for patient selection, procedural techniques, patient management and follow-up, definitions, endpoints, and research trial design: a report of the Heart Rhythm Society (HRS) Task Force on Catheter and Surgical Ablation of Atrial Fibrillation. Heart Rhythm. 2012;9(4):632–96.

6. Gage BF, Waterman AD, Shannon W, Boechler M, Rich MW, Radford MJ. Validation of clinical classification schemes for predicting stroke: results from the National Registry of Atrial Fibrillation. JAMA. 2001;285(22):2864–70.

7. Lip GY, Nieuwlaat R, Pisters R, Lane DA, Crijns HJ. Refining clinical risk stratification for predicting stroke and thromboembolism in atrial fibrillation using a novel risk factor-based approach: the euro heart survey on atrial fibrillation. Chest. 2010;137(2): 263–72.

8. Braunwald E, editor. Heart disease: a textbook of cardiovascular medicine. 3rd ed. Philadelphia: Saunders; 1988.

9. Obeyesekere MN, Leong-Sit P, Massel D, et al. Risk of arrhythmia and sudden death in patients with asymptomatic preexcitation: a meta-analysis. Circulation. 2012;125(19):2308–15.

10. Brugada P, Brugada J, Mont L, Smeets J, Andries EW. A new approach to the differential diagnosis of a regular tachycardia with a wide QRS complex. Circulation. 1991;83(5):1649–59.

11. Vereckei A, Duray G, Szénási G, Altemose GT, Miller JM. Application of a new algorithm in the differential diagnosis of wide QRS complex tachycardia. Eur Heart J. 2007;28(5):589–600.

12. Blomström-Lundqvist C, Scheinman MM, Aliot EM, et al. ACC/AHA/ESC guidelines for the management of patients with supraventricular arrhythmias – executive summary. J Am Coll Cardiol. 2003;42(8):1493–531.

CHAPTER 24

STEVEN A. LUBITZ AND CONOR D. BARRETT

Ventricular Arrhythmias and Defibrillators

CHAPTER OUTLINE

ABBREVIATIONS

AAD	Antiarrhythmic drugs
ACC	American College of Cardiology
AHA	American Heart Association
CABG	Coronary artery bypass grafting
EPS	Electrophysiology study
HRS	Heart Rhythm Society
ICD	Implantable cardioverter defibrillator
LVEF	Left ventricular ejection fraction
MI	Myocardial infarction
NSVT	Nonsustained ventricular tachycardia
NYHA	New York Heart Association
SVT	Supraventricular tachycardia
VF	Ventricular fibrillation
VT	Ventricular tachycardia

INTRODUCTION

Ventricular tachyarrhythmias have heterogeneous etiologies, clinical consequences, and treatment strategies. Distinguishing ventricular tachyarrhythmias from supraventricular tachycardia (SVT) with aberrancy clinically and on the surface electrocardiogram can be challenging, yet has substantial therapeutic implications. A wide body of randomized clinical trial data has emerged addressing the efficacy of implantable cardioverter defibrillators (ICDs) for the prevention of sudden cardiac death. In this chapter we discuss these issues as well as consensus guideline recommendations for the implantation of ICDs.

DISTINGUISHING WIDE QRS COMPLEX TACHYCARDIAS

A. **History**: A prior history of structural or coronary heart disease favors ventricular tachycardia (VT).

B. **Clinical exam**: Neither hemodynamic stability nor physical exam findings are of sufficient specificity to be relied upon in order to distinguish between wide QRS complex tachycardia etiologies.

- Jugular venous exam may reveal cannon "a" waves due to atrioventricular dissociation in patients with VT.
- A third heart sound may favor VT but is not specific enough to diagnose VT.

C. **Differential diagnosis**:

- Ventricular tachycardia
- Supraventricular tachycardia with aberrancy
- Preexcitation
- Other causes: adverse medication reactions (e.g., digitalis toxicity [specifically associated with bidirectional VT], class Ic agents), ventricular pacing with atrial arrhythmia, metabolic derangement (e.g., hyperkalemia)

D. **The 12-lead ECG may be useful to identify VT from SVT with aberrancy and should be obtained if the patient is hemodynamically stable.**
   Discrimination of VT from SVT with aberrancy:

- Helpful factors are detailed in Table 24-1
- Atrioventricular dissociation is characteristic of VT, however given the high prevalence of atrial fibrillation, the absence of evident atrioventricular dissociation does not exclude VT. In some patients with intact VA conduction VTs may have a 1:1 VA relationship, so a 1:1 relationship can not be relied upon to exclude VT and diagnose SVT.
- Additional factors favoring VT [2]:

   - QRS duration > 160 ms
     Right superior QRS axis (90° to ±180°)

	SENSITIVITY FOR VT	SPECIFICITY FOR VT
1. Absence of RS complex in all precordial leads (negative precordial concordance)	0.21	1.0
2. R to S interval > 100 ms in any precordial lead	0.66	0.98
3. AV dissociation	0.82	0.98
4. Morphology criteria for VT in V1-2 and V6	0.99	0.97
Overall algorithm	0.97	0.99

TABLE 24-1

STEPWISE ALGORITHM FOR DISCRIMINATING VT FROM SVT WITH ABERRANT CONDUCTION [1]

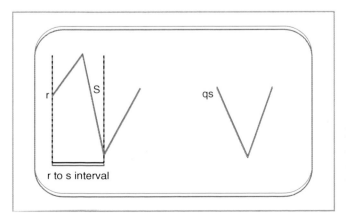

FIGURE 24-1

The *rs* interval is defined as the duration spanning the onset of the *r* wave and the trough of the *s* wave. A *qs* wave is depicted without any demonstrable *r* wave

CLASSIFICATION OF VENTRICULAR ARRHYTHMIAS

TABLE 24-2		
CLASSIFICATION OF VENTRICULAR ARRHYTHMIAS	**ARRHYTHMIA**	**ASSOCIATED FEATURES**
	Post-infarction ventricular tachycardia (Fig. 24-2)	Mechanism often reentry around scar Typically monomorphic unless associated with active ischemia Associated wall motion abnormalities and left ventricular dysfunction on imaging
	Idiopathic ventricular tachycardia	
	Outflow tract tachycardias (Fig. 24-3)	cyclic adenosine monophosphate mediated delayed afterdepolarizations, triggered activity Inferior axis, often left bundle branch block morphology during tachycardia but right bundle branch block morphology may be seen from VT from the left ventricular outflow tract More common in women, can be exacerbated with exercise and in pregnancy Adenosine, calcium channel blocker, or beta-blocker sensitive Treatable with meds or catheter ablation Benign prognosis
	Fascicular tachycardias (Fig. 24-4)	Reentry involving Purkinje tissue Commonest forms are of a right bundle branch block, left anterior fascicular block or left posterior fascicular block pattern during tachycardia More common in men Verapamil sensitive Treatable with verapamil or catheter ablation Benign prognosis
	Ventricular tachycardia and congenital heart disease	Reentry often involving surgical patch, suture lines, or scar May be amenable to ablation but ICDs often favored given structural disease
	Other ventricular tachycardias	
	Bundle branch reentrant ventricular tachycardia	Reentry involving the bundle branch fascicles Typical left or right bundle branch block pattern Associated with structural heart disease (e.g., dilated cardiomyopathy) Poor response to pharmacologic therapy; catheter ablation is first-line therapy; ICDs appropriate as typically unstable

	Arrhythmogenic right ventricular cardiomyopathy	Reentry around areas of fibrofatty tissue
		Commonly LBBB pattern
		Baseline ECG
		  May be essentially normal in some
		  1st degree atrioventricular block
		  Epsilon wave (early after depolarization)
		  T wave inversion V_{1-3}
		  Right bundle branch block or incomplete right bundle branch block, or prolonged S wave upstroke (>55 ms) in V_{1-3} in absence of right bundle branch block
		More common in young men, progressive disorder
		Associated with desmosomal mutations; genetic testing may be useful
		Typically exercise induced ventricular arrhythmias
		Sotalol useful, avoidance of competitive sports, ICD in high-risk patients

	Ventricular tachycardia in nonischemic cardiomyopathy	Reentry around deep myocardial scar or fibrosis
	Polymorphic ventricular tachycardia and fibrillation (Fig. 24-5)	Reentry, automaticity, or triggered activity Torsades de Pointes represents "twisting of the points" in context of a long QTc interval

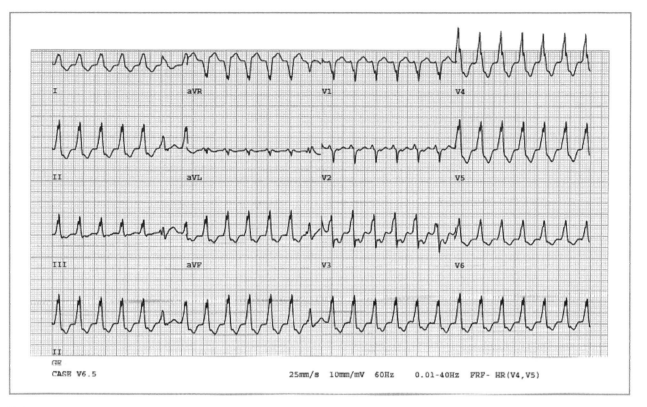

FIGURE 24-2

Exercise induced post-infraction scar-related monomorphic ventricular tachycardia in a patient with basal scar (note the fusion beats)

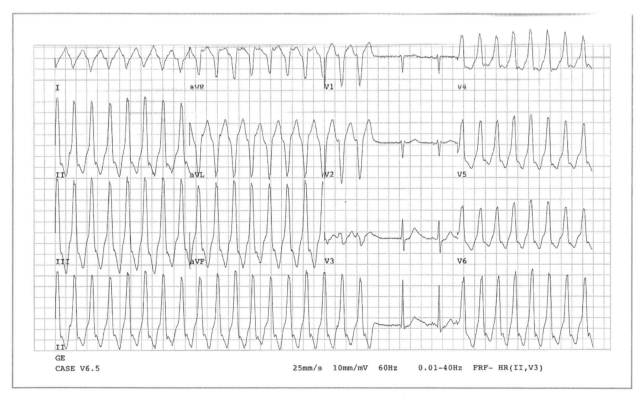

FIGURE 24-3

Exercise induced right ventricular outflow tract tachycardia manifesting with an inferior axis and left bundle branch block pattern. The tachycardia terminates and then resumes

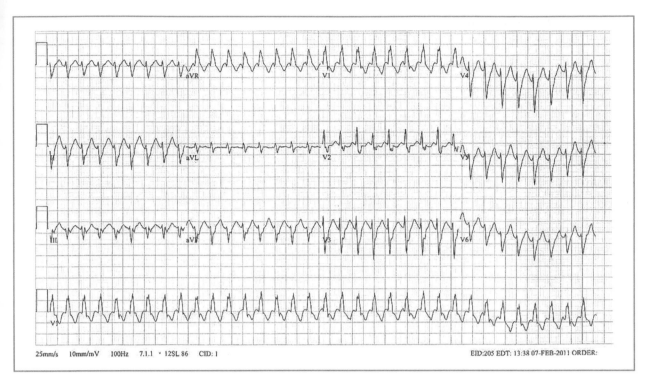

FIGURE 24-4

Fascicular ventricular tachycardia with a right bundle branch block and right superior axis pattern

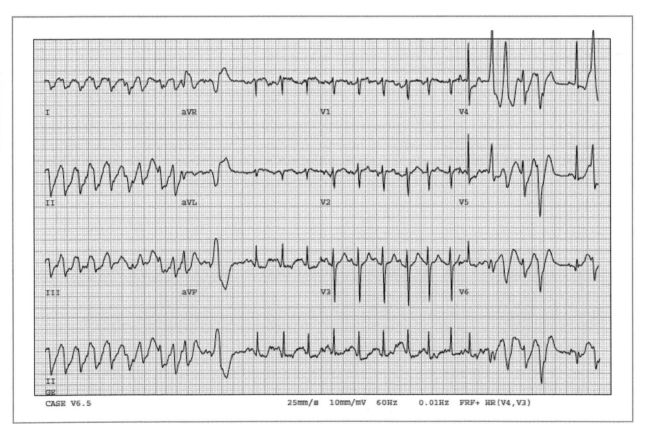

FIGURE 24-5

Exercise induced polymorphic ventricular tachycardia in a patient with left main coronary artery stenosis and myocardial ischemia

IMPLANTABLE CARDIOVERTER-DEFIBRILLATORS

A. Trials
B. Consensus guideline recommendations (Tables 24-2, 24-3 and 24-4)

TABLE 24-3

MAJOR ICD TRIALS

STUDY	YEAR	LEFT VENTRICULAR EJECTION FRACTION (LVEF) (%)	KEY TRIAL/INCLUSION CHARACTERISTICS	RELATIVE RISK FOR ICD, (95 % CONFIDENCE INTERVAL)
Primary prevention				
MADIT I [5]	1996	≤35	*ICD vs. conventional care* Prior myocardial infarction (MI) Nonsustained ventricular tachycardia (NSVT) Electrophysiology study (EPS) inducible VT/ventricular fibrillation (VF) not suppressible with antiarrhythmic drugs (AADs)	0.46 (0.26–0.82)
CABG-Patch [6]	1997	<36	*ICD vs. conventional care at time of coronary artery bypass grafting (CABG)* Scheduled CABG Abnormal signal averaged electrocardiogram	1.07 (0.87 1.42)
MUSTT [7]	1999	≤40	*EPS guided antiarrhythmic (AAD ± ICD) therapy vs. nonantiarrhythmic therapy* Coronary artery disease NSVT (≥4 days from most recent revascularization procedure) EPS-inducible VT/VF	0.80 (0.60–1.01)* EPS vs. nonantiar- rhythmic 0.45 (0.32–0.63)* ICD vs. nonantiar- rhythmic
CAT [8]	2002	≤30	*ICD vs. conventional care* Nonischemic cardiomyopathy<9 months New York Heart Association (NYHA) II or III	Not significant/ Not reported
MADIT II [9]	2002	≤30	*ICD vs. conventional care* Prior MI>(1 month prior) No coronary revascularization ≤3 months prior	0.69 (0.51–0.93)
DEFINITE [10]	2004	<36	*ICD vs. conventional care* Nonischemic cardiomyopathy NSVT, VT, or moderate number of premature ventricular contractions	0.65 (0.40–1.06)
DINAMIT [3]	2004	≤35	*ICD vs. conventional care* Recent MI (6–40 days) Impaired heart rate variability	1.08 (0.76–1.55)
SCD-HeFT [11]	2005	≤35	*ICD vs. amiodarone vs. placebo* Prior MI or nonischemic NYHA II or III	0.77 (0.62–0.96)* ICD vs. placebo
IRIS [4]	2009	Mean ~35	*ICD vs. conventional care* Recent MI (<31 days) LVEF ≤40 and heart rate >90, or NSVT	1.04 (0.81–1.35)

8. Bansch D. Primary prevention of sudden cardiac death in idiopathic dilated cardiomyopathy: the Cardiomyopathy Trial (CAT). Circulation. 2002;105:1453–8.

9. Moss AJ, Zareba W, Hall WJ, Klein H, Wilber DJ, Cannom DS, et al. Prophylactic implantation of a defibrillator in patients with myocardial infarction and reduced ejection fraction. N Engl J Med. 2002;346:877–83.

10. Kadish A, Dyer A, Daubert JP, Quigg R, Estes NAM, Anderson KP, et al. Prophylactic defibrillator implantation in patients with nonischemic dilated cardiomyopathy. N Engl J Med. 2004;350:2151–8.

11. Bardy GH, Lee KL, Mark DB, Poole JE, Packer DL, Boineau R, et al. Amiodarone or an implantable cardioverter-defibrillator for congestive heart failure. N Engl J Med. 2005;352:225–37.

12. A comparison of antiarrhythmic-drug therapy with implantable defibrillators in patients resuscitated from near-fatal ventricular arrhythmias. The Antiarrhythmics versus Implantable Defibrillators (AVID) Investigators. N Engl J Med. 1997;337: 1576–83.

13. Kuck KH, Cappato R, Siebels J, Ruppel R. Randomized comparison of antiarrhythmic drug therapy with implantable defibrillators in patients resuscitated from cardiac arrest: the Cardiac Arrest Study Hamburg (CASH). Circulation. 2000;102:748–54.

14. Connolly SJ, Gent M, Roberts RS, Dorian P, Roy D, Sheldon RS, et al. Canadian implantable defibrillator study (CIDS): a randomized trial of the implantable cardioverter defibrillator against amiodarone. Circulation. 2000;101:1297–302.

CHAPTER 25

Gaurav A. Upadhyay and Jagmeet P. Singh

Bradycardia and Pacemakers/CRT

CHAPTER OUTLINE

ABBREVIATIONS

ACC	American College of Cardiology
AF	Atrial fibrillation
AHA	American Heart Association
AV	Atrioventricular
BPEG	British Pacing Electrophysiology Group
bpm	Beats per minute
CHB	Complete heart block
CL	Cycle length
CRT	Cardiac resynchronization therapy
cSNRT	Corrected sinoatrial node recovery time
ECG	Electrocardiogram
EP	Electrophysiologic
FDA	Food and Drug Administration
HCM	Hypertrophic cardiomyopathy
HF	Heart failure
HR	Heart rate
HRS	Heart Rhythm Society
ICD	Implantable cardioverter defibrillator
LAFB	Left anterior fascicular block
LBBB	Left bundle branch block
LPFB	Left posterior fascicular block
LQT1	Long QT syndrome type 1
LV	Left ventricular
LVEF	Left ventricular Ejection fraction
MI	Myocardial infarction
NASPE	North American Society for Pacing and Electrophysiology
NYHA	New York Heart Association
PPM	Permanent pacemakers
RA	Right atrium
RBBB	Right bundle branch block
RV	Right ventricle
SA	Sinoatrial
SACT	Sinoatrial conduction time
SND	Sinus node dysfunction
SNRT	Sinoatrial node recovery time
VT	Ventricular tachycardia

- Predominant clinical manifestations of SND include:

  - Frequent sinus pauses, sinus arrest, or sinus exit block
  - Inappropriate and severe sinus bradycardia with chronotropic incompetence
  - Episodes of bradycardia alternating with atrial tachyarrhythmias (usually atrial fibrillation (AF), although may be other supraventricular arrhythmias)
  - AF with a slow ventricular response or with very slow recovery after spontaneous conversion or cardioversion to revert to sinus rhythm

- **Diagnosis**: Usually made based on elicitation of presyncopal symptoms or palpitations and confirmation on electrocardiogram (ECG). Other options include

  - Ambulatory ECG monitoring
  - Exercise testing to evaluate chronotropic competence
  - Electrophysiologic (EP) study may be diagnostic, and there is a class I indication to pursue EP study in patients with symptomatic bradycardia in whom a causal relationship between SND and symptoms has not been established [8]. Criteria evaluated include:

    - *Sinoatrial node recovery time (SNRT)*: SA node is overdrive suppressed with atrial pacing, and the time from last paced atrial beat to the first spontaneous sinus beat is measured. Centers differ on normal SNRT, although <1,500 ms is conventional. A corrected SNRT (cSNRT) is the SNRT minus the sinus cycle length (CL), and is typically < 550 ms
    - *Sinoatrial conduction time (SACT)*: is the time required for the sinus impulse to capture the atrium. Typically it is between 50 and 115 ms, and is often prolonged during SA block

- **Treatment**: Largely depends on the diagnosis of <u>symptomatic</u> bradycardia, for which the only effective treatment is permanent cardiac pacing. Guideline recommendations are presented below [4]

  - *Class I indications* for permanent pacing in SND:

    - SND with documented symptomatic bradycardia, including frequent sinus pauses that produce symptoms
    - Symptomatic chronotropic incompetence
    - Symptomatic sinus bradycardia from required drug therapy for medical conditions

  - *Class II indications* for permanent pacing in SND:

    - SND with HR < 40 bpm, when symptoms are consistent with bradycardia, although the actual presence of bradycardia has not been documented
    - Syncope of unexplained origin with abnormal EP study (class IIa)
    - HR < 40 bpm while awake with minimal symptoms (class IIb)

DISORDERS OF IMPULSE PROPAGATION

Disorders of impulse propagation may occur at any point in the conduction system. Importantly, conduction block is distinct from the normal physiologic phenomenon of *interference*, in which a preceding impulse causes a period of refractoriness due to inactivation of ion channels.

Sinoatrial Exit Block

- **Definition**: also called SA exit block, it manifests as sinus arrest of variable length on surface ECG. Prevalence is 1 % in otherwise normal subjects [9].
- **Pathophysiology**: defect of impulse propagation within the SA node

- First-degree SA exit block cannot be detected on surface ECG because sinus node depolarization is not inscribed separately from atrial depolarization (i.e., the *p* wave)
- Second-degree SA exit block

  - Type 1: progressive prolongation of conduction block within the sinus node until complete exit block occurs (surface ECG demonstrates progressive shortening of *p – p* intervals before block)
  - Type 2: spontaneous block of sinus impulse leading to sinus pause which is an *exact multiple* of the preceding *p – p* interval

- Third degree SA exit block: simply manifests as sinus arrest, usually with eventual appearance of subsidiary pacemaker (i.e., junctional escape rhythm)

- **Treatment:** Sinoatrial exit block is usually treated in the context of SND, as indicated above

Atrioventricular (AV) Block

- **Definition:** By convention, first-degree 'block' refers to impulses which are delayed, second-degree block refers to intermittent block of impulse conduction, and third-degree to complete block. Further specific terminology is described below.

  - First-degree AV block defined as PR interval > 0.20 s; generally felt due to block at the level of the AV node, although when associated with bundle branch block, may occur further down in the His-Purkinje system. Prevalence is 0.65 % in healthy adults [10]. Largely benign by itself, recent data from the Framingham cohort suggest that PR prolongation may be associated with increased risks AF, pacemaker implantation, and all-cause mortality over time [11]
  - Second-degree AV block was first classified into two types by Mobitz in 1924

    - Mobitz Type 1 (Wenkebach) AV block: characterized by progressive prolongation of the PR interval before non-conduction. Also generally associated with block at the level of the AV node.

      - Progressive shortening of *R – R* intervals prior to a dropped beat; shorter PR interval immediately after dropped beat
      - Irrespective of QRS width, usually represents an appropriate physiologic response to increasing HR through decremental conduction in the AV node

    - Mobitz Type 2: characterized by sudden non-conduction of atrial impulse without change in preceding PR interval. Usually represents infranodal disease.

      - Care should be taken to differentiate Mobitz II from a premature atrial complex (examine preceding *p – p* intervals) which causes physiologic interference and not conduction block
      - Some authors refer to multiple consecutive non-conducted impulses as 'high-degree' or 'advanced' heart block prior to true third-degree AV block
      - In the setting of AF, a prolonged pause ≥ 5 s is suggestive of underlying advanced second-degree AV block

    - 2:1 AV block: characterized by sudden non-conduction of atrial impulse without change in preceding PR interval after a single QRS complex. Based on surface ECG, it is difficult to discern whether location of block is within the AV node or below the level of the node (i.e., infrahisian). In patients with 2:1 AV block, evaluation of contemporaneous conduction disturbances (e.g., Wenkebach-type Mobitz 1) used to help infer level of block (see Fig. 25-1)

FIGURE 25-1

(**a**) Ladder diagram of 2:1 AV block and Wenkebach type block. (**b**) The rhythm strip shows a 2:1 block followed by short-stretch of Wenkebach and followed again with 2:1 block. The location of the block is inferred to be in the AV node due to the presence of Wenkebach, although cannot be determined conclusively without further information

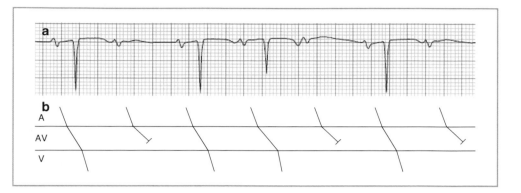

- Third-degree AV block, or complete heart block, occurs with absence of atrial impulse propagation to the ventricles and may manifest as ventricular standstill in the absence of an escape rhythm. When reversible etiologies are present (e.g., electrolyte disturbance, non-anterior ischemia), temporary pacing is usually indicated

■ **Pathophysiology**: There are numerous potential etiologies for AV block.

- Physiologic AV block (first-degree of second-degree Type 1) is commonly due to enhanced vagal tone.
- Idiopathic fibrosclerosis of the conduction system (i.e., Lev's disease affecting the old and Lenegre's affecting the young),
- Infiltrative cardiomyopathy such as amyloidosis or sarcoidosis
- Peri-AV nodal inflammation

   ■ Lyme disease
   ■ Myocarditis
   ■ Systemic lupus erythematosus
   ■ Dermatomyositis

- Endocrinologic states

   ■ Thyroid storm or myxedema

- Severe electrolyte disturbance

   ■ Hyperkalemia

- Drug toxicity or overdose, particularly when agents are added in combination or if either renal or liver insufficiency occurs, which leads to accumulation of the drugs.

   ■ β blockers
   ■ Calcium channel blockers
   ■ Amiodarone
   ■ Digoxin

- Iatrogenic etiologies of AV block are becoming increasingly common

   ■ Surgical or transcatheter aortic valve replacement
   ■ Alcohol septal ablation for hypertrophic cardiomyopathy
   ■ Transcatheter closure of ventricular septal defects
   ■ Complication of ablation during EP procedures.

- Congenital etiologies are other rare but predictable causes of AV block:

   ■ Familial AV conduction block
   ■ Sequela of neonatal lupus syndrome (particularly in babies born of mothers that are positive for antinuclear antibodies SSA/Ro and SSB/La)
   ■ Hereditary neuromuscular diseases such as myotonic dystrophy

Recommendations in acquired atrioventricular block in adults

Third-degree and advanced second-degree AV block at any anatomic level associated with bradycardia and symptoms (including heart failure) or ventricular arrhythmias presumed to be due to AV block

Third-degree and advanced second-degree AV block at any anatomic level associated with arrhythmias and other medical conditions that require drug therapy that results in symptomatic bradycardia

Third-degree and advanced second-degree AV block at any anatomic level in awake, symptom-free patients in sinus rhythm, with documented periods of asystole≥3.0 s or any escape rate less than 40 bpm, or with an escape rhythm that is below the AV node

Third-degree and advanced second-degree AV block at any anatomic level in awake, symptom-free patients with AF and bradycardia with 1 or more pauses of at least 5 s or longer

Third-degree and advanced second-degree AV block at any anatomic level after catheter ablation of the AV junction

Third-degree and advanced second-degree AV block at any anatomic level with postoperative AV block that is not expected to resolve after cardiac surgery

Third-degree and advanced second-degree AV block at any anatomic level associated with neuromuscular diseases with AV block, such as myotonic muscular dystrophy, Kearns-Sayre syndrome, Erb dystrophy (limb-girdle muscular dystrophy), and peroneal muscular atrophy, with or without symptoms

Second-degree AV block with associated symptomatic bradycardia regardless of type or site of block

Asymptomatic persistent third-degree AV block at any anatomic site with average awake ventricular rates of 40 bpm or faster if cardiomegaly or LV dysfunction is present or if the site of block is below the AV node

Second- or third-degree AV block during exercise in the absence of myocardial ischemia

Recommendations in chronic bifascicular block

Advanced second degree AV block or intermittent third-degree AV block

Type II second-degree AV block

Alternating bundle-branch block

Adapted from Epstein et al. [4]

SND sinus node dysfunction, *AV* atrioventricular, *SVT* supraventricular tachycardia, *VT* ventricular tachycardia, *MI* myocardial infarction

TABLE 25-2

ACC/AHA/HRS CLASS I RECOMMENDATIONS FOR PERMANENT PACING

- Myocardial ischemia is an important cause of AV and infranodal block

  ■ Many forms of AV block commonly seen in acute inferior MI, most often due to increased vagal tone, rarely due to AV nodal infarction
  ■ AV block and infranodal block due to acute anterior wall MI most often due to infarction of the conduction system

■ **Treatment**: the initial course of treatment is to identify and remove any potential reversible offending agents. The decision for permanent pacing is often left to the discretion of the cardiologist, based on an appreciation of the relative stability of the underlying rhythm and the risk associated with developing symptoms. Class I indications are as outlined in Table 25-2

Intraventricular Block

■ **Definition**: Failure in normal ventricular activation due to block in the His-Purkinje system.

- The left and right bundle branches are commonly divided into a trifascicular system, consisting of the right bundle branch and the left anterior and posterior fascicles [12]. Although the septal fascicle has also been identified in anatomic studies, ECG manifestations of septal conduction block are debated and remain to be defined [13].

- Beyond commonly recognized right and left bundle branch blocks (RBBB and LBBB), other commonly used terminology for intraventricular block include:

  - Bifascicular block: Block is present when either the left anterior or left posterior fascicular block (LAFB or LPFB, but not both) is associated with RBBB

    - Most often precedes third-degree AV block, although rate of progression is variable and often slow [14]

  - Trifascicular block: Evidence of disease of all three fascicles present on success ECG tracings.

    - Typically manifests as *alternating BBB*. For example, RBBB+LAFB may be seen to alternate with RBBB+LPFB
    - Care should be made to contrast true trifascicular block from patients who demonstrate first-degree AV block in association with bifascicular block. This does not constitute evidence of trifascicular disease. When symptomatic, however, bifascicular AV block and *advanced AV block* (second-degree AV block with multiple non-conducted beats) is associated with increased mortality

- **Pathophysiology**: Intraventricular block may be due to a broad array of etiologies, similar to what was described above as causes of atrioventricular block. The special case of intraventricular block in the setting of MI deserves special mention

  - Inferior MI: usually associated with varying degrees of AV block from AV nodal artery ischemia or enhanced vagal tone from exaggeration of the Bezold-Jarisch reflex, *intraventricular block is uncommon*
  - Anterior MI: can be associated with ischemia of the fascicles directly leading to true intraventricular block. In the pre-thrombolytic era, new fascicular or bundle branch blocks were common after an MI and were associated with a significantly increased risk of mortality [15]

    - A simple scoring model characterizing the risk of progression to complete heart block after MI was developed by Lamas based on ECG criteria [16].

      - The complete heart block (CHB) scoring model assigned one point to the presence of well-recognized conduction disturbances, including: first-degree AV block, second-degree block (both type I and type II), LAFB and LPFB, RBBB, or LBBB. The risk of CHB after MI was linearly correlated with the total score (or simply, the sum of number of conduction disturbances) found on their presenting ECG. For example, a patient whose ECG after MI demonstrated 1st degree AV block and right bundle branch block would have a score of 2.
      - According to Lamas' study, patients with a CHB risk score of 0 had a 1.2 % chance of developing complete heart block. CHB score of 1 was associated with 7.8 % risk, 2 with 25 % risk, and a CHB score of 3 or higher was associated 36 % risk.

- **Treatment**: Permanent pacing is considered first-line in the treatment of bifascicular block with evidence for concurrent advanced AV node block or intermittent trifascicular block (see Table 25-2).

  - Treatment of intraventricular block in the setting of symptomatic left ventricular dysfunction is a special case which will be discussed further below in the cardiac resynchronization therapy section
  - Because of the relatively common incidence of bradycardia after MI (as indicated above based on the CHB score model), the American College of Cardiology (ACC)/ American Heart Association (AHA) have clear guidelines on intervention, including the use of temporary pacing, for AV and intraventricular disturbance post MI(see Table 25-3)

Application of transcutaneous patches and standby transcutaneous pacing

Class I

> Normal AV conduction *or* first-degree AV block *or* Mobitz type I second-degree AV block with new bundle branch block
>
> Normal AV conduction *or* first-degree AV block *or* Mobitz type I second-degree AV block with fascicular block+RBBB
>
> First-degree AV block with old or new fascicular block (LAFB or LPFB) *in anterior MI only*
>
> First-degree AV block *or* Mobitz type I *or* type II second-degree AV block with old bundle branch block
>
> Mobitz type I *or* type II second-degree AV block with normal intraventricular conduction
>
> Mobitz type I *or* type II second-degree AV block with old or new fascicular block (LAFB or LPFB)

Class IIa

> First-degree AV block with old or new fascicular block (LAFB or LPFB) *in non-anterior MI only*

Class IIb

> Alternating left and right bundle branch block
>
> Normal AV conduction with old bundle branch block
>
> Normal AV conduction with new fascicular block (LAFB or LPFB)
>
> First-degree AV block with normal intraventricular conduction
>
> Mobitz type II second-degree AV block with new bundle branch block
>
> Mobitz type II second-degree AV block with fascicular block+RBBB

Class III

> Normal AV conduction with normal intraventricular conduction

Temporary transvenous pacing

Class I

> Alternating left and right bundle branch block
>
> Mobitz type II second-degree AV block with new bundle branch block
>
> Mobitz type II second-degree AV block with fascicular block+RBBB

Class IIa

> First-degree AV block *or* Mobitz type I second-degree AV block with new bundle branch block
>
> First-degree AV block *or* Mobitz type I second-degree AV block with fascicular block+RBBB
>
> Mobitz type II second-degree AV block with old bundle branch block
>
> Mobitz type II second-degree AV block with normal intraventricular conduction
>
> Mobitz type II second-degree AV block with old or new fascicular block (LAFB or LPFB) *in anterior MI only*

Class IIb

> Normal AV conduction with new bundle branch block
>
> Normal AV conduction with fascicular block+RBBB
>
> Mobitz type I *or* type II second-degree AV block with old bundle branch block
>
> Mobitz type II second-degree AV block with old or new fascicular block (LAFB or LPFB) *in nonanterior MI only*

Class III

> Normal AV conduction *or* first-degree AV block *or* Mobitz type I second-degree AV block with normal intraventricular conduction
>
> Normal AV conduction *or* first-degree AV block *or* Mobitz type I second-degree AV block with old or new fascicular block (LAFB or LPFB)
>
> Normal AV conduction with old bundle branch block

Class I recommendations for permanent pacing after the acute phase of myocardial infarction

> Persistent second-degree AV block in the His-Purkinje system with alternating bundle-branch block or third-degree AV block within or below the His-Purkinje system after ST-segment elevation MI
>
> Transient advanced second- or third-degree infranodal AV block and associated bundle-branch block. If the site of block is uncertain, an electrophysiological study may be necessary
>
> Persistent and symptomatic second- or third-degree AV block

TABLE 25-3

ACC/AHA GUIDELINES FOR TREATMENT OF ATRIOVENTRICULAR AND INTRAVENTRICULAR CONDUCTION DISTURBANCES DURING STEMIA AND ACC/AHA/HRS RECOMMENDATIONS FOR POST-MI PERMANENT PACING

Adapted from Antman et al. [30] and Epstein et al. [4]

AV atrioventricular, *BBB* bundle branch block, *BP* blood pressure, *LAFB* left anterior fascicular block, *LBBB* left bundle branch block, *LPFB* left posterior fascicular block, *MI* myocardial infarction, *RBBB* right bundle branch block

[a]Except where specified, all indications include anterior *and* nonanterior MI

FIGURE 25-2

The revised NBG coding system

The revised NASPE/BPEG generic code for antibradycardia pacing					
Position:	I	II	III	IV	V
Category:	Chamber(s) paced	Chamber(s) sensed	Response to sensing	Rate modulation	Multisite pacing
	O = None	O = None	O = None	O = None	O = None
	A = Atrium	A = Atrium	T = Triggered	R = Rate modulation	A = Atrium
	V = Ventricle	V = Ventricle	I = Inhibited		V = Ventricle
	D = Dual (A + V)	D = Dual (A + V)	D = Dual (T + I)		D = Dual (A + V)
Manufacturers' designation only:	S = Single (A or V)	S = Single (A or V)			

PERMANENT PACING

PPM utilize placement of pacing electrodes within (or to the epicardial surface of) the heart attached to a pulse generator.

■ Modern options in PPM selection include single-chamber atrial pacemaker (rarely used), single-chamber ventricular pacemaker, and dual-chamber pacemakers.

■ Selection of device is driven by indication for pacing (usually SND or AV block) and whether or not there is a desire (or substrate) for rate responsiveness.

■ As devices have become more sophisticated, the nomenclature used to define PPM functionality has been updated. A brief review is provided below

Coding/Nomenclature

■ **Background**: The first coding system for PPM was proposed in 1974 [17] and was jointly updated by the North American Society for Pacing and Electrophysiology (NASPE) and British Pacing Electrophysiology Group (BPEG) in 2002 [18].

■ The combined NASPE/BPEG generic code, or NBG code, outlines 5 distinct positions to describe PPM activity (see Fig. 25-2).

■ **Commonly used codes**:

– VVIR: also called "ventricular demand pacing"—this code is used in single-chamber ventricular lead devices in which the ventricle is paced, sensed, and inhibited in response to a sensed beat. It is commonly employed in patients with chronic atrial fibrillation and slow ventricular response. Two important caveats:

■ AV synchrony is not maintained in VVIR mode, and chronic right ventricular pacing is associated with an increased risk of heart failure (HF) hospitalization and AF due to increased ventricular dyssynchrony [19, 20]

■ In addition, some patients with chronic VVI pacing develop the pacemaker syndrome. Similar to what is seen in complete heart block, patients manifest a reduction in stroke volume, and may also demonstrate atrial contraction against a closed tricuspid or mitral valve. Reported symptoms include weakness, lightheadedness, a sensation of throat fullness, palpitations, near syncope and syncope

– DDD or DDDR: represents dual-chamber pacing which is the most "physiologic." Requiring the use of an atrial and ventricular lead, the PPM is typically programmed to maximize appropriately timed and intact native A-V conduction (i.e., through self-inhibition), add ventricular paced beats in the presence of significant AV delay or block (after allowing for native atrial depolarization), or synchronously add paced atrial and ventricular beats (in the setting of SND or asystole)

– VOO or DOO: are commonly employed "asynchronous" pacing modes in which the device paces without respect to native conduction. These modes are usually only employed for limited periods (e.g., surgeries, emergencies) in which there is high possibility for errors in sensing

■ **Special terminology:**

- Rate-modulation: also referred to as 'rate responsiveness' or 'rate adaptation,' rate modulation is a programmable device feature in which the pacing rate varies dependent upon patient activity, as detected by device sensors

- Hysteresis: also called AV-search hysteresis, this is a feature available in dual-chamber devices in the DDD mode in which the pacemaker will periodically lower its pacing rates in order to allow for potential intrinsic activity below the programmed lower rate (or sensor rate). It is often misinterpreted for oversensing with pauses.

Additional Indications

■ The most common indications for pacemaker device therapy is SND or AV block.

■ There has also been active research regarding specific indications for pacing beyond conventional SND or AV block. Some of these are briefly outlined below (see Table 25-4)

CARDIAC RESYNCHRONIZATION THERAPY (CRT)

although pacemakers have been conventionally used in the primary treatment of arrhythmia, pacing for hemodynamic indication has been recognized of increasing importance in patients with heart failure due to systolic left ventricular (LV) dysfunction

A. **Background**

   ■ CRT is the use of a biventricular pacemaker with three electrical leads to coordinate myocardial contraction.

   ■ Two leads are endocardial, placed in the right atrium (RA) and right ventricle (RV), while a third lead is placed in a tributary of the coronary sinus overlying the epicardial surface of the LV.

   ■ CRT exerts its physiological impact via synchronizing ventricular contraction, leading to improved left ventricular filling, pumping efficiency, and reducing functional mitral regurgitation.

B. **Impact**: Multiple prospective randomized studies have shown that CRT yields long-term clinical benefits, including improved quality of life, increased exercise capacity, reduced heart failure hospitalization and decreased all-cause mortality [21–26] in patients meeting traditional CRT criteria (New York Heart Association (NYHA) Class III-ambulatory class IV, LV ejection fraction (LVEF)≤35 %, QRS width≥120 ms). Recent large trials also suggest there may be similar benefit in NYHA Class II patients [27, 28]. Note: *HF symptom status should be assessed after medical therapy has been optimized for at least 3 months*.

C. **Patient-selection**: Beyond traditional criteria for CRT, there are subsets of patients who derive substantial benefit

   ■ Female patients
   ■ LBBB morphology
   ■ QRS width≥150 ms
   ■ Patients with history of nonischemic cardiomyopathy

D. **Recommendations**

   ACC/AHA/Heart Rhythm Society (HRS) Recommendations [31]

   ■ Class I

      - CRT is indicated for patients who have LVEF ≤ 35%, sinus rhythm, LBBB with a QRS duration ≥ 150 ms, and NYHA class II, III, or ambulatory IV symptoms on goal-directed medical therapy (GDMT). (*Level of Evidence [LOE]: A for NYHA class III/IV; Level of Evidence: B for NYHA class II*)

TABLE 25-4	
ACC/AHA/HRS RECOMMENDATIONS FOR PERMANENT PACING IN SPECIFIC CONDITIONS	*Recommendations for pacing **in hypersensitive carotid sinus syndrome** and **neurocardiogenic syncope*** Recurrent syncope caused by spontaneously occurring carotid sinus stimulation and carotid sinus pressure that induces ventricular asystole of≥3 s (Class I) Reasonable for syncope without clear, provocative events and with a hypersensitive *cardioinhibitory* response of≥3s (Class IIa) May be considered for significantly symptomatic neurocardiogenic syncope associated with bradycardia documented spontaneously or at the time of tilt-table testing (Class IIb)

*Recommendations for pacing after **cardiac transplantation***

Persistent inappropriate or symptomatic bradycardia not expected to resolve and for other Class I indications for permanent pacing (Class I)

May be considered when relative bradycardia is prolonged or recurrent, which limits rehabilitation or discharge after postoperative recovery from cardiac transplantation (Class IIb)

*Recommendations for pacing in **neuromuscular diseases***

Permanent pacemaker implantation may be considered in the setting of neuromuscular diseases such as myotonic muscular dystrophy, Erb dystrophy (limb-girdle muscular dystrophy), and peroneal muscular atrophy with bifasciular block or any fascicular block, with and without symptoms (Class IIb)

*Recommendations for pacing to **prevent tachycardia***

Sustained pause-dependent VT, with or without QT prolongation (Class I)

Reasonable in high-risk patients with the **congenital long-QT syndrome** (Class IIa)

May be considered for prevention of symptomatic, drug-refractory, recurrent AF in patients with coexisting SND (Class IIb)

*Recommendations for pacing in patients with **hypertrophic cardiomyopathy (HCM)***

Indicated for SND or AV block in patients with HCM per usual indications (Class I)

May be considered in medically refractory symptomatic patients with HCM and significant resting or provoked LV outflow tract gradient. When risk factors for SCD are present, consider DDD-ICD placement (Class IIb)

*Recommendations for permanent pacing in children, adolescents, and patients with **congenital heart disease***

Indicated for advanced second- or third-degree AV block associated with symptomatic bradycardia, ventricular dysfunction, or low cardiac output (Class I)

Indicated for SND with correlation of symptoms during age-inappropriate bradycardia (Class I)

Indicated for postoperative advanced second- or third-degree AV block not expected to resolve or that persists at least 7 days after cardiac surgery (Class I)

Indicated for congenital third-degree AV block with a wide QRS escape rhythm, complex ventricular ectopy, or ventricular dysfunction (Class I)

Indicated for congenital third-degree AV block in the infant with a ventricular rate $\leq$ 55 bpm or with congenital heart disease and a ventricular rate $\leq$ 70 bpm (Class I)

Adapted from Epstein et al. [4]

SND sinus node dysfunction, *AV* atrioventricular, *SVT* supraventricular tachycardia, *VT* ventricular tachycardia, *MI* myocardial infarction

■ Class IIa

– CRT can be useful for patients who have LVEF $\leq$ 35%, sinus rhythm, LBBB with a QRS duration 120 to 149 ms, and NYHA class II, III, or ambulatory IV symptoms on GDMT. (*LOE: B*)

– CRT can be useful for patients who have LVEF $\leq$ 35%, sinus rhythm, a non-LBBB pattern with a QRS duration greater than or equal to 150 ms, and NYHA class III/ambulatory class IV symptoms on GDMT. (*LOE: A*)

– CRT can be useful in patients with AF and LVEF $\leq$ 35% on GDMT if a) the patient requires ventricular pacing or otherwise meets CRT criteria and b) AV nodal ablation or pharmacologic rate control will allow near 100% ventricular pacing with CRT. (*LOE: B*)

– CRT can be useful for patients on GDMT who have LVEF $\leq$ 35% and are undergoing new or replacement device placement with anticipated requirement for significant (>40%) ventricular pacing (*LOE: C*)

■ Class IIb

- CRT may be considered for patients who have LVEF ≤ 30%, ischemic etiology of heart failure, sinus rhythm, LBBB with a QRS duration ≥ 150 ms, and NYHA class I symptoms on GDMT (*LOE: C*)
- CRT may be considered for patients who have LVEF ≤ 35%, sinus rhythm, a non-LBBB pattern with QRS duration 120 to 149 ms, and NYHA class III/ambulatory class IV on GDMT (*LOE: B*)
- CRT may be considered for patients who have LVEF ≤ 35%, sinus rhythm, a non-LBBB pattern with a QRS duration ≥ 150 ms, and NYHA class II symptoms on GDMT. (*LOE: B*)

■ Class III

- CRT is not recommended for patients with NYHA class I or II symptoms and non-LBBB pattern with QRS duration < 150 ms. (*LOE: B*)
- CRT is not indicated for patients whose comorbidities and/or frailty limit survival with good functional capacity to < 1 year (*LOE: C*)

Food and Drug Administration (FDA) expansion of approval:

■ Based on recent trials [27, 28], the FDA voted to expand indications for CRT on 3/18/10 to include:

- NYHA Class II patients *or* NYHA Class I patients with ischemic cardiomyopathy with LVEF <30 % and QRS duration >130 ms
- Selected patients must also have LBBB

QUICK REVIEW

TOPIC	KEY POINTS
Etiology of bradyarrhythmia	Can be broadly classified into (a) failure of impulse generation or (b) impulse propagation
Primary cause of bradyarrhythmias due to failure of impulse generation	Sinus node dysfunction
SND is characterized by:	1. Frequent sinus pauses, sinus arrest, or sinus exit block 2. Inappropriate sinus bradycardia with chronotropic incompetence 3. Episodes of bradycardia alternating with atrial tachyarrhythmias 4. AF with slow ventricular response or very slow recovery after conversion
Treatment of choice for SND:	PPM
Selected indications:	**Symptomatic** bradycardia **Symptomatic** chronotropic incompetence
Primary cause of bradyarrhythmias due to failure of impulse propagation	Atrioventricular block

Types of AV block:	1. First-degree AV block (usually supranodal)
	2. Second-degree AV block
	  (a) Mobitz I/Wenkebach (usually at the level of the node)
	  (b) Mobitz II (often infranodal)
	3. Third-degree AV block (usually infranodal)

Treatment of choice for AV block:	*'Advanced-AV block' or 'advanced second-degree AV block' refers to second-degree AV block with multiple nonconducted beats*
Selected indications:	Eliminate offending agent; consider PPM Advanced second- or third-degree AV block with **symptomatic** bradycardia, ≥ 3 s pauses in NSR, ≥ 5 s pauses in AF, or escape rate<40 bpm

SSS	Sick sinus syndrome
SVT	Supraventricular tachyarrhythmia
TIA	Transient Ischemic Attack
VF	Ventricular fibrillation
VT	Ventricular tachycardia
WPW	Wolff-Parkinson-White

INTRODUCTION

The word "syncope" is derived from the Greek *syn*, meaning "with" and *koptein* meaning "to cut off/interrupt" [1]. The use of the word syncope to describe the abrupt "cutting off" of consciousness has been in place for hundreds of years. No matter what term patients use: syncope, fainting, drop attacks, or spells is used, the concept transient loss of consciousness followed by spontaneous recovery has been, is and always will be a common issue for cardiologists to diagnose and manage. Many causes of syncope are outside the scope of cardiology. Due to the inherent life-threatening nature of many cardiac causes of syncope, it is important for the cardiologist to be well versed on the topic.

DEFINITION

- Sudden transient loss of consciousness (LOC) associated with a loss of postural tone followed by spontaneous recovery
- Pathophysiology: temporary inadequacy of cerebral blood flow

EPIDEMIOLOGY

- Lifetime incidence: 3 % of men and 3.5 % of women [2]
- 1–3 % of emergency room visits and 6 % of hospital admissions [3, 4]
- Increasing prevalence with age: 8/1,000 person-exams in 35–44 year-olds, ~40/1,000 person-exams in ≥75 year-olds [2]

APPROACH

- History, physical examination and ECG
- Differentiation of true syncope from others such as sudden cardiac death (SCD) or transient ischemic attacks (TIA), etc.
- Risk stratification – any high risk features that may warrant admission/workup?
- Determination of etiology with or without additional studies

ETIOLOGIES (TABLE 26-1, [5])

Neurally Mediated Syncope

Most common cause (~20 %) [5]

- **Normal physiology:** venous pooling → ↑ in Heart rate (HR), contractility, and Peripheral vascular resistance (PVR) → ↓ in venous return to right ventricle (RV) → ↓ stretch activation of cardiac mechanoreceptors (C fibers) reflexively ↑ sympathetic stimulation → ↑ HR, diastolic blood pressure (DBP), stable to ↓ systolic blood pressure (SBP) [6, 7]
- **Vasovagal pathophysiology:** sudden ↓ in venous return → vigorous ventricular contraction → large number of C fibers stimulated → ↑ neural output to brainstem → ↓ HR and PVR [6]

TABLE 26-1

CAUSES OF SYNCOPE

Etiology of syncope, *mean prevalence (Range)* *
Neurally mediated *(~20 %)*
Vasovagal *14 (8–37 %)*
Situational *3 (1–8 %)*
Micturition
Defecation
Cough
Swallow
Postprandial
Neuralgia
Trigeminal
Glossopharyngeal
Carotid Sinus Syncope *1 %*
Orthostatic hypotension *11 (4–13 %)*
Drug-induced or associated syncope *3 (0–7 %)*
Cardiac
Mechanical *3 (1–8 %)*
Obstruction to LV flow
AS, HOCM, MS, LA myxoma
Obstruction to pulmonary flow
PH, PE, Tetralogy of Fallot, PS, RA myxoma
Pump failure due to MI or advanced cardiomyopathy
Cardiac tamponade
Aortic dissection
Electrical *14 (4–26 %)*
Bradyarrhythmias
Sick sinus syndrome
Second or third degree heart block
Pacemaker malfunction
Tachyarrhythmias
Supraventricular tachycardia
Ventricular tachycardia
Torsades de Pointes
Neurologic or cerebrovascular *7 (3–32 %)*
Seizures
Transient ischemic attacks
Migraines
Subclavian steal
Psychiatric *1 (0–5 %)*
Unknown *39 (13–42 %)*

AS aortic stenosis, *LA* left atrial, *LV* left ventricular, *MI* myocardial infarct, *MS* mitral stenosis, *PE* pulmonary embolism, *PH* pulmonary hypertension, *PS* pulmonic stenosis, *RA* right atrial

* Prevalences taken from Schnipper and Kapoor Med Clin North America 2001 [5]

Vasovagal syncope (AKA Neurocardiogenic) (~18 %) [5]

■ History [1, 5, 8–12]:

- Position: usually upright
- Prodrome: fatigue, dizziness, weakness, nausea, diaphoresis, vision changes (tunnel vision), headache, abdominal discomfort, feeling of depersonalization, loss of hearing, "lack of air"LOC: usually <20 s
- Post-syncope: rapid return of alertness and orientation, fatigue or weakness may persist

■ Exam: pallor, diaphoresis, cold skin, dilated pupils, witnesses may describe motor activity **AFTER** LOC

<u>**Carotid Sinus Syncope (1 %)**</u> [5, 6]

■ History:

- Inciting factors: external pressure on carotid (e.g. tight collar, shaving, sudden head turn)
- Typical patient: usually older, men>women
- Past medical History: History of head/neck tumor, scar tissue in neck

■ Exam:

- Carotid sinus massage (CSM) (see section "Physical Examination")

<u>**Situational Syncope (5 % all types)**</u> [13]

■ History: syncope following: cough, micturition, sneeze, gastrointestinal stimulation (deglutition or defecation), airway stimulation, post-prandial,↑ intrathoracic pressure (e.g. trumpet playing, weight lifting)

<u>**Glossopharyngeal or Trigeminal Neuralgia**</u>

Orthostatic Syncope (~8 %) [5–7]

Causes

<u>**Primary autonomic disorders (synucleinopathies)**</u>

■ Multiple-system atrophy with autonomic failure (Shy-Drager), Parkinson's disease, Lewy-body dementia, Postural Orthostatic Tachycardia Syndrome (POTS) (usually does not cause syncope)

<u>**Secondary causes peripheral autonomic disorders**</u>

■ Diabetes, amyloidosis, tabes dorsalis, Sjögren's syndrome, paraneoplastic autonomic neuropathy, multiple sclerosis, spinal tumors

<u>**Hypovolemia**</u>

■ Rule out dehydration and acute blood loss

<u>**Medications**</u>

History

■ Lightheadedness, weakness, nausea, visual changes, etc. in response to sudden postural change

Cardiac Arrhythmia (~14 %) [5]

<u>**Bradyarrhythmias**</u> [1, 9, 14, 15]
<u>**Sinus node dysfunction**</u>

■ Intrinsic sinus node disease: sick sinus syndrome (SSS), sinus bradycardia, sinus pauses, sinoatrial exit block, inexcitable atrium, chronotropic incompetence
■ Associated with fibrosis or chamber enlargement
■ Drug induced: Nodal agents, e.g. beta blocker (BB) (including ophthalmic)
■ Autonomic imbalance: ↑ vagal or ↓ sympathetic tone

<u>**AV conduction disturbances**</u>

■ Syncope results usually from second or third degree atrioventricular (AV) block (risk highest at onset)
■ Congenital AV block: block usually at level of AV node, with narrow QRS

<u>**Indications for pacing**</u>

■ Syncope, dizziness, exercise intolerance

Drug effects

- antiarrhythmics, BB, calcium channel blocker (CCB), digoxin

Pacemaker malfunction

- Causes: lead malfunction, battery depletion, R on T

Tachyarrhythmias [1, 14, 15]
History: sudden onset and/or offset
Supraventricular Tachyarrhythmia (SVT)

- Factors producing syncope: rate, volume status and posture of patient at onset, presence of associated heart disease, arrhythmia mechanism (e.g. Wolff-Parkinson-White [WPW]), peripheral compensation

Ventricular Tachycardia (VT)/Ventricular Fibrillation (VF)

- Monomorphic VT usually underlying structural heart disease (SHD), e.g. prior myocardial infarction (MI), Arrhythmogenic right ventricular cardiomyopathy (ARVC)
- Long QT syndrome → Torsades de Pointes

  - Congenital: three types
  - Acquired: Drugs, www.qtdrugs.org

Structural Cardiac Disease (~4 %) [1, 5, 12, 15]

Valvular

Native Valve Issues

- Aortic stenosis (AS), mitral stenosis (MS), pulmonic stenosis (PS), myxoma

Prosthetic Valve Issues

- Thrombosis, dehiscence, malfunction

Myocardial

LVOT obstruction

- Hypertrophic obstructive cardiomyopathy (HOCM)
- Syncope ↑ risk of sudden cardiac death (SCD) (Relative Risk ~5) [12]

Pump dysfunction

- Myocardial infarction (MI) or congestive heart failure (CHF)
- Syncope may partly result from neural reflex effects

Pericardial

Potential Causes

- Tamponade, less likely constrictive etiologies

Vascular

Potential Causes

- Pulmonary Embolus (PE), Aortic dissection, Primary pulmonary hypertension
- Coronary artery anomaly: anomalous course between aorta and pulmonary artery trunk highest risk

Cerebrovascular/Neurologic (10 %) [5]

Seizure Disorders [1, 10, 16]

■ Transient LOC technically not syncope but often misdiagnosed (~16 %)

History

■ Aura, rising sensation in abdomen, déjà vu or jamais vu, tonic/clonic movement can occur **before** fall, head turning, postictal confusion or sleepiness, tongue biting

Exam

■ Focal neurologic signs may suggest mass lesion

Evaluation

■ Electroencephalogram (EEG): not for routine use, may be beneficial in history of seizures.
■ Computed tomography (CT)/magnetic resonance imaging (MRI): Low utility in routine use, consider if witnessed seizure or focal neurologic sign [17]

Transient Ischemic Attack [5, 13, 17]

■ Rarely cause syncope, vertebrobasilar TIAs/insufficiency may cause LOC, carotid TIA more likely to cause focal neurologic deficits than LOC

Exam

■ Ataxia, hemianopsia, vertigo, focal neurologic deficits on exam

Evaluation

■ CT or MRI low general utility, only 4 % diagnostic yield (patients with+scans had witnessed seizure or focal neurologic deficits)
■ Carotid TIAs not accompanied by LOC so carotid Doppler not beneficial

Subclavian Steal [4, 18]

Definition

■ Subclavian artery stenosis proximal to origin of vertebral artery results in shunt of blood through cerebrovascular system → insufficient cerebral perfusion results when demands for circulation increases such as with arm exercise

History

■ Syncope in setting of strenuous physical activity of one arm, history of Takayasu's arteritis or cervical rib

Evaluation

■ Color Doppler ultrasound, CT angiogram

Syncope Mimics (~2 %) [1, 3, 5]

Causes

Cataplexy

■ Partial or complete loss of muscular control occurs triggered by emotions, especially laughter

Psychiatric

■ Somatization disorders → conversion disorders, factitious disorder, malingering

Breath holding spells

■ Holding of breath at end expiration in response to frustration or injury, spontaneous recovery.

– Usually in children <5 years of age, 2–5 % of well patients

Metabolic

■ hypoglycemia, hypoxia, hypokalemia

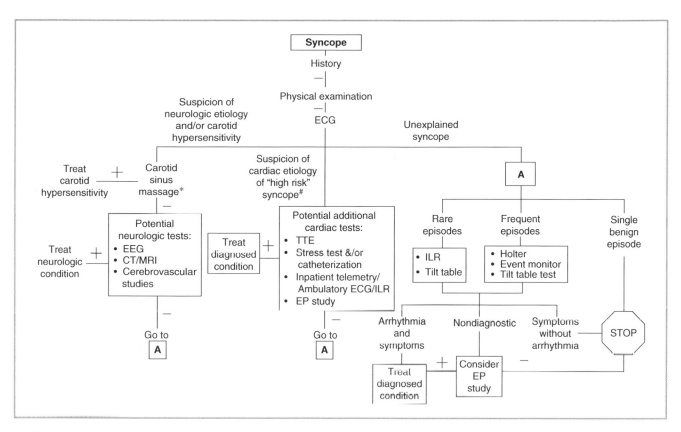

FIGURE 26-1

Approach to the evaluation of syncope. Algorithm for evaluating suspected syncope. *ECG* electrocardiogram, *ILR* implantable loop recorder, *Echo* echocardiogram, *EP* electrophysiologic, *SHD* structural heart disease. * Contraindicated in patients with prior stroke or transient ischemic attack or with bruit present. # syncope during exercise, causing injury or motor vehicle collision or in high risk occupation (e.g. pilot)

INITIAL EVALUATION (HISTORY, PHYSICAL EXAMINATION AND ECG) (FIG. 26-1)

History (To Patient and Witness If Available)

- History and physical identify cause in ~45 % of patients who are ultimately diagnosed [5]
- Initial findings suggestive of organic heart disease directed additional testing leading to diagnosis in ~8 % [5]
- Helpful to differentiate between seizure and syncope (Table 26-2) [9, 10, 16]

Basic Questions [1, 8–11, 13]

Prior to event

- Situational circumstances: position, activity prior to syncope, associated symptoms, prodrome

During Event

- Activity during LOC, length of LOC, trauma (especially to face)
- If jerking movements, specify timing in relation to LOC (seizure=prior or during LOC, NMS=after LOC)

Recovery After Event

- Assess for return of alertness and/or amnesia for event

SUGGESTIVE OF ARRHYTHMIA	SUGGESTIVE OF VASOVAGAL	SUGGESTIVE OF SEIZURE
Age >55	Usually younger age	Waking with a cut tongue
Duration of warning ≤5 s	Prodrome or warning symptoms	Déjà vu or jamais vu prior to loss of consciousness
Male>Female	Female>Male	Associated with emotional stress
≤2 prior episodes of syncope	History of syncope in childhood	Head turning during episode
Structural heart disease by history, exam, or echo	Diaphoresis prior to syncope	Unusual posturing or jerking limbs during episode
Exertional or supine syncope	Syncope with prolonged sitting or standing	Prolonged confusion or amnesia after episode
LBBB on ECG	Normal ECG	

LBBB left bundle branch block

Past Medical History
Prior syncope and presyncope

- Clarify number, frequency and circumstances of previous episodes

    - Many and more frequent episodes suggest noncardiac cause

Cardiac History

- History of SHD or arrhythmias

Neurologic history

- History of and/or risk factors for seizures, stroke/TIA

Other

- Risk factors for coronary artery disease (CAD) or PE
- Metabolic disorders (i.e. diabetes, electrolyte abnormalities)
- Recent bleeding history, trauma, dehydration

Family History
Sudden Death

- Family history of SCD especially at a young age warrants further evaluation

Assess for other cardiac diseases

- Cardiomyopathy, relatives with pacemaker or implantable cardioverter defibrillator (ICD), congenital heart disease

Drugs
Prescribed Medications

- Antihypertensives (especially in elderly)

    - BB, CCB, alpha blocker, diuretics

- Antidepressants
- Antianginals (e.g. nitrates)
- Analgesics
- Central nervous system depressants (e.g. barbiturates)
- QT prolonging agents (www.qtdrugs.org)

    - Type III antiarrhythmics, antipsychotics, antiemetics, methadone
    - Combinations may potentiate effects

Drugs of Abuse

- Alcohol, marijuana, cocaine, etc.

Physical Examination

Vital signs (INCLUDING Orthostatic Vital Signs) [7]

- **Orthostatic vital signs** Measure blood pressure (BP) and HR after standing for 3 min or head-up tilt on tilt table
- Normal response is SBP fall of 5–15 mmHg, DBP rises slightly
- Orthostatic hypotension is present if:

  - SBP↓ 20 mmHg, DBP ↓ 10 mmHg, HR ↑ > 10–20 bpm
  - Symptoms with standing

BP differential in arms

  - May suggest subclavian stenosis, aortic dissection, or coarctation of aorta

Cardiac Exam

Neck Exam

- Carotid bruit
- Carotid pulse – may suggest AS
- Jugular venous pulsation

  - Elevation may suggest CHF
  - Cannon A waves may suggest SVT

Auscultation

- S3 suggests CHF
- Pericardial rub may suggest pericardial effusion
- Murmurs including maneuvers to augment intensity

Vascular Exam

Peripheral pulses

  - Absent or diminished unilateral arm pulses may suggest subclavian steal

Neurologic Exam
Assess for focal neurologic deficits
Carotid sinus massage [1, 4, 6, 18]

  - If history suggestive of carotid sinus hypersensitivity
  - AVOID in patients with prior TIA or stroke within 3 months or if bruit present

    - Monitor patient with continuous ECG and BP measurement

  - Protocol

    - In supine and upright positions, right carotid artery is firmly massaged for 5–10 s at anterior margin of sternocleidomastoid muscle at level of cricoid cartilage, if no 'positive' result, after 1–2 min repeat on left carotid artery

  - Response

    - Cardioinhibitory – asystole of ≥3 s
    - Vasodepressive – ↓ in SBP ≥50 mmHg

Electrocardiogram (ECG)

General Information

- Diagnostic of cause of syncope in ~5 % [8]
- Abnormal in 50 % of syncope cases – may suggest cardiac cause

Suggestive ECG findings of cardiac cause of syncope (Table 26-3) [1, 15]

TABLE 26-3	
	Second (Mobitz II) or third degree AV block
ECG FINDINGS SUGGESTIVE OF CARDIAC CAUSE OF SYNCOPE	Marked sinus bradycardia (<40 beats/min) while awake
	Sinus pause ≥3 s
	Bifascicular block
	IVCD (QRS >120 ms without typical right or left bundle branch block morphology)
	Abnormal QT interval
	Preexcitation (i.e. WPW syndrome)
	Brugada pattern (Right bundle branch block with ST elevation V1–V3)
	T wave inversion V1–V3, epsilon waves and ventricular late potentials (i.e. ARVC)
	Q waves suggesting prior MI or ST or T wave abnormalities suggesting ischemia/infarction
	Evidence of pacemaker malfunction

AV atrioventricular, IVCD intraventricular conductions delay, WPW Wolff Parkinson White

ADDITIONAL DIAGNOSTIC EVALUATION

Echocardiogram [1, 5, 17]

Diagnostic Utility

- Low diagnostic yield in absence of clinical, physical or ECG findings suggestive of cardiac abnormality
- Recommended in syncopal patient when cardiac disease suspected
- Useful in risk stratification for type and severity of underlying heart disease

Echo findings suggestive of possible syncopal etiology

- Valve disease – AS most common, MS, Prosthetic valve issues
- Cardiomyopathy – decreased ejection fraction (EF), HOCM, ARVC
- Wall motion abnormalities – suggestive of prior CAD
- PE – suggestive if acute RV strain and/or pulmonary hypertension

  - Rarely can see embolus in main pulmonary artery

- Cardiac Tumor – occasionally can obstruct blood flow
- Aortic Dissection – Transthoracic echocardiogram may miss ascending aortic dissection
- Congenital heart disease

  - In young, thin patients, can identify coronary ostia to assess for anomalous coronary arteries

- Cardiac Tamponade –atrial or RV inversion, respiratory variation in inflow velocities

Exercise Testing (ETT) [1, 5, 12, 17]

Diagnostic Utility

- Low diagnostic yield in general population (<1 %)
- Recommended for patients who experience syncope during or shortly after exertion

  - *Exertional syncope patients should have echo prior to ETT to exclude HOCM*

Diagnostic ETT findings in syncope

- ECG and hemodynamic abnormalities present and syncope is reproduced during or immediately after exercise
- Mobitz II or third degree AV block during exercise even in absence of syncope
- In pt <40 years old, drop in SBP with exercise, consider HOCM or left main coronary disease
- Screen for catecholaminergic polymorphic VT

Catheterization

Recommendations [1, 12]

■ Recommended if initial history, exam, ECG or exercise testing suggestive of myocardial ischemia

Ambulatory ECG Monitoring

Holter Monitoring [1, 5, 12, 17]

<u>**Indications**</u>

■ Indicated in patients with SHD and frequent symptoms when there is a high pre-test probability of identifying an arrhythmia responsible for syncope

- Highest yield if daily symptoms
- Optimal duration is 48 h

<u>**Diagnostic Yield**</u> ≈ 19 %

■ Arrhythmia correlates with symptoms ~4 %
■ Symptoms without arrhythmia ~15 %
■ Arrhythmia without symptoms ~14 %

<u>**High risk features**</u>

■ Sinus pauses >2 s, second degree AV block (Mobitz II), complete AV block, runs of nonsustained ventricular tachycardia (NSVT)

<u>**Recommendations**</u>

■ Use Holter when symptoms suggest arrhythmia (i.e. brief LOC, no prodrome, palpitations) or in patients with unexplained cause, history of SHD or abnormal ECG

Long Term Ambulatory ECG [1, 5, 17, 19, 20]

Procedure

■ Worn for 30–60 days and patient triggering stores ECG from 1 to 4 min before and 30–60 s after activation

Indications

■ Patients with relatively frequent spells (every week to every 1–2 months) and no known SHD

- Major limitation to use is patient error and noncompliance

Ideal patient

■ Compliant, does not live alone, familiar with technology, highly motivated to achieve diagnosis

Implantable Loop Recorder (ILR) [21]

Procedure

■ Subcutaneous insertion of device capable of recording ECG signals for up to 2 years, patient uses activator to record rhythm at time of symptoms, device also automatically records bradycardia and tachycardia

Diagnostic Yield

■ In patients with unexplained syncope, ILR more likely to yield diagnosis than conventional testing (55 % vs. 19 %, p=0.0014) [21]

Length of monitoring

■ 12 month monitoring period captures >90 % of episodes in study of 167 patients with recurrent unexplained syncope of which two-thirds of patients had syncope [22]

Tilt Table Testing [1, 23, 24]

Background

■ Moving from supine to standing posture results in 15–20 % decrease in plasma volume in 10 min, can induce vasovagal syncope in susceptible individuals with or without chemical stimulation

Positive response – Syncope occurs with asystole >3 s=cardioinhibitory

Diagnostic yield

■ Sensitivity 26–80 %, Specificity 90 %

– Some studies have noted higher false positive rates with isoproterenol especially at higher angle of tilt

Indications

Class I Recommendations

■ Unexplained syncope in high risk settings (e.g. following injury or high risk occupation, e.g. pilot)
■ Recurrent episodes in absence of SHD or when SHD has been excluded
■ To demonstrate susceptibility of NMS to patient

Class III – not recommended

■ Assessment of treatment
■ Solitary episode without injury and absence of high risk setting
■ High probability of vasovagal syncope by clinical history and no change in treatment with proof of NMS

Electrophysiologic (EP) Study ([1, 15, 17], Table 26-4)

Background

■ Catheters are manipulated into heart and electrical stimulation and recording is used to assess sinus node function, AV conduction and susceptibility to SVT and VT

Diagnostic findings (Table 26-5)

TABLE 26-4	DIAGNOSTIC	INTERMEDIATE	NONDIAGNOSTIC
CLASSIFICATION OF FINDINGS IN ELECTROPHYSIOLOGY STUDY IN PATIENTS WITH SYNCOPE	Sinus bradycardia and very prolonged SNRT (>3 s)	HV interval >70 and <100 ms	Induction of polymorphic VT or VF in patients with ischemic cardiomyopathy
	HV interval ≥100 ms	Induction of polymorphic VT or VT in patients with ARVC	Induction of polymorphic VT or VF in patients with dilated cardiomyopathy
	Second or third degree HP block during Atrial pacing	Induction of NSVT	
	High-degree HP block after IV procainamide or disopyramide	Induction of SVT without hypotension or rate <180 bpm	
	Induction of sustained monomorphic VT (>150 bpm)		
	Induction of sustained SVT with hypotension or rate >180 bpm		

ARVC arrhythmogenic right ventricular cardiomyopathy, *bpm* beats per minute, *HP* His-Purkinje, *SNRT* sinus node recovery time, *NSVT* non-sustained ventricular tachycardia, *SVT* supraventricular tachycardia, *VF* ventricular fibrillation, *VT* ventricular tachycardia

ADMISSION RECOMMENDED	ADMISSION OFTEN INDICATED	POTENTIAL OUTPATIENT EVALUATION
History of and/or signs/symptoms suggesting MI, CHF, PE, aortic dissection or other SHD	Older than 65 years of age	Absence of structural heart disease and normal ECG
Exertional syncope, supine syncope, or syncope causing injury or accident	History of SHD but no active evidence of disease	History of recurrent syncope over many years
Concerning ECG abnormalities (see Table 26-3)	Frequent spells	Suspicion of syncope "mimic" (e.g. hypoglycemia, conversion disorder)
Family history of early sudden cardiac death	Lack of warning signs prior to syncope	
History of and/or signs/symptoms of stroke or focal neurologic disorder	Moderate to severe orthostatic hypotension	
Suspected malfunction of cardiac device (pacemaker, ICD, prosthetic valve)	Discontinuation or dose modification of offending drug	

CHF congestive heart failure, *ICD* implantable cardioverter defibrillator, *MI* myocardial infarction, *PE* pulmonary embolism, *SHD* structural heart disease

Diagnostic yield

■ In patients with normal initial evaluation ≈ yield 3 %

Bradyarrhythmias

■ EP study had poor sensitivity: sinus pauses ~38 %, AV block ~15 % [25]

Tachyarrhythmias

■ Assessing for induced sustained monomorphic VT

- Most useful in patients with prior MI and depressed EF

Limitations

■ High cost, invasive, poor specificity and prediction of bradyarrhythmias

Recommendations

Class I

■ Indicated when initial evaluation suggests arrhythmogenic cause of syncope (in patients with abnormal ECG and/or SHD or syncope with palpitations or family history of SCD)

Class III (Not recommended)

■ Patients with normal ECG and no heart disease or palpitations

Cardiac Imaging

■ Limited utility – consider if concern for anomalous coronary anatomy

Neurologic Studies [1, 5, 12, 17]

■ Low yield in most syncope patients unless signs and symptoms suggestive of neurologic cause

Electroencephalogram (EEG)

■ Low diagnostic yield: 1–2 % (in studies positive patients had seizure history)
■ In absence of witnessed tonic/clonic movements, prolonged confusion after LOC or known history: use of EEG not recommended

Head CT

- Low diagnostic yield in syncope: ~4 % (all studied patients had focal neurologic findings or seizure history)
- Recommended in syncope patients with focal neurologic findings, seizure activity, or in trauma patients to rule out hemorrhage

Neurovascular studies

- Carotid TIAs are not usually accompanied by LOC, so studies have not demonstrated benefit of transcranial or carotid Doppler studies in evaluating syncope
- Severe bilateral carotid or basilar artery disease can cause syncope but usually focal neurologic findings – consider carotid and/or transcranial Doppler evaluation

TREATMENT

Individualized to Underlying Etiology of Syncope

Neurally mediated syncope [6, 7, 15, 26]

Medical Therapy

- Behavioral training

  - Education on warning signs and need to lay horizontal when symptoms to prevent injury
  - Techniques for avoiding syncope
  - Liberalize salt intake and maintain hydration
  - Avoidance of triggers for situational syncope

- Physical counter-pressure maneuvers (PCM)

  - Squatting, arm-tensing, leg-crossing and leg-crossing with lower body muscle tensing
  - Shown to reduce total burden and recurrence rate of syncope in patients with recognizable warning symptoms when compared with conventional treatment (32 % vs. 51 %, $p < 0.005$) [26]

Medications

- Few randomized clinical trials so insufficient evidence to support or refute use of ANY specific agents [26]
- Potential classes

  - Volume expanders – e.g. fludrocortisone

    - Weak evidence with potential side effects: hypertension, hypokalemia

  - Beta blocker – theoretically lessen impact of adrenergic surge

    - Weak evidence: large RCT showed no benefit

  - Vaso/venoconstrictors

    - Midodrine has best evidence
    - Side effects: hypertension, urinary retention

Device Therapy

- Pacemakers have limited role in patients with "refractory" vasovagal syncope [26]

  - Mechanism of benefit thought to be prevention of severe bradycardia in cardio-inhibitory syncope
  - Strongest evidence in ISSUE-3 – 57 % relative risk reduction of syncope in patients with asystolic vasovagal syncope on ILR [27]

- Current recommendations for older patients with vasovagal syncope and documented symptomatic asystolic pauses during syncope [15]

Orthostatic syncope

- Similar to vasovagal syncope, except usually older individuals that may have issues performing PCM and may have supine hypertension

  #### Medical treatment [15, 26]

  - Education about exacerbating factors for postural hypotension (i.e. sudden postural change, polypharmacy, diminished thirst in elderly) and avoidance of triggers
  - Hydration, volume expanders with close monitoring of blood pressure to avoid hypertension, PCM
  - Vasoconstrictors

    – Midodrine has been shown to have effect in orthostatic syncope – caution with nocturnal/supine hypertension

Carotid sinus syncope [26]
  #### Medical therapy

  - Avoidance of tight collars, neckties, abrupt neck movements

  #### Device therapy

  - Cardiac pacing, especially in cardioinhibitory response to carotid sensitivity

Arrhythmias [1, 12, 15]

  #### Device Therapy

  - Benefit to pacemakers with symptomatic bradycardia or high risk for progression to heart block
  - ICD recommended in inducible sustained monomorphic VT in pt with syncope
  - ICD indications based on indications for arrhythmia and/or SHD, i.e. EF <35 % (may not prevent syncope) [15]

  #### Prolonged QT

  - Replete electrolytes (especially magnesium)
  - Avoid QT prolonging drugs

PROGNOSIS

Risk Stratification

Need for hospitalization [1, 12, 15] (Table 26-5)

- Based on multiple population studies that followed patients after emergency presentation with syncope

Risk factors predictive of arrhythmia and potential need for hospitalization [28]

- Risk factors: Abnormal ECG, prior VT, prior CHF, Age >45
- 0 risk factors: 72 h mortality 0 %, 1 year mortality 8.3 % derivation cohort and 4.4 % in validation cohort

Long term follow up

- Multiple studies in 1980s suggested cardiac syncope has higher 1 year mortality (18–33 %) than noncardiac syncope (0–12 %) or unknown cause (6 %) [5]
- Study in older hospitalized patients did not show increased mortality with cardiac syncope (RR 1.18; 95%CI 0.92–1.50) vs. unexplained syncope (RR 1.0) or noncardiac syncope (RR 0.94; 95 % CI 0.77–1.16) [29]

QUICK REVIEW (TABLE 26-6)

TABLE 26-6	
QUICK REVIEW	

FINDING ON HISTORY OR EXAM	SUGGESTED DIAGNOSES
Occurred with prolonged standing	Vasovagal syncope
Associated with pain, fear, unpleasant sight, smell or sound	Vasovagal syncope
Occur in warm or crowded environment	Vasovagal syncope
Occurs with micturition, defecation, cough or deglutition	Situational/NMS
Occurs within an hour after eating	Postprandial hypotension
Occurs with head rotation, shaving, tight collars	Carotid hypersensitivity
Tonic-clonic movements short (<15 s) and occur AFTER loss of consciousness	Vasovagal syncope
Tonic-clonic movements prolonged and initiates DURING or PRIOR TO loss of consciousness	Seizure
Syncope associated with tongue biting, aching muscles, déjà vu, olfactory sensations and prolonged confusion	Seizure
Associated with throat or facial pain (glossopharyngeal or trigeminal neuralgia)	Neurally mediated syncope
Occurs with change of position from sitting to standing	Orthostatic hypotension
Taking one or more anti-hypertensive medications (especially polypharmacy in elderly)	Drug-induced syncope
Multiple medications prolonging QT or causing bradycardia	Drug-induced syncope
Well trained athlete with structurally NORMAL heart after exertion	Vasovagal syncope
Associated with vertigo, dysarthria, diplopia	TIA, stroke, vertebro-basilar insufficiency
Blood pressure difference between arms	Subclavian steal or aortic dissection
Syncope during arm exercise (e.g. painting a fence)	Subclavian steal
Occurs with change in position (upright to supine, bending over) ± murmur that also varies with position	Atrial myxoma, thrombus
Exertional syncope	Aortic stenosis, HOCM, mitral stenosis, pulmonary hypertension, CAD, or anomalous coronary artery
Supine syncope	Arrhythmia
Family history of sudden cardiac death	Long QT, Brugada, HOCM
Deaf patient with syncope after effort or strong emotion	Long QT syndrome
Triggered by laughter or strong emotions with normal cardiac evaluation	Cataplexy
Child <5 years old after frustrating episode or injury	Breath holding spell
Diabetic who skipped meals	Hypoglycemia

CAD coronary artery disease, *HOCM* hypertrophic obstructive cardiomyopathy

REVIEW QUESTIONS

1. A 26 year-old female medical student passes out while standing up in an operating room. She states that prior to falling she felt weak, "warm all over" and sweaty. She also felt a "lack of air" but attributed it to her surgical mask. Witnesses stated she looked pale and gradually slumped to the floor. After falling the nurse noted a few jerking movements and she regained consciousness in about 5 s. The patient has no recollection for the event but states that she felt at her baseline almost immediately after awakening. She remembers passing out as a teenager, once on a hot summer day and after giving blood. She denies any medical problems, takes no medications and denies illicit drug use. Her grandfather had a heart attack at age 75 but otherwise denies family history of early coronary disease or sudden cardiac death. On physical examination, her HR is 65, BP 110/70, there is no jugular venous distention, normal pulse exam and cardiac exam. Her ECG reveals no abnormalities. Which of the following is the next appropriate step?

    (a) Echocardiogram
    (b) Admission to hospital for further evaluation, including telemetry and cardiac biomarkers
    (c) Initiate beta blockade
    (d) Educate her on physical-counter-maneuvers such as leg-crossing or squatting and fall avoidance
    (e) Arrange for an outpatient 72-h Holter monitor

2. A 65 year-old man presents with his second syncopal episode. He notes no warning symptoms prior to his episodes and he had facial trauma following the most recent episode. His initial evaluation consisted of a detailed medical and family history, physical examination, electrocardiogram and echocardiogram. Which of the following clinical findings noted on initial workup would NOT be an indication for an electrophysiologic study?

    (a) Abnormal ECG suggesting conduction system disease
    (b) Abnormal tilt table testing response
    (c) Syncope during exertion or in supine position
    (d) Family history of sudden death
    (e) Evidence of structural heart disease

3. A 35 year-old woman has a history of 5 prior episodes of syncope over the past 2 years. She occasionally has noted chest pain prior to her syncopal episodes. All of her prior episodes occurred when she was not physically active and mostly while lying in bed. She previously had been referred to a neurologist and had a negative prior neurologic workup including a normal electroencephalogram (EEG). Her family history is notable for a sister who died suddenly at age 25. She denies any other medical problems and any prescription or illicit drug use. On physical exam, her HR was 60, her BP was 115/70 and her cardiac exam reveals no murmurs or extra sounds. Her ECG is seen in Fig. 26-2. Which of the following is the most likely diagnosis?

    (a) Hypertrophic cardiomyopathy
    (b) Brugada Syndrome
    (c) Arrhythmogenic right ventricular cardiomyopathy
    (d) Long QT syndrome
    (e) Wolff-Parkinson-White syndrome

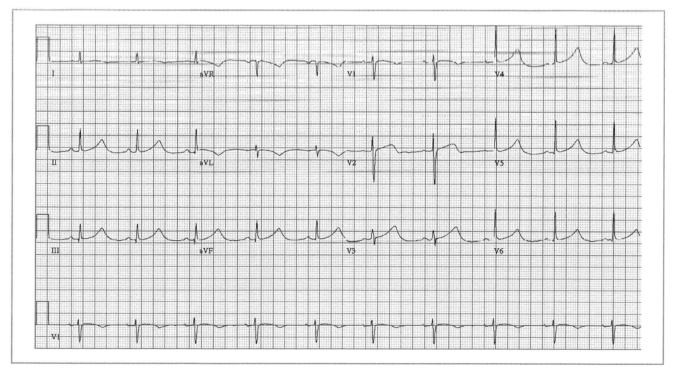

FIGURE 26-2

ECG for question 3

4. **Which of the following patients should undergo testing beyond a physical examination and ECG to establish a diagnosis?**

(a) 40 year-old female who fainted in childhood after seeing blood has syncope while standing in line at the bank

(b) 32 year-old male trumpet player who has a syncopal episode while playing a long solo

(c) 25 year-old soccer player with no prior evaluation who passes out DURING a match

(d) 28 year-old marathon runner who has prior evaluation revealing structurally normal heart on ECG and echocardiogram who loses consciousness AFTER a race

(e) 27 year-old male with pertussis who passes out during a coughing fit.

5. **All of the following findings on initial history, physical examination, or electrocardiogram should prompt hospital admission for evaluation except:**

(a) ECG demonstrating sinus pause of 2 s

(b) Physical examination demonstrating elevated jugular venous pressure, rales on lung examination, and lower extremity edema

(c) Family history of sudden cardiac death

(d) Physical examination demonstrating parvus et tardus, systolic murmur heard best at upper sternal border and absent S2

(e) ECG with Right bundle branch block and ST elevations in V1-V3

ANSWERS

1. (d) The patient and witness describe an episode of LOC and postural tone with spontaneous recovery consistent with a vasovagal episode. Factors consistent with vasovagal syncope include: standing posture, prodromal symptoms, lack of postictal confusion, and unpleasant environment. She also describes a prior history of benign syncopal episodes as a child also consistent with vasovagal syncope. Her family history, physical exam findings, and ECG also do not raise concern for a cardiac cause of syncope. A low risk young patient with vasovagal syncope can be discharged after careful discussion regarding fall avoidance and education on the importance of hydration and physical counter-maneuvers such as leg crossing with lower body muscle tensing, squatting or arm tensing to raise blood pressure. She has no high risk markers for hospital admission and there is no suspicion of CAD to justify ruling out for MI so option b is incorrect. Given the absence of known SHD and normal ECG and physical exam, an echocardiogram (option a) is unlikely to provide useful additional information. There is little evidence supporting the use of beta-blockers (option c) in vasovagal syncope. Her episodes are so infrequent that a Holter monitor would be unlikely to capture any episodes.

2. (b) The patient gives a history suspicious for syncope due to arrhythmia with lack of a prodrome and syncope causing injury suggesting lack of warning. In one study, male sex, age greater than 54, less than or equal to 2 prior syncopal episodes and less than 5 s of warning prior to syncope were predictive of syncope due to AV block or VT. In patients with concern for syncope due to cardiac arrhythmias, Class I indications for an EP study include: abnormal ECG suggesting conduction system disease (option a), syncope during exertion or in supine position (option c) or with important structural heart disease (option e), family history of sudden death (option d). Syncope with palpitations or angina-like chest pain is also a Class I indication. Class III indications for an EP study include: normal ECG, no known history of SHD and no palpitations. An abnormal tilt table testing response (option b) suggests NMS rather than arrhythmogenic syncope and is not an EP study indication.

3. (d) Several features of this patient's syncopal history are concerning of a cardiac cause of syncope including: syncope while supine and family history of sudden cardiac death. Her ECG demonstrates a prolonged QTc>480 ms. These three factors place her at high risk of long QT syndrome (option d). The remaining answers are incorrect. Hypertrophic cardiomyopathy (option a) usually presents with exertional syncope rather than supine syncope. The ECG in Brugada syndrome (option b) usually demonstrates incomplete or complete right bundle branch block and ST elevations in leads V1-V3. The ECG in Arrhythmogenic Right Ventricular Cardiomyopathy usually demonstrates T wave inversions in leads V2-V4 and an echocardiogram usually reveals right ventricular abnormalities. The ECG in Wolff-Parkinson-White syndrome demonstrates preexcited ventricular complexes.

4. (c) The scenarios described in options (a), (b), (d), and (e) all involve young individuals with neurally mediated syncope (NMS). Option (a) is consistent with vasovagal syncope, option (b) syncope while playing a brass instrument is a form of NMS. Option (d) describes POST-exertional syncope in an athlete, which is also a form of NMS. It is important to note that the athlete in question, has already had a workup revealing a structurally normal heart, as there should be a high index of suspicion when syncope occurs in athletes. Cough induced syncope (option e) is another example of situational syncope, a form of NMS. Option (c) describes syncope during exertion, which is a red flag and should be evaluated further.

5. (a) A sinus pause >3–5 s is a concerning ECG abnormality that warrants hospital stay, pauses under 3 s would be unlikely to cause syncope. Option (b) depicts the physical examination of a patient in congestive heart failure suggesting underlying cardiac etiology and should be admitted for further evaluation. A positive family history of sudden cardiac death is highly concerning in a syncopal patient and supports evaluation in a hospital. Option (d) describes a patient with severe aortic stenosis, which is a potential cause of syncope and should be further evaluated in a hospital setting. Option (e) describes a typical ECG in Brugada syndrome and any ECG with evidence of channelopathy should be admitted to the hospital for further workup.

REFERENCES

1. Brignole M, Alboni P, Benditt DG, Bergfeldt L, Blanc JJ, Thomsen PE, et al. Guidelines on management (diagnosis and treatment) of syncope-update 2004. Executive summary. Eur Heart J. 2004;25(22):2054–72.

2. Savage DD, Corwin L, McGee DL, Kannel WB, Wolf PA. Epidemiologic features of isolated syncope: the Framingham Study. Stroke. 1985;16(4):626–9.

3. Benditt DG, Remole S, Milstein S, Bailin S. Syncope: causes, clinical evaluation, and current therapy. Annu Rev Med. 1992;43:283–300.

4. Kapoor WN. Diagnostic evaluation of syncope. Am J Med. 1991;90(1):91–106.

5. Schnipper JL, Kapoor WN. Diagnostic evaluation and management of patients with syncope. Med Clin North Am. 2001;85(2):423–56, xi.

6. Goldschlager N, Epstein AE, Grubb BP, Olshansky B, Prystowsky E, Roberts WC, et al. Etiologic considerations in the patient with syncope and an apparently normal heart. Arch Intern Med. 2003;163(2):151–62.

7. Freeman R. Clinical practice. Neurogenic orthostatic hypotension. N Engl J Med. 2008;358(6):615–24.

8. Linzer M, Yang EH, Estes 3rd NA, Wang P, Vorperian VR, Kapoor WN. Diagnosing syncope. Part 1: value of history, physical examination, and electrocardiography. Clinical Efficacy Assessment Project of the American College of Physicians. Ann Intern Med. 1997;126(12):989–96.

9. Sud S, Klein GJ, Skanes AC, Gula LJ, Yee R, Krahn AD. Predicting the cause of syncope from clinical history in patients undergoing prolonged monitoring. Heart Rhythm. 2009;6(2):238–43.

10. Sheldon R, Rose S, Ritchie D, Connolly SJ, Koshman ML, Lee MA, et al. Historical criteria that distinguish syncope from seizures. J Am Coll Cardiol. 2002;40(1):142–8.

11. Calkins H, Shyr Y, Frumin H, Schork A, Morady F. The value of the clinical history in the differentiation of syncope due to ventricular tachycardia, atrioventricular block, and neurocardiogenic syncope. Am J Med. 1995;98(4):365–73.

12. Strickberger SA, Benson DW, Biaggioni I, Callans DJ, Cohen MI, Ellenbogen KA, et al. AHA/ACCF Scientific Statement on the evaluation of syncope: from the American Heart Association Councils on Clinical Cardiology, Cardiovascular Nursing, Cardiovascular Disease in the Young, and Stroke, and the Quality of Care and Outcomes Research Interdisciplinary Working Group; and the American College of Cardiology Foundation: in collaboration with the Heart Rhythm Society: endorsed by the American Autonomic Society. Circulation. 2006;113(2):316–27.

13. Kapoor WN. Syncope. N Engl J Med. 2000;343(25):1856–62.

14. Kapoor WN. Current evaluation and management of syncope. Circulation. 2002;106(13):1606–9.

15. Benditt DG, Nguyen JT. Syncope: therapeutic approaches. J Am Coll Cardiol. 2009;53(19):1741–51.

16. Hoefnagels WA, Padberg GW, Overweg J, Roos RA. Syncope or seizure? A matter of opinion. Clin Neurol Neurosurg. 1992;94(2):153–6.

17. Linzer M, Yang EH, Estes 3rd NA, Wang P, Vorperian VR, Kapoor WN. Diagnosing syncope. Part 2: unexplained syncope. Clinical Efficacy Assessment Project of the American College of Physicians. Ann Intern Med. 1997;127(1):76–86.

18. Alves C. Manual of cardiovascular medicine. 3rd ed. Philadelphia: Lippincott Williams and Wilkins; 2009.

19. Linzer M, Pritchett EL, Pontinen M, McCarthy E, Divine GW. Incremental diagnostic yield of loop electrocardiographic recorders in unexplained syncope. Am J Cardiol. 1990;66(2):214–9.

20. Gula LJ, Krahn AD, Massel D, Skanes A, Yee R, Klein GJ. External loop recorders: determinants of diagnostic yield in patients with syncope. Am Heart J. 2004;147(4):644–8.

21. Krahn AD, Klein GJ, Yee R, Skanes AC. Randomized assessment of syncope trial: conventional diagnostic testing versus a prolonged monitoring strategy. Circulation. 2001;104(1):46–51.

22. Assar MD, Krahn AD, Klein GJ, Yee R, Skanes AC. Optimal duration of monitoring in patients with unexplained syncope. Am J Cardiol. 2003;92(10):1231–3.

23. Kapoor WN, Smith MA, Miller NL. Upright tilt testing in evaluating syncope: a comprehensive literature review. Am J Med. 1994;97(1):78–88.

24. Benditt DG, Ferguson DW, Grubb BP, Kapoor WN, Kugler J, Lerman BB, et al. Tilt table testing for assessing syncope. American College of Cardiology. J Am Coll Cardiol. 1996;28(1):263–75.

25. Fujimura O, Yee R, Klein GJ, Sharma AD, Boahene KA. The diagnostic sensitivity of electrophysiologic testing in patients with syncope caused by transient bradycardia. N Engl J Med. 1989;321(25):1703–7.

26. Romme JJ, Reitsma JB, Black CN, Colman N, Scholten RJ, Wieling W, et al. Drugs and pacemakers for vasovagal, carotid sinus and situational syncope. Cochrane Database Syst Rev. 2011;(10):CD004194.

27. Brignole M, Menozzi C, Moya A, Andresen D, Blanc JJ, Krahn AD, et al. Pacemaker therapy in patients with neurally-mediated syncope and documented asystole. Third International Study on Syncope of Uncertain Etiology (ISSUE-3): a randomized trial. Circulation. 2012;125(21):2566–71.

28. Martin TP, Hanusa BH, Kapoor WN. Risk stratification of patients with syncope. Ann Emerg Med. 1997;29(4):459–66.

29. Getchell WS, Larsen GC, Morris CD, McAnulty JH. Epidemiology of syncope in hospitalized patients. J Gen Intern Med. 1999;14(11):677–87.

CHAPTER 27

Karim M. Awad and M. Brandon Westover

Ischemic Stroke, Muscular Dystrophy and Friedreich's Ataxia

CHAPTER OUTLINE

ABBREVIATIONS

ACA	Anterior cerebral artery
ACE	Angiotensin converting enzymes
ACS	Acute coronary syndrome
AF	Atrial fibrillation
ASA	Aspirin
AV	Atrioventricular
AVB	AV block
BP	Blood pressure
CMP	Cardiomyopathy
CTA	CT angiogram
DCM	Dilated cardiomyopathy
DVT	Deep venous thrombosis
ECG	Electrocardiogram
EMG	Electromyography
FA	Friedreich ataxia
HTN	Hypertension
ICA	Internal carotid artery
ICD	Implantable cardioverter defibrillator
ICH	Intracerebral hemorrhage
LBBB	Left bundle branch block
LV	Left ventricular
MAP	Arterial pressure
MCA	Middle cerebral artery
MD	Muscular dystrophy
PCA	Posterior cerebral artery
PFO	Patent foreman ovale
PVC	Premature ventricular complexes
RBBB	Right bundle branch block
RV	Right ventricle
RVH	RV hypertrophy
TIA	Transient Ischemic attacks
tPA	Recombinant tissue plasminogen activator
VF	Ventricular fibrillation
VT	Ventricular tachycardia

INTRODUCTION

Patients with stroke, coronary artery disease and peripheral vascular disease share some of the same risk factors and often live with more than one cardiovascular disease. It is increasingly important for cardiologists to be familiar with the recognition and management of stroke (whether as a co-morbidity in a cardiac patient or as a complication from cardiac disorders or procedures).

Another important connection between neurology and cardiology is the cardiac manifestation of neurological disorders such as muscular dystrophies and Friedreich's ataxia. They contribute significantly to the morbidity and mortality of such patients and often require cardiac consultation or procedures.

ISCHEMIC STROKE

Transient Ischemic Attacks (TIA)

Transient Ischemic attacks (TIA): reversible episode of focal neurologic symptoms; most last <1 h; must be <24 h by definition. Newer definition: brief, reversible episode of focal neurologic symptoms and negative MRI. Longer TIAs more likely to result from embolus, repeated similar TIAs suggest impending occlusion. Most TIAs should be worked up urgently, whether inpatient or outpatient. Early treatment and workup reduces risk of recurrent stroke by ~80 % [1] (Tables 27-1 and 27-2).

■ **Differential diagnosis for TIA/stroke**: Top two mimics are seizures and migraine. Others: syncope, conversion, malingering, prior stroke re-manifested by toxic/metabolic derangement. The following "rules" of thumb are helpful, but not absolute, guides (Table 27-3).

Helps determine urgency TIA/stroke workup				**A**ge ≥ 60 yo: 1 point
Score ≥4 should have expedited workup				**B**P ≥140/90 mmHg: 1 point
Stroke risk				**U**nilateral weakness (2 points)
Score	**Day 2** (%)	**Day 7** (%)	**Day 90** (%)	**S**peech impairment without weakness
≤4	1	1.2	3.1	(1 point)
4–5	4.1	5.9	9.8	**D**uration: >60 min (2 points), 10–59 min
				(1 point)
>5	8.1	11.7	17.8	**D**iabetes: 1 point

TABLE 27-1

ABCD2 SCORE [2]

	FACTOR	**POINTS**	**TOTAL POINTS**	**ANNUAL STROKE RISK (%)**
C	**C**HF	1	0	1.9
H	**H**TN	1	1	2.8
A	**A**ge ≥75	1	2	4.0
D	**D**iabetes	1	3	5.9
S₂	**S**troke or TIA	2	4	8.5
	Total possible	**6**	5	12.5
			6	18.2

TABLE 27-3	DX	PTS	SYMPTOMS	DURATION
DIFFERENTIATING TIA FROM SEIZURES AND MIGRAINES	TIA	Older, male, risk factors (HTN, DM)	Negative. If multiple modalities (e.g. sensory, motor) usually occur all at once Sometimes headache with symptoms	Brief (usually 15 min, can be longer)
	Seizures	Younger	Begins with positive symptoms. (e.g. tingling). Negative symptoms (e.g. paresis, aphasia) may follow	Very brief (sec – min). Postictal sx can last hours
	Migraines	Younger, female, + FH	Headache after attack. Often associated with nausea, vomiting, photo/phonophobia. Begin with positive sx (e.g. seeing stars), then Negative sx. Sx evolve slowly (e.g. tingling slowly spreads up arm)	Longer (30 min up to hours)

Ischemic Stroke

- **Basic Mechanisms**:

  - Embolic: Sudden symptom onset, usually *maximal at onset*.
  - Thrombotic: Main deficit sometimes preceded by warning signs (TIAs or minor symptoms) or stuttering/progressive course over several hours.

- **Common etiologies**: Main subtypes of ischemic stroke (Table 27-4).

- **Uncommon stroke etiologies**: (~2 %)

  - **Vasculitis**: Due to autoimmune disease, arteritis (temporal, Takayasu), infectious (tuberculosis, syphilis, varicella zoster virus) or primary central nervous system vasculitis.
  - **Dissections**: Strokes in younger patients (age 35–50).
  - **Fibromuscular dysplasia**: Uncommon, affects women age 30–50. Imaging: segmental arterial narrowing and dilation ('string of beads'). Arteries affected: renal, internal carotid artery (ICA) > vertebral > intracranial. Stenosis causes thrombosis or dissection.
  - **Subcortical vascular dementia**: Multiple subcortical infarctions cause dementia. Risk: chronic hypertension (HTN).
  - **Drugs**: Amphetamines, cocaine cause acute HTN or drug induced vasculopathy

- **Evaluation of ischemic stroke**:

  - **Urgent (in emergency department)**: CBC, BMP, PT, PTT, Cardiac Enzymes, non-contrast head CT to rule out intracerebral hemorrhage, (ICH) if considering treatment with IV tissue plasminogen activator (tPA).
  - **Studies for secondary prevention**:

    - Labs: Lipid panel, including lipoprotein(a), Hemoglobin A1c, homocysteine, TSH (looking for hyperthyroidism – increases risk of atrial fibrillation [AF]), ESR if suspecting vasculitis or endocarditis; Hypercoagulable panel for patients <50 years old (antiphospholipid antibodies, lupus anticoagulant, prothrombin G20210A gene mutation, factor V Leiden, protein C/protein S/antithrombin deficiencies) (Table 27-5).

Large artery atherosclerosis (~18 %)	Most common sites: carotid bifurcation, vertebrals at origin or at the vertebro-basilar junction, MCA at stem/bifurcation. Plaques rarely occur beyond first branching point. Risk factors: HTN, DM, dyslipidemia, smoking	**TABLE 27-4** MAJOR SUBTYPES OF ISCHEMIC STROKE
Cardioembolic (~21 %)	AF, MI, HF, prosthetic valves, rheumatic heart disease Most often lodges in MCA (especially superior division) or PCA territory Small embolus: cortical or penetrating arteries; large embolus: main branches	
Small vessel (lacune) (24 %)	Due to severe atherosclerosis→thrombosis of small penetrating vessels Infarcts up to 2 cm in size. Often associated with HTN	
'Unknown' (~34 %)	Paradoxical embolism. Falls under cryptogenic strokes: not lacunar, without evidence of cardioembolic (e.g. AF), or large artery source (e.g. carotid stenosis). Many are due to PFO	

AF atrial fibrillation, *DM* diabetes mellitus, *HF* heart failure, *HTN* hypertension, *MCA* middle cerebral artery, *MI* myocardial infarction, *PCA* posterior cerebral artery, *PFO* patent foramen ovale

Association with ischemic stroke/cerebral venous thrombosis in younger pts <50 years. Strongest association with antiphospholipid antibody syndrome. Most guidelines recommend testing in pts <50 years old with *venous* thrombosis, no recommendations for acute ischemic stroke. Treatment: controversial, usually for *venous* thromboembolism: anticoagulation; for arterial thrombus (ischemic stroke) aspirin v. anticoagulation (except for Antiphospholipid antibody syndrome: anticoagulate)	**TABLE 27-5** HYPERCOAGULABLE STATES THAT MAY LEAD TO ISCHEMIC STROKE
Antiphospholipid Antibody Syndrome: Acquired, associated with autoimmune disease (e.g. lupus). Symptoms: recurrent pregnancy loss/thrombotic events. Diagnosis: Clinical event+1 Lab abnormality: Antibodies against: cardiolipin and Beta 2 glycoprotein I lupus anticoagulant. If test abnormal, recheck in 12 weeks. Treatment: life-long anticoagulation	
Prothrombin G20210A Gene Mutation: Causes ↑ liver synthesis of prothombin. Mostly in Caucasians	
Factor V Leiden: Mutation in Factor V: becomes resistant to degradation (by activated protein C)	
Protein C, Protein S, or Antithrombin deficiencies: Very uncommon. Diagnosis is difficult due to false positives, especially acutely after acute stroke. All three ↓ in acute thrombosis/surgery, or due hepatic dysfunction (i.e. decreased production), heparin decreases antithrombin, warfarin/OCPs decrease protein C/S	

- **Brain Imaging**: CT angiogram (CTA): for endovascular intervention/medical therapy (e.g. dissection, atherosclerosis, vasculitis), comparable to ultrasound for ICA stenosis; MRI/MR angiogram (MRA): very sensitive within first few hours; Carotid ultrasound if CTA or MRA not done.
- 24 h Holter for AF (longer if high suspicion).
- Echocardiogram: rule out PFO or atrial septal aneurysm (in cryptogenic stroke), severe HF, thrombus, left atrial dilatation (increases risk for AF).
- CT-Venogram of lower extremities: for+PFO and cryptogenic stoke, to rule out deep venous thrombosis (DVT)'s (Lower extremity ultrasound does not assess for DVT in iliac veins).

- **Early management of ischemic strokes**

  - **Urgent Treatment**:

    - Thrombolysis: tPA in first 3 h of symptom; number needed to treat for improvement: 3, number needed to harm: 30. Not used with minor/mild or rapidly resolving

TABLE 27-6			
GENERAL MEDICAL CARE IN ISCHEMIC STROKE	Blood pressure	HTN: >60 % of stroke pts have SBP >160 mmHg. Treat BP>220/120 mmHg in pts *not* receiving tPA, or if end-organ damage (kidney, heart, eye); treat BP>185/110 mmHg if receiving tPA. Don't ↓BP more than 15 %. Initiate oral anti-HTN meds within 24 h of stroke	Hypotension: Worse outcomes, esp. if <100/70 mmHg. Treat underlying cause (volume depletion, arrhythmia, blood loss, sepsis); raise BP with fluids, pressors
	Blood glucose	Hyperglycemia: Goal BG 80–140, treat with insulin sliding scale or insulin drip. Recommendation extrapolated from other scenarios (Medical/Surgical ICU)	Hypoglycemia: Promptly correct hypoglycemia (may mimic strokes)
	Temperature	Fever Increases mortality. Seek cause of fever and reduce temperature with antipyretic	Hypothermia: insufficient data for use of cooling in stroke
	Oxygenation	Keep O_2 Sats ≥92 %. Patients needing intubation have 50 % mortality at 30 days, aspiration pneumonia important complication and leading cause of death	

HTN hypertension, *BG* blood glucose, *BP* blood pressure, *ICU* intensive care unit, *SBP* systolic blood pressure

symptoms. Sooner treatment→better outcome. Contraindications: severe HTN, recent surgery. tPA carries risk of ICH.

- ■ Heparin: Not recommended by guidelines, though, some centers consider it for large artery atherosclerosis or embolizing carotid (some evidence) or AF (little evidence); others: left ventricular (LV) thrombus, mechanical heart valve, dissection, cerebral venous thrombosis. Do not give heparin if: Coma, large territory of infarction, mass effect or hemorrhage on CT, mean arterial pressure (MAP) >130 mmHg.

- ■ Endovascular treatments: intra-arterial thrombolysis; mechanical disruption+retriever; EKOS catheter (delivers ultrasonic pulses). Generally (with exceptions) reserved for within 6 h of onset (if within 3 h and eligible can give IV tPA bridge).

- ■ Other Acute Treatments: aspirin (ASA) 81 mg daily (full dose not proven to be more effective): two large trials showed small reduction in death or disability in pts treated with ASA within 48 h.

- ■ Statins: Some centers give high dose statin (same as in acute coronary syndrome [ACS]) acutely. Weak evidence of benefit. Evidence of harm from abrupt withdrawal of already-prescribed statin (fivefold increase in death/dependence, larger infarct volume); withdrawal postulated to trigger pro-thrombotic/inflammatory response.

- ■ Induced HTN: Used in select patients with caution. Possibly ↑blood pressure (BP) restores perfusion to penumbra (Table 27-6).

■ **Complications of ischemic stroke**

- – **Ischemic brain swelling**: Most common in middle cerebral artery (MCA) main stem occlusion and large cerebellar infarcts (less common in anterior cerebral artery [ACA]/ posterior cerebral artery [PCA] infarcts). Herniation occurs between day 2–5 (but up to 25 % can herniated in <24 h). Treatment: osmotic therapy, hypothermia, surgical decompression.

■ **Secondary prevention of ischemic stroke** (Tables 27-7, 27-8, 27-9, 27-10, 27-11, and 27-12)

TABLE 27-7

ANTIPLATELET AGENTS USED FOR
ISCHEMIC STROKE RISK REDUCTION

ASA	High and low-dose equal efficacy
	Increasing ASA dose doesn't reduce risk of stroke but increases risk of bleeding
Dipyridamole and ASA	French Toulouse Study/AICLA: no benefit of adding dipyridamole to ASA
	ESPS-2 trial: ASA reduced relative risk of stroke by 18 %, ASA/ extended-release dipyridamole by 37 %; neither affected mortality [3]
	Headache is a most common side effect of dipyridamole
Clopidogrel	Used if allergic to ASA. No evidence clopidogrel better than ASA in patients with prior strokes. No added benefit of combining with ASA but greater risk of bleeding [4]
	CAPRIE: Clopidogrel more effective vs. ASA in *composite* risk of stroke, MI, or vascular death; but with prior strokes, benefit was *not* statistically significant [5]
	CHARISMA: ASA v. ASA+Clopidogrel, no difference in composite risk stroke, MI, or vascular death [6]

ASA aspirin, *MI* myocardial infarction

Carotid endarterectomy (CEA)	Indications: (1) Symptomatic: stenosis 50–99 %. (2) Asymptomatic: stenosis 60–99 % (if 5 year life expectancy). Most benefit for recent stroke (rather than TIA), severe stenosis, >75 years old, male. One trial showed ↑ benefit in with TIA or nondisabling strokes if done within 2 weeks. Unclear if CEA alone or in combination better than new/more aggressive treatments
Carotid artery stenting (CAS)	Few trials, mixed results (negative results due to lack of technical expertise), no evidence CAS better than CEA. May be appropriate for high risk pts not fit for surgery. Current guidelines: CAS for high risk surgical pts with symptomatic stenosis >70 %
Extracranial/intracranial bypass	Superficial temporal artery anastomosed to MCA. Used only in highly selected cases of carotid disease (e.g. Moyamoya disease)

TABLE 27-8

TREATMENT/PREVENTION FOR
ISCHEMIC STROKE CAUSED BY
EXTRACRANIAL ATHEROSCLEROSIS

MCA middle cerebral artery, *TIA* transient ischemic attack

Medical treatment	Carotid stenosis: Antiplatelets or warfarin or other oral anticoagulant. ASA is usually given; may consider anticoagulation with severe flow-limiting stenosis consider to prevent progression
	Intracranial stenosis: *WASID Trial* [7] concluded warfarin no better than ASA to prevention ischemic stroke
Angioplasty/stenting	Consider if >50 % intracranial stenosis (intracranial ICA, MCA, vertebrobasilar), after failed optimal medical therapy (i.e. get TIA and ischemic strokes)
	3 days prior to procedure to at least 6 weeks after stenting: clopidogrel 75 mg daily and ASA (continue for life). Re-stenosis is common

TABLE 27-9

TREATMENT/PREVENTION FOR
ISCHEMIC STROKE CAUSED BY
INTRACRANIAL ATHEROSCLEROSIS

ASA aspirin, *ICA* internal carotid artery, *MCA* middle cerebral artery, *TIA* transient ischemic attack

MUSCULAR DYSTROPHIES (MD)

Includes a variety of genetic disorders. The following directly involve cardiac muscle: (1) Duchenne muscular dystrophy and Becker muscular dystrophy; (2) myotonic dystrophies; (3) Emery-Dreifuss muscular dystrophy; (4) Limb-girdle muscular dystrophy; (5) Facioscapulohumeral muscular dystrophy

TABLE 27-10 TREATMENT/PREVENTION FOR ISCHEMIC STROKE CAUSED BY CARDIOEMBOLISM	Atrial fibrillation	Both paroxysmal and persistent AF causes 75,000 strokes per year. Anticoagulate with warfarin INR (2–3) within 2 weeks of stroke/TIA. Warfarin superior to ASA in pts with AF and recent stroke/TIA
	HF	Causes stasis + increased risk of thromboembolism. Anticoagulation is controversial; sometimes used with very low ejection fraction, though most guidelines don't recommend unless DVT/PE, mobile LV thrombus, or AF. No conclusive evidence of benefit
	LV thrombus	Warfarin (goal INR 2–3) 3 months to 1 year in pts with acute stroke/TIA. Add ASA if CAD

AF atrial fibrillation, *ASA* aspirin, *CAD* coronary artery disease, *DVT* deep venous thrombosis, *LV* left ventricular, *PE* pulmonary embolism, *TIA* transient ischemic attack

TABLE 27-11 OTHER CARDIAC ABNORMALITIES THAT MAY CAUSE OR CONTRIBUTE TO ISCHEMIC STROKE	Atrial septal abnormalities	PFO: fetal anomaly, allowing communication between atria
		Atrial Septal Aneurysm : redundant tissue in the region of the fossa ovalis, acts as a nidus for thrombus formation. Association between cryptogenic strokes in pts ≥55 years old and PFO ± atrial septal aneurysm in one study In pts aged <55, PFO + atrial septal aneurysm > atrial septal aneurysm > PFO significantly associated with an ischemic stroke. One study showed association with PFO/ cryptogenic strokes and older pts [8]
		Four main treatment modalities: antiplatelet, anticoagulation, surgical closure, percutaneous closure. PICSS found no difference between ASA and warfarin [9]. Guidelines: Atrial anomalies with ischemic stroke: Antiplatelets (use anticoagulation if high risk or has concomitant DVT or PE). PFO closure: considered after failed medical therapy (i.e. get recurrent cryptogenic strokes)
		Clinical trials of medical vs. closure therapy ongoing
	Valvular heart diseases	Rheumatic Mitral Valve disease: Warfarin (INR 2–3) recommended. If recurrent embolism despite adequate warfarin, add ASA
		Prosthetic heart valves: (1) Modern mechanical valve and ischemic stroke/TIA: Warfarin (INR 2.5–3.5); consider adding ASA if pt has another stroke despite adequate warfarin treatment. (2) Bioprosthetic heart valve with ischemic stroke, consider anticoagulation (e.g. warfarin, INR goal 2–3. (3) Other valvular disease: Antiplatelet

ASA aspirin, *DVT* deep venous thrombosis, *PE* pulmonary embolism, *PFO* patent foramen ovale, *TIA* transient ischemic attack

Duchenne Muscular Dystrophy and Becker Muscular Dystrophy

■ **Genetics**: X-linked recessive; mutation in dystrophin gene → loss of dystrophin → degeneration of cardiac & skeletal muscle. Almost absent in Duchenne MD; only reduced in Becker MD (hence more benign course).

■ **Neurological presentation**:

– Duchenne MD: most common inherited neuromuscular disorder (1/3,500 male births). Symptom develop <5 years old. Natural history: progressive skeletal muscle weakness → wheelchair-bound usually by age 13, death by age 25 from respiratory failure dysfunction, or less commonly heart failure. Intensive treatment with steroids, cardiac therapy, ventilatory support prolongs survival.

– Becker MD: less common (1/33,000 male births), variable weakness at presentation, most live to 40–50 years.

		TABLE 27-12
HTN	Reducing BP→40 % reduction in stroke risk BP goal <140/90 or for DM/chronic kidney disease <130/80 mmHg	MODIFIABLE MEDICAL RISK FACTORS FOR ISCHEMIC STROKE
Diabetes	HgA$_{1C}$ goal ≤7 %. BP <130/80 with ACE-I or ARBs (which decreases progression of renal disease). LDL ≤70mg/dL. Glucose control never shown to prevent macrovascular events (stroke, MI) only microvascular ones (Neuropathy)	
Lipids	First goal is to ↓LDL, then ↓TG. If history of stroke, target LDL <100mg/dL (for DM, LDL as low as ≤70). Treatment: statin. Goal TG <150. If TG <200: Treatment: lifestyle modification; TG 200–499: lifestyle ± fibrate or nicotinic acid; TG ≥500: fibrate or nicotinic acid). Goal HDL>40: treat only after LDL and TG goals achieved (use fibrates/nicotinic acid). Statins ↓stroke risk with and without CAD	
Lipoprotein(a)	An LDL, lowered by nicotinic acid. Risk factor for stroke [10]	
Hyperhomocys teinemia	Associated with two times greater risk of stroke. No evidence that reducing serum homocysteine levels has any effect on strokes, but given low risk, if levels >10 μmol/L give folate 1 g daily (if normal level not achieved, add Vitamin B12 and B6)	
Smoking	Doubles risk of stroke, risk decreases after quitting and disappears after 5 years	
Alcohol	Light drinking (1–2 drinks/day): protective (↑s HDL, ↓s platelet aggregation, ↓ serum fibrinogen). Heavy drinking (>5 drinks/day): increased risk (due to alcohol induced HTN, AF, ↓ in cerebral perfusion, and coagulopathies)	
Obesity	Losing weight not shown to reduce stroke risk, but obesity contributes to other risk factors for stroke including diabetes, dyslipidemia, HTN	
Physical activity	Moderately/highly active people have a reduced risk of stroke (30 min of daily moderate intensity exercise recommended)	

ACE-I angiotensin converting enzyme inhibitor, AF atrial fibrillation, ARB angiotensin II receptor blocker, BP blood pressure, CAD coronary artery disease, DM diabetes mellitus, HTN hypertension, MI myocardial infarction, TG triglycerides

■ Cardiovascular Manifestations

– Duchenne MD: most get cardiomyopathy; becomes clinically apparent by age 10, 90 % have dilated cardiomyopathy (DCM) by age 18.
– Becker MD: variable cardiac effects (none to severe). Cardiac involvement may occur without significant skeletal weakness. Progression is common. May involve right ventricle (RV) early.
– Female carriers of Duchenne MD and Becker MD have higher risk of dilated cardiomyopathy.

■ ECG:

– Duchenne MD: Classically: distinctive tall R waves, increased R/S amplitude in V1, deep narrow Q waves in left precordial leads; may be due to posterolateral LV involvement. Other findings: short PR, RV hypertrophy (RVH).
– Becker MD: ECG abnormalities in 75 %: tall R waves, increased R/S amplitude in V1, incomplete right bundle branch block (RBBB) (due to early RV involvement). LBBB is common with CHF.

■ Echocardiography

– Abnormalities occur in Duchenne MD & Becker MD. Diastolic dysfunction & regional wall motion abnormalities may precede global systolic dysfunction. Posterobasal & lateral wall abnormalities usually occur first. Mitral regurgitation may follow dystrophic changes in the posterior leaflet papillary muscles.

- **Arrhythmias**:

  - Duchenne MD: most common is sinus tachycardia. AF or atrial flutter. Atrial arrhythmias occur late ('preterminal rhythms'). Atrioventricular (AV) conduction abnormalities: ↓ or ↑ PR. Ventricular arrhythmias in 30 %, mainly premature ventricular complexes (PVC)'s. Complex ventricular arrhythmias & sudden death can occur in patients with severe skeletal disease.
  - Becker MD: Function of severity of structural cardiomyopathy. Distal conduction system disease with complete heart block and bundle branch reentry ventricular tachycardia (VT) may occur.

- **Treatment and Prognosis**

  - Duchenne MD: progressive disorder→death from respiratory or cardiac causes. Steroids delay muscle disease deterioration, stunt progression of DCM. Cardiac death (due to sudden cardiac death or heart failure) in 25 % of patients; % increasing due to improved respiratory care. Commence annual imaging to assess LV function at age 10. Angiotensin converting enzymes (ACE) inhibitors and beta blockers improve LV function when started early, though no clear evidence of improved long-term outcome.
  - Becker MD: ACE inhibitors, beta blockers also improve LV function. Begin screening LV imaging at age 10.
  - Females with Duchenne MD & and Becker MD do not get cardiomyopathy (CMP) during childhood; screening can begin in adolescence.

Myotonic Dystrophies

- **Genetics**: Autosomal dominant. Present with reflex & percussion myotonia (delayed muscle relaxation), distal limb muscle atrophy and weakness, endocrine abnormalities, cataracts, cognitive impairment, cardiac involvement.

  - Type 1: earlier onset, increased neuromuscular and cardiac involvement (conduction disease and arrhythmias).
  - Type 2: (a.k.a. proximal myotonic dystrophies): less severe skeletal and cardiac muscle involvement; no congenital presentation or cognitive impairment.

- **Clinical Presentation**: myotonic dystrophies are the most common inherited neuromuscular disorders presenting in adulthood.

  - Type 1 is most common (vs. Type 2). Age of diagnosis typically 20–25. Initial symptoms/signs: facial, neck, and distal extremity muscle weakness; myotonia (grip, tongue). Electromyography (EMG) and genetic testing may aid diagnosis. Usually cardiac symptoms occur after skeletal muscle weakness begins.
  - Type 2 presents similarly to Type 1, but at an older age. Also presents with myotonia, muscle weakness, cataracts, endocrine abnormalities, as in Type 1.

- **Cardiovascular Manifestations**: Fibrosis, degeneration, fatty infiltration of conduction tissue (sinus node, AV node, His-Purkinje system); no clear differences between Type 1 and 2. Rarely progresses to DCM. Main cardiac functional problems are arrhythmias.

- **ECG**:

  - Type 1: most adults (65 %) have abnormal ECG, e.g. first degree AV block (AVB), RBBB, left bundle branch block (LBBB). Abnormalities worsen with age.
  - Type 2: ECG abnormalities less common (20 % of adults).

- **Echocardiography**:

  - Type 1: LV and diastolic dysfunction, LVH, mitral valve prolapse, regional wall motion abnormalities, left atrial dilation all moderately common. HF occurs in only 2 %.
  - Type 2: LVH, ventricular dilation are most common.

- **Arrhythmias**:
  - Type 1: various arrhythmias, including: prolonged His-ventricular interval (can→symptomatic AVB); AF, atrial flutter. High risk of VT because of reentry in dysfunctional distal conduction system (manifest by bundle branch reentry, interfascicular reentry tachycardia). RBBB or fascicular radiofrequency ablation can correct this problem. Sudden death due to arrhythmias is common.
  - Type 2: Arrhythmias, sudden are less common, but do occur.

- **Treatment and Prognosis**: Neuromuscular course is variable; may be minimally symptomatic or progress to death from respiratory failure. Optimal cardiac management is uncertain. However, workup should include: echocardiogram (→ ACE inhibitor and beta blocker in case of DCM). Annual ECGs, 24-h holter monitoring often recommended to monitor asymptomatic patients. Significant/progressive ECG abnormalities alone (without symptoms) probably should prompt consideration of prophylactic pacing. Significant ECG conduction pathology or atrial arrhythmias signal risk for sudden cardiac death; unclear whether pacemakers are protective, or whether implantable cardioverter defibrillator (ICD) would be more appropriate. Anesthesia in myotonic dystrophies patients may provoke AVB/other arrhythmias – careful perioperative monitoring is essential.

Emery-Dreifuss Muscular Dystrophy

- **Genetics**: Rare. Often with mild skeletal muscle symptoms but severe/life threatening cardiac involvement. Usually X-linked recessive but can be variable. Sometimes called 'benign X-linked muscular dystrophy' to differentiate from Duchenne MD. Affects membrane structural support proteins including emerin, lamins A and C. Diagnose with genetic testing & muscle biopsy with anti–emerin antibody staining.
- **Presentation**: Triad (1) early contractures (elbow, Achilles tendon, posterior cervical muscles); (2) slowly progressive muscle atrophy & weakness (mainly humeroperoneal muscles); (3) cardiac involvement.
- **Cardiovascular Manifestations**: Mainly arrhythmias & DCM

  - X-linked recessive Emery-Dreifuss MD: impaired impulse generation & conduction (e.g. first degree AVB) by age 20–30. AF, atrial flutter, atrial standstill, junctional bradycardia are all common. Pacing often required by age 35. Sustained VT, ventricular fibrillation (VF) may occur. Sudden cardiac death before age 50 is common.
  - Female carriers of X-linked skeletal muscle disease but may develop cardiac abnormalities similar to males.
    DCM may rarely develop.

- **Treatment and Prognosis**: Monitor for ECG abnormalities. AVB may occur with anesthesia. Recommend permanent pacing in X-linked recessive Emery-Dreifuss MD. Prophylactic ICD rather than pacing alone often recommended for Emery-Dreifuss MD with lamin A and C mutations and significant ECG conduction disease. Cardiac imaging is recommended for all patients with Emery-Dreifuss MD to assess for LV dysfunction; if found, treat with standard heart failure regimen. Heart transplant in appropriate case is beneficial. Routine ECG monitoring is appropriate for Female carriers of X-linked recessive Emery-Dreifuss MD, because of risk for conduction disease.

Limb-Girdle Muscular Dystrophies

- **Genetics**: Group of dystrophies with limb–pelvic girdle distribution of weakness. Various genetic causes, usually autosomal recessive (Type 2); sporadic and autosomal dominant (Type 1) also occur.
- **Clinical Presentation**: Variable age of onset of muscle weakness; usually occurs by age 30. Commonly present with difficulty walking or running (due to pelvic girdle weakness). Later, involves shoulder muscles then distal muscles, sparing facial muscles. Slow progression to death can occur.

■ **Cardiovascular Manifestations**: Heterogeneous degree of cardiac involvement.

– Types 2C–F: autosomal recessive sarcoglycanopathies. Manifest as DCM. ECG: similar to Duchenne MD and Becker MD.
– Type 2I: autosomal recessive, age of onset & severity of skeletal muscle involvement is variable. Many develop DCM.
– Type 1B: Autosomal dominant. Presentation similar to Emery-Dreifuss MD: mild muscle symptoms, more severe cardiac involvement, especially arrhythmias. AV block by early middle age. Sudden cardiac death is common. DCM can occur.

■ **Treatment and Prognosis**: Recommendations differ by genetic cause. Genetic testing can detect Types 2C–F, 2I, and 1B, which pose highest risk for cardiac morbidities. Cardiac evaluation for arrhythmias and ventricular dysfunction for these patients and their families is recommended. For DCM: standard heart failure therapy. If conduction disease occurs: prophylactic ICD instead of a pacemaker.

FRIEDREICH ATAXIA (FA)

FA is the most common inherited spinocerebellar degenerative disease, with a prevalence of 1/50,000. Involves prominent signs of cerebellar and spinal cord degeneration, and cardiac dysfunction.

Genetics

■ Autosomal recessive neurodegenerative disease affecting primarily the spinal cord and cerebellum.
■ Gene mutation: in a mitochondrial protein used in iron homeostasis & respiratory function; highly expressed in the heart, *frataxin* (GAA amplified trinucleotide repeat: normal <33; FA: 66–1,500). GAA repeat → severely decreased frataxin synthesis → mitochondrial dysfunction, poor cellular response to oxidative stress, apoptosis. Larger GAA triplet size → earlier symptom onset, increased neurologic symptom severity, worse left ventricular hypertrophy.
■ Abnormal cardiac function is from abnormal respiratory function & iron handling.

Presentation

■ Symptoms typically start at puberty with progressive neuromuscular deficits → wheelchair-bound 10–20 years after symptom onset. Neurologic symptoms precede cardiac symptoms in most cases.
■ **Neurologic abnormalities**: Limb + trunk ataxia, dysarthria, loss of reflexes & sensation
■ **Cardiac abnormalities**:

– Concentric hypertrophic cardiomyopathy; less often: asymmetric septal hypertrophy; rare: dilated cardiomyopathy (occurs as progressive transition from hypertrophic cardiomyopathy).
– Hypertrophy is more common with younger diagnosis and higher GAA trinucleotide repeat length.
– 95 % patient with neurological symptomatic have abnormal on ECG and echocardiogram.

   ■ Most findings stem from ventricular hypertrophy.
   ■ Widespread T wave inversions are common
   ■ Arrhythmias:

– Atrial (e.g. AF, atrial flutter) develop with progression to dilated cardiomyopathy.
– Ventricular tachycardia (related to dilated cardiomyopathy).
– Cardiac hypertrophy in FA is usually <u>not</u> associated with more serious ventricular arrhythmias.

- Myocardial fiber disarray is <u>uncommon</u> in FA.
- Sudden death: reported; not common; unexplained.
- **Endomyocardial biopsies**: find myocyte hypertrophy, interstitial fibrosis.
- **Histopathologic findings**: myocyte hypertrophy/degeneration, interstitial fibrosis, muscle necrosis, pleomorphic nuclei, periodic acid-Schiff–positive deposition in large and small coronary arteries, degeneration+fibrosis in cardiac nerves, deposition of calcium salts and iron.
- **Other associated morbidities**: Skeletal deformities, diabetes.

Treatment

- **Idebenone**: Free radical scavenger. Modestly ↓'s LV hypertrophy & in FA patients; a free radical scavenger. No effect on neurological deficits/progression.

Prognosis

- Natural history is progressive neurologic deterioration → death from respiratory failure or infection, typically in 30s or 40s.
- Cardiac death: DCM → rapid progression to end-stage HF.
- No compelling evidence that medical or ICD improves outcomes in FA and DCM.

REVIEW QUESTIONS

1. A 75 year old man with a history of AF, HTN, and mild DM type II presents with shortness of breath and fatigue for a 'cardiac workup'. An echocardiogram shows LV dysfunction, with an ejection fraction of 35 %. During a review of systems, he mentions a recent episode of transient garbled speech lasting 30 min, which subsequently resolved completely. What is your best estimate of his risk of experiencing an ischemic stroke in the next year?
   (a) 2 %
   (b) 4 %
   (c) 6 %
   (d) 8 %
   (e) >10 %

2. The following often occur in embolic TIAs originating from the ICA, except:
   (a) Transient blindness in one eye.
   (b) Transient aphasia.
   (c) Transient double vision.
   (d) Transient hemiparesis.

ANSWERS

1. (e) This patient with AF has a CHADS2 risk score of 6, because he has all risk factors included in the CHADS2 risk score for predicting embolic stroke in patients with atrial fibrillation: HF (1 point), HTN (1 point), Age ≥75, DM (1 point), previous Stroke or TIA (2 points). A score of 6 carries an approximately 18 % annual risk of ischemic stroke.

2. (c) Transient monocular blindness (a) results from an embolus (e.g. forming on an atherosclerotic plaque or arterial dissection) travels from the ICA to occlude the ipsilateral ophthalmic or retinal artery. Transient aphasia (b) may occur when an ICA embolus travels to the MCA territory in the dominant (typically left) hemisphere. Transient hemiparesis (d) typically occurs contralateral to an embolic event from the ICA to an MCA artery territory. By contrast, ischemic diplopia typically results from an ischemic event to the 'posterior circulation', e.g. due to restricted flow through (due to stenosis, embolus, or thrombus) the vertebral or basilar arteries, rather than the ICA.

REFERENCES

1. Rothwell PM, Giles MF, Chandratheva A, Marquardt L, Geraghty O, Redgrave JNE, et al. Effect of urgent treatment of transient ischaemic attack and minor stroke on early recurrent stroke (EXPRESS study): a prospective population-based sequential comparison. Lancet. 2007;370(9596):1432–42.

2. Johnston SC, Rothwell PM, Nguyen-Huynh MN, Giles MF, Elkins JS, Bernstein AL, et al. Validation and refinement of scores to predict very early stroke risk after transient ischaemic attack. Lancet. 2007;369(9558):283–92.

3. Diener HC, Cunha L, Forbes C, Sivenius J, Smets P, Lowenthal A. European Stroke Prevention Study. 2. Dipyridamole and acetyl-salicylic acid in the secondary prevention of stroke. J Neurol Sci. 1996;143(1–2):1–13.

4. Diener H-C, Bogousslavsky J, Brass LM, Cimminiello C, Csiba L, Kaste M, et al. Aspirin and clopidogrel compared with clopidogrel alone after recent ischaemic stroke or transient ischaemic attack in high-risk patients (MATCH): randomised, double-blind, placebo-controlled trial. Lancet. 2004;364(9431):331–7.

5. CAPRIE Steering Committee. A randomised, blinded, trial of clopidogrel versus aspirin in patients at risk of ischaemic events (CAPRIE). CAPRIE Steering Committee. Lancet. 1996;348(9038):1329–39.

6. Bhatt DL, Fox KAA, Hacke W, Berger PB, Black HR, Boden WE, et al. Clopidogrel and aspirin versus aspirin alone for the prevention of atherothrombotic events. N Engl J Med. 2006;354(16):1706–17.

7. Chimowitz MI, Lynn MJ, Howlett-Smith H, Stern BJ, Hertzberg VS, Frankel MR, et al. Comparison of warfarin and aspirin for symptomatic intracranial arterial stenosis. N Engl J Med. 2005;352(13):1305–16.

8. Handke M, Harloff A, Olschewski M, Hetzel A, Geibel A. Patent foramen ovale and cryptogenic stroke in older patients. N Engl J Med. 2007;357(22):2262–8.

9. Homma S, Sacco RL, Di Tullio MR, Sciacca RR, Mohr JP. Effect of medical treatment in stroke patients with patent foramen ovale: patent foramen ovale in Cryptogenic Stroke Study. Circulation. 2002;105(22):2625–31.

10. Smolders B, Lemmens R, Thijs V. Lipoprotein (a) and stroke: a meta-analysis of observational studies. Stroke. 2007;38(6):1959–66.

CHAPTER 28

M. Brandon Westover, Brian L. Edlow, and David M. Greer

Coma After Cardiac Arrest: Management and Neurological Prognostication

CHAPTER OUTLINE

ABBREVIATIONS

ACLS	Advanced cardiac life support
BP	Blood pressure
cEEG	Continuous electroencephalography
CPR	Cardiopulmonary resuscitation
DPD	Delayed posthypoxic demyelination
ECS	Electrocerebral silence
EEG	Electroencephalography
EMS	Emergency medical services
ESE	Electrographic/subtle status epilepticus
FPR	False positive rate
GPEDs	Generalized periodic epileptiform discharges
ICP	Intracranial pressure
LAS	Lance adams syndrome
MSE	Myoclonic status epilepticus
NSE	Neuron-specific enolase
PEA	Pulseless electrical activity
PED	Periodic epileptiform discharges
PMSE	Postanoxic myoclonic status epilepticus
PSE	Postanoxic status epilepticus
PVS	Persistent vegetative state
ROSC	Return of spontaneous circulation
SPECT	Single-photon emission computed tomography
SSEP	Somatosensory evoked potentials
TCD	Transcranial doppler ultrasound
TH	Therapeutic hypothermia
VF	Ventricular fibrillation
VT	Ventricular tachycardia

- Reduces excitotoxic neuronal injury
- Minimizes free radical release
- Suppresses inflammation

B. **Evidence**
- Protocols & inclusion/exclusion criteria vary, but mortality and neurological recovery benefits demonstrated by multiple, randomized trials [6, 7].
- Data exist only for out-of-hospital, ventricular fibrillation (VF)/ventricular tachycardia (VT) cardiac arrest; no data for pulseless electrical activity (PEA), asystolic arrest, or in-hospital arrest → therapeutic cooling for these types of cardiac arrest may be applied at the discretion of the clinician [8].
- TH NOT proven beneficial for coma after isolated respiratory arrest without cardiac arrest
- Elevated temperature (*hyperthermia*) is detrimental (odds ratio for unfavorable outcome >2) for each 1 °C increase in temperature after arrest [9].

C. **Basic principles of TH**
- Initiate cooling rapidly; cooling must be initiated within 6 h of Return Of Spontaneous Circulation (ROSC).
- Multiple methods may be required to meet temperature goal of 32–34 °C (89–93 °F)
- Total cooling period is 24 h; begins when cooling is initiated, NOT upon reaching target temperature
- <u>Shivering</u> generates heat → neuronal injury by increasing cerebral metabolism; sedation and paralysis may be necessary for duration of cooling to prevent shivering

D. **Preparation for hypothermia:**
- Laboratory evaluation: Complete metabolic panel, CBC, PT/PTT, fibrinogen, d-dimer
- Place arterial line for blood pressure (BP) monitoring
- Place temperature monitor for continuous assessment of core temp → bladder temp probe, or pulmonary artery temp probe if oliguric (bladder temp probe requires presence of urine in bladder)

E. **Eligibility and exclusion criteria for TH** (Table 28-2)

F. **Therapeutic Hypothermia Protocol** (Table 28-3)

TABLE 28-2 INCLUSION CRITERIA AND CONTRAINDICATIONS FOR THERAPEUTIC HYPOTHERMIA AFTER CARDIAC ARREST	*Inclusion*:
	Comatose (the state of unresponsiveness) Time <6 h since cardiac arrest Hemodynamically stable without significant pressor requirement after CPR
	Relative contraindications (hypothermia may carry increased risk):
	Major head trauma: rule out intracranial hemorrhage (ICH) by head CT prior to cooling if clinical suspicion for head trauma at time of arrest Recent major surgery (within 14 days) Systemic infection/sepsis (hypothermia interferes with immune function) Other etiology for coma (e.g. drug/EtOH intoxication, pre-existing coma prior to arrest) Active bleeding (hypothermia impairs clotting factor activity)
	Not grounds for exclusion: Administration of thrombolytic, anti-platelet, or anticoagulation meds for cardiac condition is NOT a contraindication to hypothermia

---

TABLE 28-3 THERAPEUTIC HYPOTHERMIA (PROTOCOLS MAY DIFFER BY INSTITUTION)	***External cooling with cooling blankets and ice***: Obtain two cooling blankets and cables (one machine) to "sandwich" the patient; place sheets between blankets and patient to protect skin Use additional cooling methods as needed to bring patient to goal temperature Pack ice in groin, sides of chest, axillae, and/or side of neck Infuse cold (4 ° C) normal saline via peripheral or femoral central venous line (but *not* via a subclavian or IJ central line) (30 cc/kg over 30 min) Medicate for shivering with sedating and paralyzing agents (see below) Once goal temperature is reached, remove ice bags and maintain temp using cooling blankets **Avoid** packing ice on top of chest → may impair ventilation

TABLE 28-3

(CONTINUED)

External cooling with cooling vest devices:
Set target temperature goal on device
Medicate for shivering with sedation and paralyzing agents (see below)
Consider secondary temperature monitor. Record patient temperature on cooling vest
  device, secondary temperature source, and follow water temperature of the cooling device.
  Water temperature indicates the work the device must perform to keep patient at target
  body temp

Paralysis and sedation
Paralyze with cisatracurium: 150 mcg/kg bolus, then continuous infusion of 2 mcg/kg/min
Sedate with propofol: bolus (optional) 0.3–0.5 mg/kg then continuous infusion of 1 mg/kg/h
OR:
Midazolam: bolus (optional) 0.05 mg/kg then continuous infusion of 0.125 mg/kg/h.

Monitoring and supportive therapy during hypothermia:
No indication for BIS or train-of-four monitoring during TH
EEG use at clinician's discretion; consider to detect subclinical seizure activity
MAP >90 mmHg to maximize cerebral perfusion; potentially additive neuroprotective effects of
  high perfusion pressure with hypothermia
MAP goal may be lowered at discretion of clinician, depending on cardiac effects of high afterload
  or coronary vasoconstriction
If serious cardiac dysrhythmias, hemodynamic instability or bleeding develops during cooling, stop
  the cooling process, and actively re-warm the patient
Osborn waves (positive deflection between QRS complex and ST segment; see Fig. 28-2 below) or
  bradycardia may develop during cooling. No indication for specific therapy, but this may impair
  the ability to detect Brugada syndrome
Check blood cultures at 12 and 24 h after initiation of cooling (TH may mask infection)
Check electrolytes, CBC, and glucose at 12 and 24 h (TH may cause hypokalemia, esp. during
  concurrent insulin administration; rewarming may cause hyperkalemia due to K+ efflux from
  intracellular compartment)
Hyperglycemia and increases in serum amylase and lipase may occur during cooling
Goal CO_2 35–45 mmHg: analyze all ABGs at pt's body temperature
Examine skin for burns q2 h if using cold blankets

Rewarming:
Basic principles:
Do NOT rewarm faster than 0.25 °F/h; passive or controlled rewarming should take 8–12 h
Shunting of cardiac output to re-opening peripheral vascular beds may cause hypotension
Monitor closely for hypotension, hyperkalemia
Aim for normothermia once rewarming phase is completed
Maintain paralytic and sedative therapy until temperature of 36 °C (96.8 °F) is reached
  First stop paralytic, then sedative once patient shows motor activity or train of 4 on ulnar
  nerve stimulation

Rewarming after cooling blankets ± ice:
Remove cooling blankets (and ice if still in use)

Rewarming after cooling vest use:
Program device for controlled rewarming over 8–12 h. Dial in desired warming rate on
  machine, keep device in place and program for target temp of 37 °C (98.6 °F) for the next
  48 h (72 h total).

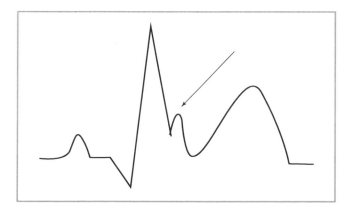

FIGURE 28-2

An Osborn wave on
electrocardiogram

NEUROPHYSIOLOGICAL FINDINGS IN POSTANOXIC COMA

Brain activity in comatose cardiac arrest patients is assessed using electroencephalography (EEG) recorded from electrodes placed on the scalp, and somatosensory evoked potentials (SSEP). Common EEG and SSEP findings are described in this section. Their quantitative prognostic significance is described in Tables 28-4 and 28-5 in the following section.

A. **EEG patterns in postanoxic coma (Fig. 28-3):** Common EEG patterns in this setting, in order from most abnormal (suggesting severe cortical injury) to least abnormal (suggesting milder cortical injury) are: electrocerebral silence > burst suppression > epileptiform activity > diffuse voltage attenuation > generalized slowing. Low voltage patterns (diffuse attenuation and electrocerebral silence) and burst suppression can be reversibly

TABLE 28-4

FALSE POSITIVE RATES OF UNIVARIATE PREDICTORS OF POOR NEUROLOGICAL OUTCOMEA

PREDICTOR	TIMING	FPR: NO TH	FPR: TH
Non-VF Cardiac arrest			15 (6–30)%
ROSC >25 min			24 (13–40)%
Low voltage[b] EEG – early on	Before TH		47 (35–60)%
Low voltage[b] EEG – upon rewarming	Day 1[c]		5 (2–14)%
Discontinuous EEG (burst suppression pattern)	Day 1[c]		7 (2–23)%
Seizure activity on first EEG[b]	Day 1–3		9 (2–21)%
Unreactive EEG background	Day 1–3[c]		7 (1–18)%
Early myoclonus	Day 1[c]	0 (0–8.8)%	3 (0–11)%
Bilaterally absent N20 on SSEP	Day 1–3[c]	0.7 (0–3.7)%	0 (0–8)%
Serum Neuron-specific Enolase (NSE)>33 μg/L	Day 1–3[c]	0 (0–3)%	11 (4–27)%
Absent or Extensor only motor response to pain	Day 3[c]	0 (0–3)%	24 (14–39)%
≥1 brainstem reflexes absent (pupillary, oculocephalic, corneal)	Day 3[c]	0 (0–3)%	4 (1–15)%
Head CT diffuse hypodensity+GCS ≤8	Day 1–3[c]	0 (0–48)%	0 (0–27)%
MRI: Any diffusion restriction	Day 1–3[c]	54 (26–80)%[d]	54 (26–80)%[d]

After cardiac arrest, with and without therapeutic hypothermia [10–16]
Note: grayed-in boxes indicate data not available
[a]Poor neurological outcome = death, unconsciousness, or severe disability at >1 month
[b]"*Seizure activity*"=epileptiform discharges of any kind (e.g. spikes, lateralized periodic discharges (PLEDs) or generalized epileptiform discharges (GPEDs)) or electrographic seizures; "*Low voltage*"=<10 mv (but not meeting criteria for electrocerebral silence)
[c]Assessed after rewarming and discontinuation of sedation
[d]Patients who did and did not undergo TH were analyzed as one group

TABLE 28-5

MULTIVARIATE PREDICTORS OF OUTCOME IN POSTANOXIC COMA

Prognostic value of <u>A COMBINATION OF AT LEAST TWO</u> of the following negative findings (measured after completion of re-warming following TH, between 36 and 72 h post cardiac arrest) [16]
Bilaterally absent SSEP
Unreactive EEG background
Early myoclonus
Incomplete recovery of brainstem reflexes

Prediction:	In-hospital mortality	Poor 3–6 month neurological outcome
Sensitivity (95 % CI)	79 (67–88)%	62 (51–72) %
False positive rate (95 % CI)	0 (0–8)%	0 (0–14)%
PPV (95 % CI)	100 (93–100)%	100 (93–100)%
NPV (95 % CI)	76 (63–86)%	44 (31–58) %

Statistics are based on outcomes in 111 comatose survivors of cardiac arrest treated with TH
PPV positive predictive value, *NPV* negative predictive value, *Spec* specificity, Poor outcome: defined as severe disability/dependency, coma, or death

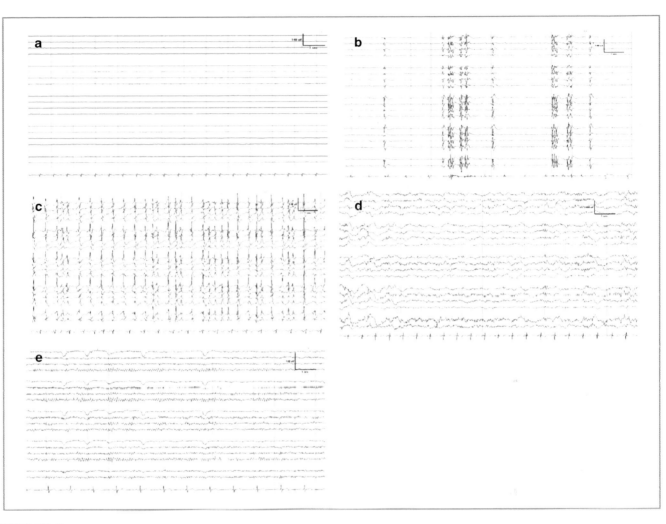

FIGURE 28-3

Examples of key EEG patterns in postanoxic coma (**a–d**), compared with normal EEG (**e**). Each panel displays 10 s of EEG data from 16 channels (sampling different regions of the scalp), and single-lead EKG (*bottom*). Patterns: (**a**) Electrocerebral silence; (**b**) burst-suppression; (**c**) electrographic status epilepticus; (**d**) diffuse irregular slowing; (**e**) normal awake EEG, with a sinusoidal-appearing signal emanating from the back of the head ('posterior alpha rhythem')

induced by cooling and/or anesthesia in undamaged brains; hence, these patterns must be interpreted with caution in the setting of ongoing cooling and/or anesthetic administration.

■ **Electrocerebral silence (ECS)**: Complete absence of detectable cortical EEG activity. Suggests brain death, but not technically sufficient for the diagnosis (see below).

■ **Burst suppression**: Alternating periods of diffuse voltage attenuation ('suppressions', or 'flats') alternating with brief periods of higher amplitude EEG activity or 'bursts'. The burst suppression pattern is also referred to as "discontinuous".

■ **Epileptiform activity**: Includes (1) <u>sporadic epileptiform discharges</u> (e.g. spikes, sharp waves, spike-and-wave complexes, polyspikes), (2) <u>periodic epileptiform discharges</u> (PEDs), i.e. epileptiform discharges which occur in a regular/periodic fashion (e.g. with a frequency of 1-3 Hz), characteristically appearing to start simultaneously over the entire cortex (hence 'GPEDs', generalized periodic epileptiform discharges; PEDs may also occur exclusively or more prominently on one side of the brain, in which case they are often called 'PLEDs', periodic lateralized epileptiform discharges); (3) <u>discrete seizures</u>, i.e. transient periods of high frequency, repetitive epileptiform or rhythmic EEG activity, with a discrete beginning and end; and (4) <u>status</u>

epilepticus: continuous high frequency (usually defined as >3Hz) epileptiform activity or frequently recurring discrete seizures. The distinction between GPEDs and status epilepticus is controversial in this setting, and probably largely semantic in nature, as both have similar prognostic value. Note that all forms of epileptiform activity may occur with or without obvious clinical manifestations.

■ **Diffuse attenuation**: Low voltage EEG pattern (but not complete absence of EEG activity).

■ **Generalized slowing**: EEG rhythms lack the high frequency (>8Hz) activity characteristic of normal wakefulness, but brain activity is continuous (i.e. not burst-suppressed), with voltages in the normal range, and lacks epileptiform activity.

■ **Alpha coma**: Diffuse, low amplitude alpha EEG activity (i.e. oscillations of 8-10Hz). This pattern superficially resembles brain activity in the normal awake state, but unlike normal alpha activity is not reactive to / modulated by eye opening or closure or to noxious stimulation. This pattern is relatively rare in postanoxic coma.

■ **EEG Reactivity**: Any reproducible change (excluding the appearance of seizure activity) in the EEG background activity in response to stimulation, e.g. acceleration or slowing of background rhythms, or modulation of background amplitude. *Absence of reactivity is a poor prognostic sign.*

B. **Myoclonus, with and without epileptiform EEG activity:** Up to 44 % of patients after cardiac arrest develop myoclonus [3, 17]. Myoclonus may occur with or without seizures or other epileptiform EEG abnormalities. Prognostic implications of myoclonus after cardiac arrest range from near-certain poor neurological outcome (e.g. with reticular myoclonus) to good chance of only mild disability (e.g. with Lance Adams Syndrome), depending on clinical context.

■ **Myoclonic status epilepticus (MSE)**: Confident diagnosis requires both clinical and EEG features (1) Clinical: Continuous or frequently recurring repetitive myoclonic movements of head, extremities, and trunk; (2) EEG: Spontaneous occurrence of repetitive, rhythmic (>2Hz), focal or generalized epileptiform discharges, or periodic or rhythmic waves with clear evolution in morphology, distribution, or frequency over time, lasting at least 5 min. Whether GPEDs or other EEG patterns containing abundant epileptiform activity should be considered seizures (and hence might merit aggressive treatment) is controversial. For abnormal patterns of uncertain significance, clinical improvement upon resolution of the abnormality (spontaneously or after treatment) supports the diagnosis of status epilepticus. Before TH, MSE was thought to imply an invariably poor prognosis; however, recent reports in patients treated with TH suggest good neurological outcome is possible in some cases (see below).

■ **Electrographic/subtle status epilepticus (ESE)**: Seizures on EEG only (defined as in (2) above) without any or with only subtle motor manifestations. MSE may evolve over time into ESE. Prognostic significance is similar to that of MSE.

■ **Reticular myoclonus**: Massive continuous clinical myoclonus without EEG correlate. Thought to be of brainstem origin in cases where cortical anoxic damage is too severe to support seizure activity. Limited data suggest no chance of good outcome with reticular myoclonus; however, diagnostic criteria are not well established. *Must be carefully distinguished from Lance Adams Syndrome.*

■ **Lance Adams Syndrome (LAS)**: Persistent myoclonus in patients who survive and recover consciousness after anoxia. See description below in the Sect. 28.7

■ **Postanoxic Status Epilepticus (PSE)**: An inclusive term, which includes MSE and ESE (defined above), as well as status epilepticus with clinical manifestations other than myoclonus, e.g. tonic-clonic or focal convulsive movements. PSE requires EEG for diagnosis. Clinical manifestations are not necessary for the diagnosis, i.e. PSE may be 'non-convulsive' or 'subclinical' or 'subtle' (synonyms).

C. **Somatosensory evoked potentials (SSEP)**: Assesses integrity of thalamo-cortical connections by electrically stimulating the median nerve at the wrist and quantifying the evoked EEG response recorded over the primary somatosensory cortex approximately 20 ms after stimulation. The cortical evoked response is known as the 'N20' peak.

FIGURE 28-4

Somatosensory evoked potentials (Used with permission from Young [18])

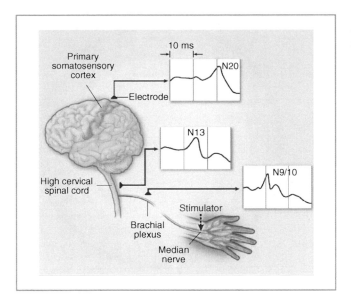

Additional waveforms are recorded as controls to ensure that the sensory pathway leading to the cortex is intact, including a waveform over the posterior columns of the high cervical spinal cord (N13 peak), and over the brachial plexus (N9/10 response). When the N20 waveform is absent, there is no upward deflection 20 ms after stimulation. Bilateral absence of N20 SSEP waveforms suggests severe cortical anoxic injury and is associated with poor neurological prognosis. See Fig. 28-4.

ACUTE PROGNOSTICATION: PREDICTING NEUROLOGICAL OUTCOME IN POSTANOXIC COMA

A. **Predicting *poor* neurological outcome:**
   ■ Table 28-4 summarizes the false positive rate (FPR) associated with using a variety of clinical features as a basis for predicting *poor* neurological outcome. At present, no specific combination of findings is known to predict *good* neurological outcome.

   – FPR values hold for each predictor *used in isolation*, whereas in practice all clinical data should be integrated before prognostication
   – Most data, particularly pertaining to prognostication *after* TH, are from small or retrospective trials and should be used with caution. Finally, most studies to date have been biased by the "self-fulfilling prophecy" fallacy, i.e. early withdrawal of life-sustaining therapies in cases with indicators of poor prognosis inflates the apparent statistical reliability of these indicators. There is growing evidence (see Table 28-4) that many indicators previously thought to be universally indicative of poor neurological outcome are, when used in isolation, subject to unacceptable rates of false positives (i.e. incorrectly pronouncing a poor prognosis).

   ■ Further information about particular findings (e.g. EEG, imaging, SSEPs) is provided in subsequent sections. One attempt to provide a quantitative multimodal (integrative) approach to prognostication is provided in Table 28-5.

   – Some factors may confound the reliability of the clinical exam and ancillary tests. Major confounders include current or recent use of sedatives or neuromuscular blocking agents, induced hypothermia therapy, presence of organ failure (e.g., acute renal or liver failure) and shock (e.g., cardiogenic shock requiring inotropes). Studies in comatose patients have not systematically addressed the role of these confounders in neurologic assessment.

– Note that duration of anoxia and duration of CPR are *not* recommended as a useful parameter in neurological prognostication for coma after cardiac arrest. The reason is that these durations are often difficult to accurately estimate in clinical practice, hence potentially misleading.

– Neuroimaging has shown promise as a helpful auxiliary test in evaluating patients with coma after cardiac arrest. For example, in some cases dramatic, devastating neurological damage apparent on an MRI or CT may strongly support a poor neurological prognosis; and absence of evident MRI or CT abnormalities in a still-comatose patient may in some cases warrant continued observation before definitively declaring a poor prognosis. The optimal use of neuroimaging in post-anoxic coma prognostication is an area of active research [10, 11].

– Appreciation of the prognostic value of continuous EEG monitoring in postanoxic coma is a relatively recent development. While postanoxic myoclonic status epilepticus has been recognized as a poor prognostic sign for decades, EEG reactivity, continuity, and the pattern of evolution over time are an increasingly integral component of the overall evaluation [19].

B. Predicting *favorable* neurological outcome:
No agreed-upon criteria currently exist for predicting favorable neurological outcome in the setting of postanoxic coma. However, small studies in the post-TH era suggest that many findings previously believed invariably to imply a poor neurological outcome should be interpreted with caution, as suggested by the false positive rates listed in Tables 28-4 and 28-5.

PUTTING IT ALL TOGETHER: RECOMMENDED APPROACH TO PROGNOSTICATION IN POSTANOXIC COMA

A. **Guidelines for evaluation:** The following guidelines, based on a synthesis of the information summarized above, are intended for cardiac arrest patients in whom neurological prognosis is in question. Patients who are awakening rapidly, who are brain dead, or who have suffered an isolated respiratory arrest are not appropriate for these guidelines. Consultation of the neurology service, or clinical neurophysiology service in particular (for assistance with EEG and SSEP interpretation) is recommended. Suggested timing of tests, to maximize accuracy and prognostic utility, is summarized in Table 28-6.

■ **Daily clinical neurological examination**, with particular attention to pupillary responses, corneal reflexes, oculocephalic reflexes, and motor responses. Document exams daily while coma persists for at least 2 weeks or until a decision to withdraw

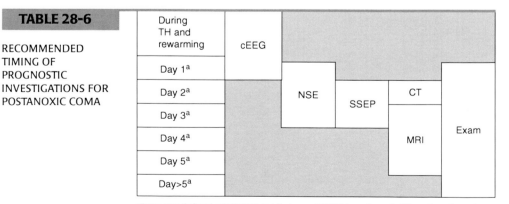

TABLE 28-6							
RECOMMENDED TIMING OF PROGNOSTIC INVESTIGATIONS FOR POSTANOXIC COMA	During TH and rewarming	cEEG					
	Day 1[a]						
	Day 2[a]		NSE		CT		
	Day 3[a]			SSEP			
	Day 4[a]				MRI		Exam
	Day 5[a]						
	Day>5[a]						

[a]Days are defined relative to cardiac arrest if TH is not used. Otherwise, days above are relative to completion of rewarming. In case of burst suppression undertaken for seizures, days are relative to the end of the initial 24-h burst suppression period

care. Declaration of a poor neurological prognosis (negligible chance of functional recovery) may be made on <u>day 3</u> (post-arrest if no TH, or 3 days post-rewarming after TH) *if all data are* concordant in pointing to a poor outcome.

- **Continuous EEG (cEEG) monitoring** should be considered in all patients with postanoxic coma for a minimum of 24 h. For patients undergoing TH, cEEG should begin during cooling and continue for at least the first 24 h after completion of rewarming. Presence or absence of EEG reactivity should be documented after rewarming (off sedation) based on direct bedside examination.
- **Seizure activity**: Patients found to have seizures on EEG should be treated with anticonvulsants, targeting seizure control. Patients found to have status epilepticus on EEG, with or without myoclonus, should be considered for treatment with IV antiepileptic drugs targeting electrographic burst suppression for 24 h, in which case exam & testing which would otherwise take place during the period of burst suppression should be postponed until after at least 24 h of burst suppression, and then performed off sedation.
- **SSEPs** should be performed no earlier than 48 h post-arrest, or 48 h post-rewarming if the patient underwent TH.
- **Serum neuron-specific enolase (NSE)** may be sent on day 1–3 post arrest, or on day 1–3 after rewarming in patients who have undergone TH. Note that while higher values generally correlate with worse prognosis, and a value of 33 is often cited as indicating poor prognosis, no definitive "cutoff" value is known, and cases of good neurological outcome have been reported with NSE >33, e.g. [12]; see false positive rate in Table 28-4. Also, cooling may artificially lower NSE values, decreasing the sensitivity of NSE testing. Thus NSE values must be interpreted within the global context of the other data.
- **Brain CT**: Consider CT at 48 h post-arrest or 48 h post-rewarming. If obvious widespread injury is absent, consider proceeding with brain MRI.
- **Brain MRI**: Consider brain MRI on day 3–5 if coma persists and no widespread injury on CT.

B. **The decision to withdraw life-sustaining therapies**

The decision to withdraw life-sustaining therapies is ultimately based on the clinician's and family's judgment, but factors to consider include:

1. Age
2. Comorbidities (either pre-existing or subsequent to the arrest)
3. Prior wishes of the patient
4. Take into account all available data, including the clinical examination, EEG and SSEP findings, serum biomarkers and neuroimaging findings.
5. Many patients have a delayed recovery of meaningful neurological function. When in doubt about the prognosis, particularly in younger patients, consider allowing more time (e.g. 2–3 weeks) to determine if recovery appears more likely (e.g. improving neurological exam).

LONG TERM PROGNOSIS OF ANOXIC BRAIN INJURY AFTER CARDIAC ARREST

A. **Vegetative states and persistent vegetative state (PVS)** [20]
- **Definition**

  - *Vegetative state*: Wakefulness without detectable awareness of self or environment. Accompanied by intact sleep-wake cycles and complete or partial preservation of brain stem reflexes/functions, hypothalamic functions, and autonomic functions. Patient may show subcortical or reflexive movements, including: spontaneous nonpurposeful limb movements, random conjugate eye movements (but not tracking), stereotyped/automatic emotional facial expressions; startle myoclonus (twitching/jerking in response to loud noises).

- *Persistent vegetative state (PVS)*: Vegetative state lasting > 1 month. Recovery of consciousness from PVS is possible but rare and nearly always associated with moderate to severe disability.
- *Permanent vegetative state*: PVS that has lasted at least 3 months after cardiac arrest.

- **Pathophysiology**: Severe cortical and/or thalamic and/or bihemispheric white matter damage with preserved brainstem function, due to differential susceptibility to ischemia.
- **Natural history of PVS**: In a review of 169 patients in VS after 1 month: By 3 months: 11 % regained consciousness. By 12 months: 15 % regained consciousness, only 1 with good functional recovery (independence), 53 % died. Authors suggested that "permanent vegetative state" be defined as PVS lasting at least 3 months. Very rare exceptions exist (case reports) of more delayed recovery.

B. **Lance Adams Syndrome (LAS; aka 'posthypoxic myoclonus')**
- **Definition**: A syndrome in survivors of anoxic brain injuries who *regain consciousness*. The syndrome is defined by myoclonic jerks caused by rapid active muscle contractions during voluntary action or by attempts to move ('action myoclonus'). Jerks may disappear during relaxation; can be triggered by emotion, startle, sounds, touch (esp. noxious stimulation). Patients may also have negative myoclonus (lapses of tone, followed by a compensatory jerk of antagonist muscles); can lead to falls. Associated signs may include incoordination, dysarthria, and tremor.
- **Pathophysiology**: Arises from damage to cortical or subcortical brain structures damaged by anoxia.
- **Natural history of LAS**: Up to half of patients with LAS eventually have no neurological deficits except isolated action myoclonus. Resolution of incoordination, dysarthria, and tremor may be gradual. Functional recovery may continue for several years.
- **Distinguishing LAS from myoclonic status epilepticus (MSE)**: *Requires EEG* in the acute stage after cardiac arrest, while coma persists (MSE shows seizures; the EEG of patients who ultimately regain consciousness but continue to have myoclonus (LAS) may show discharges preceding jerks, but not seizures). Clinical distinction can be difficult, but generally in LAS myoclonus is stimulus-dependent and may spare the face or trunk, whereas MSE typically shows repetitive twitching of the bilateral trunk and face and is typically not stimulus-dependent. Recovery of consciousness with persistent myoclonus rules out MSE.
- **Treatment**: Myoclonus may respond to clonazepam, valproate, or levetiracetam.

C. **Movement disorders**
- **Types**: Survivors of cerebral anoxia may develop a variety of movement disorders, including Parkinsonism, dystonia, chorea, tics, tremor, athetosis, akinetic rigidity, 'person in a barrel syndrome' (brachial diplegia).
- **Pathophysiology**: Damage to the basal ganglia, e.g. putamen or globus pallidus. Person in a barrel syndrome typically follows watershed infarcts due to profound hypotension.
- **Natural history**: Delayed onset is common; may occur up to 3 months post-cardiac arrest

D. **Cognitive & functional deficits**
- **Types**: Deficits range from transient encephalopathy lasting hours, days, or weeks, to global dementia with impaired memory, attention, insight, and judgment. Memory impairment is the most common isolated persistent cognitive deficit in survivors of cardiac arrest.
- **Pathophysiology**: Isolated memory deficits follow bilateral damage to the hippocampi, which are particularly vulnerable to anoxia.

E. **Delayed encephalopathy (delayed posthypoxic demyelination, DPD)**
- **Definition**: A 'lucent' period after apparent complete clinical recovery from coma after anoxic brain injury, followed (usually 1–4 weeks later) by rapid neurological

deterioration. Typical triad of delayed deficits include rapid cognitive decline, urinary incontinence, and gait instability. DPD is rare.

■ **Pathophysiology**: Delayed development of extensive cerebral demyelination and basal ganglia degeneration. Pathogenesis is uncertain; hypothesized mechanisms include delayed vascular injury, impairment of myelin metabolism, delayed hypersensitivity reaction.

■ **Natural history**: Unknown. Case reports describe occasional complete or partial recovery.

REVIEW QUESTIONS

1. A 62-year-old woman is found unconscious in her apartment hallway by a neighbor. Emergency medical services (EMS) personnel called to the scene find her pulseless and not breathing. Ventricular fibrillation is the initial recorded cardiac rhythm. Advanced cardiac life support (ACLS) measures including intubation, 2 mg of epinephrine (total dose), and 4 defibrillation attempts, restore spontaneous circulation 15 min after EMS arrival on the scene. Upon arrival in the emergency department, she is hemodynamically stable, but comatose. You consider initiation of your hospital's therapeutic hypothermia (TH) protocol. Which additional factors would make her ineligible for TH?
   (a) Major head trauma
   (b) Repetitive twitching movements
   (c) No pupillary, corneal, and oculocephalic reflexes, and no motor response to noxious stimulation.
   (d) Time of arrival to the emergency department is 8 h after initial resuscitation.

2. A 32-year old male cardiac arrest patient is hemodynamically stable but remains comatose 3 days after rewarming after 24 h of therapeutic hypothermia. During the first 24 h, he had diffuse, rhythmic twitching movements involving the trunk and bilateral face, trunk, arms and legs, accompanied by EEG findings of seizure activity, diagnostic of postanoxic myoclonic status epilepticus (PMSE). Currently, noxious stimulation and loud sounds elicit myoclonic jerks, but none occur spontaneously; each jerk is accompanied on EEG by a brief discharge, though it is not possible to determine whether the discharge is epileptiform or simply the result of muscle activity (myogenic artifact). On neurological exam, corneal reflexes are equivocal (not definitely absent), and pupillary responses to light are minimal and sluggish but present. His wife is asking whether there is 'any chance' of regaining consciousness and returning to work. Which additional data would support a prognostic statement that there is essentially no chance of return to functional independence?
   (a) No additional data is necessary.
   (b) Assessment of the N20 response on SSEP
   (c) Assessment of EEG reactivity
   (d) Finding out that the time before return of spontaneous circulation as >25 min.
   (e) Serum NSE measurements of >33 μg/L.
      Interpretation of myoclonus [reactivity, continuous background]
   (f) Documentation of absent or extensor only (i.e. no flexion or withdrawal) to pain.

3. A 75-year old woman with a history of coronary artery disease and hypertension is treated with hypothermia after an out-of-hospital cardiac arrest that caused coma. Upon completion of rewarming, the patient experiences diffuse twitching (myoclonus) with an epileptiform correlate on EEG, suggesting the diagnosis of postanoxic myoclonic status epilepticus (PMSE). She is treated with intravenous valproic acid, midazolam, and levetiracetam for 3 days, after which time the clinical and electrographic features of myoclonus abate. The midazolam drip is weaned over 24 h, and valproic acid and levetiracetam are continued for seizure prevention. One hour after cessation of the midazolam drip, the patient experiences an episode of hypotension (blood pressure = 70/40 mmHg for 10 min), requiring the initiation of intravenous vasopressor medications. Neurological examination after the hypotensive episode reveals absence of all brainstem reflexes, no movement of the extremities to deep nailbed pressure, and bilateral Babinski's signs (extensor plantar responses). The patient is not initiating respirations on the ventilator. On a continuous infusion of 10 mcg/min norepinephrine, the blood pressure is 110/78 mmHg, heart rate is 65 beats/min, and urine output is 25 cc over the past hour. Laboratory evaluation reveals normal electrolytes, mild anemia, and acute elevation of the liver transaminase levels (ALT = 1,450 U/L [normal = 10–50 U/L], AST = 1,600 U/L [normal = 10–50 U/L]). Which of the following is the most appropriate management with regard to a possible brain death evaluation in this patient?
   (a) Proceed to apnea testing for confirmation of brain death since the neurological exam reveals no brainstem reflexes, limb movement, or initiation of respirations.
   (b) The patient does not meet criteria for brain death since Babinski's sign is present bilaterally.
   (c) The patient does not meet criteria for brain death since the serum sodium concentration is normal and urine output is inconsistent with diabetes insipidus.
   (d) Apnea testing cannot be used to confirm brain death, because the patient recently received midazolam and the elevated transaminase levels suggest impaired hepatic clearance of this medication. Ancillary testing for confirmation of brain death should be pursued.
   (e) Apnea testing cannot be used to confirm brain death, because the patient is requiring a vasopressor medication to maintain SBP > 90 mmHg. Ancillary testing for confirmation of brain death should be pursued.
   (f) (d) and (e) are both correct.

4. A 24-year-old woman with a history of congenital disease has a cardiac arrest and is comatose upon arrival to the hospital 30 min later. Therapeutic hypothermia is initiated in the emergency department and the patient is admitted to the cardiac intensive care unit. Which of the following statements regarding the rewarming of this patient is true?

   (a) If she develops Osborn waves (positive deflection between QRS complex and ST segment) on the EKG while being treated with hypothermia, she should be actively rewarmed because of the risk of ventricular tachycardia.

   (b) If the patient develops severe bleeding causing hemodynamic instability during therapeutic hypothermia, she should be rewarmed at a rate of 0.5 °F/h.

   (c) The patient should be monitored closely for hyperkalemia during the rewarming process, since the increase in temperature may cause an efflux of K+ from the intracellular compartment

   (d) Once the 24-h period of hypothermia is completed, rewarming should be performed in a controlled manner, with an increase in core body temperature of 1.0 °F/h.

ANSWERS

1. (d) TH is not recommended for patients arriving >6 h after cardiac arrest; TH in this setting is believed to cause more risk than potential benefit. (c) may be correct, since absence of brainstem reflexes and absent motor responses suggest the possibility of brain death; however, a diagnosis of brain death must be made with extreme caution in the acute setting, as e.g. the key findings needed for the diagnosis can be influenced by the recent administration of paralytics and anesthetics, and most recommend a waiting period of at least 6 h. (a) is incorrect, because recent major head trauma, active bleeding, or recent major surgery are relative, not absolute, contraindications to TH. The reason for caution in this setting is that hypothermia may impair clotting factor activity. If recent major head trauma is suspected, a head CT should be considered prior to cooling to rule out intracranial hemorrhage. (b) is incorrect: twitching (myoclonus) immediately after cardiac arrest suggests possible seizure activity (though reticular myoclonus and Lance Adams syndrome are other possibilities); acute myoclonus should prompt initiation of EEG monitoring for seizure activity, but is not a contraindication to and should not delay initiation of TH.

2. The best responses are (b) and (c). The presence of early myoclonic status epilepticus *in combination with* either bilaterally absent N20 SSEP waveforms or absent EEG reactivity would support minimal chance of meaningful neurological recovery (see Table 28-5). (a) is probably incorrect: While evidence before the widespread use of TH did suggest that MSE invariably carried a poor neurological prognosis, several recent publications document cases in patients treated with TH who subsequently regained partial or complete functional independence, invalidating the claim that MSE has a 'zero false positive rate' for predicting poor neurological outcome. The presence on day 3 of myoclonus in the absence of clear-cut epileptiform activity on EEG which is provoked by stimulation is most suggestive of the development of Lance Adams syndrome, which does not significantly influence the chances of awakening and functional recovery. The *definite* absence of one or more brainstem reflex (among: pupillary response to light, corneal reflex, and oculocephalic reflex) in combination with early myoclonus would provide sufficient data on day 3 to justify rendering a confident poor neurological prognosis (see Table 28-5). Answers (e), (d), and (f) are incorrect, since these findings appear to have unacceptably high false positive rates for predicting poor neurological outcome in patients treated with TH (see Table 28-4). Ethical considerations mandate that, in approaching prognosis to postanoxic coma, any "discordant" data (i.e. data suggesting brain function compatible with good or improving neurological recovery) should prompt consideration of re-evaluation and further waiting before declaring no chance or good neurological outcome.

3. The best response is (f) since (d) and (e) are both correct. (a) would be correct if the patient were not requiring vasopressors and if she did not recently receive 3 days of continuous intravenous midazolam. However, the patient's pressor requirement precludes the use of apnea testing as a confirmatory test for brain death (hence, (e) is correct). Similarly, the recent administration of midazolam precludes apnea testing as a confirmatory test for brain death, especially since the elevated transaminase levels (likely due to hepatic hypoperfusion during the hypotensive episode) indicate impaired hepatic clearance of midazolam (hence, (f) is correct as well). (b) is incorrect because Babinski's sign is consistent with a diagnosis of brain death. (c) is incorrect because a normal serum sodium concentration and the absence of diabetes insipidus are also consistent with brain death. The most appropriate next step in the management of this patient would be to pursue an ancillary test to confirm brain death, such as with a single-photon emission computed tomography (SPECT) brain perfusion scan, an EEG, a 4-vessel cerebral angiogram, or a transcranial Doppler ultrasound (TCD).

4. (c) Serum potassium should be monitored closely during the rewarming period, since a temperature-related efflux of K+ from the intracellular compartment may cause hyperkalemia. Of note, total body potassium should not be affected by the temperature changes that occur during the hypothermia and rewarming processing. (a) is incorrect because Osborn waves are not considered to be reflective of a predisposition to serious arrhythmias. Osborn waves are typically best seen in the inferior and lateral precordial leads on EKG. (b) is incorrect because if a patient develops severe bleeding and/or hemodynamic instability during hypothermia, she should be actively rewarmed, not rewarmed at a rate of 0.5 °F/h. (d) is incorrect because the controlled rewarming that is performed upon completion of therapeutic hypothermia should occur at rate of no more than 0.5 °F/h. This slow rate of rewarming minimizes the risk of complications that may occur with rapid rewarming, such as hypotension due to peripheral shunting of cardiac output.

REFERENCES

1. Callans DJ. Out-of-hospital cardiac arrest – the solution is shocking. N Engl J Med. 2004;351(7):632–4.
2. Peberdy MA, Kaye W, Ornato JP, Larkin GL, Nadkarni V, Mancini ME, et al. Cardiopulmonary resuscitation of adults in the hospital: a report of 14720 cardiac arrests from the National Registry of Cardiopulmonary Resuscitation. Resuscitation. 2003; 58(3):297–308.
3. Khot S, Tirschwell DL. Long-term neurological complications after hypoxic-ischemic encephalopathy. Semin Neurol. 2006;26(4): 422–31.
4. Rogove HJ, Safar P, Sutton-Tyrrell K, Abramson NS. Old age does not negate good cerebral outcome after cardiopulmonary resuscitation: analyses from the brain resuscitation clinical trials. The Brain Resuscitation Clinical Trial I and II Study Groups. Crit Care Med. 1995;23(1):18–25.
5. Wijdicks EF, Varelas PN, Gronseth GS, Greer DM. Evidence-based guideline update: determining brain death in adults: report of the Quality Standards Subcommittee of the American Academy of Neurology. Neurology. 2010;74(23):1911–8.
6. Hypothermia after Cardiac Arrest Study Group. Mild therapeutic hypothermia to improve the neurologic outcome after cardiac arrest. N Engl J Med. 2002;346(8):549–56.
7. Bernard SA, Gray TW, Buist MD, Jones BM, Silvester W, Gutteridge G, et al. Treatment of comatose survivors of out-of-hospital cardiac arrest with induced hypothermia. N Engl J Med. 2002;346(8):557–63.
8. Nolan JP, Morley PT, Vanden Hoek TL, Hickey RW, Kloeck WG, Billi J, et al. Therapeutic hypothermia after cardiac arrest: an advisory statement by the advanced life support task force of the International Liaison Committee on Resuscitation. Circulation. 2003;108(1):118–21.
9. Zeiner A, Holzer M, Sterz F, Schorkhuber W, Eisenburger P, Havel C, et al. Hyperthermia after cardiac arrest is associated with an unfavorable neurologic outcome. Arch Intern Med. 2001; 161(16):2007–12.
10. Wu O, Batista LM, Lima FO, Vangel MG, Furie KL, Greer DM. Predicting clinical outcome in comatose cardiac arrest patients using early noncontrast computed tomography. Stroke. 2011; 42(4):985–92.
11. Greer D, Scripko P, Bartscher J, Sims J, Camargo E, Singhal A, et al. Clinical MRI interpretation for outcome prediction in cardiac arrest. Neurocrit Care. 2012;17:240–4.
12. Rossetti AO, Carrera E, Oddo M. Early EEG correlates of neuronal injury after brain anoxia. Neurology. 2012;78(11): 796–802.
13. Rossetti AO, Oddo M, Logroscino G, Kaplan PW. Prognostication after cardiac arrest and hypothermia: a prospective study. Ann Neurol. 2010;67(3):301–7.
14. Wijdicks EF, Hijdra A, Young GB, Bassetti CL, Wiebe S. Practice parameter: prediction of outcome in comatose survivors after cardiopulmonary resuscitation (an evidence-based review): report of the Quality Standards Subcommittee of the American Academy of Neurology. Neurology. 2006;67(2):203–10.
15. Oddo M, Rossetti AO. Predicting neurological outcome after cardiac arrest. Curr Opin Crit Care. 2011;17(3):254–9.
16. Rundgren M, Westhall E, Cronberg T, Rosen I, Friberg H. Continuous amplitude-integrated electroencephalogram predicts outcome in hypothermia-treated cardiac arrest patients. Crit Care Med. 2010;38(9):1838–44.
17. Wijdicks EF, Parisi JE, Sharbrough FW. Prognostic value of myoclonus status in comatose survivors of cardiac arrest. Ann Neurol. 1994;35(2):239–43.
18. Young GB. Clinical practice. Neurologic prognosis after cardiac arrest. N Engl J Med. 2009;361(6):605–11.
19. Rossetti AO, Urbano LA, Delodder F, Kaplan PW, Oddo M. Prognostic value of continuous EEG monitoring during therapeutic hypothermia after cardiac arrest. Crit Care. 2010;14(5):R173.
20. Medical aspects of the persistent vegetative state (2). The Multi-Society Task Force on PVS. N Engl J Med. 1994;330(22): 1572–9.

CHAPTER 29

EMILY P. HYLE, ROCÍO M. HURTADO, AND RAJESH TIM GANDHI

Infective Endocarditis, Device Infections, and Cardiac Manifestations of HIV

CHAPTER OUTLINE

ABBREVIATIONS

Abx	Antibiotics
AIDS	Acquired immunodeficiency syndrome
ART	Antiretroviral therapy
AZT	Zidovudine
BCx	Blood cultures
CAD	Coronary artery disease
CHF	Congestive HF (Heart Failure)
CIED	Cardiac implantable electronic devices
CNS	Central nervous system
CT	Computed tomography
CVD	Cardiovascular disease
ECG	Electrocardiography
HIV	Human immunodeficiency virus
ICD	Implantable cardioverter defibrillator
IDU	Intravenous drug user
IE	Infective endocarditis
JVP	Jugular venous pressure
LVAD	Left ventricular assist device
NSTEMI	Non-ST elevation myocardial infarction
NVE	Native valve endocarditis
NYHA	New York Heart Association
PAH	Pulmonary arterial hypertension
PCR	Polymerase chain reaction
PPM	Permanent pacemaker
PVE	Prosthetic valve endocarditis
TEE	Trans-esophageal echocardiography
TIMI	"Thrombolysis in myocardial infarction" research group
TPN	Total parenteral nutrition
TTE	Trans-thoracic echocardiography

INTRODUCTION

Infective endocarditis (IE) is a highly morbid infection with a diversity of clinical presentations and etiologies that is best managed with a multidisciplinary team. Similarly, cardiac device infections are occurring at increasing rates and require a high index of suspicion, careful workup, and a multidisciplinary treatment plan.

HIV-infected patients not on antiretroviral therapy (ART) or with low CD4 cell counts (<200 cells/mm^3) are at risk for a broad array of opportunistic conditions (infections and cancers). HIV-infected patients on ART with normal CD4 cell counts are not at risk for opportunistic conditions but have an increased rate of atherosclerosis and cardiovascular events, probably because of ongoing inflammation. Drug interactions with antiretroviral medications should be considered before prescribing commonly used cardiac medications, including statins.

INFECTIVE ENDOCARDITIS

An infection of the endocardium, which most frequently involves the heart valves but can also include chamber walls, chordae, and prosthetic tissue [1]

A. **Epidemiology and Risk Factors**
  - 10–20 % of IE cases occur in those without prior cardiac disease [1, 2]
  - Degenerative valvular heart disease is a common predisposing condition in the modern era [2]
  - Up to 25 % of IE cases in a large international cohort have been linked to nosocomial exposure [2]
  - IE continues to be common among intravenous drug users (IDU) and account for ~10 % of hospital admissions [3]

    - *Staphylococcus aureus* is most common pathogen
    - Polymicrobial or unusual pathogens are also more common in IDU with IE
    - Right-sided IE is particularly common in IDU with presentation of tricuspid insufficiency and/or pleuritic chest pain from septic emboli

B. **Clinical Presentation and Diagnosis**
  - IE is a heterogeneous disease with a wide range of clinical presentations, so a high index of suspicion and thorough, multidisciplinary diagnostic evaluation is often needed
  - **Clinical signs and symptoms**: Most common findings in international cohort of IE [2].

    - Fever (96 %)
    - New murmur (48 %)
    - Worsening of old murmur (20 %)

  - **Echocardiography**: Characteristics suggestive of vegetation [1]

    - Location: amidst high velocity jet or on "upstream" side of regurgitant valve
    - Motion: chaotic
    - Shape: amorphous
    - Texture: grey scale in comparison to calcification on myocardium
    - Associated abnormalities, such as leaks, fistula, or abscess

  - Serial echocardiograms may be useful in the setting of high pre-test probability and an initially negative study (Table 29-1)

	SENSITIVITY (%)	SPECIFICITY (%)
Native valve		
TTE	60–65	90–98
TEE	85–95	90–98
Prosthetic valve		
TTE	<50	90–98
TEE	82–90	90–98

TABLE 29-1

TEST CHARACTERISTICS OF ECHOCARDIOGRAPHY FOR DIAGNOSIS OF IE [1]

TABLE 29-2	Definite infective endocarditis
DEFINITION OF IE ACCORDING TO THE MODIFIED DUKE CRITERIA, ADOPTED WITH PERMISSION FROM [64]	Pathologic criteria (1) Microorganisms demonstrated by culture or histologic examination of a vegetation, a vegetation that has embolized, or an intracardiac abscess specimen; or (2) Pathologic lesions; vegetation or intracardiac abscess confirmed by histologic examination showing active endocarditis Clinical criteria (1) Two major criteria; or (2) One major criterion and three minor criteria; or (3) Five minor criteria
	Possible infective endocarditis (1) One major criterion and one minor criterion; or (2) Three minor criteria
	Rejected (1) Firm alternate diagnosis explaining evidence of infective endocarditis; or (2) Resolution of infective endocarditis syndrome at surgery or autopsy, with antibiotic therapy for ≤4 days; or (3) No pathologic evidence of infective endocarditis at surgery or autopsy, with antibiotic therapy for ≤4 days; or (4) Does not meet criteria for possible infective endocarditis, as above

TABLE 29-3	**Major criteria**

DEFINITION OF TERMS USED IN THE MODIFIED DUKE CRITERIA FOR THE DIAGNOSIS OF INFECTIVE ENDOCARDITIS (IE), ADOPTED WITH PERMISSION FROM [64]	Blood culture positive for IE:
	    Typical microorganisms consistent with IE from 2 separate blood cultures: Viridans streptococci, *Streptococcus bovis,* HACEK group, *Staphylococcus aureus;* or community-acquired enterococci in the absence of a primary focus
	or
	    Microorganisms consistent with IE from persistently positive blood cultures, defined as follows: At least two positive cultures of blood samples drawn > 12 h apart or single positive blood culture for *Coxiella burnetii* or IgG antibody titer > 1:800
	Evidence of endocardial involvement:
	    Echocardiogram positive for IE, defined as follows:
	        Oscillating intracardiac mass on valve or supporting structures, in the path of regurgitant jets, or on implanted material in the absence of an alternative anatomic explanation
	        or
	        Abscess
	        or
	        New partial dehiscence of prosthetic valve
	    New valvular regurgitation (worsening or changing of pre-existing murmur not sufficient)

	Minor criteria
	Predisposition, predisposing heart condition, or IDU
	Fever (temperature >38 °C)
	Vascular phenomena:
	    Major arterial emboli, septic pulmonary infarcts, mycotic aneurysm, intracranial hemorrhage, conjunctival hemorrhages, and Janeway lesions
	Immunologic phenomena
	    Glomerulonephritis, Osler's nodes, Roth spots, and rheumatoid factor
	Microbiological evidence: positive blood culture but does not meet a major criterion as noted above or serologic evidence

C. **Microbiology and pathology:**

■ Blood cultures <u>prior</u> to antimicrobial initiation are imperative for diagnosis

■ Optimally, three sets of blood cultures will be obtained over 24 h

■ Minimum of 10 cc in each blood culture bottle for improved yield in adults

■ Histologic findings on cardiac valves after surgical resection can be diagnostic [4], including the specific pattern of inflammation [5]

– However, positive histopathology stains can persist in sterile vegetations; tissue culture can be helpful [6] but must be interpreted with caution as there can be high rates of contamination [4]

Current standard of care for diagnosis is the modified Duke criteria (Tables 29-2, 29-2, and 29-3)

PATHOGEN	ANTIMICROBIAL (S)	DURATION (WEEKS)
Streptococcus (viridans group or bovis) (dosing depends on MIC to PCN) If MIC for PCN >0.5 ug/mL	PCN or Ceftriaxone OR	4
	PCN or Ceftriaxone + Gentamicin OR	2
	Vancomycin (PCN-allergic) use Enterococcal IE guidelines	4
Staphylococci		6
If oxacillin-susceptible[a]	Nafcillin or Oxacillin ± Gentamicin	3–5 days
If oxacillin-resistant or for PCN-allergic patients	Vancomycin ± Gentamicin (or PCN-allergic)	6
Enterococcus (if susceptible to PCN, Gentamicin, and	Ampicillin or PCN + Gentamicin OR	4–6
Vancomycin (in cases of resistance, ID consultation)	Vancomycin + Gentamicin	6
HACEK[b]	Ceftriaxone OR Ampicillin-sulbactam OR Ciprofloxacin (PCN-allergy)	4
Culture-negative	Ampicillin-sulbactam + Gentamicin OR Vancomycin + Gentamicin + Ciprofloxacin	4–6
Culture-negative (suspected *Bartonella*)	Ceftriaxone + Gentamicin ± Doxycycline (Gentamicin can be discontinued at 2 weeks)	6

[a]Oxacillin-susceptibility should be confirmed with the microbiology lab as some staphylococcal or *Staphylococcus* spp have heteroresistance and require screening for *mecA* gene
[b]*Haemophilus parainfluenza*, *Haemophilus aphrophilus*, *Actinobacillus actinomycetemcomitans*, *Cardiobacterium hominis*, *Fikenella corrodens*, and *Kingella kingae*

D. Treatment

Prompt initiation of parenteral antimicrobials is the mainstay of treatment, in conjunction with surgical evaluation when indicated (Table 29-4)

E. Complications

IE can pursue a fulminant or subacute clinical course that depends on host, pathogen and the rapidity of diagnosis, treatment initiation, and presence of complications from the endovascular infection.

■ **Heart failure (HF)** [3]

- Most common and feared complication of IE given increased rates of morbidity and mortality
- Frequency of acute HF depends on location of IE: 29 % (aortic), 20 % (mitral), versus 8 % (tricuspid)
- All patients with IE and in clinical HF should be considered for immediate surgical evaluation
- Timing of surgical intervention depends on clinical status; surgery earlier in clinical course is often better tolerated [7]
- Worse outcomes when surgical intervention is performed in patients with advanced age, in renal failure or in NYHA Class III or IV heart failure

■ **Embolization**

- Evident in 22–50 % of IE cases and associated with increased morbidity and mortality
- 65 % of emboli involve the central nervous system (CNS), especially in the middle cerebral artery distribution
- Uncertain clinical significance to asymptomatic CNS emboli incidentally found on imaging [8]
- After initial 2–3 weeks of antimicrobials, embolic events are much less likely
- Risk factors for embolization may include: vegetation size, mitral valve involvement, staphylococcal species, prior emboli [9, 10]

TABLE 29-5	COMPLICATION	CLINICAL FEATURES	DIAGNOSTIC TESTING (SENSITIVITY/ SPECIFICITY)	TREATMENT RECOMMENDATIONS
ADDITIONAL COMPLICATIONS OF IE [1, 3]	Valvular extension	Heart block	ECG to assess for conduction abnormalities (sensitivity 45 %) TEE (sensitivity 76–100 %; specificity 95 %)	Surgical evaluation
	Splenic abscess	Abdominal pain Pleuritic or shoulder pain Persistent fever	CT or MRI (sensitivity and specificity: 90–95 %)	Percutaneous drainage or splenectomy
	Mycotic aneurysm (intracranial or extracranial)	Focal neurologic findings or mental status deterioration	CT or MRA (sensitivity and specificity: 90–95 %)	Antimicrobials with surgical or endovascular treatment if progression or rupture

TABLE 29-6	VEGETATION	VALVULAR DYSFUNCTION	PERIVALVULAR EXTENSION
ECHOCARDIOGRAPHIC FINDINGS THAT SHOULD PROMPT CONSIDERATION OF SURGICAL EVALUATION [3]	Persistent vegetation after systemic embolization	Acute aortic or mitral insufficiency with signs of ventricular failure	Valvular dehiscence, rupture, or fistula
	Anterior mitral leaflet vegetation, particularly if >10 mm	CHF that is unresponsive to medical management	New heart block
	≥1 embolic events during first 2 weeks of antimicrobial therapy	Valve perforation or rupture	Large abscess or extension of abscess despite appropriate antimicrobial therapy
	Increase in vegetation size despite appropriate antimicrobial therapy		

- Timing of surgery in patient with CNS emboli and/or use of anticoagulation remain a controversial topic [9, 11]
- Intracranial hemorrhage remains a devastating complication (~5 %) and contraindication to surgical intervention [8, 12] (Table 29-5)

F. **Surgery for IE**
   Although surgical interventions must always be individualized with input from the medical and surgical teams, guidelines suggest specific indications for careful consideration of surgical intervention [1, 3]. Importantly, post-operative infection of new prostheses is rare (2–3 %) even when surgical intervention is performed in active IE [3] (Table 29-6).
   ■ Class I, Level of Evidence: B

   - HF
   - Valvular dehiscence, rupture, or perforation
   - Perivalvular abscess or periannular extension
   - Fungal IE or multidrug-resistant aggressive pathogens
   - Persistently positive blood cultures after >1 week of targeted antimicrobials
   - ≥1 embolic event during the initial 2 weeks of antimicrobials

   ■ Class IIa, Level of Evidence: B

   - Anterior mitral leaflet vegetation, especially if >10 mm

   ■ Class IIb, Level of Evidence: C

   - Increased vegetation size despite targeted antimicrobials

G. **Outcomes and follow-up**
- Almost 50 % of patients with IE require surgical intervention [2]
- Inpatient mortality remains 15–20 % in the twenty first century [2]

    – Risk factors for death include increasing age, HF, paravalvular complications, prosthetic valve endocarditis, and *Staphylococcus aureus* as the causative organism

- Many patients with IE on stable parenteral antimicrobial therapy can be managed in the outpatient setting with careful monitoring and follow-up [13]

    – TTE should be obtained as a new baseline after treatment; if cardiac windows are inadequate, then a TEE should be performed
    – IE prophylaxis should be prescribed for appropriate procedures in patients who have recovered from IE [14]

SPECIAL TOPIC – PROSTHETIC VALVE ENDOCARDITIS (PVE)

- Distinguished by early and late presentation (≤ or >1 year post-valve surgery); clinical course and causative organisms can be different [15]

    – Most often requires surgical intervention because frequently complicated by perivalvular abscess, leak or other valvular dysfunction
    – *S. aureus* and coagulase-negative staphylococcus are the most common etiologies, especially in early PVE; nosocomial pathogens are also more common than in NVE [16]

- Antimicrobial treatment algorithms are available for PVE [3] but should be used in conjunction with Infectious Disease consultation given complexities of diagnosis and treatment in this patient population

    – Multidisciplinary collaboration is essential; combined medical-surgical management yields the best outcomes
    High morbidity and mortality persist despite improved diagnosis, medical-surgical collaboration, and prompt treatments [16, 17]

SPECIAL TOPIC: CULTURE NEGATIVE ENDOCARDITIS

- Causes [18]

    – Receipt of antimicrobials prior to collection of blood cultures
    – Right-sided endocarditis
    – Endocarditis with cardiac device
    – Non-bacterial pathogen (e.g., fungi, mycobacteria) or non-infectious etiology (e.g., neoplastic or auto-immune phenomenon)
    – Fastidious organisms (often intracellular) that require different diagnostic tools

        - *Coxiella burnetii* ("Q fever")
        - *Bartonella* spp
        - *Brucella* spp
        - *Mycoplasma* spp
        - *Tropheryma whipelii*
        - Nutritionally deficient streptococci (non-intracellular org)
        - HACEK organisms (haemophilus spp; *Actinobacillus* spp; *Cardiobacterium hominis*; *Eikenella corrodens*; *Kingella kingae*)

- Diagnosis [19]

    – Specialized culture techniques
    – Serology
    – 16S and 18S ribosomal PCR (serum, valve tissue)

- Treatment: in conjunction with Infectious Diseases consultation

SPECIAL TOPIC: FUNGAL ENDOCARDITIS

- Fungal IE is a rare (<10 %) but increasingly prevalent form of IE
    - Most commonly *Candida* spp
    - *Aspergillus* spp, Histoplasmosis and other fungi have been reported to cause IE especially in immunocompromised hosts
- Risk factors: prosthetic valves, nosocomial exposures, short-term catheters [21], immunocompromise, antibiotic use, IDU, TPN [20]
- Complications: most commonly embolization and large vegetations. HF is less common [21]
- Treatment: medical ± surgical
    - Antifungals [22]:
        - Liposomal amphotericin B ± 5-flucytosine
        - IV echinocandin may be an option
- Recurrence rates are extremely high, so secondary prophylaxis with oral fluconazole is recommended for at least 2 years if not life-long [21–23]
- ID Consultation is strongly advised

SPECIAL TOPIC: ENDOCARDITIS PROPHYLAXIS (TABLES 29-7, 29-8, AND 29-9)

- Antibiotic prophylaxis is indicated in patients with cardiac conditions with the highest risk of adverse outcome from IE (Table 29-7) undergoing certain procedures (Table 29-8)

TABLE 29-7 CARDIAC CONDITIONS AT HIGHEST RISK FOR IE [14]	
	Prosthetic cardiac valve or prosthetic material in valve repair
	History of prior IE
	Specific forms of congenital heart disease (CHD)
	Completely repaired CHD if prosthetic material or device was placed within past 6 months
	Repaired CHD with residual defects at or adjacent to site of prosthetic material or device
	Unrepaired cyanotic CHD
	Cardiac transplant with valvulopathy

TABLE 29-8 PROCEDURES FOR WHICH THERE ARE GUIDELINES ON IE PROPHYLAXIS [9]	
	Dental procedures: Any procedure that involves manipulation of gingival tissue or the periapical region of teeth or perforation of the oral mucosa.
	Respiratory procedures: If procedure is invasive with incision or biopsy. Not indicated in bronchoscopy.
	GI/GU procedures: No prophylaxis indicated. Active treatment of GI or GU infection (if present) prior to procedure is recommended.

TABLE 29-9 RECOMMENDED ANTIBIOTIC PROPHYLACTIC REGIMEN [9]	REGIMEN	ANTIBIOTICS
	Preferred	Amoxicillin 2 g PO
	PCN allergy	Clindamycin 600 mg PO OR Azithromycin 500 mg PO
	Unable to take oral medication	Ampicillin 2 g IV OR Cefazolin 1 g IM or IV
	Unable to take oral and PCN allergy	Cefazolin 1 g IM or IV OR Clindamycin 600 mg IM or IV

Note: all regimens are single doses to be given 30–60 min prior to procedure

HOST FACTORS	PROCEDURAL FACTORS	PATHOGEN FACTORS
Immunosuppression, including renal failure and steroids	"Peri-procedural factors" such as periprocedure ppx	Specific microbiology of any blood stream infection in patient with CIED
Oral anticoagulation	"Operator experience"	
Patient co-morbidities	Device exchange	
Other "indwelling hardware"		

TABLE 29-10

RISK FACTORS FOR ALL CIED INFECTIONS [24]

SPECIAL TOPIC: DEVICE INFECTIONS

A. Cardiovascular implantable electronic device infection (CIED): includes ICD and PPM
B. **Epidemiology:** CIED infections is a growing problem that is out of proportion to the increased rates of device implantation
   - Over past 20 years, there have been more infections and more hospitalizations
   - Risk of infection is higher among patients with ICD as opposed to PPM
   - Increase risk of in-hospital death by >2-fold (Table 29-10)
C. **Clinical presentation:**
   - Superficial infection
   - Local inflammatory changes without evidence of device involvement
   - Local inflammatory changes that can progress to erosion

     – Systemic symptoms frequently absent

   - Endocarditis

     – Less common but most feared
     – ~10–20 % of all CIED infections

D. **Diagnosis** [24, 25].
   - Two sets of blood cultures prior to antibiotic initiation in all patients with possible CIED infection
   - TEE much higher yield and should be performed even if vegetations evident on TTE, as imaging of left-side of heart is considerably improved
   - At time of device removal:

     – Gram stain and culture of generator-pocket-site tissue and lead tips
     – Fungal and mycobacterial cultures, if indicated by epidemiology or if original cultures are unrevealing

   - Aspiration of device pocket is not recommended because it is unlikely to be high yield and risks introducing infection
E. **Management**: (Table 29-11)
   - Complete device removal should be completed as soon as possible after CIED infection is confirmed
   - Given high rates of relapse, even localized device infections should still be treated with complete device removal
   - Duration of antibiotics is listed in Table 29-11 and begun from time of device removal
   - Blood cultures to be drawn after device removal to document sterilization

     – If blood cultures are no growth in the setting of recent antibiotics, treat as though blood culture is positive

   - Management of device re-implantation:

     – Assess whether the patient still requires the device: 33–50 % of patients with prior CIED will no longer need CIED at time of consideration of reimplantation
     – Contralateral placement, if possible
     – At least 72 h of negative blood cultures prior to reimplantation, if possible

TABLE 29-11	TYPE OF INFECTION	MINIMUM DURATION OF ANTIBIOTICS	DEVICE
TREATMENT OF CIED INFECTION [24]	Superficial or incisional infx	7–10 days	Can be retained
	Pocket infection	10–14 days	Complete removal of all hardware
	CIED with erosion	7–10 days	
	CIED with BCx+[a]	≥ 2 weeks of IV abx (minimum)	
	Valve vegetation on TEE[a]	IE guidelines	
	Lead vegetation on TEE[a]	2–6 weeks depending on pathogen and complications	

[a]ID Consultation is strongly recommended

TABLE 29-12	**Local infection**	
DEFINITIONS OF DIFFERENT LVAD-ASSOCIATED INFECTIONS [28]	Driveline	Purulent drainage from exit site (abdominal wall) with ≥ 1 pathogen on microbiologic culture
	Device pocket	Purulence in subcutaneous space surrounding device with ≥ 1 pathogen on microbiologic culture
	Systemic infection	
	LVAD endocarditis	Microbiologic culture of a pathogen from > 1 blood culture and histopathologic evidence of infection from the device
	LVAD-associated bloodstream	Microbiologic culture of the same pathogen from > 1 blood culture and from exit site, device or pocket in the absence of histopathologic evidence of infection from the device

■ **Suppressive antibiotics**: in setting of inability or high morbidity of device removal

  – Not recommended unless the following are all present:

    ■ Stable clinical status
    ■ Clinical improvement after initiation of antimicrobials
    ■ Sterilization of blood cultures
    ■ Pursued in consultation with Infectious Disease specialists and with careful follow-up

SPECIAL TOPIC: LEFT VENTRICULAR ASSIST DEVICE (LVAD) INFECTIONS

■ Infection is a leading cause of morbidity and mortality in patients with LVADs, although rates and outcomes are improving [26, 27] (Table 29-12)

■ **Microbiology** [28, 29]

  – Most commonly staphylococcus species
  – Also *Candida* spp and *Pseudomonas aeruginosa*

■ **Management** [30]

  – Surgical incision and drainage
  – Parenteral antimicrobials, often followed by oral antimicrobial suppression while device remain in place
  – Varied opinions on duration of antimicrobials: patients treated with limited antimicrobials seem to have higher relapse rates but those treated with continuous antimicrobials have high risk of multi-drug resistant organisms such as Vancomycin-resistant *Enterococcus* (VRE)
  – History of LVAD infection does not appear to affect post-transplant outcomes

CARDIOVASCULAR COMPLICATIONS IN HIV-INFECTED PATIENTS

■ Pericarditis in HIV

- Pericardial effusion is common in immunosuppressed HIV-infected patients not on antiretroviral therapy (ART) [31]
- Dramatically reduced prevalence in HIV patients on ART [32]
- Historically pericardial effusions have been associated with overall increased mortality, even when asymptomatic [31]
- Specific etiology depends on degree of immunosuppression, exposures, and acuity of clinical presentation (Table 29-13)
  Clinical presentation [31, 33]

  - Frequently asymptomatic
  - When symptomatic, typically presents with dyspnea and edema
  - Rarely progresses to cardiac tamponade

- **Diagnosis**

  - If symptomatic, pericardiocentesis for pericardial fluid cytology/culture
  - If pericardial fluid analysis non-diagnostic, pericardial biopsy may be necessary

- **Treatment**

  - Depends on specific etiology
  - ART to control virus, block viral replication and restore immune system is key to improving outcome

■ Myocarditis in HIV

- Most data are from case reports or autopsy in patients not on ART
- Broad differential diagnosis: HIV itself or a variety of opportunistic infections can cause myocarditis [34] or direct invasion of the myocardium
- Acute HIV may lead to myocarditis

HIV AND ATHEROSCLEROSIS

■ Epidemiology

- HIV infection is associated with premature atherosclerosis and increased incidence of cardiovascular events [35, 36]

  - Rate of ischemic stroke may be increasing in HIV patients [37]
  - HIV-infected patients may present with acute coronary syndrome (ACS) at younger ages with lower TIMI scores and may be less likely to have multi-vessel disease [38, 39] than HIV-negative patients

TABLE 29-13

COMMON ETIOLOGIES OF PERICARDIAL EFFUSION IN HIV PATIENTS [31, 65]

ETIOLOGY	COMMENTS
TB	Most common cause in endemic regions or high-risk populations
Bacterial	*Staphylococcus* or *Streptococcus* spp are most common
Viral	CMV, HSV, HIV (capillary leak syndrome from cytokine release)
Parasitic	*Toxoplasma gondii*
Fungal	*Cryptococcus neoformans, Histoplasma capsulatum*
Malignancy	Lymphomas, especially non-Hodgkin's; primary effusion lymphoma (HHV-8-related); Kaposi's sarcoma; other solid tumors

- Observational data suggests subclinical atherosclerosis (based on carotid intimal medial thickening, coronary CT, ECG [40–42]) may be more prevalent in HIV-infected patients
- Clinical significance and optimal risk reduction is uncertain

– Increased atherosclerosis risk likely due to [43, 44]

- Increased prevalence of traditional risk factors in HIV-infected patients (e.g. smoking)
- Dyslipidemia (related to HIV itself and some antiretroviral medications)
- Body-fat abnormalities (increased visceral adiposity)
- Impaired glucose homeostasis
- Adverse effect of antiretroviral medications, including particular protease inhibitors [45] and abacavir (the latter is controversial)
- Chronic inflammation due to HIV infection [46] and viremia [47]

- **Management of ACS in HIV-infected patients**

– Acute management of the HIV patient with ACS is the same as for those without HIV infection

- Drug-drug interactions should be carefully considered for medication dosing
- PCI has excellent short-term and long-term outcomes; restenosis may be more common in HIV-infected patients but data is variable [38, 48, 49]
- Good results with CABG in HIV-infected patients [50]

- **Prevention of CHD events in HIV**

– Aggressive risk reduction:

- Smoking cessation
- Diet
- Lipid lowering agents [51]
- Blood pressure control [52]

– Guidelines recommend initiation of ART in HIV-infected patients at high risk for CAD [54]

CARDIOMYOPATHY AND HEART FAILURE IN HIV-INFECTED PATIENTS

- In the pre-ART era, prevalence was 10–30 % in HIV patients; less common among patients on ART

– Even among HIV patients without CAD, heart failure is more prevalent [55] than among HIV-negative individuals. Role of the possible contributing etiologies is under ongoing investigation:

- Chronic inflammation
- Nutritional deficiencies
- ART (especially AZT and other meds with mitochondrial toxicity)

– Asymptomatic cardiomyopathy with decreased exercise tolerance and diastolic dysfunction is evident in HIV patients on ART [56]; long term consequences of such findings are not yet known

– HIV-infected patients with dyspnea should have prompt and careful cardiopulmonary workup [56, 57]

– Management of heart failure in the HIV-infected patient is the same as in non-infected patient. Because HIV may cause cardiomyopathy, ART should be initiated.

PULMONARY ARTERIAL HTN (PAH) IN HIV-INFECTED PATIENTS

■ **Epidemiology** [58, 59]

- Infrequent complication of HIV infection (prevalence ~ 0.5 %) but with high mortality even in the ART era
- Risk of developing PAH does not seem to be directly related to immunosuppression
- May be more common in injection drug users
- All patients with new diagnosis of PAH should be tested for HIV
- Conflicting literature regarding whether ART reduces incidence

■ **Pathophysiology** [60]

- Evidence of chronic inflammation
  Uncertain if caused by a direct viral effect or interactions with HIV-associated proteins
- Histopathology similar to idiopathic PAH

  ■ Medial hypertrophy and proliferation of endothelium

■ **Clinical presentation** [57]

- Dyspnea (85 %)
- Non-productive cough (19 %)
- Fatigue (13 %)
- Syncope (12 %)

■ **Physical exam** [25]

- Signs of right heart failure, e.g., loud P2, right-sided S3, murmur of tricuspid regurgitation, increased JVP, pedal edema

■ **Diagnosis** [57]

- ECG: evidence of right ventricular hypertrophy, right heart strain
- TTE: elevated right-sided pressures, tricuspid regurgitation
- Right heart catheterization demonstrates pulmonary hypertension
  Other modifiable causes of PAH (e.g. chronic thromboembolic disease) excluded

■ **Therapy**

- Although benefit of ART for reversing PAH is not certain [61], most patients with HIV-associated PAH should initiate ART

PAH THERAPY	RECOMMENDATIONS	NOTES
Supplemental oxygen	All Recommended	
Digitalis	All Recommended	
Diuretics	All Recommended	
Anticoagulation (PO)	Recommended, if no medical contraindication	Benefit is not clear in HIV patients
Calcium channel blockers (CCB)	Rarely effective given vasoreactivity testing is usually negative in HIV-PAH, so seldom recommended	Low dose if used; HIV protease inhibitors (PIs) can increase CCB levels
Prostacyclins (IV or SQ)	Recommended [66]	No drug-drug interactions noted
PDE-5 Inhibitors (PO)	Can be used with caution	Dose adjust and use with caution in patients on PIs. No interaction with HIV non-nucleoside reverse transcriptase inhibitors (NNRTIs), such as efavirenz, or raltegravir
Endothelin receptor antagonists (PO)	Recommended [67]	Contraindicated in advanced liver disease. Use with caution in patients on PI therapy as drug-interactions exist.

- Because of absence of large trials in HIV-infected patients, treatment of PAH extrapolated from guidelines for HIV-negative patients [62]
- Note: several PAH drugs interact with antiretroviral medications (see Tables 29-15 and 29-14).

CARDIOVASCULAR DRUG INTERACTIONS IN HIV-INFECTED PATIENTS

■ Nucleoside reverse transcriptase inhibitors (NRTIs) and integrase inhibitors seldom have drug-drug interactions

■ Ritonavir and other HIV PIs are strong CYP 34A inhibitors (Table 29-15)

■ HIV patients may have QTc prolongation [53], so co-administration of drugs such as fluconazole, fluoroquinolones, and macrolides should be carefully monitored

Acknowledgements Many thanks to Elke Backman, Pharm D, of the Department of Pharmacy, Massachusetts General Hospital.

TABLE 29-15

A SELECTION OF IMPORTANT CARDIOVASCULAR AND ANTIRETROVIRAL DRUG-DRUG INTERACTIONS; THIS LIST IS NOT COMPLETE OR COMPREHENSIVE [54, 63]

	PROTEASE INHIBITOR	EFAVIRENZ	ETRAVIRINE	CCR5-ANTAGONIST
Statins [68]	Increased levels statin Simvastatin, lovastatin contraindicated Pravastatin OK Pitavastatin OK Atorvastatin and rosuvastatin: start at low dose, titrate up slowly; see reference for maximum dose with particular PIs	Decreased levels statin Simvastatin levels especially decreased; consider alternative	Decreased levels statin	No change expected
PDE-5 inhibitors	Increased levels PDE5; dose adjust with cautious titration	Decreased levels PDE-5 inhibitor	Decreased levels PDE-5 inhibitor	No change expected
Beta-blockers	Additive PR prolongation with ritonavir	No change expected	No change expected	No change expected
Calcium-channel blockers	Increased levels CCB; dose adjust Specifically dose-reduce 50 % with ATV and monitor ECG	Decreased levels CCB; dose adjust	No change expected	No change expected
Warfarin	Can increase or decrease INR	Can increase or decrease INR	Increased INR	No change expected
Clopidogrel	Potent CYP3A4 inhibitors have been shown to decrease the antiplatelet activity of clopidogrel	No change expected	Decreased levels clopidogrel	No change expected
Nonthienopyridine platelet inhibitors (e.g., Ticagrelor, Prasugrel)	Increased levels ticagrelor so contraindicated Prasugrel can be used	Decreased levels of ticagrelor	Decreased levels of ticagrelor	No change expected
Endothelin receptor antagonists (e.g., Bosentan, Ambrisentan)	Increased levels bosentan; dose adjust Initiate bosentan only if pt on PIs for ≥ 10 days. For pts stable on bosentan needing to start ART, discontinue for 36 h prior to starting PI, then reinstitute after 10 days Do not give with unboosted ATV	Bosentan levels may increase or, more likely, may decrease	Bosentan levels may increase or, more likely, may decrease	Decreased levels maraviroc; dose adjust
Prostacyclins (e.g., Epoprostenol, Treprostinil)	No change expected	No change expected	No change expected	No change expected
Amiodarone	Decreased levels amiodarone Contraindicated but can still be used in treatment of life-threatening arrhythmia	Amiodarone levels can increase or decrease	Amiodarone levels can increase or decrease	No change expected

REVIEW QUESTIONS

1. A 45 year old man with a history of unrepaired bicuspid aortic valve is scheduled for an upcoming extraction of several teeth. When he was a child, he had a rash (not hives) after taking amoxicillin for an ear infection. In anticipation of the upcoming dental extraction, he should receive:
    (a) Amoxicillin 2 g PO 30–60 minutes prior to the procedure
    (b) Clindamycin 600 mg PO
    (c) Azithromycin 500 mg PO ×1 now followed by 250 mg PO until the procedure
    (d) Cefazolin 1 g IM
    (e) No prophylaxis

2. A 76 year old male with recent uncomplicated hospitalization for non-ST elevation MI presents to his cardiologist for follow-up at post-discharge week 2. He has had increasing fatigue over the past week. In the clinic, he is febrile (101.0 F) and is ill-appearing with a stable II/VI harsh systolic murmur loudest at the right upper sternal border consistent with his previously diagnosed mild aortic stenosis. A careful physical exam reveals one new non-tender nodular lesion on the sole of his right foot. He is re-admitted to the hospital where two sets of blood cultures are drawn and methicillin-resistant *S aureus* (MRSA) grows in 3/4 bottles at 14 h. He has a TTE followed by a TEE that reveal no vegetation. Given clinical improvement with IV Vancomycin and assuming no additional complications, what is the diagnosis and basic treatment plan?
    (a) Possible endocarditis; 6 weeks of IV Vancomycin
    (b) Possible endocarditis; 2 weeks of IV Vancomycin
    (c) Definite endocarditis; 6 weeks of IV Vancomycin
    (d) Definite endocarditis; 4 weeks of IV Linezolid
    (e) Not endocarditis; 2 weeks of IV Vancomycin

3. A 68 year old female with a permanent pacemaker (PPM) implanted 6 years ago presents with fevers to 100.5 and cough to her primary care physician. She is prescribed 5 days of azithromycin for tracheobronchitis but experiences no improvement in her fevers. On return to her PCP, she notes slight erythema of the soft tissue overlying the PPM site. Given concern for a late device infection, she is admitted to the hospital where blood cultures are obtained. Given her CIED, a TEE is appropriately ordered and demonstrates a vegetation on one of the PPM leads. What are the next steps in therapeutic management?
    (a) Device removal alone
    (b) Antimicrobials; no indication for device removal
    (c) Device removal with concurrent antimicrobials and immediate reimplantation of CIED
    (d) Device removal with concurrent antimicrobials and reimplantation of CIED after 2 weeks
    (e) Device removal with concurrent antimicrobials and evaluation to determine if reimplantation of CIED is indicated

4. A 39 year old man with HIV treated with antiretroviral medications presents to the hospital with substernal chest pain that is brought on by exertion. On admission, workup reveals an MI and he undergoes cardiac catheterization with a drugeluting stent placed to the left circumflex artery. His low-density lipoprotein (LDL) was elevated at 170 mg/dL. What is one of the next steps in his management?
    (a) Prescribe atorvastatin 80 mg daily
    (b) Prescribe simvastatin 40 mg daily
    (c) Confirm his antiretroviral regimen; if he is prescribed a regimen that includes a protease inhibitor, then prescribe atorvastatin 10–20 mg daily
    (d) Confirm his antiretroviral regimen; if he is prescribed a regimen that includes a protease inhibitor, then prescribe simvastatin 40 mg daily
    (e) Statins are contraindicated in HIV infected patients; no statin can be prescribed

ANSWERS

1. (e) By the updated endocarditis prophylaxis guidelines, the patient does not have any of the cardiac pathologies that are most at risk for IE and as a result he does not require antimicrobial prophylaxis prior to a higher risk dental procedure. However, if he did need IE prophylaxis, then oral clindamycin would be the agent of choice with instructions to be taken 30–60 min prior to the procedure. Because of his documented allergy to penicillin (rash not hives after amoxicillin), he should not receive the standard preferred regimen of amoxicillin 2 g. A full course of azithromycin is not recommended, although a single dose of azithromycin can be used in penicillin-allergic patients who require prophylaxis. Cefazolin could be used in this patient if he could not take oral medications given that his prior allergy to penicillin resulted in rash, so cephalosporins are not contraindicated.

2. (c) Despite the absence of echocardiographic evidence, his clinical presentation meets criteria for definite IE by the modified

Duke criteria given the positive blood cultures for *S Aureus* (major criteria) and fever with predisposing heart condition and a non-tender nodular lesion consistent with a Janeway lesion (three minor criteria). Janeway lesions are microabscesses in the dermis that result from small septic emboli and are vascular phenomenon seen in IE. As a result, he should be treated with appropriate parenteral antibiotics with close clinical follow-up. Vancomycin remains the drug of choice in MRSA endovascular infections; linezolid is not FDA-approved for treatment of endovascular infection except for VRE.

3. (e) This patient presents with a late-onset CIED infection which requires both antimicrobial management and immediate device removal. Although the blood cultures do not reveal an organism, they were obtained after initiation of antimicrobials and thus the patient required further evaluation for a CIED with a TEE. After CIED is confirmed by echocardiographic evidence, the patient required immediate device removal as well as ongoing parenteral antimicrobial therapy. Given that many patients will no longer require CIED support after explanation (13–52 % in several series), she should undergo careful evaluation regarding whether she requires reimplantation of a CIED [24, 25].

4. (c) Statins are an essential class of drugs for HIV-infected patient and are indicated to manage the frequent dyslipidemias evident in this population. However, drug-drug interactions are important to acknowledge so that medications can be dosed as safely as possible. Close follow-up of patients prescribed both a statin and protease inhibitor is essential, as they are at higher risk for rhabdomyolysis. Atorvastatin can be used in patients who take ritonavir, but it must be used at lower doses given that serum levels of atorvastatin will be higher because ritonavir inhibits CY P 34A; 80 mg of atorvastatin is too high a dose to be used in a patient also prescribed ritonavir. Simvastatin is contraindicated in patients who are receiving ritonavir, which is a frequent component of proteaseinhibitor regimens, because drug-drug interactions cause markedly elevated levels of simvastatin when co-prescribed.

REFERENCES

1. Lester SJ, Wilansky S. Endocarditis and associated complications. Crit Care Med. 2007;35(8 S):S384–91.
2. Murdoch DR, Corey GR, Hoen B, Miro JM, Fowler Jr VG, Bayer AS, et al. Clinical presentation, etiology, and outcome of infective endocarditis in the 21st century: the International Collaboration on Endocarditis-Prospective Cohort Study. Arch Intern Med. 2009;169(5):463–73.
3. Burns JC, Falace DA, Newburger JW, Pallasch TJ, Takahashi M, Taubert KA, et al. Infective endocarditis: diagnosis, antimicrobial therapy, and management of complications: a statement for healthcare professionals from the Committee on Rheumatic Fever, Endocarditis, and Kawasaki Disease, Council on Cardiovascular Disease in the Young, and the Councils on Clinical Cardiology, Stroke, and Cardiovascular Surgery and Anesthesia, American Heart Association: endorsed by the Infectious Diseases Society of America. Circulation. 2005;111(23):e394–434.
4. Durack DT, Lukes AS, Bright DK. New criteria for diagnosis of infective endocarditis: utilization of specific echocardiographic findings. Duke Endocarditis Service. Am J Med. 1994;96(3):200–9.
5. Lepidi H, Casalta JP, Fournier PE, Habib G, Collart F, Raoult D. Quantitative histological examination of mechanical heart valves. Clin Infect Dis. 2005;40(5):655–61.
6. Morris AJ, Drinkovic D, Pottumarthy S, Strickett MG, MacCulloch D, Lambie N, et al. Gram stain, culture, and histopathological examination findings for heart valves removed because of infective endocarditis. Clin Infect Dis. 2003;36(6):697–704.
7. Kiefer T, Park L, Tribouilloy C, Cortes C, Casillo R, Chu V, et al. Association between valvular surgery and mortality among patients with infective endocarditis complicated by heart failure. JAMA. 2011;306(20):2239–47.
8. Snygg-Martin U, Gustafsson L, Rosengren L, Alsio A, Ackerholm P, Andersson R, et al. Cerebrovascular complications in patients with left-sided infective endocarditis are common: a prospective study using magnetic resonance imaging and neurochemical brain damage markers. Clin Infect Dis. 2008;47(1):23–30.
9. Thuny F, Avierinos JF, Tribouilloy C, Giorgi R, Casalta JP, Milandre L, et al. Impact of cerebrovascular complications on mortality and neurologic outcome during infective endocarditis: a prospective multicentre study. Eur Heart J. 2007;28(9):1155–61.
10. Vilacosta I, Graupner C, San Roman JA, Sarria C, Ronderos R, Fernandez C, et al. Risk of embolization after institution of antibiotic therapy for infective endocarditis. J Am Coll Cardiol. 2002;39(9):1489–95.

11. Thuny F, Habib G. When should we operate on patients with acute infective endocarditis? Heart. 2010;96(11):892–7.

12. Angstwurm K, Borges AC, Halle E, Schielke E, Einhaupl KM, Weber JR. Timing the valve replacement in infective endocarditis involving the brain. J Neurol. 2004;251(10):1220–6.

13. Tice AD, Rehm SJ, Dalovisio JR, Bradley JS, Martinelli LP, Graham DR, et al. Practice guidelines for outpatient parenteral antimicrobial therapy. IDSA guidelines. IDSA guidelines. Clin Infect Dis. 2004;38(12):1651–72.

14. Wilson W, Taubert KA, Gewitz M, Lockhart PB, Baddour LM, Levison M, et al. Prevention of infective endocarditis: guidelines from the American Heart Association: a guideline from the American Heart Association Rheumatic Fever, Endocarditis, and Kawasaki Disease Committee, Council on Cardiovascular Disease in the Young, and the Council on Clinical Cardiology, Council on Cardiovascular Surgery and Anesthesia, and the Quality of Care and Outcomes Research Interdisciplinary Working Group. Circulation. 2007;116(15):1736–54.

15. Lopez J, Revilla A, Vilacosta I, Villacorta E, Gonzalez-Juanatey C, Gomez I, et al. Definition, clinical profile, microbiological spectrum, and prognostic factors of early-onset prosthetic valve endocarditis. Eur Heart J. 2007;28(6):760–5.

16. Wang A, Athan E, Pappas PA, Fowler Jr VG, Olaison L, Pare C, et al. Contemporary clinical profile and outcome of prosthetic valve endocarditis. JAMA. 2007;297(12):1354–61.

17. Alonso-Valle H, Farinas-Alvarez C, Garcia-Palomo JD, Bernal JM, Martin-Duran R, Gutierrez Diez JF, et al. Clinical course and predictors of death in prosthetic valve endocarditis over a 20-year period. J Thorac Cardiovasc Surg. 2010;139(4):887–93.

18. Houpikian P, Raoult D. Blood culture-negative endocarditis in a reference center: etiologic diagnosis of 348 cases. Medicine (Baltimore). 2005;84(3):162–73.

19. Fournier PE, Thuny F, Richet H, Lepidi H, Casalta JP, Arzouni JP, et al. Comprehensive diagnostic strategy for blood culture-nega-tive endocarditis: a prospective study of 819 new cases. Clin Infect Dis. 2010;51(2):131–40.

20. Baddley JW, Benjamin Jr DK, Patel M, Miro J, Athan E, Barsic B, et al. International Collaboration on Endocarditis-Prospective Cohort Study Group (ICE-PCS). Candida infective endocarditis. Eur J Clin Microbiol Infect Dis. 2008;27(7):519–29.

21. Ellis ME, Al-Abdely H, Sandridge A, Greer W, Ventura W. Fungal endocarditis: evidence in the world literature, 1965–1995. Clin Infect Dis. 2001;32(1):50–62.

22. Pappas PG, Kauffman CA, Andes D, Benjamin Jr DK, Calandra TF, Edwards Jr JE, et al. Clinical practice guidelines for the man-agement of candidiasis: 2009 update by the Infectious Diseases Society of America. Clin Infect Dis. 2009;48(5):503–35.

23. Pappas PG, Rex JH, Sobel JD, Filler SG, Dismukes WE, Walsh TJ, et al. Guidelines for treatment of candidiasis. Clin Infect Dis. 2004;38(2):161–89.

24. Baddour LM, Epstein AE, Erickson CC, Knight BP, Levison ME, Lockhart PB, et al. Update on cardiovascular implantable electronic device infections and their management: a scientific statement from the American Heart Association. Circulation. 2010;121(3): 458–77.

25. Sohail MR, Uslan DZ, Khan AH, Friedman PA, Hayes DL, Wilson WR, et al. Management and outcome of permanent pacemaker and implantable cardioverter-defibrillator infections. J Am Coll Cardiol. 2007;49(18):1851–9.

26. Rose EA, Gelijns AC, Moskowitz AJ, Heitjan DF, Stevenson LW, Dembitsky W, et al. Long-term use of a left ventricular assist device for end-stage heart failure. N Engl J Med. 2001; 345(20):1435–43.

27. Slaughter MS, Rogers JG, Milano CA, Russell SD, Conte JV, Feldman D, et al. Advanced heart failure treated with continuous-flow left ventricular assist device. N Engl J Med. 2009;361(23): 2241–51.

28. Simon D, Fischer S, Grossman A, Downer C, Hota B, Heroux A, et al. Left ventricular assist device-related infection: treatment and outcome. Clin Infect Dis. 2005;40(8):1108–15.

29. Schaffer JM, Allen JG, Weiss ES, Arnaoutakis GJ, Patel ND, Russell SD, et al. Infectious complications after pulsatile-flow and continuous-flow left ventricular assist device implantation. J Heart Lung Transplant. 2011;30(2):164–74.

30. Topkara VK, Kondareddy S, Malik F, Wang IW, Mann DL, Ewald GA, et al. Infectious complications in patients with left ventricular assist device: etiology and outcomes in the continuous-flow era. Ann Thorac Surg. 2010;90(4):1270–7.

31. Khunnawat C, Mukerji S, Havlichek Jr D, Touma R, Abela GS. Cardiovascular manifestations in human immunodeficiency virus-infected patients. Am J Cardiol. 2008;102(5):635–42.

32. Pugliese A, Isnardi D, Saini A, Scarabelli T, Raddino R, Torre D. Impact of highly active antiretroviral therapy in HIV-positive patients with cardiac involvement. J Infect. 2000;40(3): 282–4.

33. Mishra RK. Cardiac emergencies in patients with HIV. Emerg Med Clin North Am. 2010;28(2):273–82. Table of Contents.

34. Barbaro G, Di Lorenzo G, Grisorio B, Barbarini G. Cardiac involvement in the acquired immunodeficiency syndrome: a mul-ticenter clinical-pathological study. Gruppo Italiano per lo Studio Cardiologico dei pazienti affetti da AIDS Investigators. AIDS Res Hum Retroviruses. 1998;14(12):1071–7.

35. Bozzette SA, Ake CF, Tam HK, Chang SW, Louis TA. Cardiovascular and cerebrovascular events in patients treated for human immunodeficiency virus infection. N Engl J Med. 2003;348(8):702–10.

36. Triant VA, Lee H, Hadigan C, Grinspoon SK. Increased acute myocardial infarction rates and cardiovascular risk factors among patients with human immunodeficiency virus disease. J Clin Endocrinol Metab. 2007;92(7):2506–12.

37. Ovbiagele B, Nath A. Increasing incidence of ischemic stroke in patients with HIV infection. Neurology. 2011;76(5):444–50.

38. Hsue PY, Giri K, Erickson S, MacGregor JS, Younes N, Shergill A, et al. Clinical features of acute coronary syndromes in patients with human immunodeficiency virus infection. Circulation. 2004;109(3):316–9.

39. Boccara F, Ederhy S, Janower S, Benyounes N, Odi G, Cohen A. Clinical characteristics and mid-term prognosis of acute coronary syndrome in HIV-infected patients on antiretroviral therapy. HIV Med. 2005;6(4):240–4.

40. Mangili A, Polak JF, Skinner SC, Gerrior J, Sheehan H, Harrington A, et al. HIV infection and progression of carotid and coronary atherosclerosis: the CARE study. J Acquir Immune Defic Syndr. 2011;58(2):148–53.

41. Lo J, Abbara S, Shturman L, Soni A, Wei J, Rocha-Filho JA, et al. Increased prevalence of subclinical coronary atherosclerosis detected by coronary computed tomography angiography in HIV-infected men. AIDS. 2010;24(2):243–53.

42. Carr A, Grund B, Neuhaus J, El-Sadr WM, Grandits G, Gibert C, et al. Asymptomatic myocardial ischaemia in HIV-infected adults. AIDS. 2008;22(2):257–67.

43. Calza L, Manfredi R, Verucchi G. Myocardial infarction risk in HIV-infected patients: epidemiology, pathogenesis, and clinical management. AIDS. 2010;24(6):789–802.

44. Grinspoon S, Carr A. Cardiovascular risk and body-fat abnormalities in HIV-infected adults. N Engl J Med. 2005;352(1):48–62.

45. Friis-Møller N, Sabin CA, Weber R, d'Arminio Monforte A, El-Sadr WM, Reiss P, et al. Combination antiretroviral therapy and the risk of myocardial infarction. N Engl J Med. 2003;349(21):1993–2003.

46. Hsue PY, Hunt PW, Schnell A, Kalapus SC, Hoh R, Ganz P, et al. Role of viral replication, antiretroviral therapy, and immunodeficiency in HIV-associated atherosclerosis. AIDS. 2009;23(9):1059–67.

47. Strategies for Management of Antiretroviral Therapy (SMART),Study Group, El-Sadr W, Lundgren J. CD4+ count-guided interruption of antiretroviral treatment. N Engl J Med. 2006;355:2283–96.

48. Boccara F, Teiger E, Cohen A, Ederhy S, Janower S, Odi G, et al. Percutaneous coronary intervention in HIV infected patients: immediate results and long term prognosis. Heart. 2006;92(4):543–4.

49. Ren X, Trilesskaya M, Kwan DM, Nguyen K, Shaw RE, Hui PY. Comparison of outcomes using bare metal versus drug-eluting stents in coronary artery disease patients with and without human immunodeficiency virus infection. Am J Cardiol. 2009;104(2):216–22.

50. Boccara F, Cohen A, Di Angelantonio E, Meuleman C, Ederhy S, Dufaitre G, et al. Coronary artery bypass graft in HIV-infected patients: a multicenter case control study. Curr HIV Res. 2008;6(1):59–64.

51. Dube MP, Stein JH, Aberg JA, Fichtenbaum CJ, Gerber JG, Tashima KT, et al. Guidelines for the evaluation and management of dyslipidemia in human immunodeficiency virus (HIV)-infected adults receiving antiretroviral therapy: recommendations of the HIV Medical Association of the Infectious Disease Society of America and the Adult AIDS Clinical Trials Group. Clin Infect Dis. 2003;37(5):613–27.

52. Chobanian AV, Bakris GL, Black HR, Cushman WC, Green LA, Izzo Jr JL, et al. The seventh report of the joint national committee on prevention, detection, evaluation, and treatment of high blood pressure: the JNC 7 report. JAMA. 2003;289(19):2560–72.

53. Soliman EZ, Princas RJ, Roediger MP, Duprez DA, Boccara F, Boesecke C, et al. Prevalence and prognostic significance of ECG abnormalities in HIV-infected patients: results from the Strategies for Management of Antiretroviral Therapy study. J Electrocardiol. 2011;44(6):779–85.

54. Thompson MA, Aberg JA, Cahn P, Montaner JS, Rizzardini G, Telenti A, et al. Antiretroviral treatment of adult HIV infection: 2010 recommendations of the International AIDS Society-USA panel. JAMA. 2010;304(3):321–33.

55. Butt AA, Chang CC, Kuller L, Goetz MB, Leaf D, Rimland D, et al. Risk of heart failure with human immunodeficiency virus in the absence of prior diagnosis of coronary heart disease. Arch Intern Med. 2011;171(8):737–43.

56. Schuster I, Thoni GJ, Ederhy S, Walther G, Nottin S, Vinet A, et al. Subclinical cardiac abnormalities in human immunodeficiency virus-infected men receiving antiretroviral therapy. Am J Cardiol. 2008;101(8):1213–7.

57. Sitbon O. HIV-related pulmonary arterial hypertension: clinical presentation and management. AIDS. 2008;22 Suppl 3:S55–62.

58. Degano B, Guillaume M, Savale L, Montani D, Jais X, Yaici A, et al. HIV-associated pulmonary arterial hypertension: survival and prognostic factors in the modern therapeutic era. AIDS. 2010;24(1):67–75.

59. Opravil M, Sereni D. Natural history of HIV-associated pulmonary arterial hypertension: trends in the HAART era. AIDS. 2008;22 Suppl 3:S35–40.

60. Almodovar S, Cicalini S, Petrosillo N, Flores SC. Pulmonary hypertension associated with HIV infection: pulmonary vascular disease: the global perspective. Chest. 2010;137(6 Suppl):6S–12.

61. Panel on antiretroviral guidelines for adults and adolescents. Guidelines for the use of antiretroviral agents in HIV-1 infected adults and adolescents. 2011. Available at: http://www.aidsinfo.nih.gov/contentfiles/AdultandAdolescentGL.pdf. Accessed 13 Aug 2011.

62. McLaughlin VV, Archer SL, Badesch DB, Barst RJ, Farber HW, Lindner JR, et al. ACCF/AHA. ACCF/AHA 2009 expert consensus document on pulmonary hypertension: a report of the American College of Cardiology Foundation Task Force on Expert Consensus Documents and the American Heart Association: developed in collaboration with the American College of Chest Physicians, American Thoracic Society, Inc., and the Pulmonary Hypertension Association. Circulation. 2009;119(16):2250–94.

63. Fisher SD, Kanda BS, Miller TL, Lipshultz SE. Cardiovascular disease and therapeutic drug-related cardiovascular consequences in HIV-infected patients. Am J Cardiovasc Drugs. 2011;11(6):383–94.

64. Li JS, Sexton DJ, Mick N, Nettles R, Fowler VG, Ryan T, et al. Proposed modifications to the Duke criteria for the diagnosis of infective endocarditis. Clin Infect Dis. 2000;30:633–8.

65. Chen Y, Brennessel D, Walters J, Johnson M, Rosner F, Raza M. Human immunodeficiency virus-associated pericardial effusion: report of 40 cases and review of the literature. Am Heart J. 1999;137(3):516–21.

66. Aguilar RV, Farber HW. Epoprostenol (prostacyclin) therapy in HIV-associated pulmonary hypertension. Am J Respir Crit Care Med. 2000;162(5):1846–50.

67. Degano B, Yaici A, Le Pavec J, Savale L, Jais X, Camara B, et al. Long-term effects of bosentan in patients with HIV-associated pulmonary arterial hypertension. Eur Respir J. 2009;33(1):92–8.

68. FDA. FDA drug safety communication: interactions between certain HIV or hepatitis C drugs and cholesterol-lowering statin drugs can increase the risk of muscle injury. 2012. Available at: http://www.fda.gov/Drugs/DrugSafety/ucm293877.htm#dose. Accessed 27 Apr 2012.

CHAPTER 30

Andreas C. Mauer and Shawn A. Gregory

Perioperative Cardiovascular Management

CHAPTER OUTLINE

ABBREVIATIONS

ACE	Angiotensin converting enzyme
CAD	Coronary artery disease
CVD	Cardiovascular disease
ECG	Electrocardiography
ICD	Implantable cardioverter defibrillator
INR	International normalized ratio
LAD	Left anterior descending
LV	Left ventricular
LVEF	Left ventricular ejection fraction
MI	Myocardial infarction
PAD	Peripheral artery disease
PCI	Percutaneous coronary intervention

INTRODUCTION

The cardiologist is frequently called upon to assist in the management of patients with cardiovascular disease in the perioperative setting. Questions surrounding risk stratification, risk management, diagnostic testing, management of cardiovascular medications, and revascularization, among others, are germane to the optimal management of such patients. The cardiovascular consultant must be prepared to approach these questions in a systematic and evidence-based fashion.

GENERAL APPROACH [1, 2]

- Define the question
- Establish urgency
- Gather primary data
- Provide concise recommendations
- Offer contingency plans
- Offer narrow recommendations within consultant's purview
- Educate, when appropriate
- Communicate directly
- Follow up on recommendations
- For the cardiovascular consultant:

    - Conduct history and physical examination
    - Consider ancillary testing
    - Stratify risk based on the above
    - Weigh strategies to reduce risk

RATIONALE FOR PERIOPERATIVE CARDIOVASCULAR CONSULTATION

A. Over one million cardiac complications, including 50,000 perioperative myocardial infarctions (MI), occur annually [3].

- Cardiac complications cause over 50 % of perioperative deaths
- Cardiac complications prolong hospitalization by a mean of 11 days
- Total cost: Over $20,000,000,000 annually [4]

HISTORY – ASSESS

- Personal and family history of cardiovascular disease
- Risk factors for cardiovascular disease

    - Hypertension
    - Hyperlipidemia
    - Smoking

- Symptoms suggestive of cardiovascular disease: chest pain; dyspnea; palpitations; syncope; edema
- Functional capacity (Fig. 30-1):
- Co-morbid disease

    - Pulmonary disease
    - Diabetes mellitus
    - Renal disease
    - Hematologic disorders

- Urgency and risk of procedure

    - If emergency noncardiac surgery is required (e.g., death or major complications are very likely or certain without surgery), proceed to surgery without further cardiovascular evaluation (Class IC)
    - If noncardiac surgery is not emergent, assess risk of surgery (Table 30-1):

- Further testing and/or therapy and as described below

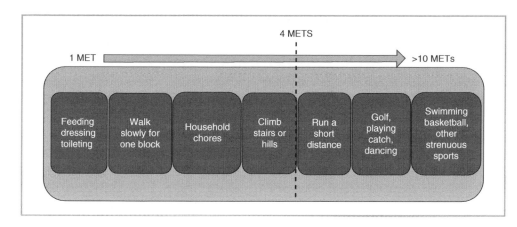

FIGURE 30-1

Functional capacity (Adapted from Fleisher et al. [2] and Hlatky et al. [5])

RISK CATEGORY	EXAMPLE
Vascular (reported cardiac risk often more than 5 %)	Aortic and other major vascular surgery Peripheral vascular surgery
Intermediate (reported cardiac risk generally 1–5 %)	Intraperitoneal and intrathoracic surgery Carotid endarterectomy Head and neck surgery Orthopedic surgery Prostate surgery
Low (reported cardiac risk generally less than 1 %)	Endoscopic procedures Superficial procedure Cataract surgery Breast surgery Ambulatory surgery

TABLE 30-1

RISK OF SURGERY

Adapted from Fleisher et al. [6]

PHYSICAL EXAMINATION (TABLE 30-2)

TABLE 30-2

PHYSICAL EXAMINATION IN PERI-OPERATIVE ASSESSMENT

EXAMINATION COMPONENT	FINDINGS THAT SHOULD PROMPT ADDITIONAL INVESTIGATION
Vital signs	Hypotension, hypertension, tachycardia, bradycardia
Carotid pulse	Bruits, abnormal pulse contour
Jugular venous pressure/pulse	Elevation or abnormal contour
Pulmonary auscultation	Crackles, wheezing; dullness to percussion suggestive of pleural effusion
Cardiac auscultation	Murmurs (particularly if loud, harsh, or associated with other findings suggestive of heart failure or other pathology), irregular rhythm
Peripheral pulses	Diminished (particularly if associated with bruits and/or limb discoloration)
Edema	If severe, unilateral, or associated with other findings of heart failure

PREOPERATIVE CARDIOVASCULAR TESTING

A. Electrocardiography (ECG)

- ■ Provides prognostic information in patients with active cardiac conditions, e.g., ischemia, arrhythmia
- ■ Preoperative 12-lead ECG is recommended for:
  - – Patients with known coronary artery disease (CAD), peripheral artery disease (PAD), or cardiovascular disease (CVD) undergoing intermediate-risk surgery (Class I)
  - – Patients with at least one clinical risk factor undergoing vascular surgery (e.g., hypertension, hyperlipidemia, smoking; Class I) [6]
- ■ Preoperative 12-lead ECG is NOT recommended for asymptomatic patients undergoing low-risk procedures (Class III) [7]

B. Noninvasive (Stress) Testing

- ■ Provides an objective measure of functional capacity; identifies myocardial ischemia; and estimates perioperative cardiac risk and long-term prognosis
- ■ Patients with active cardiac issues do <u>not</u> require testing; they should be treated for the active condition (Class I)
- ■ Noninvasive testing should <u>NOT</u> be performed in patients without clinical risk factors undergoing intermediate-risk surgery or in patients undergoing low-risk surgery (Class III)
- ■ Exercise stress test favored over other modalities, if possible; choice of adenosine/regadenason/dobutamine/dipyridamole and/or imaging depends on local expertise and patient characteristics (e.g., avoidance of dobutamine in patients with ventricular arrhythmia, avoidance of adenosine in patients with bronchospasm) [8]

C. Echocardiography

- ■ Provides a measure of left ventricular (LV) function; identifies and characterizes valvular disease

  - – May be indicated if:

    - ■ Physical examination or other data are suggestive of worsening or previously undiagnosed heart failure and/or valvular disease

- ■ Routine perioperative evaluation of LV function is of limited utility and is NOT recommended (Class III) [9]

PERIOPERATIVE MEDICATIONS

A. Beta-blockers

- ■ Initially thought to decrease perioperative ischemia in high-risk patients

  - – In early trials, dramatic reduction in early events [10]
  - – No difference for in-hospital morbidity/mortality but decreased morbidity/mortality at 2 years [11]

- ■ Subsequent studies less promising

  - – POBBLE, MaVS, DIPOM trials: no benefit [12–14]
  - – POISE: Largest study, high risk patients undergoing intermediate-to-high risk surgery; metoprolol reduced non-fatal MI but *increased* stroke and total mortality [15]

- ■ Salutary effects in patients with arrhythmia (e.g., rate control) and cardiomyopathy (e.g., neurohormonal blockade)
- ■ Beta -blockers are indicated in patients who:

  - – Are already receiving beta-blockers (Class I)
  - – Are high risk and undergoing vascular surgery (Class I)

- Beta -blockers are NOT indicated in patients with:

  - Absolute contraindication(s) to beta blockade (Class III)

B. Antiplatelet Agents

- Aspirin

  - Indicated in patients with known CVD, unless absolutely contraindicated
  - Should not be routinely discontinued prior to surgery

- Thienopyridines (Clopidogrel, Prasugrel, Ticagrelor; ADP receptor/P2Y12 blockade)

  - Should not be discontinued for: 4 weeks after percutaneous balloon angioplasty; 4–6 weeks after bare metal stent deployment; 12 months after drug eluting stent deployment
  - In the event that surgery is required earlier, bridging can be instituted with an intravenous glycoprotein IIa/IIIb inhibitor

C. Anticoagulation

- In patients with atrial fibrillation/flutter, mechanical valves, or known cardiac or systemic thrombi
- Aspirin should be continued
- Warfarin should be discontinued at least 5 days before surgery and the international normalized ratio (INR) should be monitored before surgery

  - Reversal with fresh frozen plasma (acutely) and/or vitamin K (subacutely)

- Newer agents, e.g., dabigatran, apixaban, should be discontinued at least two half-lives before surgery

  - If bridging is necessary, low molecular weight or unfractionated heparin can be used

- Preoperative bridging with low molecular weight heparin or unfractionated heparin depending on thrombotic risk and outpatient/inpatient setting

  - Bridging should be strongly considered in patients with mechanical valve replacements and/or prior thromboembolic stroke

- Postoperative resumption depending on postsurgical bleeding risk

  - In the event of epidural anesthesia, anticoagulation should not be resumed until epidural catheter has been removed

D. Statins

- Have been associated with significant reduction in perioperative reduction; magnitude of benefit likely greatest in high-risk patients [16, 17]

  - Benefit extends to patients not previously on statins [18]
  - Important caveat: above studies are retrospective or from small trials

- Should be continued in patients already taking statins (Class I)

E. Angiotensin converting enzyme (ACE)-inhibitors/Angiotensin II receptor blockers (ARB)

- Should be continued in patients already taking these agents, unless prohibited by hypotension
- Caution is advised when epidural anesthesia is used due to profound hypotension

CORONARY REVASCULARIZATION

A. Indications = same as if patient were not going to surgery, i.e.:

- Stable angina with significant left main coronary stenosis (Class I)
- Stable angina with 3-vessel disease (Class I)

■ Stable angina with 2-vessel disease with significant proximal left anterior descending (LAD) stenosis and either left ventricular ejection fraction (LVEF) <50 % or ischemia on noninvasive testing (Class I)

■ Patients with high-risk unstable angina, non-ST elevation MI, or ST-elevation MI (Class I)

■ In observational studies, patients with recent revascularization for standard indications (i.e., not perioperative) reduces risk for subsequent surgery [19, 20]

B. NOT indicated for:

■ Routine prophylactic revascularization in patients with stable CAD (Class III)

- Increased risk of in-stent thrombosis and sequelae when surgery is performed in immediate post-percutaneous coronary intervention (PCI) period [21, 22]

- CARP trial demonstrated no immediate or long-term benefit to revascularization for stable CAD (>70 % stenosis of at least one coronary artery) [23]

C. Elective surgery is NOT recommended within 4 weeks of balloon angioplasty, 4–6 weeks of bare metal stent implantation, or 12 months of drug-eluting stent implantation (Class III)

■ Thienopyridines can be discontinued after the above times have elapsed

■ Aspirin should NOT be discontinued before elective surgery in patients with CAD

SPECIAL TOPICS

A. Arrhythmia

■ Supraventricular Arrhythmia

- In stable supraventricular arrhythmia, rate-control strategy with digoxin, beta-blockers or calcium channel blockers

- Cardioversion (and/or rarely, electrophysiology study with catheter ablation) in selected patients with hemodynamic instability particularly for easily ablatable arrhythmias, such as atrial flutter.

■ Ventricular Arrhythmia

- Routine therapy not indicated in the absence of high-grade arrhythmia, hemodynamic compromise or ongoing ischemia

- Consider assessment of LVEF

- Consider initiation of beta blockade, if patient is not already taking

B. Heart Failure/Cardiomyopathy

■ Judicious use of intra- and post-operative intravenous fluids

■ Diuresis as needed; patients with longstanding diuretic use may require higher doses of loop diuretics

■ Continued use or early resumption of afterload reduction and beta blockade when hemodynamically stable

- Particular caution is advised with re-initiation of vasodilators when epidural anesthesia is used

■ Consider preoperative placement of pulmonary artery catheter in patients with severe and/or unstable heart failure (Class IIb)

C. Valvular Heart Disease

■ Routine assessment of valvular function and/or intervention is not indicated

■ In patients with severe aortic and/or mitral regurgitation, LV afterload should be optimized with vasodilators

■ In patients with severe aortic and/or mitral stenosis, percutaneous catheter balloon valvulotomy may be considered as a bridge to definitive treatment

■ Consider invasive hemodynamic monitoring (e.g., pulmonary artery catheter) in patients with significant valvular heart disease (Class IIb)

D. Implantable cardioverter defibrillators (ICD) and pacemakers

■ Routine preoperative pacemaker implantation not indicated in the absence of standard indications

■ Electrocautery may interfere with devices, leading to:

– Device reset to default mode
– Inhibition of pacemaker output
– False sensing with increased pacemaker rate
– ICD firing
– Myocardial injury with lead failure

■ Recommendations

– Devices should be evaluated/interrogated preoperatively
– Pacemakers should be reprogrammed to asynchronous mode or a magnet should be placed over the device during surgery to create VOO mode.
– For ICD's, tachyarrhythmia algorithms should be deactivated during surgery, with reactivation postoperatively
– Bipolar electrocautery should be used and its use minimized.
– The distance between electrocautery and implanted device should be maximized.

INTEGRATED APPROACH (FIG. 30-2)

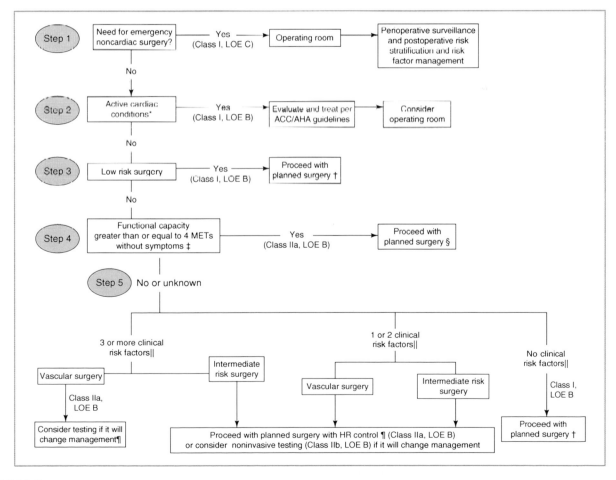

FIGURE 30-2

Integrated approach to peri-operative assessment (From Fleisher et al. [2])

POSTOPERATIVE MANAGEMENT

A. MI surveillance

- An ECG should be performed immediately postoperatively and on postoperative days 1 and 2 [24]
- Troponin measurement

    - Indicated with typical chest pain or ECG changes (Class I)
    - NOT indicated in asymptomatic patients after low-risk surgery (Class III)

B. Arrhythmia

- Standard diagnostic algorithms apply
- Treatment directed at underlying cause
- Electrolyte, acid/base, and volume abnormalities more common in immediate postoperative period

REVIEW QUESTIONS

1. You are asked to consult on a 75-year-old woman with a past medical history of hypothyroidism and hypertension who is now presenting with a hip fracture and will be taken to the operating room for urgent open reduction and internal fixation. At baseline, she has no dyspnea or chest pain and walks two city blocks to the grocery store several times a week. Her blood pressure is 125/70 mmHg and the heart rate is 75 bpm. Cardiovascular auscultation discloses a soft, non-radiating, II/VI systolic ejection murmur at the base. Her medications include levothyroxine and hydrochlorothiazide. Laboratory studies are notable for an LDL of 110 mg/dL, HDL 55 mg/dL. What is the next step?
    (a) Initiate metoprolol.
    (b) Initiate atorvastatin.
    (c) Order an echocardiogram.
    (d) Order a pharmacologic stress test.
    (e) Allow her to proceed to surgery without any additional interventions.

2. You are asked to consult on a 66 year old man with a history of CAD, hypertension, hyperlipidemia, and ischemic cardiomyopathy with a LVEF of 30 % who has been newly diagnosed with PAD after ankle-brachial indices were performed due to claudication with exertion. He is scheduled to undergo femoral-popliteal bypass surgery. He underwent cardiac catheterization for a non-ST elevation MI 9 months ago with implantation of a drug-eluting stent. His medications include carvedilol, losartan, pravastatin, furosemide, clopidogrel, and aspirin. On physical examination, he appears euvolemic without lower extremity edema has a regular rate and rhythm without murmurs, and has an ICD. He does not have any angina, but his activity is limited to ambulating about two blocks due to lower extremity pain. Laboratory studies are notable for HDL 40 mg/dL and LDL 130 mg/dL. What do you recommend?
    (a) Order a pharmacologic stress test.
    (b) Order an exercise stress test with perfusion imaging.
    (c) Delay surgery for at least 3 months.
    (d) Delay surgery for at least 6 months.
    (e) Allow him to proceed to surgery without any additional interventions.

3. The above patient's surgery is delayed due to a death in the family, and he returns to your office a year later requesting "clearance" for surgery next month. What is the most important modification to make in the immediate preoperative period?
    (a) Discontinue aspirin.
    (b) Discontinue clopidogrel.
    (c) Discontinue losartan.
    (d) Intensify statin therapy.
    (e) Turn off his ICD.

ANSWERS

1. (e) Allow her to proceed to surgery without additional interventions. This patient has one risk factor for coronary artery disease (hypertension). However, her surgery is urgent, and she is able to routinely perform activities in excess of 4 METS. Therefore, additional testing is not indicated, especially since it may delay her needed surgery. Initiation of perioperative metoprolol is not likely to be beneficial. Statins may be beneficial in high-risk patients, and should be continued in patients who are already taking this class of medication, but there is no convincing evidence that this relatively low-risk patient would benefit.

2. (c) Delay surgery for at least 3 months. This patient has recently revascularized CAD without evidence of ongoing ischemia; therefore, there is no indication for additional testing. He is on an appropriate medical regimen, his heart failure is well-compensated, and an ICD has (appropriately) been placed. However, a drug-eluting stent was placed 9 months ago, mandating at least an additional 3 months of clopidogrel. Though his indication for surgery (claudication) is not urgent, it is not necessary to delay surgery for 6 additional months.

3. (b) Discontinue clopidogrel. Since more than a full year has elapsed since stenting was performed, clopidogrel can be safely discontinued, thereby reducing the patient's bleeding risk during surgery. Aspirin should not be routinely discontinued prior to surgery. ACE inhibitors and ARB's are typically discontinued the day of surgery, but there is no need to discontinue losartan a month before surgery. The patient's LDL is not at goal for a patient with known coronary artery disease, but intensifying statin therapy is less important than discontinuing clopidogrel in the preoperative period. The patient's device should be interrogated and tachyarrhythmia treatment algorithms should be turned off on the day of surgery.

REFERENCES

1. Goldman L, Lee T, Rudd P. Ten commandments for effective consultations. Arch Intern Med. 1983;143(9):1753–5

2. Fleisher LA, Beckman JA, Brown KA, Calkins H, Chaikof E, Fleischmann KE, et al. ACC/AHA 2007 guidelines on perioperative cardiovascular evaluation and care for noncardiac surgery: executive summary: a report of the American College of Cardiology/American Heart Association Task Force on Practice Guidelines. Circulation. 2007;116(17):e418–99. Epub 2007 Sep 27.

3. Fleischmann KE, Goldman L, Young B, Lee TH. Association between cardiac and noncardiac complications in patients undergoing noncardiac surgery: outcomes and effects on length of stay. Am J Med. 2003;115(7):515–20.

4. Mangano DT. Perioperative cardiac morbidity. Anesthesiology. 1990;72(1):153–84.

5. Hlatky MA, Boineau RE, Higginbotham MB, Lee KL, Mark DB, Califf RF, et al. A brief self-administered questionnaire to determine functional capacity (the Duke Activity Status Index) Am J Cardiol. 1989;64:651–4.

6. Landesberg G, Einav S, Christopherson R, et al. Perioperative ischemia and cardiac complications in major vascular surgery: importance of the preoperative twelve-lead electrocardiogram. J Vasc Surg. 1997;26:570–8.

7. Liu LL, Dzankic S, Leung JM. Preoperative electrocardiogram abnormalities do not predict postoperative cardiac complications in geriatric surgical patients. J Am Geriatr Soc. 2002; 50:1186–91.

8. Kertai MD, Boersma E, Bax JJ, Heijenbrok-Kal MH, Hunink MG, L'talien GJ, et al. A meta-analysis comparing the prognostic accuracy of six diagnostic tests for predicting perioperative cardiac risk in patients undergoing major vascular surgery. Heart. 2003;89(11):1327–34.

9. Rohde LE, Polanczyk CA, Goldman L, Cook EF, Lee RT, Lee TH. Usefulness of transthoracic echocardiography as a tool for risk stratification of patients undergoing major noncardiac surgery. Am J Cardiol. 2001;87(5):505–9.

10. Poldermans D, Boersma E, Bax JJ, Thomson IR, van de Ven LL, Blankensteijn JD, et al. The effect of bisoprolol on perioperative mortality and myocardial infarction in high-risk patients undergoing vascular surgery. N Engl J Med. 1999;341(24):1789–94.

11. Mangano DT, Layug EL, Wallace A, Tateo I. Effect of atenolol on mortality and cardiovascular morbidity after noncardiac surgery. N Engl J Med. 1996;335(23):1713–20.

12. Brady AR, Gibbs JS, Greenhalgh RM, Powell JT, Sydes MR. POBBLE Trial Investigators. Perioperative beta-blockade (POBBLE) for patients undergoing infrarenal vascular surgery: results of a randomized double-blind controlled trial. J Vasc Surg. 2005;41(4):602–9.

13. Yang H, Raymer K, Butler R, Parlow J, Roberts R. The effects of perioperative beta-blockade: results of the Metoprolol after Vascular Surgery (MaVS) study, a randomized controlled trial. Am Heart J. 2006;152(5):983–90.

14. Juul AB, Wetterslev J, Gluud C, Kofoed-Enevoldsen A, Jensen G, Callesen T, et al. Effect of perioperative beta blockade in patients with diabetes undergoing major non-cardiac surgery: randomised placebo controlled, blinded multicentre trial. BMJ. 2006; 332(7556):1482.

15. POISE Study Group, Devereaux PJ, Yang H, Yusuf S, Guyatt G, Leslie K, et al. Effects of extended-release metoprolol succinate in patients undergoing non-cardiac surgery (POISE trial): a randomised controlled trial. Lancet. 2008;371(9627):1839–47.

TABLE 31-1

CARDIAC INVOLVEMENT IN RHEUMATIC DISEASES

Disease frequency

Common ↕ Rare

	Pericarditis	Myocarditis/ CHF	Conduction disease	Valvular disease	Aortic disease	Pulmonary HTN	CAD
Lyme	Occasional	Occasional	Common				
Rheumatoid arthritis	Rare	Rare					Common
SLE	Common	Occasional		Occasional			Common
Giant cell arteritis							
Ankylosing spondylitis			Rare	Occasional			
Scleroderma	Rare	Common	Occasional			Common	
Sarcoidosis			Occasional				
Kawasaki		Occasional		Occasional			Common
Takayasu's	Occasional				Common		Occasional
Adult onset still's disease	Common						
Churg strauss syndrome	Rare	Common					Rare

LYME DISEASE

A. **Clinical presentation**
   - Early localized disease – erythema migrans rash, arthralgias (without joint effusions) and constitutional symptoms.
   - Early disseminated disease – cranial neuropathies, meningitis and peripheral neuropathy.
   - Late disseminated disease – large joint arthritis (with effusions), encephalopathy, peripheral neuropathy.

B. **Cardiac manifestations – occur in early disseminated disease (1–2 months after the onset of symptoms) in 1.5–10 % of untreated patients [1].**
   - Atrioventricular (AV) block is most common, present in 20–50 % of patients, with up to 30 % of symptomatic patients requiring temporary pacing.
   - Myopericarditis may be present but tends to be relatively mild with <15 % of patients demonstrating signs of heart failure and only mild left ventricular systolic dysfunction.

C. **Diagnosis**
   - Lyme antibody confirmed by Western blot.

D. **Treatment**
   - Mild manifestations (First degree AV block) – Doxycycline for 4 weeks.
   - Severe manifestations (Second or Third degree AV block) – Ceftriaxone for 4 weeks.

RHEUMATOID ARTHRITIS (RA)

A. **Clinical presentation**
   - Women>men, incidence highest 50–70 years old.
   - Articular manifestations – symmetric, polyarticular arthritis.
   - Extra-articular manifestations – nodules (skin and lung), pleuritis, interstitial lung disease (ILD), scleritis.

B. **Cardiac manifestations**
   - Coronary artery disease (CAD) – patients with RA have increased incidence of MI and mortality from cardiovascular disease [2].
   - Pericarditis and myocarditis – occur in <1 % of patients, usually in those with seropositive, erosive disease.

C. **Diagnosis**
   - Rheumatoid factor (RF; less specific) or anti-cyclic citrullinated peptide antibody (anti-CCP; more specific). Combined sensitivity ~80 %.
   - Joint erosions on radiographs.

D. **Treatment**
  - CAD – treatment of RA may improve cardiovascular outcomes [3].
  - Pericarditis/myocarditis – prednisone 1 mg/kg ± steroid sparing immunomodulator.

SYSTEMIC LUPUS ERYTHEMATOSUS (SLE)

A. **Clinical Presentation**
  - Women > men, incidence highest 30–50 years old
  - Skin disease – malar rash, photosensitivity, discoid rash
  - Oral ulcers
  - Arthritis – two or more swollen and tender joints
  - Serositis – pleuritis or pericarditis
  - Renal involvement – proteinuria
  - Neurologic involvement – seizures or psychosis
  - Hematologic – leucopenia, thrombocytopenia or hemolytic anemia
  - Antiphospholipid syndrome – arterial or venous thrombosis, thrombocytopenia, second-trimester pregnancy losses

B. **Cardiac manifestations**
  - CAD – patients at increased risk for myocardial infarction (MI) and cardiovascular mortality independent of traditional risk factors [4].
  - Pericarditis – most common cardiac manifestation occurring in 20–50 % of patients. Tamponade is rare (<10 %) [5].
  - Valvulitis – manifests as nodules or sterile vegetations (Libman-Sacks endocarditis) on aortic and mitral valves in 3–19 % of patients undergoing echocardiography [5]. Patients with high-titer antiphospholipid antibodies are at higher risk.
  - Myocarditis – <10 % of patients [6]. Typically occurs with other disease manifestations. Rarely initial manifestation.

C. **Diagnosis**
  - Clinical diagnosis. Most patients meet 4 of 11 classification criteria which include clinical manifestations (listed above) and the following:

    Antinuclear antibody (ANA) positivity (>95 % of patients)
    - Positive antibodies – anti-Smith or double-stranded DNA antibody or positive tests for antiphospholipid antibodies (aPL).

      - Optimal testing for aPL includes:

        - Anticardiolipin antibodies
        - Lupus anticoagulant assay
        - Anti-beta-2-glycoprotein I antibodies

It is worth noting that the classification criteria are not diagnostic criteria, and some patients have SLE without fulfilling the classification criteria. Conversely, other patients fulfill classification criteria but do not have SLE.

D. **Treatment**
  - Pericarditis – Non-steroidal anti-inflammatory drugs (NSAIDs) and low dose corticosteroids if NSAID refractory.
  - Valvulitis – anticoagulation if thrombotic events.
  - Myocarditis – high dose corticosteroids ± another immunosuppressive agent.

GIANT CELL ARTERITIS

A. **Clinical manifestations**
  - Occurs in individuals >50 years old.
  - Fever, headache, visual changes, jaw claudication, shoulder/hip girdle stiffness and pain.

FIGURE 31-1

Conventional angiogram from a patient with giant cell arteritis. There are several long, smooth stenoses of the left subclavian artery. Multiple collateral blood vessels are seen in the region of the shoulder. Such a patient will have greatly diminished or absent pulses in the arm but ample blood flow even to the distal extremity because of the collaterals. Re-vascularization attempts are usually not indicated, ineffective, and ill-advised

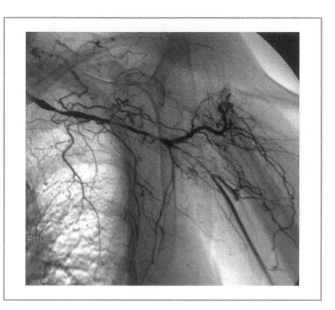

B. **Cardiac manifestations**
- Aortitis – 18 %, thoracic > abdominal, 5 % with dissection [7].
- Large vessel vasculitis – 13 %, leading to symptomatic stenosis (most commonly arm claudication) [7] (Fig. 31-1).
- Coronary ischemia due to ostial left main and/or right coronary obstruction.

C. **Diagnosis**
- Temporal artery biopsy demonstrating granulomatous vasculitis.
- Erythrocyte sedimentation rate elevated in 96 % [8].

D. **Treatment**
- Prednisone 1 mg/kg. ± Aspirin 81mg

ANKYLOSING SPONDYLITIS

A. **Clinical presentation**
- Men > women, incidence highest 20–30 years old.
- Axial symptoms – low back/buttock pain due to sacroiliitis (worse with rest).
- Peripheral symptoms – asymmetric lower extremity oligoarthritis and enthesitis.
- Extraarticular symptoms – uveitis, inflammatory bowel disease.

B. **Cardiac manifestations**
- Aortic regurgitation – 5–13 % of patients (typically mild) [5].
- Conduction abnormalities – ECG abnormalities in up to 20 %, but symptomatic AV block rare [5].

C. **Diagnosis**
- Sacroiliitis on radiographs (less sensitive) or magnetic resonance imaging MRI (more sensitive).
- 90 % are human leukocyte antigen (HLA) B27 positive.

D. **Treatment**
- Immunosuppression has no role in treating cardiac manifestations.

SYSTEMIC SCLEROSIS (SCLERODERMA)

A. **Clinical presentation**
- Women > men, incidence highest 30–50 years old.
- Diffuse form: skin thickening involves trunk, face and extremities. Raynaud's phenomenon, interstitial lung disease, renal and gastrointestinal (GI) dysmotility.

■ Limited form (CREST syndrome): skin thickening limited to extremities, Raynaud's phenomenon, GI dysmotility, interstitial lung disease, calcinosis.

B. Cardiac manifestations

■ Pulmonary hypertension – most common in limited disease (8–20 %).

■ Conduction disease – ECG abnormalities in 25–75 %, but symptomatic AV block is rare (<2 %) [9].

■ Diastolic dysfunction in ~30 % due to myocardial fibrosis [10].

■ Pericarditis – clinically significant pericarditis is uncommon (0–15 %) [5].

C. Diagnosis

■ Skin thickening in the proper clinical setting.

■ Diffuse form – positive ANA, anti-topoisomerase 3 (Scl-70) present in 30 % [11].

■ Limited form– positive ANA, anti-centromere present in 70–80 % [11].

D. Treatment

■ Symptomatic treatment only. Immunomodulatory agents are unlikely to benefit cardiac manifestations.

SARCOIDOSIS

A. Clinical manifestations

■ Incidence highest 20–40 years old, more often African Americans.

■ Can involve any organ but pulmonary symptoms (up to 90 %), arthritis, skin lesions and ocular inflammation are most common.

B. Diagnosis

■ Typically a tissue diagnosis.

■ Hilar lymphadenopathy ± interstitial lung disease present in the majority of patients.

■ Histology demonstrating non-caseating granulomas (endomyocardial biopsy not sensitive as cardiac involvement is patchy and frequently in the region of the mitral or tricuspid annulus, where biopsy frequently cannot reach) (Fig. 31-2).

■ Serum angiotensin converting enzyme concentrations have poor sensitivity and specificity and do not supplant tissue diagnosis as the gold standard for diagnosis.

■ Echocardiography may show thickened myocardium, LV systolic and diastolic dysfunction.

■ Cardiac MRI may reveal diffusely increased myocardial signal on T2 weighted images with heterogenous distribution.

■ [67]Gallium or [201]thallium scans have been traditionally used to identify the presence of sarcoid lesions in the myocardium, although neither is specific to the diagnosis. [18]Fluoro-2-deoxy-d-glucose positron emission tomography may be of use.

C. Cardiac manifestations

■ 5 % have AV block or ventricular arrhythmias [12].

■ Sudden death from myocardial and conduction system disease is a substantial cause of morbidity and mortality.

D. Treatment

■ Prednisone 1 mg/kg or other immunomodulatory for refractory disease.

■ Anti tumor necrosis alpha (TNF) agents for refractory disease.

■ Automatic implantable cardioverter-defibrillator placement prophylactically can be considered in patients with known myocardial involvement.

KAWASAKI DISEASE [13]

A. Clinical manifestations

■ Initial illness is typically self-limited but can be severe.

■ Fever, mucositis (strawberry tongue), bilateral conjunctivitis and erythematous rash on hands and feet are present in the majority of patients. Cervical lymphadenopathy may be present.

B. Cardiac manifestations

■ Coronary artery aneurysms occur in up to 25 % of untreated patients leading to acute coronary syndrome, arrhythmias and sudden death.

FIGURE 31-2

Granulomatous inflammation within the myocardium of a patient with sarcoidosis. Several multinucleated giant cells without caseating features are shown

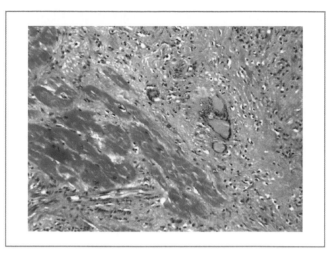

- Coronary artery aneurysms formed during the acute childhood illness sometimes thrombose later in life, leading to myocardial infarction.
- Less common manifestations not related to CAD include mitral regurgitation due to valvulitis and heart failure with impaired ejection fraction in the acute setting.

C. **Diagnosis**
- Clinical diagnosis based on findings of fever, mucosal involvement, conjunctivitis, rash and lymphadenopathy.

D. **Treatment**
- Intravenous immune globulin (IVIG) prevents cardiac complications.
- Benefit of corticosteroids is unproven.

TAKAYASU'S ARTERITIS [14]

A. **Clinical manifestations**
- 90 % are women less than 40 years old. Most prevalent in Asian populations.
- Fever, arthralgias, fatigue, and increased acute phase reactants during the "inflammatory" phase.
- Claudication and long-term complications of vascular stenosis during the "stenotic" phase.

B. **Cardiac manifestations**
- Vasculitis leading to stenosis >> aneurysm.

  - The classic lesion in Takayasu's is a long, smooth narrowing of the subclavian arteries.
  - Thoracic aortic branch vasculitis may lead to arm claudication and diminished or absent distal pulses in the upper extremities, although lower extremity involvement is possible.
  - Abdominal aortic involvement may lead to renovascular hypertension or occlusion of the abdominal aorta.
  - Carotid and vertebral artery involvement leads to central nervous system (CNS) symptoms, including retinal arterial occlusions, which may lead to characteristic changes.
  - Pulmonary artery involvement may occur in <5 %, leading to pulmonary infarction.

- Aortic insufficiency due to AV root dilatation (20 %).
- Angina (~10 %) due to coronary artery vasculitis or obstruction involving the ostia of the left main or right coronary artery.
- Hypertension may be extremely difficult to detect because involvement of the arteries to all four limbs can make peripheral blood pressure measurements inaccurate. Central aortic catheterization may be required to assess blood pressure accurately.

■ Heart failure due to severe hypertension and/or valvular/coronary involvement.
■ Pericarditis (<1 %).

C. **Diagnosis**
■ Vascular imaging demonstrating narrowing and occlusion of large arteries not explained by other causes (such as fibromuscular dysplasia, Ehlers-Danlos syndrome or segmental arterial mediolysis).
■ Histologically similar in appearance to giant cell arteritis.

D. **Treatment**
■ Prednisone 1 mg/kg.
■ ~50 % require addition of another immunomodulator.
■ Angioplasty or surgical intervention may be required.

ADULT ONSET STILL'S DISEASE [15]

A. **Clinical manifestations**
■ Disease onset typically 16–35 years old.
■ Cyclic (quotidian) fever, salmon-colored rash with fevers, arthritis, hepatitis and serositis.

B. **Cardiac manifestations**
■ Pericarditis in 25 % of patients.

C. **Diagnosis**
■ Clinical diagnosis. Markedly elevated ferritin (70 %) and elevated hepatic aminotransferases (75 %) are typically present.

D. **Treatment**
■ Prednisone 1 mg/kg
■ Interleukin-1 receptor or interleukin-6 receptor blockade if refractory to prednisone.

CHURG STRAUSS SYNDROME (CSS)

A. **Clinical manifestations**
■ Occurs primarily in patients with asthma and eosinophilia.
■ Fever, arthralgias, peripheral neuropathy and skin lesions (Fig. 31-3).

B. **Cardiac manifestations [16]**
■ Cardiac abnormalities are the most common cause of morbidity in CSS, affecting 40–60 % of patients.
■ Heart failure is the most common cardiac manifestation – ~60 % have endomyocarditis, ~70 % have valvular abnormalities.
■ Pericardial effusions can be seen in ~40 % but are frequently asymptomatic.
■ Coronary artery vasculitis (<1 %).

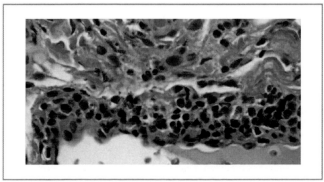

FIGURE 31-3

Skin biopsy from a patient with Churg-Strauss syndrome who presented with focal areas of palpable purpura and ulceration on the lower extremities. The biopsy demonstrates extensive eosinophilic infiltration of the blood vessel wall

C. **Diagnosis**
   ■ Eosinophilia (100 % of patients) and positive anti-neutrophil cytoplasmic antibodies (ANCA) (~50 % of patients) or tissue diagnosis.
D. **Treatment**
   ■ Significant cardiac involvement requires high-dose corticosteroids and cyclophosphamide.
   ■ Rituximab may be useful if corticosteroid or cyclophosphamide refractory.

REVIEW QUESTIONS

1. 35 year old man with chronic low back pain is referred by his primary care physician for an evaluation of a murmur. Physical examination reveals a heart rate of 80 beats per minute (bpm) and blood pressure 116/74 mmHg. A III/VI early diastolic murmur with a blowing, decrescendo quality is heard over the left lower sternal border. There are no gallops. There is no joint pain, laxity or swelling. Examination of the back reveals loss of the normal lumbar lordosis and tenderness of both sacroiliac joints. The erythrocyte sedimentation rate is 28 mm/h (normal < 15). Complete blood count and chemistry profile are unremarkable. Which of the following is likely to confirm the diagnosis?
   (a) Blood cultures
   (b) HLA-B27 testing
   (c) Ambulatory blood pressure monitoring
   (d) Slit lamp eye exam
   (e) Fluorescent treponemal antibody testing

2. A 66 year-old man with a history of asthma presents to the Emergency Department with dyspnea. His temperature is 100.8 °F, pulse is 110 bpm, blood pressure 106/48 mmHg, and oxygen saturation 98 % on 4 l nasal cannula. Examination reveals a jugular venous pressure of 11 cm, bibasilar crackles, a purpuric rash on both lower extremities, and decreased sensation in the right hand up to the wrist. Laboratory evaluation is as follows:

WBC	9.4 th/cmm
Hgb	10 g/dL
Hct	30.6 %
Platelets	468 th/cmm
Neutrophils	55 %
Lymphocytes	20 %
Eosinophils	25 %
Monoctyes	0 %
Basophils	0 %
Sodium	140 mmol/L
Potassium	4.2 mmol/L
Chloride	106 mmol/L
Carbon Dioxide	24 mmol/L
BUN	38 mg/dL
Creatinine	1.7 mg/dL

Urinalysis – 3+ blood, 2+ protein, nitrite and leukocyte esterase negative

What diagnostic test is most likely to confirm the diagnosis?
(a) Echocardiography
(b) Cardiac catheterization with myocardial biopsy
(c) ANCA testing
(d) Skin biopsy
(e) Nerve conduction studies

3. A 67 year old woman with a history of hypertension and hyperlipidemia presents with right arm pain. Over the past several months she has experienced arm pain with activity that resolves with rest. She denies chest pain and shortness of breath. She has also noticed headaches and bilateral hip pain. Examination reveals temperature 99.2 °F, pulse 68 bpm, and blood pressure 95/66 on the right arm and 130/68 on the left arm. Cardiac examination is unremarkable. No bruits are audible. Radial and brachial pulses are absent on the right. Erythrocyte sedimentation rate is 68 mm/h. Angiography reveals stenosis of the right subclavian artery and a 3.5 cm thoracic aortic aneurysm. Which of the following is the most likely diagnosis?
(a) Atherosclerosis
(b) Takayasu's arteritis
(c) Segmental arterial mediolysis
(d) Giant cell arteritis
(e) Ehlers-Danlos syndrome

4. A 45 year old female with a history of gastroesophageal reflux disease and constipation presents to the Emergency Department with dyspnea. Heart rate is 95 bpm, blood pressure 145/76 and oxygen saturation 94 % on 2 l nasal cannula. Examination reveals jugular venous pressure of 12 cm, an S4 gallop, bibasilar crackles and thickened skin over both hands, extending up to the elbows. There is also tight skin over her chest and abdomen. The patient is unable to close her hands completely. Laboratories reveal troponin I 0.1 (ref < 0.06). ECG demonstrates left ventricular hypertrophy and t-wave inversions in leads II, II, V4 and V5. What is the likely etiology of her heart failure?
(a) Acute coronary syndrome
(b) Hypertension
(c) Myocardial fibrosis
(d) Myocarditis
(e) Constrictive pericarditis

ANSWERS

1. (b) Chronic back pain with bilateral sacroiliac tenderness in a young man raises suspicion for ankylosing spondylitis (AS). Aortic regurgitation is seen in up to 13 % of patients with AS. 90 % of patients with AS are HLA-B27 positive. Sacroiliitis on plain film or MRI would also be suggestive AS.

2. (d) This patient's heart failure is likely due to myocarditis from Churg Strauss syndrome as evidence by petechial rash, neurologic findings, renal disease, eosinophilia and history of asthma. Anti-neutrophil cytoplasmic antibodies (ANCA) are positive in some patients with Churg-Strauss, but less than 50 % in some series. A skin biopsy of the purpuric lesions would demonstrate leukocytoclastic vasculitis with intensive eosinophil infiltration confirming the diagnosis.

3. (d) Headaches, hip pain and elevated inflammatory markers in a patient older than 50 years of age is suggestive of giant cell arteritis (GCA) which can lead to large vessel vasculitis in up to 20 % of patients with the disease. Takayasu's arteritis, which can cause a similar large vessel vasculitis to GCA, is made less likely by the patient's age.

4. (c) This patient is likely suffering from scleroderma as evidenced by skin thickening and gastrointestinal dysmotility. Diastolic dysfunction is a well-described manifestation of scleroderma, and occurs most commonly due to myocardial fibrosis.

REFERENCES

1. Rostoff P, Gajos G, Konduracka E, Gackowski A, Nessler J, Piwowarska W. Lyme carditis: epidemiology, pathophysiology, and clinical features in endemic areas. Int J Cardiol. 2010;144(2): 328–33.

2. Maradit-Kremers H, Crowson CS, Nicola PJ, et al. Increased unrecognized coronary heart disease and sudden deaths in rheumatoid arthritis: a population-based cohort study. Arthritis Rheum. 2005; 52(2):402–11.

3. Greenberg JD, Kremer JM, Curtis JR, et al. Tumour necrosis factor antagonist use and associated risk reduction of cardiovascular events among patients with rheumatoid arthritis. Ann Rheum Dis. 2011;70:576–82.

4. Esdaile JM, Abrahamowicz M, Grodzicky T, et al. Traditional Framingham risk factors fail to fully account for accelerated atherosclerosis in systemic lupus erythematosus. Arthritis Rheum. 2001;44:2331–7.

5. Roman MJ, Salmon JE. Cardiovascular manifestations of rheumatologic diseases. Circulation. 2007;116(20):2346–55.

6. Wijetunga M, Rockson S. Myocarditis in systemic lupus erythematosus. Am J Med. 2002;113:419–23.

7. Nuenninghoff DM, Hunder GG, Christianson TJ, McClelland RL, Matteson EL. Incidence and predictors of large-artery complication (aortic aneurysm, aortic dissection, and/or large-artery stenosis) in patients with giant cell arteritis: a population-based study over 50 years. Arthritis Rheum. 2003;48:3522–31.

8. Smetana GW, Shmerling RH. Does this patient have temporal arteritis? JAMA. 2002;287:92–101.

9. Seferović PM, Ristić AD, Maksimović R, et al. Cardiac arrhythmias and conduction disturbances in autoimmune rheumatic diseases. Rheumatology (Oxford). 2006;45 Suppl 4:iv39–42.

10. Meune C, Avouac J, Wahbi K, et al. Cardiac involvement in systemic sclerosis assessed by tissue-Doppler echocardiography during routine care: a controlled study of 100 consecutive patients. Arthritis Rheum. 2008;58(6):1803–9.

11. Reveille JD, Solomon DH. Evidence-based guidelines for the use of immunologic tests: anticentromere, Scl-70, and nucleolar antibodies. Arthritis Rheum. 2003;49(3):399–412.

12. Statement on sarcoidosis. Joint Statement of the American Thoracic Society (ATS), the European Respiratory Society (ERS) and the World Association of Sarcoidosis and Other Granulomatous Disorders (WASOG) adopted by the ATS Board of Directors and by the ERS Executive Committee, February 1999. Am J Respir Crit Care Med. 1999;160:736–55.

13. Newburger JW, Takahashi M, Gerber MA. Diagnosis, treatment, and long-term management of Kawasaki disease: a statement for health professionals from the Committee on Rheumatic Fever, Endocarditis and Kawasaki Disease, Council on Cardiovascular Disease in the Young, American Heart Association. Circulation. 2004;110(17):2747–71.

14. Kerr GS, Hallahan CW, Giordano J, et al. Takayasu arteritis. Ann Intern Med. 1994;120(11):919–29.

15. Bagnari V, Colina M, Ciancio G, Govoni M, Trotta F. Adult-onset Still's disease. Rheumatol Int. 2010;30(7):855–62.

16. Neumann T, Manger B, Schmid M, et al. Cardiac involvement in Churg-Strauss syndrome: impact of endomyocarditis. Medicine (Baltimore). 2009;88(4):236–43.

CHAPTER 32

Nancy J. Wei and J. Carl Pallais

Cardiovascular Disease in Endocrine Disorders

CHAPTER OUTLINE

ABBREVIATIONS

ACTH	Adrenocorticotropic hormone
AF	Atrial fibrillation
AI	Adrenal insufficiency
AIT	Amiodarone-induced thyrotoxicosis
BMD	Bone mineral density
CAD	Coronary artery disease
CHF	Congestive heart failure
CMV	Cytomegalovirus
CO	Cardiac output
CV	Cardiovascular
CVD	Cardiovascular disease
DBP	Diastolic blood pressure
DTR	Deep tendon reflexes
EKG	Electrocardiogram
GH	Growth hormone
HIV	Human immunodeficiency virus
HR	Heart rate
HTN	Hypertension
IGF-1	Insulin-like growth factor - 1
IV	Intravenous
LV	Left ventricular
OGTT	Oral glucose tolerance test
PAC	Plasma aldosterone concentration
PE	Physical exam
PRA	Plasma renin activity
PTH	Parathyroid hormone
PTU	Propylthiouracil
PVR	Peripheral vascular resistance
RAI	Radioactive iodine
RAIU	Radioactive iodine uptake
SBP	Systolic blood pressure
SSKI	Supersaturated potassium iodide
SV	Stroke volume

SVR   Systemic vascular resistance
T3   Triiodothyronine
T4   Thyroxine
TB   Tuberculosis
TFT   Thyroid function tests
TSH   Thyroid stimulating hormone
TTE   Trans-thoracic echocardiography
WNL   Within normal limits

INTRODUCTION

Cardiovascular symptoms are often the first signs and symptoms of underlying endocrinopathies. This chapter reviews endocrine disorders with a focus on cardiovascular changes and presentations.

THYROID (TABLE 32-1)

Hyperthyroidism/Thyrotoxicosis

Hyperthyroidism/Thyrotoxicosis – physiologic manifestations of excessive quantities of thyroid hormones (endogenous or exogenous) [1]

■ Signs/Symptoms:

 – General – weight loss, tremors, insomnia, heat intolerance, warm moist skin, hyperreflexia, hyperdefecation. Goiter may be present. Proptosis may occur in Graves' disease.
 – Cardiovascular (CV) – ↑ sympathetic tone (tachycardia, palpitations, atrial fibrillation [AF]), ↑ cardiac output [CO] (from ↑ heart rate [HR], in severe cases ↑ stroke volume [SV]), ↑ inotropy, ↑ circulatory demand from hypermetabolism, ↓ peripheral vascular resistance (PVR), ↑ pulse pressure

    ■ Physical exam (PE) findings: dynamic precordium, systolic ejection murmur, enhanced S_1, Means-Lerman scratch (systolic pleuropericardial friction rub)
    ■ Arrhythmia: 2–20 % of patients will have AF. Cardioversion is not indicated when thyrotoxicosis is present. 60 % revert spontaneously within 4 months after normalization of thyroid function tests (TFT). Anticoagulation is recommended in patients with AF who are at moderate risk for stroke on the basis of identified risk factors [2]. Patients with newly diagnosed AF with clearly reversible hyperthyroidism and no risk factors for thromboembolism do not warrant long-term anticoagulation.

■ Laboratory testing:

 – ↓ Thyroid stimulating hormone (TSH), ↑ thyroid hormones (free thyroxine [T4] and/or triiodothyronine [T3]); ↑ thyroid antibodies in Graves' disease
 – Radioactive iodine uptake (RAIU)/thyroid scan – in the setting of a suppressed TSH, RAIU measures autonomous activity of the thyroid gland; thyroid scan measures the pattern of distribution of iodine trapping within the gland (homogeneous, heterogeneous, focal)

CV PARAMETER	HYPERTHYROID	HYPOTHYROID
Systemic vascular resistance	Decreased	Increased
Heart rate	Increased	Decreased
Cardiac output	Increased	Decreased
Blood volume	Increased	Decreased

TABLE 32-1

CARDIOVASCULAR CHANGES WITH THYROID DISEASE

- Causes:

  - ↑ RAIU (thyroid scan pattern): Graves' disease (homogeneous), toxic multinodular goiter (heterogeneous), toxic adenoma (focal), TSH-secreting pituitary tumors (homogenous)
  - ↓ RAIU: Iodide-induced thyrotoxicosis, thyroiditis (autoimmune, post-viral/subacute, drug induced [amiodarone, lithium, interferon-alpha, interleukin-2, granulocyte macrophage colony-stimulating factor]), exogenous thyroid hormone ingestion, struma ovarii

- Treatment:

  - β-blockers (preferably propranolol, atenolol, or metoprolol which also ↓ T4 to T3 conversion), methimazole, ± inorganic iodine (after methimazole) to ↓ release of pre-formed thyroid hormone (Wolff-Chaikoff effect), ± glucocorticoids (↓T4 to T3 conversion)
  - RAI ablation, thyroidectomy

Special Cases of Hyperthyroidism

1. **Thyroid Storm** – accelerated hyperthyroidism. Precipitants usually infection, trauma, surgery [3].

   - Signs/Symptoms: Fever, sweating, marked tachycardia, arrhythmias, pulmonary edema, high-output congestive heart failure (CHF), tremulousness, delirium, psychosis, abdominal pain, jaundice. Can be fatal if not treated.
   - Treatment: Intensive care, propylthiouracil (PTU), super-saturated potassium iodide (SSKI) after PTU, dexamethasone. ±β-blocker depending on cardiac state

2. **Subclinical Hyperthyroidism** – biochemical findings of low TSH with normal T4 and T3 levels

   - Increased risk for AF if TSH <0.1 mU/L (2 × ↑ risk over 10 years), and ± ↓ bone mineral density (BMD) [4]
   - Treatment impacts hemodynamic parameters (↓HR, ↓CO, ↑systemic vascular resistance [SVR], ↓ premature atrial or ventricular contractions, ↓ left ventricular [LV] mass) and improve BMD, especially in older adults [5]
   - Assessment of cause and appropriate treatment recommended for elderly, postmenopausal osteoporosis, cardiac disease (left atrial enlargement, AF, CHF, angina), and infertility

Hypothyroidism

- Signs/Symptoms: Dry/coarse skin, peri-orbital puffiness, delayed relaxation phase of deep tendon reflexes (DTR), hair loss, fatigue, weight gain [6, 7]

  - CV Signs/Symptoms: ↓ CO (↓ SV & ↓HR), ↑ PVR at rest with possible diastolic hypertension (HTN), narrow pulse pressure, ↓ blood volume, ↓ circulation → coolness, pallor; pericardial effusion
  - Labs: ± ↑CK and LDH (skeletal muscle source), ↑ LDL
  - Electrocardiogram (EKG) changes: sinus bradycardia, prolonged PR, low voltage, non-specific ST-segment changes, flattened/inverted T-waves
  - Trans-thoracic echocardiogram (TTE): resting LV diastolic dysfunction

- Diagnosis: Primary hypothyroidism = ↑ TSH, ↓ T4 & T3. Central hypothyroidism = low/normal TSH, ↓ T4 & T3.
- Causes: Primary hypothyroidism is much more common than central hypothyroidism

  - **Primary hypothyroidism** – Hashimoto's thyroiditis, infiltrative disease (sarcoid, hemochromatosis, etc.), thyroid resection, post-radioiodine therapy, iodine deficiency, drugs (lithium, thionamides, sulfonamides, iodine, tyrosine kinase inhibitors)

– Thyroiditis (painless/subacute/postpartum) can cause transient hyperthyroidism followed by transient hypothyroidism

– **Central hypothyroidism** – pituitary tumor, pituitary surgery, radiation therapy

■ <u>Treatment:</u> Thyroid hormone replacement; start at low replacement dose and slowly titrate up if coronary artery disease (CAD) suspected (thyroid hormone replacement may exacerbate angina)

Note: Hypothyroidism decreases the metabolism of many cardiac drugs. Care must be exercised when treating cardiovascular disease (CVD) in hypothyroid patients or initiating thyroid hormone replacement in these patients.

Special Cases of Hypothyroidism

1. **Myxedema coma** – condition seen with severe long-standing hypothyroidism, primarily in older patients. High mortality rate [8]

    ■ <u>Signs/Symptoms:</u> Comatose state, hypothermia, bradycardia, hypotension, delayed DTR/areflexia, seizures, hypoventilation, hyponatremia, hypoglycemia

    ■ Risk factors: Age, exposure to cold, infection, trauma, central nervous system depressants, anesthetics

    ■ <u>Diagnosis:</u> Clinical diagnosis, delay of treatment worsens prognosis. Treatment should be initiated while awaiting thyroid function test results.

    ■ <u>Treatment:</u> Intravenous (IV) levothyroxine 500 mcg load, 100 mcg IV daily, hydrocortisone 100 mg IV q8h to cover for relative adrenal insufficiency; correction of metabolic derangements (hyponatremia, hypoglycemia), as well as respiratory failure (mechanical ventilation), and work-up for coexisting disease

2. **Euthyroid Sick Syndrome (Non-Thyroidal Illness Syndrome)** – Abnormalities of circulating TSH, T4, and T3 levels without underlying thyroid disease. Occurs in fasting and illness [9] (Table 32-2)

    ■ Replacement of T3 or T4 does not improve outcomes
    ■ Normalization of TFTs expected 1–2 months after recovery

Other Thyroid Disorders

1. **Iodine-induced thyroid dysfunction**

    ■ Hyperthyroidism (Jod-Basedow effect) – iodine administration can result in hyperthyroidism in patients with autonomous thyroid function (autonomous nodules, Graves' disease, endemic goiter in setting of iodine deficiency) and rarely in patients with normal glands (iodine-induced thyroiditis) [10]

    ■ Hypothyroidism – can occur in patients with underlying thyroid dysfunction who fail to escape from the Wolff-Chaikoff effect (thyroiditis, s/p RAI treatment, s/p subtotal thyroidectomy) [11]

TABLE 32-2

STAGES OF EUTHYROID SICK SYNDROME

STAGE	SEVERITY OF ILLNESS	T3 OR FREE T3	T4 OR FREE T4	REVERSE T3	TSH
Stage 1	Mild (ex. URI)	↓	Normal	↑	Normal
Stage 2	Moderate (ex. NSTEMI)	↓↓	Normal, ↓, ↑	↑↑	Normal, ↓
Stage 3	Severe (ex. STEMI in ICU)	↓↓↓	↓	↑↑	↓↓
Recovery	Convalescence	↓	↓	↑	↑

2. **Amiodarone-induced thyroid disease** – Amiodarone contains 37 % iodine by weight and has a long $t_{1/2}$ (50–60 days). Excess iodine load can precipitate hypo- or hyper-thyroidism (see above). Can also have direct cytotoxic effect causing subacute thyroiditis or precipitating autoimmune thyroid disease (Graves' and Hashimotos') [12, 13]

   ■ Measure TFTs every 3 months on amiodarone therapy
   ■ If TSH >10 → amiodarone induced hypothyroidism. Start thyroid hormone replacement (25–50 mcg/day) and titrate up every 6 weeks until TSH WNL.
   ■ If TSH <0.1 → Amiodarone-induced thyrotoxicosis (AIT). More common in iodine-deficient regions

   – Type 1 AIT: Occurs in pts with pre-existing thyroid disease. Goiter, hypervascular thyroid on ultrasound, ± thyroid auto-antibodies

   ■ Treat with methimazole.

   – Type 2 AIT: Destructive thyroiditis. Hypovascular thyroid on ultrasound

   ■ Treat with glucocorticoids. Clinical benefit takes 2–4 weeks.

   – Mixed AIT: treat with both methimazole and glucocorticoids
   – Surgery if medical treatment unsuccessful
   – Stopping amiodarone does not hasten resolution given long $t_{1/2}$ and lipid-soluble stores. Discontinuation of amiodarone has not been shown to improve clinical outcomes [14].

ADRENAL GLAND DISORDERS

Adrenal Insufficiency

1. **Primary adrenal insufficiency (Addison's disease)** – adrenal gland disorder resulting in glucocorticoid AND mineralocorticoid deficiency [15]

   ■ <u>Signs/Symptoms</u>: Weakness, anorexia (weight loss), nausea/vomiting/diarrhea/abdominal pain, salt craving, postural dizziness (hypotension), muscle/joint pain, hyperpigmentation. With autoimmune etiology, may have findings of other autoimmune disorders.
   ■ <u>Lab abnormalities:</u> Hyponatremia, hyperkalemia, hypercalcemia, anemia, eosinophilia
   ■ <u>Diagnosis:</u> Low baseline serum cortisol (ideally early morning between 6 and 8 AM given diurnal variation) and elevated adrenocorticotropic hormone (ACTH) levels. Confirmed with failure to achieve peak plasma >18 mcg/dL after 250 mcg ACTH stimulation.
   ■ <u>Causes:</u> Autoimmune; infections (TB, fungal, HIV, CMV), metastatic tumor, infiltrative disease (amyloid, hemochromatosis); hemorrhage (Waterhouse-Friderichsen syndrome) from meningococcal or bacterial sepsis, anticoagulants, hypercoagulable / thromboembolic disease (antiphospholipid syndrome, heparin-induced thrombocytopenia), trauma; drugs (etomidate, ketoconazole); adrenoleukodystrophies; congenital adrenal hyperplasia; surgical resection
   ■ <u>Treatment:</u> Glucocorticoid (hydrocortisone 15–20 mg in AM, 5–10 mg in early PM or prednisone 4–5 mg in AM) AND mineralocorticoid replacement (fludrocortisone 0.05–0.2 mg daily) at physiologic doses

2. **Secondary adrenal insufficiency (ACTH deficiency)** – More common than primary adrenal insufficiency (AI). Chronic ACTH deficiency results in adrenal atrophy and impaired glucocorticoid production.

   ■ <u>Signs/Symptoms:</u> Same as primary adrenal insufficiency but notably no hyperpigmentation or hypokalemia

- ■ Causes: Most commonly caused by sudden cessation of exogenous glucocorticoid therapy. Other drugs (megestrol, opiates); hypopituitarism (tumors, infarct, surgery, radiation, granulomatous disease, autoimmune/infiltrative disease); hypothalamic disorders (trauma, tumors, surgery, radiation, infiltrative disease)
- ■ Diagnosis: In chronic AI cases – ACTH-stimulation test with failure to achieve peak cortisol >18 mcg/dL. In acute cases, low morning cortisol with simultaneous low ACTH levels. Insulin tolerance test is the gold standard for diagnosing central AI but is generally not performed in patients with CV and cerebrovascular disease.
- ■ Treatment: Glucocorticoid (hydrocortisone 15–20 mg in AM, 5–10 mg in early PM, or prednisone 4–5 mg in AM)

3. **Adrenal crisis**

- ■ Signs/symptoms: Dehydration, hypotension, shock out of proportion to concurrent illness, nausea/vomiting, abdominal pain, hypoglycemia, fever, delirium/confusion, hyponatremia, hyperkalemia, renal failure, hypercalcemia
- ■ Treatment: Hydrocortisone 100 mg IV q6h, supportive measures (IV fluid resuscitation)

Cushing's/Hypercortisolism

Cushing's/Hypercortisolism – excess cortisol secretion [16, 17]

- ■ Signs/Symptoms: Easy bruising, weight gain, proximal muscle weakness, wide purple/violaceous striae, hirsutism, facial plethora, hypokalemia

  - CV: Increased risk for CV morbidity/mortality, accelerated atherosclerosis, HTN, LV hypertrophy, impaired contractility, dilated cardiomyopathy, increased risk of thromboembolic events
  - Other comorbidities: obesity, diabetes/impaired glucose tolerance/insulin resistance, platelet dysfunction, osteopenia/osteoporosis, kidney stones

- ■ Diagnosis: Elevated 24 h urine free cortisol collection, or midnight salivary cortisol × 2, or overnight 1 mg dexamethasone suppression test with 8 AM serum cortisol >1.8 mcg/dL

  - Drugs that can interfere with dexamethasone suppression test: exogenous glucocorticoids, diltiazem, anti-epileptics, rifampin, fluoxetine
  - Drugs that can interfere with serum cortisol measurement: exogenous glucocorticoids, estrogen, mitotane
    Drugs that increase urine free cortisol results: exogenous glucocorticoids, licorice, fenofibrate, carbamazepine

- ■ Causes: Excess ACTH secretion (pituitary adenoma or ectopic source) or functional adrenal gland adenoma

  - ACTH producing adenoma (65 %)
  - Ectopic ACTH (10 %) – Small cell carcinoma, carcinoid tumors, pancreatic islet cell tumors, medullary thyroid cancer
  - Adrenal adenoma (25 %) with suppressed ACTH
  - Carney complex – triad of hypercortisolism (micronodular adrenal lesions), cardiac myxoma, and pigmented dermal lesions (monogenic autosomal dominant disorder due to mutations in *PKAR1A* tumor suppressor gene)

- ■ Treatment: Surgical (pituitary surgery, adrenalectomy, resection of carcinoid/tumor), medical (ketoconazole, metyrapone, octreotide, pasireotide, cabergoline, mifepristone), radiation to destroy tumor

Pheochromocytoma/Paraganglioma

Pheochromocytoma/paraganglioma – Rare catecholamine-secreting tumors, estimated incidence 1/125,000 per year, <0.2 % of HTN patients [18]

■ Signs/Symptoms: Anxiety, diaphoresis, chest pain, headache, nausea/vomiting, pallor, fever, tremor, lid lag, hyperglycemia, hypercalcemia, hemoconcentration

– CV: HTN, paroxysmal palpitations, orthostatic hypotension

■ Diagnosis: Screen with plasma metanephrine levels (sensitivity 96–100 %, specificity 85–89 %). Confirm with 24 h urine catecholamine and metanephrine levels (± dopamine). If elevated, then imaging to localize tumor.

– Drugs that may increase catecholamine/metanephrine levels – tricyclic antidepressants, levodopa, decongestants, amphetamines, buspirone, prochlorperazine, reserpine, clonidine withdrawal, alcohol, acetaminophen (depending on assay) norepinephrine epinephrine, cocaine
– Major physical stress (MI, CVA, etc.) can also cause false elevation in catecholamine or metanephrine measurements

■ Treatment: Surgical resection. Perioperative management – alpha-blockade (i.e. phenoxybenzamine) 7–10 days prior to surgery, high sodium diet (>5 g/day) and aggressive volume repletion to control orthostasis. Add beta-blocker (i.e. propanolol) once α-blockade is at goal to control tachycardia.

– Watch for CHF after starting beta-blocker, from underlying cardiomyopathy from chronic catecholamine excess

Primary Aldosteronism

Primary aldosteronism – hypertension, increased plasma aldosterone concentration (PAC) AND suppressed plasma renin activity (PRA). Present in approximately 5 % of hypertensive patients [19].

■ Signs/Symptoms: Screening recommended for hypertensive patients with any of the following features: early onset hypertension (<30 years of age), resistant hypertension ($\geq$3 drugs with poor control), moderate/severe hypertension (SBP $\geq$ 160 or DBP $\geq$ 100), hypokalemia, adrenal incidentaloma, family history of early strokes (<40 years). Other possible findings: mild hypernatremia, periodic paralysis (in Asians), polyuria/nocturia

■ Diagnosis: Morning (8–10 AM) ambulatory paired random PAC and PRA [some centers measure plasma renin concentration]

– Positive screening test – PAC$\geq$15 ng/dL AND PAC/PRA ratio $\geq$20 (with PRA usually<1.0 ng/mL/h)$\rightarrow$perform confirmatory test
– Confirmatory tests – Evaluate for inappropriate aldosterone secretion by oral sodium loading test, 2 L normal saline infusion test, or fludrocortisone suppression test
– Adrenal imaging if confirmatory test is positive. However, imaging studies cannot determine if adrenal adenoma is functioning and may miss unilateral hyperaldosteronism.
– If unilateral adrenalectomy is an option, consider adrenal venous sampling to confirm unilateral disease and rule out a non-functional adrenal incidentaloma that would not benefit from surgery
– For any of the functional tests, aggressive potassium repletion is required. Must also be off aldosterone receptor antagonists (i.e. spironolactone, eplerenone) and amiloride.

■ Causes:

– Unilateral disease: Aldosterone-producing adenoma (35 %), primary adrenal hyperplasia (2 %), aldosterone-producing adrenocortical carcinoma (<1 %)
– Bilateral disease (more common): Bilateral idiopathic hyperplasia (60 %), familial hyperaldosteronism (2 %)
– Other: ectopic aldosterone-producing adenoma or carcinoma (<0.1 %)

■ Treatment: Depends on the cause. Surgery for unilateral or ectopic disease. Medical management (mineralocorticoid receptor blockade, low sodium diet) for bilateral disease and certain cases of familial hyperaldosteronism (Table 32-3).

DISORDERS ASSOCIATED WITH NORMAL K	DISORDERS ASSOCIATED WITH LOW K	TABLE 32-3
Hyperthyroidism Hypothyroidism Pheochromocytoma/paraganglioma Hyperparathyroidism Acromegaly	Primary aldosteronism Cushing's syndrome Congenital adrenal hyperplasia Hyperdeoxycorticosteronism/apparent mineralocorticoid excess	ENDOCRINE CAUSES OF HYPERTENSION

OTHER ENDOCRINE DISORDERS

Acromegaly

Acromegaly – Growth hormone (GH) excess from hyperfunctioning pituitary adenoma [20]

■ Signs/Symptoms: Enlarging hands/feet/head, coarsening of facial features, frontal skull bossing, arthralgias/arthritis, carpal tunnel, prognathism, sleep apnea, skin tags, hyperhidrosis, visceromegaly, tumor mass effects (headaches, vision changes, cranial nerve palsy)

  – CV: ~20 % have symptomatic cardiac disease; CVD is cause of ~60 % of deaths. Short term (<5 years): increased LV mass index, increased SVR. Untreated: hypertension, cardiac hypertrophy→global LV diastolic dysfunction/LV hypertrophy, cardiomyopathy, CHF

    ■ EKG abnormalities: L axis deviation, septal Q waves, ST-T segment depression, abnormal QT dispersion, and conduction defects (premature atrial/ventricular contractions, sick sinus syndrome, supraventricular tachycardia/ventricular tachycardia). 4 × increased risk for complex ventricular arrhythmias

  – Other comorbidities: diabetes/impaired glucose tolerance/insulin resistance, hypertriglyceridemia, hypogonadism

■ Diagnosis: Elevated insulin-like growth factor – 1 (IGF-1) levels, or GH nadir >1 mcg/L after oral glucose tolerance test (OGTT)

■ Treatment: Manage pituitary mass and suppress GH and IGF-1 hypersecretion to prevent long-term effects of hypersomatotropism. Surgical resection of pituitary tumor + radiation therapy. Medical therapy with dopamine agonists, somatostatin receptor ligands, or growth hormone receptor antagonists.

Calcium Disorders

Primary hyperparathyroidism – excess parathyroid hormone (PTH) resulting in hypercalcemia [21]

■ Signs/Symptoms: Majority of patients are asymptomatic. Renal stones, renal failure, osteitis fibrosa cystic, osteoporosis, lethargy, CNS dysfunction, muscle weakness, vague abdominal discomfort

  – CV effects: HTN is common but does not generally improve with surgical resection

    ■ PTH has direct effect on the heart, smooth muscle and endothelial cells
    ■ Hypercalcemia – increase cardiac contractility, shortening of ventricular action potential, calcific deposits on valve cusps/annuli
    ■ EKG: shortened QT interval, shortened PR interval

■ Diagnosis: Elevated PTH with concomitant hypercalcemia
■ Treatment: Surgical resection of parathyroid adenoma or cinacalcet. Watchful waiting may be an option for some patients.

Other endocrine disorders associated with hypercalcemia: Paraneoplastic syndrome with PTHrP secretion, granulomatous disease (TB, sarcoid, HIV immune reconstitution syndrome) with increase in 1,25-vitamin D synthesis

REVIEW QUESTIONS

1. A 30-year-old man is referred for hypertension, not currently on treatment. The patient is a non-smoker, non-drinker and there is no family history of hypertension. Physical examination was significant for a blood pressure of 161/96, BMI 24, and otherwise normal. Lab studies: Na = 140 mEq/L, K = 3.5 mEq/L, Cr = 0.8 mg/dL, PAC = 35 ng/dL, PRA = 0.8 ng/mL/h. What is the next step?
   (a) Order a magnetic resonance angiogram of the renal arteries
   (b) Order a CT scan of the adrenal glands
   (c) Schedule adrenal venous sampling for aldosterone
   (d) Start spironolactone
   (e) Perform a saline suppression test

2. A 56-year-old man with monomorphic ventricular tachycardia is started on amiodarone. Baseline thyroid hormone levels were checked and were normal. Three months later, his TSH is 13.2 (normal range 0.4–5.0 µ/mL) and free T4 is 0.6 ng/mL (normal range 0.8–1.8 ng/mL). What is the next step?
   (a) Order radioactive iodine uptake scan
   (b) Discontinue amiodarone therapy
   (c) Start levothyroxine replacement therapy
   (d) Obtain thyroid ultrasound
   (e) Start methimazole therapy

ANSWERS

1. (e) The patient has early onset hypertension with normokalemia. His PAC is elevated, PRA is suppressed and PAC/PRA ratio is >20, consistent with primary aldosteronism. Confirmation with a saline suppression test should be done prior to any adrenal imaging or adrenal venous sampling. Spironolactone will interfere with confirmatory testing.

2. (c) The patient has amiodarone-induced hypothyroidism, likely due to the iodine load from amiodarone causing the Wolff-Chaikoff effect. The appropriate next step is to start levothyroxine replacement therapy at low doses and titrate up every 4–6 weeks until TSH is between 0.4 and 5 mIU/L. Thyroid ultrasound and RAIU scans are not useful in this situation as he is not hyperthyroid. Amiodarone has a long $t_{1/2}$ so even if it were to be discontinued, iodine-related effects will persist for many months. Methimazole is used to suppress thyroid hormone production in hyperthyroid states.

REFERENCES

1. Franklyn JA. The management of hyperthyroidism. N Engl J Med. 1994;330(24):1731–8.
2. Fuster V, Ryden LE, Cannom DS, Crijns HJ, Curtis AB, Ellenbogen KA, et al. 2011 ACCF/AHA/HRS focused updates incorporated into the ACC/AHA/ESC 2006 guidelines for the management of patients with atrial fibrillation: a report of the American College of Cardiology Foundation/American Heart Association Task Force on practice guidelines. Circulation. 2011;123(10):e269–367.
3. Nayak B, Burman K. Thyrotoxicosis and thyroid storm. Endocrinol Metab Clin North Am. 2006;35(4):663–86, vii.
4. Sawin CT, Geller A, Wolf PA, Belanger AJ, Baker E, Bacharach P, et al. Low serum thyrotropin concentrations as a risk factor for atrial fibrillation in older persons. N Engl J Med. 1994;331(19):1249–52.
5. Sgarbi JA, Villaca FG, Garbeline B, Villar HE, Romaldini JH. The effects of early antithyroid therapy for endogenous subclinical hyperthyroidism in clinical and heart abnormalities. J Clin Endocrinol Metab. 2003;88(4):1672–7.
6. Cooper DS. Clinical practice. Subclinical hypothyroidism. N Engl J Med. 2001;345(4):260–5.
7. Devdhar M, Ousman YH, Burman KD. Hypothyroidism. Endocrinol Metab Clin North Am. 2007;36(3):595–615, v.
8. Wartofsky L. Myxedema coma. Endocrinol Metab Clin North Am. 2006;35(4):687–98, vii–viii.
9. Adler SM, Wartofsky L. The nonthyroidal illness syndrome. Endocrinol Metab Clin North Am. 2007;36(3):657–72, vi.
10. Roti E, Uberti ED. Iodine excess and hyperthyroidism. Thyroid. 2001;11(5):493–500.
11. Markou K, Georgopoulos N, Kyriazopoulou V, Vagenakis AG. Iodine-Induced hypothyroidism. Thyroid. 2001;11(5):501–10.
12. Martino E, Bartalena L, Bogazzi F, Braverman LE. The effects of amiodarone on the thyroid. Endocr Rev. 2001;22(2):240–54.
13. Bogazzi F, Bartalena L, Martino E. Approach to the patient with amiodarone-induced thyrotoxicosis. J Clin Endocrinol Metab. 2010;95(6):2529–35.
14. Osman F, Franklyn JA, Sheppard MC, Gammage MD. Successful treatment of amiodarone-induced thyrotoxicosis. Circulation. 2002;105(11):1275–7.
15. Bornstein SR. Predisposing factors for adrenal insufficiency. N Engl J Med. 2009;360(22):2328–39.
16. Tritos NA, Biller BM, Swearingen B. Management of Cushing disease. Nat Rev Endocrinol. 2011;7(5):279–89 [Review].
17. Sharma ST, Nieman LK. Cushing's syndrome: all variants, detection, and treatment. Endocrinol Metab Clin North Am. 2011;40(2):379–91, viii–ix.
18. Young Jr WF. Adrenal causes of hypertension: pheochromocytoma and primary aldosteronism. Rev Endocr Metab Disord. 2007;8(4):309–20.
19. Rossi GP. Diagnosis and treatment of primary aldosteronism. Endocrinol Metab Clin North Am. 2011;40(2):313–32, vii–viii.
20. Melmed S. Medical progress: acromegaly. N Engl J Med. 2006;355(24):2558–73.
21. Walker MD, Silverberg SJ. Cardiovascular aspects of primary hyperparathyroidism. J Endocrinol Invest. 2008;31(10):925–31.

CHAPTER 33

Emily J. Karwacki Sheff and James L. Januzzi, Jr.

Pharmacology

CHAPTER OUTLINE

ABBREVIATIONS

ACE	Angiotension converting enzyme
AV	Atrioventricular
CCB	Calcium channel blocker
ED50	Median effective dose
IM	Intramuscular
IV	Intravenous
PO	By mouth 'per os'
SC	Subcutaneous

INTRODUCTION

Pharmacology is the detailed study of drugs – their chemical and physical properties, biochemical and physiological effects, and pharmacokinetics (alterations of the drug on the body) and phamacodynamics (the mechanism of actions). As there is no ideal drug in existence, it is the responsibility of every member of the healthcare team to promote therapeutic effects and minimize drug-induced harm to each patient. This section discusses the pharmacokinetic processes and pharmacodynamic principles, along with a selection of cardiac medication pearls to help the prescriber carry out the therapeutic objective-to provide maximum benefit with minimum harm to each patient with each medication prescribed.

GENERAL PHARMACOLOGY

Pharmacokinetics: Action of the Body to the Drug

<u>Absorption</u>: the movement of a drug into the bloodstream

- Variability in absorption and bioavailability based on route of administration (PO, IM, IV, SC, mucosal, etc.)
- Factors affecting absorption: dose administered, percentage of dose that is 'active' and bioavailability of drug
- Bioavailability: the rate or percentage of drug dose reaching systemic circulation. 100 % bioavailability with IV administration, but variable bioavailability with other routes of administration.

    – Factors affecting bioavailability: characteristics of medication dosage form, solubility, administration route, metabolism in the gut wall or liver (first-pass effect) and the permeability of the gastrointestinal tract (i.e. edematous tract due to heart failure may not be able to absorb as much drugs through the gut wall).

<u>Distribution</u>: the process of the dispersion of the drug into the bloodstream and surrounding tissues

- Influenced by lipid solubility (i.e. in general, water-soluble drugs are limited to the vascular space and cannot easily cross the blood–brain barrier while lipid-soluble drugs are distributed more widely and can better cross the blood–brain barrier), degree of ionization, blood flow and binding affinities to proteins in plasma and specific tissues
- During constant infusion or multiple doses of a medication, drug levels rise in the blood and tissue until they reach a plateau, or **steady state**

    – At steady state, the rate of drug administration equals rate of drug elimination
    – Generally takes 4–5 half-lives to reach desired steady-state drug concentration

- Volume of distribution (the volume of body fluid that the medication is distributed in) can help to estimate loading dose (i.e. large volume of distribution = low concentration of the drug)
- Protein binding

    – Describes a drug's affinity for plasma protein
    – Drugs are either bound or unbound
    – The less bound a drug is the more drug circulating throughout the body that is "active"
    – Only unbound drug undergoes metabolism in liver and elimination
    – Coumadin is 97 % protein bound. Dramatic implications may ensue when another medication is added that is protein bound as well

        - Protein-bound medications compete for proteins, resulting in larger amounts of both medications' free drug concentrations and risk for side effects.

<u>Metabolism</u>

- Complex or lipid-soluble drugs undergo hepatic metabolism to a water-soluble metabolites which can then be excreted. These metabolites can be biologically active or inactive leading to either therapeutic effects or increase toxic side effects related to the medication administered

    – i.e. procainamide is metabolized into NAPA in the body, a Class III antiarrhythmic with a therapeutic level of 10–20 mcg/mL. Toxic levels of NAPA can manifest in the prolongation of action potential, prolonged QT interval and ultimately Torsades de Pointes. Even if procainamide level is not toxic, NAPA level may be

- Phase 1 (mainly oxidation of the drug to make it more water-soluble) and Phase 2 (mainly conjugation of the drug)
- Oxidation is mainly through the cytochrome P450 (CYP450) system. The most drugs are metabolized by CYP3A (>50 %), CYP2D6 (genetic polymorphism leads to decreased

TABLE 33-1

MEDICATIONS THAT AFFECT HEPATIC METABOLISM

CYP450 FAMILY	CARDIOVASCULAR DRUGS METABOLIZED BY THE CYTOCHROME FAMILY	INHIBITORS	INDUCERS
CYP3A	Statins (except for pravastatin), CCB, amiodarone, cyclosporine, tacrolimus, quinidine, mexiletine	Grapefruit juice, CCB, amiodarone, antivirals, erythromycin, clarithromycin, itraconazole, ketoconazole	Rifampin, St. John's wort, phenytoin, pioglitazone, efavirenz, nevirapine, barbiturates
CYP2D6	b-blockers, propafenone	Amiodarone, quinidine, fluoxetine, paroxetine	Rifampin
CYP2C9	Irbesartan, losartan, warfarin, carvedilol	Amiodarone, zafirlukast	Rifampin

CCB calcium channel blocker

enzyme levels in up to 25 % in Caucasian and African population resulting in hypersensitivity to medications such as b-blockers, propafenone), CYP2C9 and CYP1A2 families of the CYP450 system (Table 33-1). Note that CYP450 activity can decrease with increasing age and lead to increased drug levels/toxicity.

■ Clearance of a drug is one of the most important factors to understand, as it helps in dosing the patient to maintain a therapeutically effective level of the drug.
■ Drug clearance occurs through both metabolism (biotransformation) and excretion.

– Genetics (polymorphism), concurrent disease, age or drug-drug interactions can affect drug clearance

■ First-pass effect (important drugs are listed in Table 33-2)

– Concentration of drug is greatly reduced before it reaches systemic circulation, typically metabolized during absorption in the liver
– Greatly reduces bioavailability of the drug
– Suppositories, IV, IM, sublingual and inhaled medications bypass first-pass effect

Elimination

■ Final route of exit from the body; expressed in terms of half life or clearance.
■ Excretion occurs through the kidneys primarily, but also through bile, sweat, saliva, breast milk and exhalation.
■ Renal Drug Excretion is the net effect of glomerular filtration, secretion, and passive reabsorption

– With renal dysfunction, may need to decrease medication doses if renally cleared (i.e. digoxin)

■ Half-life: time for serum concentration of drug to decrease by 50 % (hours)

– Determined by clearance and volume of distribution
– Poor indicator of the efficacy of drug elimination and plasma drug concentration at steady state
– Typically takes 4–5 half lives to clear medication from system
– Clearance: volume of serum from which drug is removed per time (mL/min or L/h)

Pharmacodynamics: The Drug's Effect on the Body

Dose–response relationship

■ the effect of a drug based on the concentration that is present at the site of action
■ In most cases a maximum value is approached where a further increase in concentration is not effective
■ ED50=dose producing a response that is 50 % of the maximum value
■ Depends on both exposure time and exposure route

TABLE 33-2	Diltiazem, verapamil
DRUGS WITH A SIGNIFICANT FIRST PASS EFFECT	Labetalol, metoprolol, propranolol
	Hydralazine
	Nitroglycerin

TABLE 33-3	**Increases anticoagulation effects:**
DRUGS WITH IMPORTANT INTERACTIONS WITH WARFARIN SODIUM	Cimetidine
	Alcohol
	Disulfiram
	Many antibiotics, notably including sulfa agents
	Decreases anticoagulant effects:
	Vitamin K
	Barbiturates
	Rifampin

Drug toxicity
■ reduced clearance=drug accumulation and toxicity

Drug-Drug Interactions
■ Most common with cardiac medications, and may result in increased absorption, additive or antagonistic effects, as well as induced or inhibited metabolism.

CARDIAC MEDICATION PEARLS

Anticoagulants

Heparin: accelerates the action of antithrombin III which rapidly inactivates the clotting factors
■ Oral bioavailability 0 %, thus IV or subcutaneous route is mandatory
■ Adverse effects: bleeding, heparin induced thrombocytopenia
■ Action can be reversed by protamine sulfate

Warfarin sodium: Vitamin K antagonist (prevents formation of new clotting factors in liver)
■ Oral bioavailability is >95 %
■ Onset of action=8–12 h
■ Effects can be reversed by Vitamin K, but take 24 h
■ Oral vitamin K (5–10 mg) is as effective as subcutaneous for reversing excessive anticoagulation.
■ Intravenous vitamin K may be slightly faster, though this is debated.
■ Contraindicated in pregnancy

- May result in aplasia cutis congenita

■ Numerous drug-drug interactions to remember (Table 33-3).

Non-warfarin oral anticoagulants
■ Dabigatran

- Direct thrombin inhibitor
- Rapidly effective, high oral bioavailability
- No monitoring generally necessary, though dose reduction recommended in elderly patients and in those with reduced renal function.

- – Cleared via P-glycoprotein pumps, thus may be used in patients with moderately impaired renal function (though risk for bleeding increases in end-stage renal disease).
- – More reliable anticoagulation with lower risk for bleeding compared to warfarin in clinical trials of non-valvular atrial fibrillation.
- – Down sides: twice daily dosing, no specific antidote, high incidence of dyspepsia (related to acidic preparation).

■ Rivaroxaban

- – Factor Xa inhibitor
- – Rapidly effective, high oral bioavailability, once-daily dosing.
- – As with dabigatran, rivaroxaban may be as effective as warfarin with lower risk for bleeding.
- – As with dabigatran, rivaroxaban has predictable dose responsiveness, predictable anti-coagulation, and lacks an antidote.

■ Apixaban

- – Factor Xa inhibitor
- – Rapidly effective, high oral bioavailability, twice daily dosing
- – As with dabigratran, apixaban may be as effective as warfarin, with lower risk for bleeding
- – As with dabigatran, apixaban has predictable dose responsiveness, predictable antico-agulation, and lacks an antidote

Antiplatelet Agents

Aspirin
■ Works via irreversible inactivation of cyclo-oxygenase-1 (lasts for life of the platelet)
■ Enteric coating reduces gastrointestinal intolerance, but may retard absorption of drug
■ While clearly indicated for those with coronary artery disease and acute coronary syndrome, debate exists about use of aspirin for primary prevention.

Clopidogrel, prasugrel
■ Thienopyridines that work via irreversible blockade of ADP-mediated platelet activation via the P2Y12 receptor.
■ Prasugrel is more potent. Both are taken with aspirin.
■ Metabolism of clopidogrel is through the liver, requiring modification to active drug; prasugrel does not require such processing.
■ Some patients show genetically-based impaired activation of clopidogrel, which may result in inadequate antiplatelet effects.
■ Certain drugs that affect cytochrome P450 3A4 may affect metabolic activation of clopidogrel. Among these are proton pump inhibitors. Despite this biological basis, clinical data are heavily conflicting as to whether proton pump inhibitors truly result in a clinical impairment of clopidogrel effectiveness, and thus this topic is best viewed as a hypothesis.
■ Prasugrel may have an edge for those resistant to clopidogrel effects, and is indicated for those intolerant to clopidogrel.
■ Prasugrel is contraindicated in patients with low body weight and/or a history of cerebrovascular disease, given the higher risk for bleeding.

Ticagrelor
■ Non-thienopyridine, reversible P2Y12 inhibitor.
■ Does not require hepatic activation like clopidogrel.
■ In the PLATO study, twice daily ticagrelor was superior to clopidogrel in patients with acute coronary syndromes [1].
■ Approved for use with low-dose aspirin only.

Angiotensin Converting Enzyme (ACE) Inhibitors

Inhibit ACE and prevents the inactivation of bradykinin
- Venous tone and total peripheral resistance is decreased
- Side effects

  - Postural hypotension
  - Dry cough (as a result of bradykinin accumulation in the lungs)
  - Hyperkalemia
  - Azotemia
  - Angioedema
  - Changes in taste (ageusia, dysgeusia).

- Contraindications

  - Pregnancy (see below)
  - Severe aortic stenosis
  - Severe renal insufficiency
  - Hyperkalemia
  - History of angioedema

Angiotensin II Receptor Blockers

Inhibit binding of angiotensin II to its receptor
- Venous tone and total peripheral resistance is decreased
- Side effects

  - Postural hypotension
  - Hyperkalemia
  - Azotemia

- Contraindications

  - Pregnancy (see below)
  - Severe aortic stenosis
  - Severe renal insufficiency
  - Hyperkalemia
  - Concomitant use of ACE inhibitor in the context of chronic kidney disease

Thiazide Diuretics

- Initial hypotensive effect (related to reduction of blood volume and cardiac output)

  - Resolves after 6–8 weeks when blood volume normalizes

- Peripheral vascular resistance decreases

  - Slow loss of sodium leads to decreased intracellular fluid smooth muscle sodium, resulting in decrease in intracellular fluid muscle calcium and ultimately vascular tone decreases.

- Adverse effects

  - Hypokalemia
  - Hyponatremia
  - Hyperuricemia, gout
  - Hyperglycemia
  - Rarely, erectile dysfunction

- Contraindications

  - Use with caution in the elderly
  - Pregnancy

α Blockers

- Block effects of epinephrine and norepinephrine at the level of the α receptor
- Side effects

  - Orthostatic hypotension
  - Peripheral edema

- Contraindications

  - History of intolerance

Central α agonist (clonidine)

- Acts as an α2 agonist
- Side effects

  - Lightheadedness, fatigue, dizziness, constipation
  - Rebound hypertension if abruptly stopped

- Contraindications

  - Category C in pregnancy

β Adrenergic Blockers

- Decrease cardiac output and inhibit renin
- Side effects

  - Bradycardia, hypotension (rare)
  - Fatigue, particularly centrally acting agents such as propranolol or nadolol
  - Erectile dysfunction
  - Bronchospasm; a history of asthma is not a contraindication to beta blocker use
  - Peripheral vasospasm

- Contraindications

  - History of severe bronchospasm to beta blockers
  - Severe bradycardia; use caution when combining with calcium channel blockers
  - Renal failure (nadolol, atenolol), hepatic failure (metoprolol)
  - In later pregnancy may lead to intrauterine growth retardation and neonatal hypoglycemia

Calcium Channel Blockers

- Two general classes: dihydropyridines and non-dihydropyridines.

  - Dihydropyridine examples include nifedipine, amlodipine, and felodipine.
  - Non-dihydropyridines include diltiazem and verapamil

- Calcium channel blockers block calcium influx from activated and inactivated calcium channels and lowers blood pressure as a result

  - Total peripheral resistance is also reduced
  - Myocardial inotropy is reduced, particularly by non-dihydropyridines
  - Non-dihydropyridines also result in bradycardia and PR interval increases (verapamil>diltiazem).

- Side effects

  - Edema (predominantly dihydropyridines)
  - Hypotension
  - Bradycardia, heart block (non-dihydropyridines)
  - Headache
  - Rash

■ Contraindications

  – Severe renal failure
  – Heart failure

Oral Vasodilators

Hydralazine
■ Direct effect on arterial tone
■ Short acting preparations necessitate frequent dosing, which limits utility
■ Adverse effects include a lupus-like syndrome due to autoantibodies against histone proteins, and myocardial ischemia due to reflex tachycardia

Minoxidil
■ Direct effect on arterial tone
■ Effective antihypertensive but side effects (hirsuitism) limit use.

Intravenous Vasodilators

Nitroprusside
■ Arteriolar and venous dilator
■ Red blood cells metabolize medication, releasing cyanide that is ultimately metabolized to thiocyanate
■ Adverse reactions: accumulation of cyanide (metabolic acidosis, arrhythmias and potential for fatality); accumulation of thiocyanate (confusion, increased reflexes, psychosis, and convulsions)

Diazoxide
■ Dilation of arterioles which open potassium channels in smooth muscles. Once the membrane stabilizes contraction is less likely
■ Contraindicated in patients with diabetes due to adverse effect of hyperglycemia (50 %)

Fenoldopam
■ Selective D1 receptor antagonist
■ Dilation of arteries and arterioles, reduces afterload, and promotes sodium excretion
■ Side effects include headache, flushing, nausea, reflex tachycardia, and increased ocular pressure (thus contraindicated in patients with glaucoma).

Antiarrhythmics

■ May be divided into classes (Table 33-4)

  – Class IA: Sodium channel blockers that affect QRS width by lengthening the action potential.
  – Class IB: Sodium channel blockers that do not affect QRS width; shorten action potential.
  – Class IC: Sodium channel blockers that do not affect QRS width or action potential
  – Class II: Block sympathetic nervous system function
  – Class III: Prolong repolarization by effecting potassium efflux
  – Class IV: Calcium channel blockers

■ *Use dependent*: when medications have stronger effects at increased heart rates-i.e. flecainide and propafenone. In order to monitor for side effects such as QRS widening, use a test that increase heart rate such as treadmill exercise stress test.
■ *Reverse use dependent*: when medications have stronger effects at decreased heart rates-i.e. sotalol, dofetilide
■ Adverse effects (Table 33-4)

TABLE 33-4

ANTI-ARRHYTHMIC DRUGS

CLASS	EXAMPLES	MECHANISM(S)	IMPORTANT SIDE EFFECTS
IA	Quinidine Procainamide Disopyramide	Sodium channel blockade with intermediate association/ dissociation (Increases defibrillation threshold)	Thrombocytopenia (quinidine) Lupus like syndrome (procainamide) Anticholinergic symptoms (disopyramide)
IB	Lidocaine Mexiletine	Sodium channel blockade with fast association/dissociation (Increases defibrillation threshold)	Confusion, agitation (typically in the elderly with renal insufficiency and in the context of elevated drug levels)
IC	Flecainide Propafenone	Sodium channel blockade with slow association/dissociation (Increases defibrillation threshold)	Pro-arrhythmia in the context of ischemic heart disease; incessant ventricular tachycardia; accelerated ventricular response from atrial flutter in the context of use without nodal agents (due to slowing of flutter rates together with anticholinergic effects on AV node)
II	b blockers	Blocking of sympathetic nervous system effects	Bradycardia, hypotension, bronchospasm, fatigue, erectile dysfunction
III	Amiodarone, sotalol, dofetilide, dronedarone	Potassium channel blocker (sotalol is also a Class II agent, while amiodarone has class I-IV effects) (Decreases defibrillation threshold, except for amiodarone which increases defibrillation threshold)	Bradycardia, heart block, pro-arrhythmia (all) Amiodarone may also cause hypo- or hyper-thyroidism, acute or chronic pulmonary injury, hepatotoxicity, renal failure, skin changes, bone marrow suppression, neuropathy
IV	Calcium channel blockers	Block calcium channels	Bradycardia, hypotension, constipation, peripheral edema

■ Contraindications

– Commonly include renal failure, hepatic failure

Statins

■ Inhibit rate limiting step of cholesterol biosynthesis. The liver then compensates and increases the low density lipoprotein (LDL) receptors, which decreases the amount of LDL circulating in the blood and decreases hepatic very low density lipoprotein production.
■ Up to 55 % reduction in LDL, 35 % reduction in triglycerides, and small increase (10 %) of HDL.
■ First pass metabolism
■ Adverse effects

– Hepatotoxicity: reversible and generally benign.
– Myopathy: reversible, typically without evidence of muscle injury on testing.
– Rhabdomylosis (risk increased if taking concurrently with fibric acid derivatives, niacin, or compounds that inhibit the cytochrome P450 system, such as grapefruit juice). Especially an issue for simvastatin at 80 mg dose.
– Gastrointestinal upset
– Neuropathy
– Insomnia, memory loss

TABLE 33-5		A	B-1	B-2
IMPORTANT INOTROPIC AGENTS	Dobutamine	None	++	+
	Dopamine	+	++	+
	Adrenaline	++	+++	++
	Noradrenaline	+++	+	None

- Contraindications

  - Hepatic disease, jaundice, cholestasis
  - Pregnancy (Category X; see section "Special Topics: Pregnancy")
  - Dose reductions for rosuvastatin recommended in Asians (starting dose of 5 mg), due to genetic predisposition to higher concentrations of active drug, and hence higher risk for adverse effects.
  - Due to drug-drug interactions, simvastatin should be avoided entirely when using antifungals, erythromycin, clarithromycin, HIV drugs, or nefazodone.
  - Due to drug-drug interactions, dose of simvastatin should be reduced if concomitantly used with calcium blockers, amiodarone, and cyclosporine.

Inotropic Agents (Table 33-5)

- Agents that increase or decrease the force of the heart's contractions and/or stimulate vascular constriction or dilation.
- Act on α, β-1 and β-2 receptors

  - α: peripheral vasoconstriction and increased vascular resistance
  - β-1: increased heart rate, ventricular contractility and atrioventricular conduction velocity
  - β-2: peripheral vasodilation and bronchodilation

Special Topics: The Elderly Patient

- The elderly may be at higher risk for drug toxicities due to changes in pharmacokinetics:

  - Absorption rate may be delayed; delayed time to peak concentration
  - Changes in hepatic first-pass metabolism
  - Metabolic clearance may be reduced (examples = metoprolol, propranolol, verapamil)
  - Reduced renal function may reduce elimination.

    - Decreased lean body mass

      - Results in decreased volume of distribution

    - Decreased plasma protein (albumin) → increase percentage of unbound or free drug (example = warfarin)
- The elderly may be at higher risk for drug toxicities due to changes in pharmacodynamics:

  - Examples:

    - Decreased heart rate response to β blockers
    - Increased cardiac sensitivity to digoxin

Special Topics: Pregnancy

- General recommendations

  - Avoid medication use in first trimester when possible.
  - Topical route preferred over systemic agents.

Class B: No risk reported in animal studies and human use

Anticoagulants: Heparins

Antihypertensive: methyldopa

Antiarrhythmic: sotalol (First trimester only)

Diuretic: torsemide, amiloride

Lipid lowering: cholestyramine

Class C: Small risk reported in controlled animal studies and human use

Antiplatelet: clopidogrel, persantine

Antihypertensive: hydralazine, clonidine, prazosin, all calcium channel blockers, most beta blockers during first trimester (some controversy exists regarding beta blockers in second/third trimester causing intrauterine growth retardation)

Antiarrhythmic: atropine, digoxin, disopyramide, lidocaine, procainamide, quinidine, amiodarone

Diuretic: furosemide

Lipid lowering: niacin, gemfibrozil

Class D: Strong evidence for risk to the human fetus

Anticoagulants: warfarin

Antihypertensive: ACE inhibitors, angiotensin receptor blockers, beta blockers in second/third trimester

Diuretics: ethacrynic acid, bumetanide, hydrochlorothiazide, spironolactone

Class X: Very high risk to the human fetus

Statins

TABLE 33-6

CARDIOVASCULAR DRUGS AND PREGNANCY

- Effect of pregnancy on pharmacokinetics is substantial:

  - Absorption: Gastric emptying time prolonged
  - Distribution: Increased volume of water in body and hemodynamic changes result in dilutional hypoalbuminemia, particularly in last trimester

    - Results in decreased drug-binding capacity and increased distribution rates

      - Metabolism: Biotransformation largely depends on hepatic blood flow, drug metabolizing enzymes and hormonal influence- all in altered states during pregnancy
      - Excretion: increases in glomerular filtration affect concentrations of drug.

- Choice of drugs, including contraindicated medications in pregnancy are listed in Table 33-6

Special Topics: Drugs That Increase QT Interval and Risk for Torsades des Pointes (For More See www.qtdrugs.org)

- Antiarrhythmics: Class IA (quinidine, procainamide, disopyramide), Class III (sotalol, NAPA, ibutilide, dofetilide, amiodarone, azimilide)
- Antimicrobials: erythromycin, trimethoprim/sulfamethoxazole, itraconazole, ketoconazole, cloroquine, pentamidine, amantadine
- Antihistamine: terfenadine, astemizole
- Antidepressants: tricyclics
- Psych medications: haloperidol, droperidol, phenothiazines
- Others: vasopressin, organophosphate poisoning

REVIEW QUESTIONS

1. A 68 year old woman is admitted with dyspnea, chest heaviness, and confusion. She has a past medical history notable for hypertension, chronic kidney disease, glaucoma, coronary artery disease, and diabetes mellitus. She admits to having missed doses of her "heart medications" due to recent problems with gout and feeling unwell. She also notes that she has been taking increased doses of non-steroidal anti-inflammatory drugs for the pain she is suffering. Medications on presentation include lisinopril 40 mg daily, clonidine 0.2 mg twice daily, metoprolol 50 mg twice daily, aspirin 325 mg daily, and simvastatin 20 mg at bedtime.

   On physical examination, she is confused, sleepy, and unable to give more history. Her heart rate is 50 bpm, and her blood pressure is 210/82 mmHg. Her exam is notable for arteriolar nicking of the vessels in her eye grounds, rales on pulmonary exam, and a loud S3 gallop. Laboratory examinations include a serum creatinine of 3.8 mg/dL (baseline of 1.6 mg/dL), normal liver functions, potassium of 4.9 mmol/L, and an electrocardiogram shows diffuse non-specific ST and T wave abnormalities.

   An intravenous line is started, and the patient is admitted to the intensive care unit.

   All of the following are true about this patient EXCEPT:
   (a) The cause of her bradycardia is increased accumulation of metoprolol from acute renal failure
   (b) Fenoldopam is contraindicated due to her history of glaucoma
   (c) Withdrawal from a centrally acting a2 agonist may explain her hypertension
   (d) Extended use of sodium nitroprusside may result in thiocyanate toxicity
   (e) Lisinopril should be discontinued until her renal function and potassium are stabilized

2. A 27 year old woman in the second trimester of pregnancy develops progressive hypertension. She has no prior history of medical problems, and other than a blood pressure of 168/92 mmHg, she is physically well.

   All of the following are true about this patient EXCEPT:
   (a) Calcium channel blockers are reasonable choices for her hypertension
   (b) b blockers are to be avoided in mid- to late pregnancy
   (c) An angiotensin converting enzyme inhibitor is a reasonable choice for her hypertension
   (d) Alpha methyl dopa is a reasonable choice for her hypertension
   (e) Hydralazine is a reasonable choice for her hypertension

3. A 42 year old man develops a rapid pulse. Soon after, he loses consciousness, without prodrome. After waking, he is fully conscious, but dizzy. On arrival of the Emergency Medical Service, he is noted to have a heart rate of 300 bpm and blood pressure of 70/30 mmHg. Before a rhythm strip can be obtained, his heart rate drops to 50 bpm.

   He has a past medical history notable for atrial fibrillation, for which he takes flecainide 100 mg twice daily; aspirin is taken for stroke prophylaxis. He has no other medical history, is an avid marathon runner, and denies any anginal symptoms.

   What is the most likely cause of his rapid heart rhythm?
   (a) Incessant ventricular tachycardia from flecainide
   (b) Ventricular flutter due to coronary ischemia and the concomitant use of a Ib agent
   (c) A Stokes-Adams attack from atrial fibrillation
   (d) Atrioventricular reentrant tachycardia through a concealed pathway, potentiated by flecainide
   (e) Atrial flutter with 1:1 conduction

ANSWERS

1. (a) Metoprolol is cleared hepatically. All other answers are true.

2. (c) Angiotensin converting enzyme inhibitors are strictly contraindicated in pregnancy.

3. (e) Flecainide has dual effects to promote such a scenario: it slows the flutter rate, and has anti-cholinergic effects on the atrioventricular node, potentially promoting rapid conduction. Class Ic agents should never be employed without concomitant use of an agent that slows conduction.

REFERENCE

1. Wallentin L, Becker RC, Budaj A, Cannon CP, Emanuelsson H, Held C, et al. Ticagrelor versus clopidogrel in patients with acute coronary syndromes. N Engl J Med. 2009;361:1045–57.

CHAPTER 34

ANNE M. BORDEN AND HANNA K. GAGGIN

ACLS

CHAPTER OUTLINE

ABBREVIATIONS

ABC	Airway Breathing, Circulation
ACLS	Advanced Cardiac Life Support
AED	Automated external defibrillator
AHA	American Heart Association
BLS	Basic Life Support
CAB	Circulation Airway and Breathing
CPR	Cardiopulmonary resuscitation
ETT	Endotracheal tube
IV	Intravenous
PEA	Pulseless electrical activity
PETCO$_2$	Partial pressure of end-tidal carbon dioxide
ROSC	Return Of Spontaneous Circulation
VF	Ventricular fibrillation
VT	Ventricular tachycardia

INTRODUCTION

Successful resuscitation relies on a foundation of good Basic Life Support (BLS) and integration of Advanced Cardiac Life Support (ACLS) guidelines. Changes in ACLS from the American Heart Association (AHA) guidelines that all providers should be familiar with were introduced in 2010. Changes covering the basic elements of Circulation Airway and Breathing (CAB) have also been expanded to include post-cardiac arrest care and the Return Of Spontaneous Circulation (ROSC). Teamwork and closed-loop feedback communication solidify an integrated approach. This section summarizes the current adult recommendations highlighting the changes in guidelines.

Key Changes in the 2010 AHA Guidelines [1, 2]

- Circulation, Airway, Breathing (CAB). This is the new sequence replacing the Airway, Breathing and Circulation (ABC). The priority is to decrease the time to first chest compression. Greatest survival rates happen with witnessed cardiac arrest, ventricular fibrillation (VF) and pulseless ventricular tachycardia (VT) [3].
- Compression-only cardiopulmonary resuscitation (CPR) for the lay rescuer. If a sole lay rescuer is present or multiple lay rescuers are reluctant to perform mouth-to-mouth ventilation.
- Adenosine was added for the diagnosis and treatment of stable undifferentiated regular and monomorphic wide complex tachycardia.
- Atropine is no longer recommended in the use for pulseless electrical activity (PEA)/ asystole.
- Symptomatic unstable bradycardia. Intravenous (IV) chronotropic agents such as epinephrine and dopamine are recommended as they are equally effective as external pacing when atropine is ineffective.

Basic Life Support (BLS)=CAB D

(A) **Circulation**
- Chest compressions: **at least 100/min** and **at least 2 inches** in depth
- **30**:**2** compressions to ventilation ratio

(B) **Airway**
- Open airway: head-tilt, chin lift
- Continuous quantitative waveform capnography (Class I recommendation) if available
- If partial pressure of end-tidal carbon dioxide ($PETCO_2$) <10 mmHg, confirm airway and monitor the endotracheal tube (ETT) placement if applicable

(C) **Breathing**
- 8–10 breaths per minute
- Avoid hyperventilation

(D) **Defibrillation**
- Automated external defibrillator (AED) as soon as possible

ACLS Algorithms

(A) **The unresponsive patient (Fig. 34-1)**
(B) **Cardiac arrest (VF/ VT or Asystole/PEA) (Fig. 34-2)**
(C) **Post-cardiac arrest care (Fig. 34-3)**
(D) **Tachycardia (with pulse) (Fig. 34-4)**
(E) **Bradycardia (with pulse) (Fig. 34-5)**

Clinical Pearls

(A) **Reversible causes of cardiac arrest (Table 34-1)**
(B) **Defibrillation and cardioversion**
- Monophasic vs biphasic waveforms

  — Biphasic waveforms, at the manufacturer's recommended energy level (Class I recommendations, level of evidence=B) is associated with a more effective defibrillation at lower energy levels than monophasic waveforms [4], but no conclusive data on any difference in clinical outcomes such as survival-to-discharge rate with either waveform.

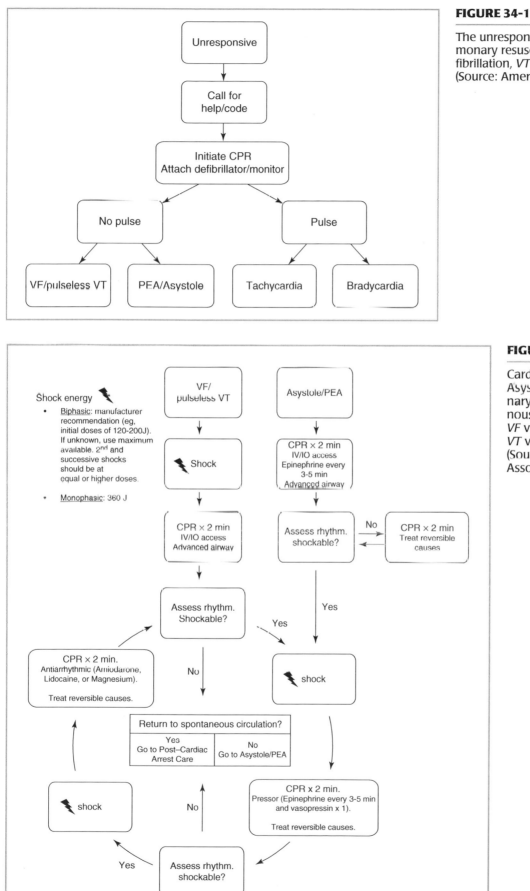

FIGURE 34-1

The unresponsive patient. *CPR* cardiopulmonary resuscitation, *VF* ventricular fibrillation, *VT* ventricular tachycardia (Source: American Heart Association, Inc)

FIGURE 34-2

Cardiac Arrest (VF/pulseless VT or Asystole/PEA). *CPR* cardiopulmonary resuscitation, *IV* intravenous, *IO* intraosseous, *VF* ventricular fibrillation, *VT* ventricular tachycardia (Source: American Heart Association, Inc)

FIGURE 34-3

Post-cardiac arrest care.
BP blood pressure, *PETCO₂*
End-tidal carbon dioxide tension,
ROSC return of spontaneous
circulation (Source: American
Heart Association, Inc)

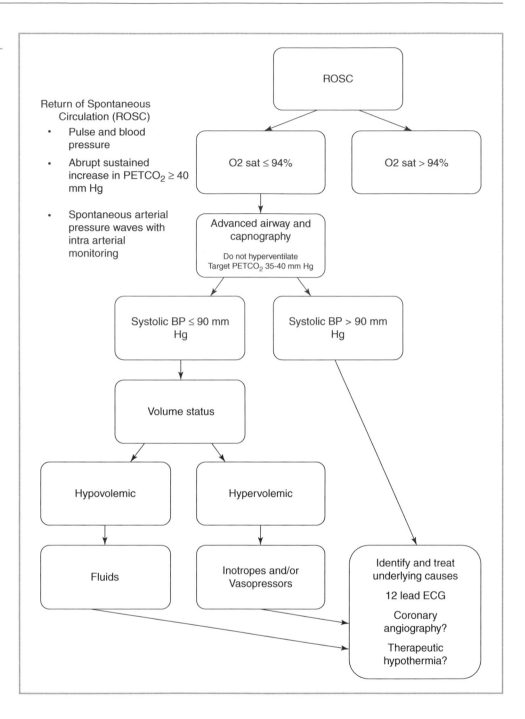

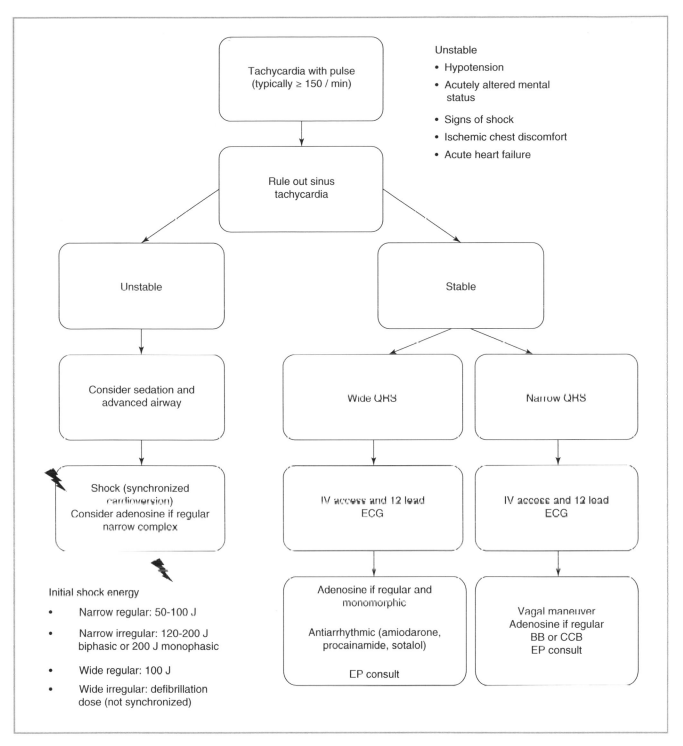

FIGURE 34-4

Tachycardia (with pulse). *BB* beta blockers, *CCB* calcium channel blocker, *EP* electrophysiology, *IV* intravenous (Source: American Heart Association, Inc)

FIGURE 34-5

Bradycardia (with pulse).
EP electrophysiology
(Source: American Heart
Association, Inc)

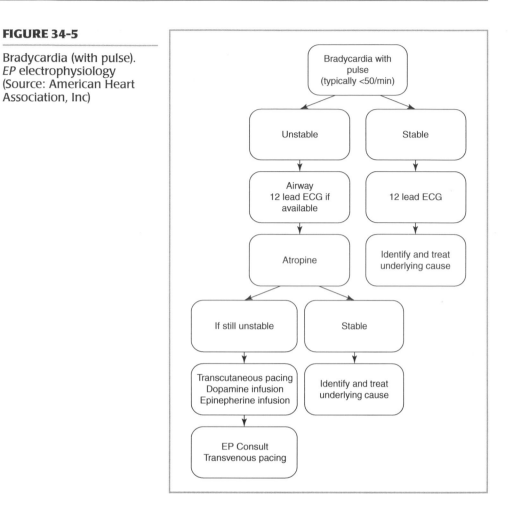

TABLE 34-1

H'S AND T'S

H'S	T'S
Hypo(hyper) kalemia	Tamponade (cardiac)
Hypovolemia	Tension pneumothorax
Hypoxia	Thrombosis (cardiac)
Hydrogen ion (acidosis)	Thrombosis (pulmonary)
Hypothermia	Toxins
Hypoglycemia	

■ **Contraindication for defibrillation or cardioversion**

— Sinus tachycardia
— Multifocal atrial tachycardia
— Digitalis toxicity–associated tachycardia
— Junctional tachycardia

■ Indications for synchronized cardioversion (Table 34-2)
■ Implanted pacemaker or defibrillator:

— If possible, place defibrillator pads away from the implanted device, not directly on top of them. But operate normally otherwise.

TABLE 34-2

INDICATIONS FOR SYNCHRONIZED CARDIOVERSION

SYNCHRONIZED CARDIOVERSION	NOT APPROPRIATE FOR SYNCHRONIZED CARDIOVERSION
Atrial fibrillation	Ventricular fibrillation
Atrial flutter	Pulseless ventricular tachycardia
Atrial tachycardia	Polymorphic ventricular tachycardia
Supraventricular tachycardia	
Regular monomorphic ventricular tachycardia with a pulse	

TABLE 34-3

KEY MEDICATIONS

MEDICATION	DOSE
Atropine	0.5 mg IV every 3–5 min, max dose 3 mg
Adenosine	Rapid 6 mg IV push. Chase with 20 mL saline
	If no response: Repeat with 12 mg
Amiodarone	Cardiac Arrest: 300 mg IV/IO push, second dose 150 mg IV/IO push
	Arrhythmias: 150 mg IV over 10 min, may repeat as needed
	Maintenance infusion: 1 mg/min × 6 h
Dopamine	Bradycardia: 2–10 mcg/kg/min IV, titrate as needed
Epinephrine	Cardiac Arrest: 1mg IV/IO (10 mL of 1:10,000 solution) every 3–5 min
	Alternatively 2–2.5 mg ETT (1:1,000 solution)
	Bradycardia: 2–10 mcg/min IV infusion, titrate as needed
Lidocaine	Cardiac Arrest: 1–1.5 mL/kg IV/IO. Repeat at half the dose every 5–10 min, max 3 mg/kg
	Alternatively 2–4 mg/kg ETT
Magnesium	Cardiac Arrest: 1–2 g (2–4 mL of 50 % solution diluted in10 mL of D_5W) IV/IO over 5–20 min
Procainamide	Arrhythmias: 20–50 mg/min IV until arrhythmia is suppressed, hypotension, QRS duration increases >50 % or max dose of 17 mg/kg given
	Maintenance infusion: 1–4 mg/min
	Avoid if prolonged QT or CHF
Sotalol	Arrhythmias: 100mg (1.5 mg/kg) IV over 5 min
	Avoid if prolonged QT
Vasopressin	Cardiac arrest: 40 units IV/IO × 1 only
	May replace first or second dose of epinephrine

— If the analysis and shock cycles of the implanted device conflict with the external defibrillator, then wait 30–60 s for the implanted device to complete the treatment cycle before delivering a shock with the external defibrillator.

■ Know the equipment: cables get disconnected, batteries may not be charged, paper runs out and sync button may be engaged inadvertently.

Key ACLS Medications (Table 34-3)

■ Medications that can go down an endotracheal tube: (LEAV)

— Lidocaine, Epinephrine, Atropine, Vasopressin

■ Torsade de pointes: try magnesium first

■ Medications for the treatment of hyperkalemia: (CBIG)

— Calcium chloride has more effective than calcium gluconate IV but high risk of tissue necrosis if extravasates. 1–2 amps IV.
— Bicarbonate 1–3 amps IV
— Regular insulin 10 units IV with 1–2 amps dextrose 50 % water ($D_{50}W$)

References

1. Neumar RW, Otto CW, Link MS, Kronick SL, Shuster M, Callaway CW, et al. Part 8: adult advanced cardiovascular life support: 2010 American Heart Association Guidelines for Cardiopulmonary Resuscitation and Emergency Cardiovascular Care. Circulation. 2010;122(18 Suppl 3):S729–67.

2. Field JM, Hazinski MF, Sayre MR, Chameides L, Schexnayder SM, Hemphill R, et al. Part 1: executive summary: 2010 American Heart Association Guidelines for Cardiopulmonary Resuscitation and Emergency Cardiovascular Care. Circulation. 2010;122 (18 Suppl 3):S640–56.

3. Rea TD, Cook AJ, Stiell IG, Powell J, Bigham B, Callaway CW, et al. Predicting survival after out-of-hospital cardiac arrest: role of the Utstein data elements. Ann Emerg Med. 2010;55(3): 249–57.

4. Schneider T, Martens PR, Paschen H, Kuisma M, Wolcke B, Gliner BE. Multicenter, randomized, controlled trial of 150-J biphasic shocks compared with 200- to 360-J monophasic shocks in the resuscitation of out-of-hospital cardiac arrest victims. Optimized Response to Cardiac Arrest (ORCA) Investigators. Circulation. 2000;102(15):1780–7.

CHAPTER 35

Marcello Panagia and Malissa J. Wood

Imaging Studies Section (Echocardiograms, Ventriculograms, Aortograms and Angiograms)

CHAPTER OUTLINE

ABBREVIATIONS

A3C	Apical 3 chamber or apical long axis
A4C	Apical 4 chamber
A5C	Apical 5 chamber
Ao	Aorta
ASD	Atrial septal defect
AV	Aortic valve
CW	Continuous wave
DT	Deceleration time
Ef	Effusion
HOCM	Hypertrophic obstructive cardiomyopathy
LA	Left atrium
LAD	Left anterior descending artery
LAO	Left anterior oblique
LCx	Left circumflex coronary artery
LIMA	Left internal mammary artery
LM	Left main coronary artery
LV	Left ventricle
LVOT	Left Ventricular outflow track
MR	Mitral regurgitation
MV	Mitral valve
OM	Obtuse marginal
PA	Pulmonary artery
PFO	Patent foramen ovale
PLAX	Parasternal long axis
PSAX	Parasternal short axis
Pulm	Pulmonary
PW	Pulsed wave
RA	Right atrium
RAO	Right anterior oblique
RCA	Right coronary artery
RPA	Right pulmonary artery
RV	Right ventricle
RVOT	Right ventricular outflow track
SAM	Systolic anterior motion
SVG	Saphenous vein graft

TEE   Transesophageal echo
ToF   Tetralogy of Fallot
TTE   Transthoracic echo
TV   Tricuspid valve
VSD   Ventricular septal defect

To prepare for the imaging studies section of the board exam, **you MUST know the answer option lists for the section INSIDE AND OUT**. You can find the answer option lists on the American Board of Internal Medicine (ABIM) official website, http://www.abim.org/, under the tab, "take the exam *your complete guide*," then under the "Prepare for the Exam: Take the Tutorial" section, near the bottom is a pdf file called "**Sample Cases - Electrocardiograms and Imaging Studies (pdf).**" **Pay extra attention** to the last page, which explains the scoring of sample cases.

In this section, we have put heavy emphasis on the specific diagnoses that are on the answer option lists to complement bread and butter clinical training in imaging. **We have included still-frame images with illustrate key findings, however, the actual exam contains moving images and will require COMPLETE CODING OF ALL YOU SEE RATHER THAN JUST THE KEY FINDINGS. All of the still-frame images in this chapter are available as moving images on our multi-media website.** See Fig. 35-1 for an example of complete coding. *The number of each key finding corresponds to the number of the diagnosis on the answer option sheet, but be mindful that the exact number may change over time as the answer option list evolves.* We recommend that you try viewing the movies on the website with ABIM answer options list and code each and every case in a timed manner first.

Please note that ventriculograms and aortograms are no longer covered in the Imaging Studies section of the board. However, they will be continued to be covered under the multiple choice questions section and are briefly covered here.

Acknowledgements: We would like to acknowledge Dr. Michael Fifer for his assistance in selecting cardiac catheterization images.

QUICK INDEX WITH FIGURE NUMBERS

Echocardiograms

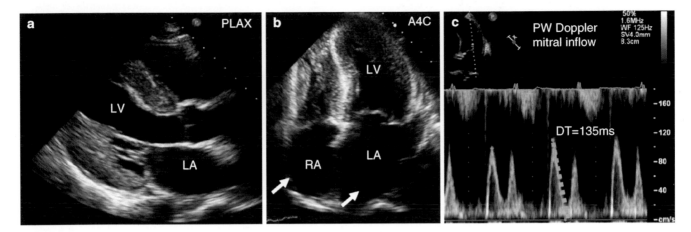

FIG. 35-1

A 47 year-old man with renal failure and syncope. Cardiac amyloidosis. 2D TTE images show biventricular hypertrophy, increased myocardial reflectivity, as well as biatrial enlargement (*arrows*) (**a**, **b**). Panel (**c**) showing PW Doppler at the mitral valve leaflet tips revealing a steep deceleration slope characteristic of a restrictive filling pattern. Key findings: 7. Grade 3 (restrictive) diastolic dysfunction, 16. Concentric LV wall thickness, 68. Enlarged left atrium, 69. Enlarged right atrium, 121. Amyloid. Complete coding: (in addition to above) 1. Normal LV size, 8. Normal WM, 12. Normal to hyperdynamic (≥50 %), 61. RV Normal size and function, 137. Pericardial effusion

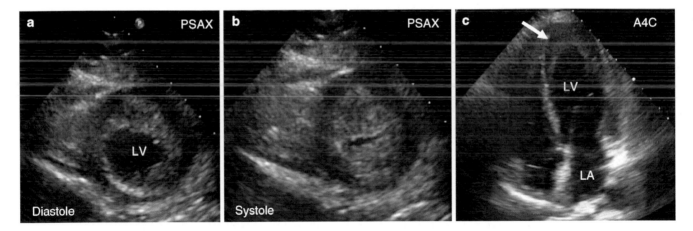

FIG. 35-2

A 45 year-old man with eczema and dyspnea. Hypereosinophilic syndrome. 2D TTE images showing PSAX in diastole (**a**) and systole (**b**) with significant LV soft tissue/eosinophils and thrombus deposition (*arrow*) at the apex of the heart (usually obliterating the apex), and no underlying wall motion abnormality. Panel (**c**) showing apical 4 chamber view of the same process. Make sure to be able to differentiate this from apical hypertrophic cardiomyopathy (which maintains a slitlike opening in the apex). Key findings: 19. LV mass or thrombus, 122. Hypereosinophilia

FIG. 35-3

A 35 year-old woman with stroke-like symptoms. LV Non-compaction. 2D TTE showing a thickened myocardium with a deeply trabeculated (*arrow*) appearance with intramyocardial sinusoids. Apical long axis (**a**) and PSAX (**b**) views are shown. Key findings: 119. Noncompaction

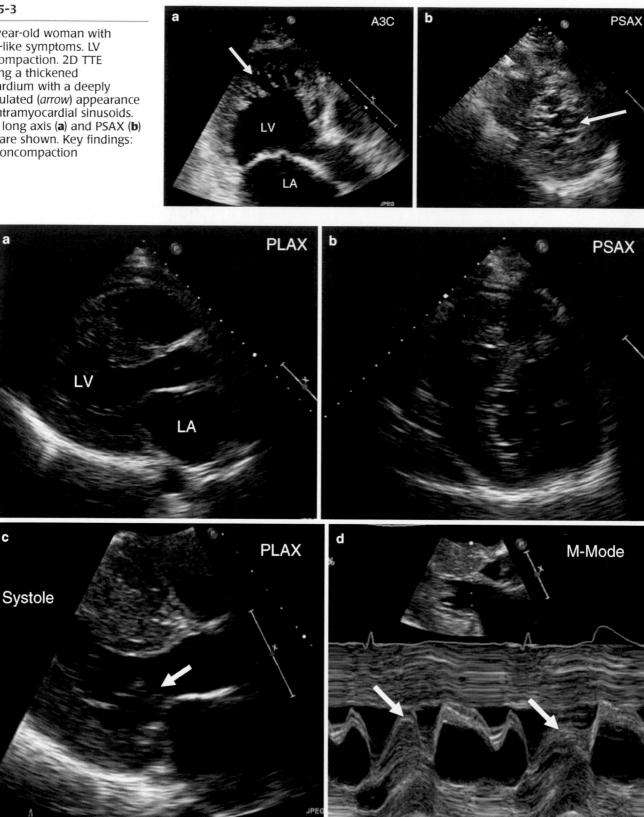

FIG. 35-4

A 45 year-old woman with syncope. HOCM. 2D TTE showing asymmetric septal hypertrophy in PLAX (**a**) and PSAX (**b**). Panel (**c**) showing SAM (*arrows*) also evident by MMODE in panel (**d**). Key findings: 17. Asymmetric septal hypertrophy, 18. LVOT obstruction/SAM, 114. Hypertrophic cardiomyopathy

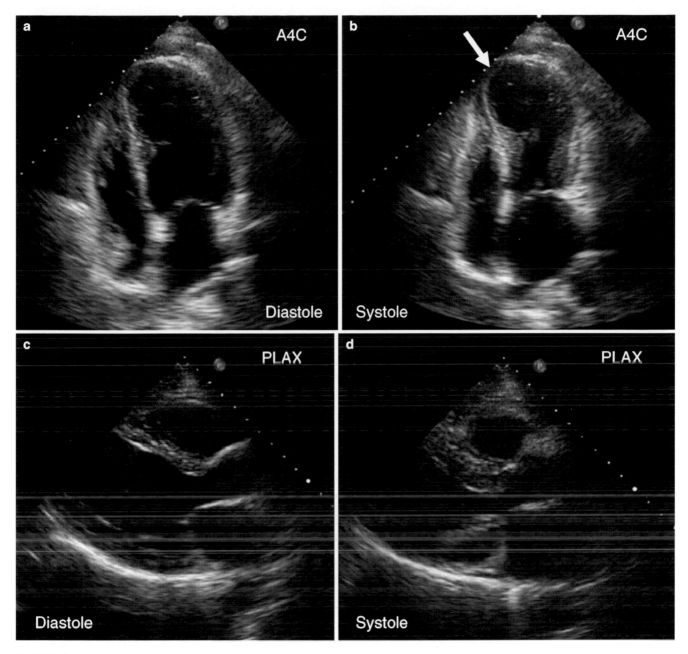

FIG. 35-5

A 77 year-old woman with chest pain at her husband's funeral. Stress induced (Takotsubo's) cardiomyopathy. 2D TTE showing an apical 4 chamber diastolic (**a**) and systolic (**b**) frames with apical hypokinesis (*arrow*) and preserved function at the base. PLAX diastolic (**c**) and systolic (**d**) frames are also shown. Key findings: 13. Mild to moderately reduced EF, 30. Apical hypokinesis, 120. Takotsubo (stress induced) cardiomyopathy

FIG. 35-6

A 65 year-old diabetic with crushing sub-sternal chest pain 1 year ago. Myocardial scar. 2D TTE apical 4 chamber showing a thinned and echo-bright septum (*arrow*) characteristic of scar formation. Key findings: 2. Enlarged LV size, 37. Septal thinning and/or scar

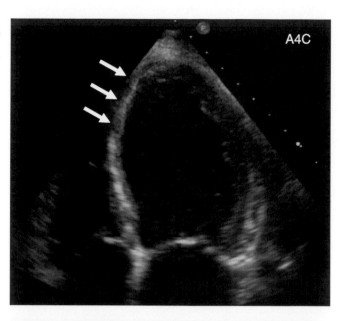

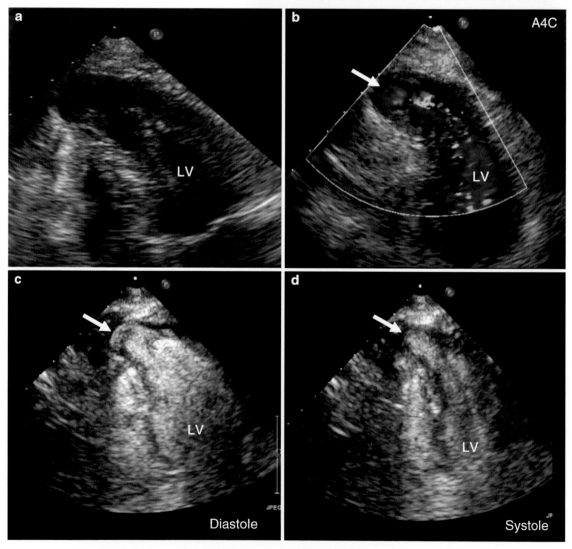

FIG. 35-7

A 76 year-old man with history of prior infarction. LV apical aneurysm. 2D TTE. Panel (**a**) shows an apical 4 chamber view of the aneurysm with color Doppler flow (**b**) into the aneurysm (*arrow*). Diastolic (**c**) and systolic (**d**) frames with LV contrast clearly show myocardial contraction in the aneurysmal segment (*arrows*). Key findings: 45. Apical aneurysm

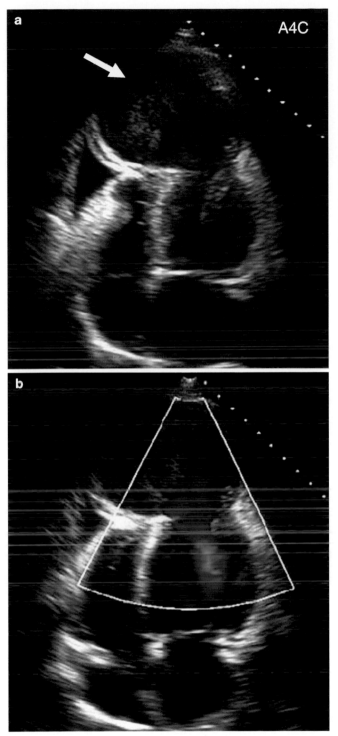

FIG. 35-8

A 75 year-old woman with coronary artery disease. LV pseudoaneurysm. 2D TTE. Panel (**a**) shows an apical 4 chamber view at end systole with a large (72 × 73 mm) akinetic space containing spontaneous echo contrast at the apex of the LV suggestive of pseudoaneurysm (*arrows*). Panel (**b**) shows color Doppler with flow into the pseudoaneurysm. Key findings: 50. Apical pseudoaneurysm

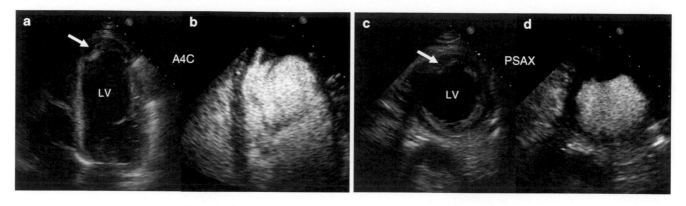

FIG. 35-9

A 45 year-old man with gangrene of his toe. LV thrombus. 2D TTE. Apical 4 chamber view (**a**) suggestive of a laminar apical thrombus (*arrow*) which is subsequently confirmed with LV contrast (**b**). PSAX views with (**d**) and without (**c**) LV contrast highlighting its utility in identifying ventricular thrombus. Key findings: 2. Enlarged LV size, 9. Global hypokinesis, 14. Severely reduced EF, 19. LV mass or thrombus

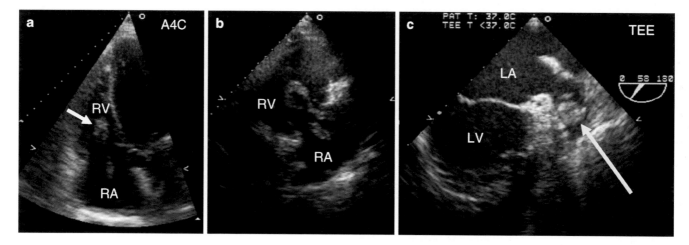

FIG. 35-10

A 50 year-old man with Factor V Leiden deficiency. RV thrombus. 2D TTE. Apical 4 chamber view (**a**) of a patient with an intracardiac thrombus (*arrow*) visible as it prolapses from the right atrium (*RA*) to the right ventricle (*RV*). Panel (**b**) shows the same serpiginous thrombus which likely originated from a vein. Panel (**c**) shows a TEE of a different patient with atrial fibrillation and a left atrial appendage containing thrombus (*arrow*). Key findings (**a**, **b**): 2. Enlarged LV, 9. Global hypokinesis, 14. Severely reduced EF, 63. Global RV dysfunction, 21. Atrial thrombus, 67. RV thrombus present

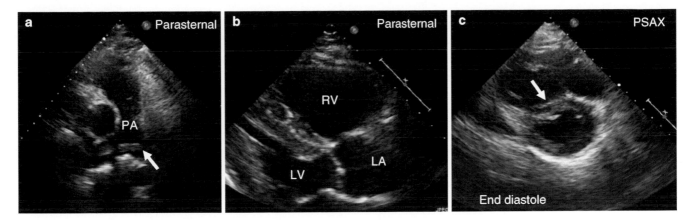

FIG. 35-11

A 45 year-old woman with shortness of breath after a long flight. Pulmonary emoblism. 2D TTE. Parasternal view (**a**) of the main pulmonary artery at the bifurcation revealing a saddle pulmonary embolism (*arrow*). Parasternal view (**b**) at end systole showing a dilated and hypokinetic RV. PSAX view (**c**) of the LV at end diastole showing interventricular septal flattening (*arrow*) consistent with volume overload. Key finding: 123. Findings consistent with acute pulomary embolism, 63. Global RV dysfunction, 62. Enlarged RV, 64. Septal motion suggests volume overload

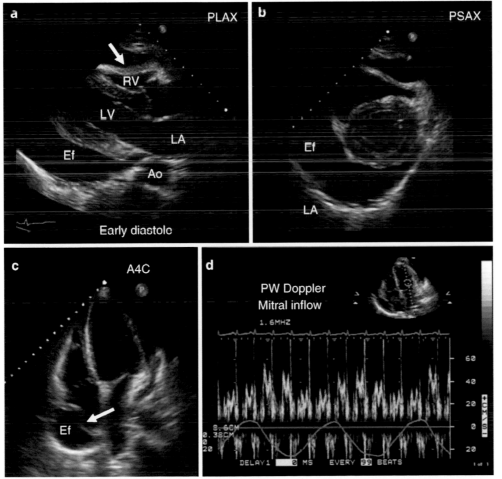

FIG. 35-12

A 35 year-old woman with metastatic breast cancer and shortness of breath. Cardiac tamponade. 2D TTE. PLAX (**a**) and PSAX (**b**) showing a large circumferential pericardial effusion with RV inversion (*arrow*) during early diastole. Apical 4 chamber view (**c**) showing RA inversion (*arrow*) and PW Doppler (**d**) at the mitral valve leaflet tips showing respirophasic variation of Doppler flow across the mitral valve. Key findings: 137. Pericardial effusion, 136. Pericardial tamponade

FIG. 35-13

A 67 year-old woman from India with exertional dyspnea. Rheumatic mitral stenosis. 2D TTE. PLAX view (**a**) showing thickened MV leaflet tips in a "hockey stick" (*arrow*) and domed appearance. Panel (**a**) also shows a dilated LA. PSAX view (**b**) in diastole showing a restricted MV orifice which can be planimetered. Panel (**c**) is a typical MMODE tracing showing thickening leaflets (*arrow*). Panel (**d**) is a transmitral continuous wave (*CW*) Doppler tracing showing a relatively flat pressure decay and variability of the spectral profile influenced by the diastolic filling time. Key findings: 77. Rheumatic MV, 68. Enlarged LA, 101. Severe MV stenosis

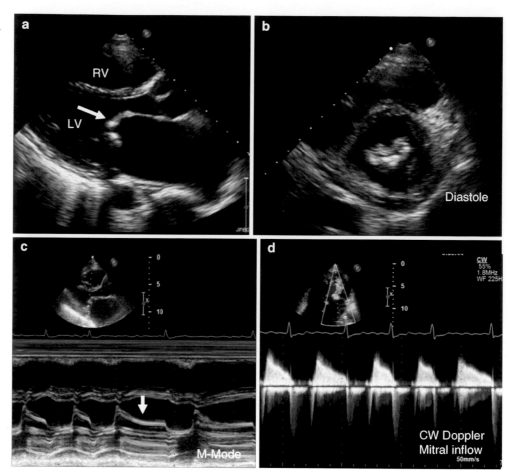

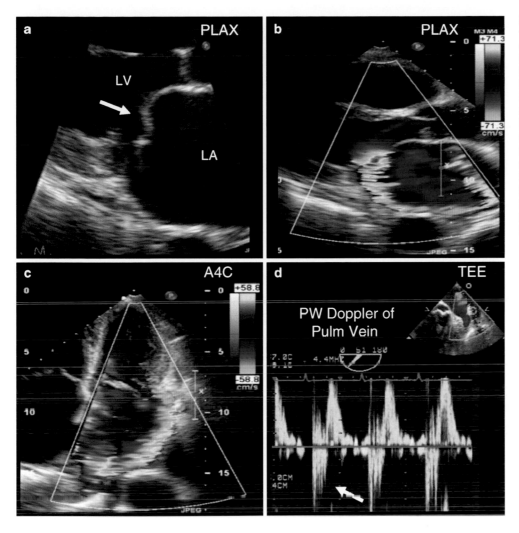

FIG. 35-14

A 65 year-old woman with dyspnea and lower extremity edema. Flail MV leaflet. 2D TTE. PLAX view (**a**) showing anterior leaflet flail (*arrow*) resulting in eccentric, posteriorely directed MR by color Doppler (**b**). Apical 4 chamber view (**c**) again showing eccentric MR resulting from flail anterior MV leaflet. Pulsed wave Doppler of the pulmonary vein (**d**) by TEE showing systolic flow reversal (*arrow*). Key findings: 81. Flail MV, 109. Severe MR, 68. Enlarged LA

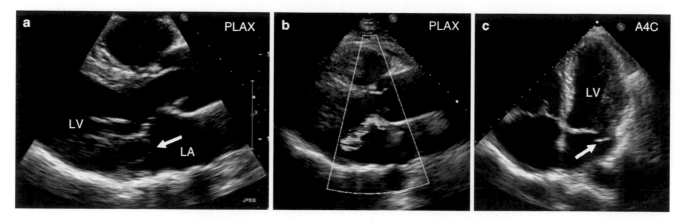

FIG. 35-15

A 52-year old woman with a new holosystolic murmur. MV prolapse. 2D TTE. PLAX view (**a**) showing posterior leaflet prolapse resulting in an anteriorely directed jet of MR seen by color Doppler (**b**). Apical 4 chamber view (**c**) also showing posterior leaflet MV prolapse. Key findings: 80. MV prolapse, 108. Mild/moderate MR

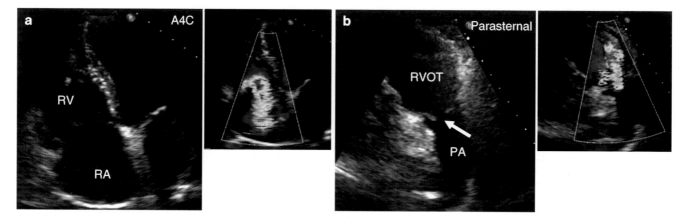

FIG. 35-16

A 65 year-old man with lower extremity edema and elevated liver enzymes. Carcinoid. 2D TTE. Apical 4 chamber view (**a**) systolic frame showing thickened TV leaflets with failure of coaptation resulting in severe TR seen by color Doppler. Parasternal view (**b**) showing pulmonary valve (*arrow*) involvement and leaflet thickening resulting in severe pulmonary insufficiency. Key findings: 69. Enlarged RA, 84. TV carcinoid, 103. Severe TR, 89. PV carcinoid, 113. Severe PR

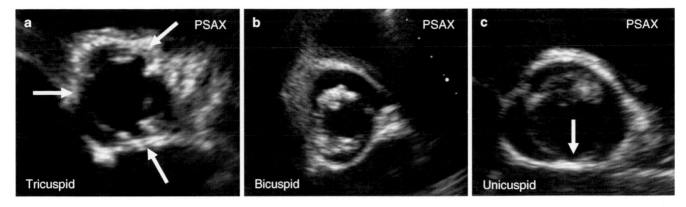

FIG. 35-17

A 35 year-old man with a crescendo-decrescendo systolic ejection murmur. Tricuspid (**a**), bicuspid (**b**), and unicuspid (**c**) AV. 2D TTE. PSAX views of the AV in systole. Notable is the elliptical shape of the bicuspid valve orifice in systole as well as the thickened valve leaflets. The unicuspid valve showing only one commissure reaching the annulus at the 6 o'clock position (*arrow*) whereas the tricuspid valve has all three commissures reaching the annulus (*arrows*). Key findings for figure (**b**): 72. Bicuspid AV

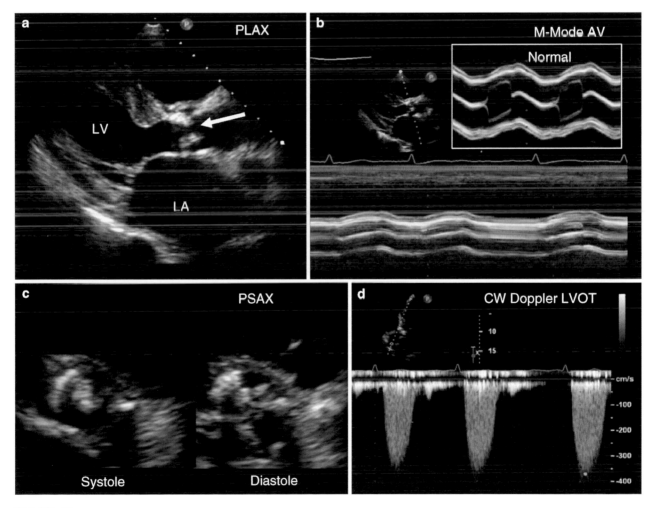

FIG. 35-18

An 84 year-old man with exertional dyspnea and syncope. Calcific aortic stenosis. 2D TTE. PLAX view (**a**) showing calcified AV leaflets (*arrow*) and LV hypertrophy. In addition to thickened leaflets, reduced excursion is evident by MMODE across the AV (**b**). *Inset* shows MMODE across normal AV leaflets. PSAX view in systole and diastole (**c**) showing reduced orifice opening size. Aortic stenosis resulted in increased transvalvular flow velocity measured by CW Doppler (**d**). Key findings: 16. Concentric LV wall thickness, 68. Enlarged LA, 70. Calcific AV, 99. Severe aortic stenosis

FIG. 35-23

A 75 year-old man with worsening dyspnea. Thrombus on mechanical MV. 2D TEE. A mid-esophageal TEE view of a St. Jude mechanical valve in the mitral position in systole (**a**) and diastole (**b**). Notable is thrombus (*arrow*) on the valve leaflet obstructing opening of that leaflet resulting in only one valve leaflet functioning properly. Color Doppler (**c**) shows flow through the only functioning orifice and no flow across the obstructed orifice resulting in mitral stenosis evident by increased mitral valve gradients seen with CW Doppler (**d**). Key findings: 93. Prosthetic valve present, elevated gradients, 94. Prosthetic valve present, obstruction due to thrombus or pannus

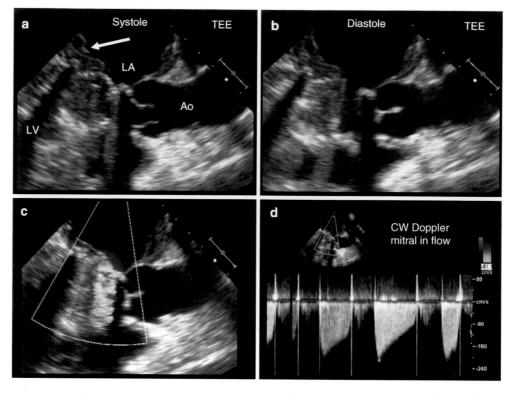

FIG. 35-24

A 24 year-old man with fevers, malaise and stroke. Endocarditis. 2D TTE. PLAX view (**a**) showing an echo-density on the non-coronary leaflet of the AV likely representing vegetation. Color Doppler (**b**) showing severe aortic regurgitation resulting from the vegetation. Key findings: 73. Aortic valve, vegetation. 107. Severe aortic regurgitation

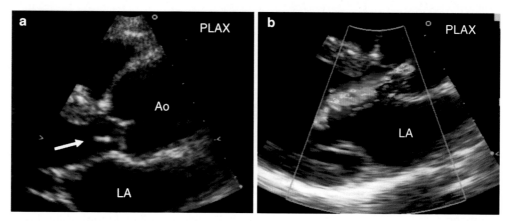

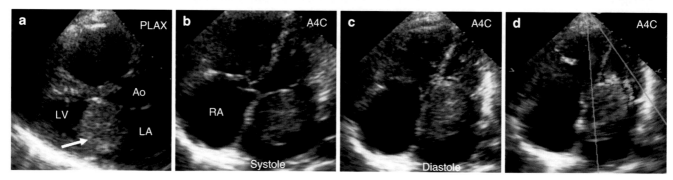

FIG. 35-25

A 20 year-old man with exertional dyspnea and left arm weakness. Atrial myxoma. 2D TTE. PLAX view (**a**) of the myxoma (*arrow*). Apical 4 chamber view in systole (**b**) and diastole (**c**) showing the mass prolapsing into the MV orifice resulting in significant obstruction to flow across the MV seen by color Doppler (**d**). Key findings: 20. Atrial myxoma, 101. Severe MS

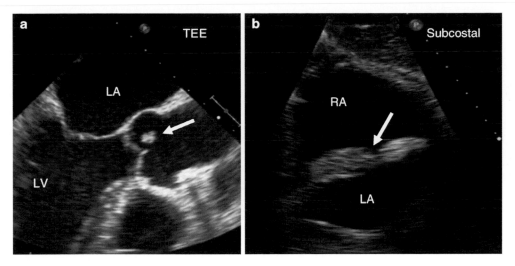

FIG. 35-26

A 20 year-old woman with an ST elevation infarction. Papillary fibroelastoma (**a**) and Lipomatous hypertrophy of the interatrial septum (**b**). Mid-esophageal TEE long axis view (**a**) of the AV showing a small spherical mass attached via a pedicle to the aortic side of the valve leaflets suspicious for a papillary fibroelastoma. Subcostal view (**b**) by 2D TTE showing lipomatous hypertrophy of the interatrial septum with characteristic sparing (thinning) of the fossa ovalis (*arrow*). Key findings: (**a**) 25. Fibroelastoma. (**b**) 23. Atrial septal lipomatous hypertrophy

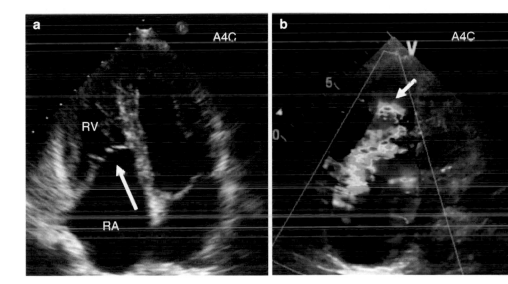

FIG. 35-27

A 20 year-old woman with palpitations. Ebstein's anomaly. 2D TTE. Apical 4 chamber view (**a**) showing an apically displaced TV (*arrow*) as compared with the MV annulus resulting in a smaller and distorted true right ventricle as well as a larger and distorted "atrialized" right ventricle. Panel (**b**) is an apical 4 chamber color Doppler of another patient with Ebstein anomaly where the TV is even further apically displaced. Poor coaptation of the leaflets (*arrow*) results in severe tricuspid regurgitation. Key findings: 153. Ebstein's anomaly, 111. Severe TR

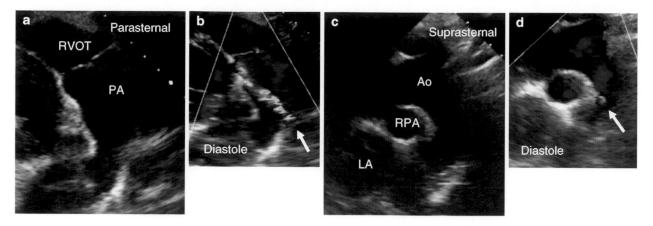

FIG. 35-28

A 12 year-old boy with a continuous murmur. Patent ductus arteriosus. 2D TTE. Parasternal view of the main pulmonary artery (**a**) with color Doppler (**b**) showing diastolic flow (*arrow*) into the vessel. Suprasternal view (**c**) with color Doppler (**d**) showing high velocity diastolic flow originating in the aorta. Key findings: 132. PDA

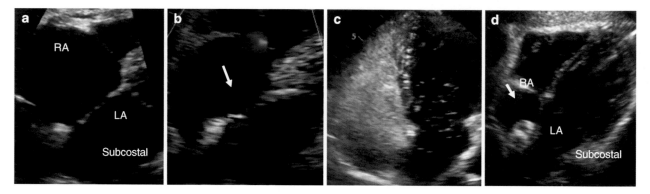

FIG. 35-29

A 30 year-old man with cryptogenic stroke. Patent foramen ovale. 2D TTE. Subcostal view (**a**) with color Doppler (**b**) showing a jet of high velocity flow (*arrow*) across the interatrial septum consistent with a PFO. A bubble study (**c**) with numerous bubbles crossing the septum by the third heart beat confirms the diagnosis. Panel (**d**) shows an Amplatzer closure device (*arrow*) placed in the interatrial septum. Key findings: 125. Patent foramen ovale

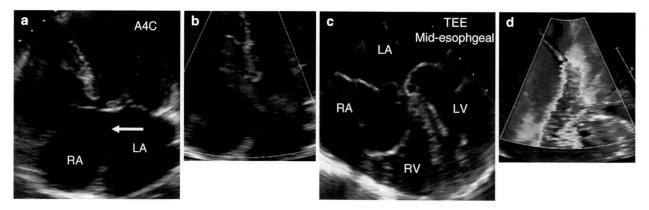

FIG. 35-30

A 19 year-old woman with palpitations and shortness of breath. Primum atrial septal defect. 2D TTE and 2D TEE. Apical 4 chamber 2D TTE (**a**) showing the absence of any tissue at the most inferior portion of the atrial septum (*arrow*, at level of A-V valve insertion). Color Doppler (**b**) confirms flow across the defect. Mid-esophageal 4 chamber view (**c**) with color Doppler (**d**) further characterizes the defect. Key findings: 126. Primum ASD

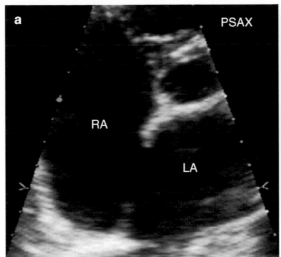

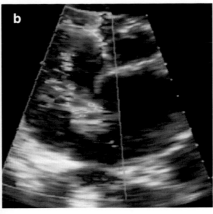

FIG. 35-31

A 27 year-old man with new onset atrial fibrillation. Secundum atrial septal defect. 2D TTE. PSAX view (**a**) of the interatrial septum showing a small ridge of tissue at the inferior edge of the septal defect consistent with a secundum ASD. Color Doppler (**b**) confirms flow across the defect. Key findings: 69. Enlarged RA, 127. Secundum ASD

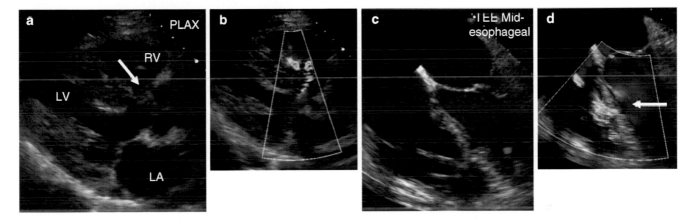

FIG. 35-32

A 15 year-old boy with fatigue and dyspnea. Membranous and muscular ventricular septal defects. 2D TTE and 2D TEE. PLAX view (**a**) showing a VSD in the membranous basal septum (*arrow*) resulting in high velocity and turbulent flow into the right ventricle seen on color Doppler (**b**). Mid-esophageal 2D TEE (**c**) showing a muscular VSD again resulting in turbulent flow across the defect (*arrow*) (**d**). Key findings: (**a**, **b**) 130. Membranous VSD, (**c**, **d**) 129 Muscular VSD

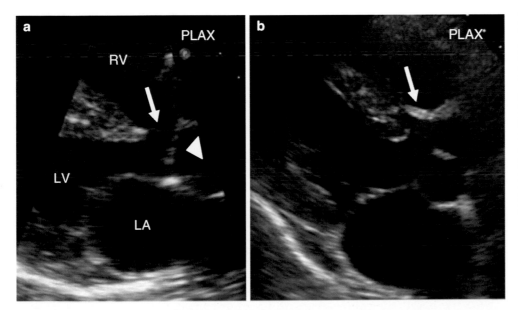

FIG. 35-33

A 30 year old woman with a history of multiple heart surgeries from birth. Tetralogy of Fallot. 2D TTE. PLAX view (**a**) showing a significant subaortic VSD (*arrow*) in combination with an overriding or anterior displaced aorta (*arrowhead*). Right ventricular outflow tract obstruction and right ventricular hypertrophy not shown. PLAX view (**b**) of a patient with ToF after a patch repair (*arrow*). Key findings: 152. Tetralogy of Fallot

Angiograms

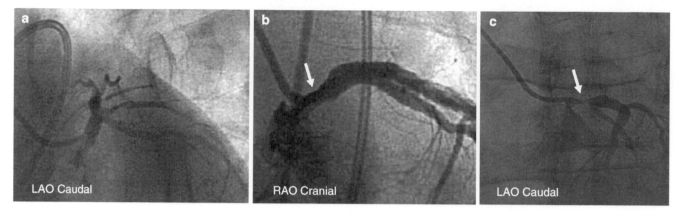

FIG. 35-34

Coronary angiography of two patients with ostial LM lesions. LAO Caudal (**a**) and RAO Cranial (**b**) view of a patient with an ostial 50 % LM lesion (*arrow*) and LAO Caudal (**c**) view of a patient with a 95 % LM lesion (*arrow*). Key findings: (**a**) and (**b**) 7. LM moderate stenosis, (**c**) 12. LM severe stenosis, for the exam, don't forget to code other findings such as other vessels with stenosis

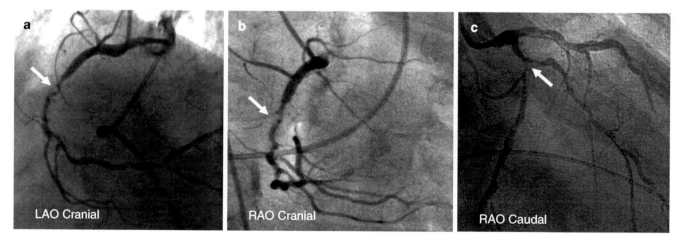

FIG. 35-35

Coronary angiogram of a patient with a long irregular 95 % right coronary artery (RCA) lesion in LAO Cranial (**a**) and RAO Cranial (**b**) views. Panel (**c**) shows an RAO Caudal view of a patient with a left circumflex artery-obtuse marginal artery (LCx-OM) bifurcation lesion. Key findings: (**a**) and (**b**) 15. RCA severe stenosis, (**c**) 14. LCx severe stenosis

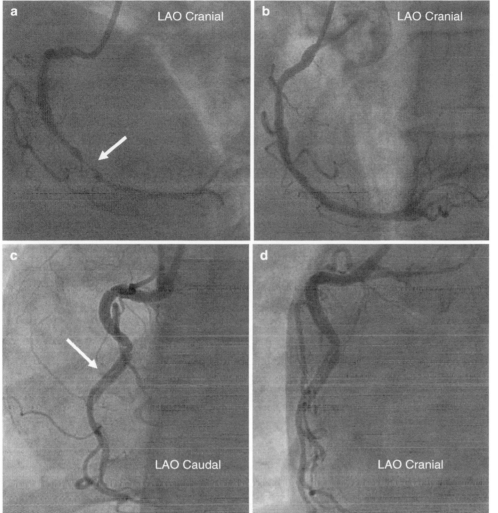

FIG. 35-36

Coronary angiography of two patients one with a coronary thrombus and another patient with a coronary dissection. Panel (**a**) shows an LAO Cranial view of the RCA containing thrombus material (*arrow*). Coronary flow is improved (**b**) after thrombus aspiration and stenting. Panel (**c**) shows an LAO Caudal view of the RCA of a patient with a coronary dissection (*arrow*). Panel (**d**) is an LAO Cranial view of the same process. Key findings: (**a**) 15. RCA severe stenosis and 32. RCA thrombus present, (**b**) 61. RCA stent:patent, (**c**) and (**d**) 56. RCA dissection

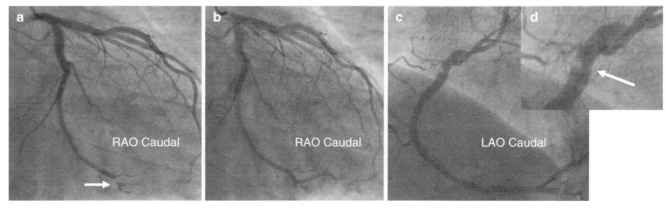

FIG. 35-37

Coronary angiography of a patient with coronary vasospasm and of a patient with an air embolism. RAO Caudal view (**a**) showing obstruction to coronary flow distal in the LCx (*arrow*) which improves after administration of intracoronary nitroglycerine (**b**). Panel (**c**) is an LAO Caudal view of the RCA containing an air embolism (*arrow*) which is seen in close-up in panel (**d**). Key findings: (**a**) and (**b**) 27. LCx spasm

FIG. 35-38

Coronary angiography of a patient with left to right collateral blood flow. LAO Caudal view (**a**) showing a chronically occluded RCA. Panel (**b**) shows an LAO Caudal view of the left system early in the injection and subsequently late in the injection (**c**). Notable is the collateral blood flow (*arrow*) supplying the RCA territory evident in panel (**c**) as well in the RAO Caudal view (**d**). Key findings: (**a**) 20. RCA complete occlusion, (**b**), (**c**) and (**d**) 24. RCA filled by collaterals

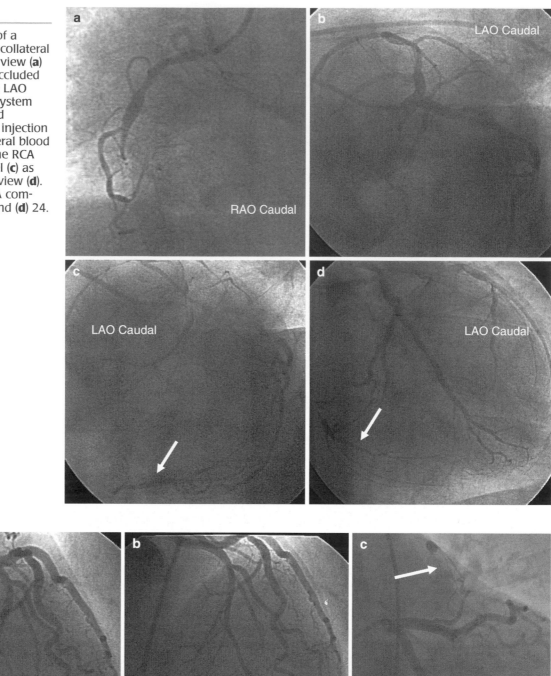

FIG. 35-39

Coronary angiography of a patient with a myocardial bridge and a patient with a LAD to PA fistula. Panel (**a**) shows a RAO Cranial view in systole and diastole (**b**) of a patient with a myocardial bridge of the mid LAD (*arrow*). LAO Caudal view (**c**) of a patient with an LAD to PA fistula. Key findings: (**a**) and (**b**) 34. LAD myocardial bridge, (**c**) 42. LAD coronary fistula

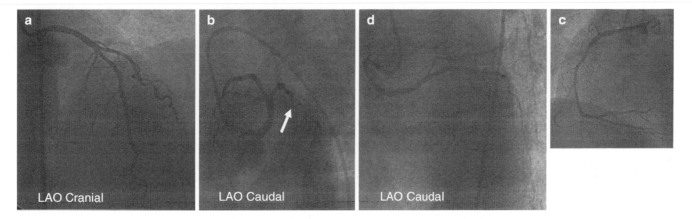

FIG. 35-40

Coronary angiography of a patient with LCx arising from the right coronary cusp. LAO Cranial (**a**) and LAO Caudal (**b**) view of the left system. Notable is the absence of the LCx (*arrow*). LAO Cranial (**c**) view showing a normal RCA. Panel (**d**) is an LAO Caudal view that shows a coronary vessel supplying the LCx territory. This vessel was engaged via a separate ostium in the right coronary cusp. Key findings: 39. LCx anomalous origin

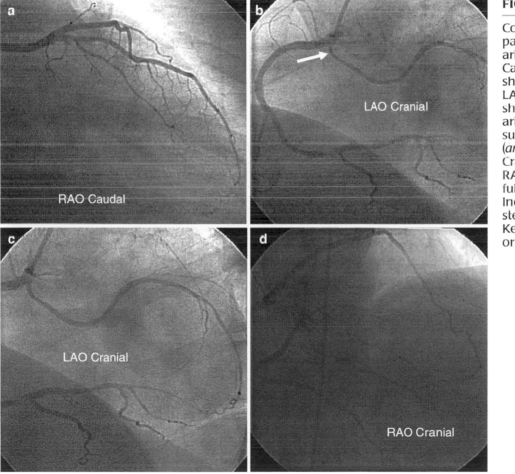

FIG. 35-41

Coronary angiography of a patient with an anomalous LCx arising from the RCA. RAO Caudal (**a**) view of the left system showing the absence of the LCx. LAO Cranial (**b**) view of the RCA showing an anomalous vessel arising from the RCA and supplying the LCx territory (*arrow*). Panel (**c**) is an LAO Cranial view and panel (**d**) is an RAO Cranial view showing the full course of the anomalous LCx. Incidentally, a discrete 70 % RCA stenosis is also visible mid-vessel. Key findings: 39. LCx anomalous origin, 10. RCA moderate stenosis

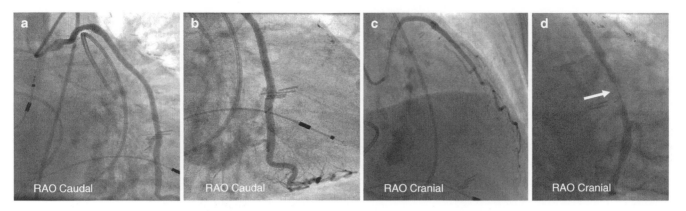

FIG. 35-42

Coronary angiography of venous bypass grafts. RAO Caudal view early (**a**) and late (**b**) in the injection showing a patent SVG to diagonal branch bypass graft. RAO Cranial view (**c**) of the same patient showing a patent SVG to OM branch bypass graft. Panel (**d**) shows a patient with in-stent restenosis (*arrow*) of a venous bypass graft. Notable is the outline of the stent containing a thin line of contrast flow. Key findings: (**a**) and (**b**) 50. Bypass graft to LAD, (**c**) 51. Bypass graft to LCx, (**d**) 67. Bypass graft stent: occluded

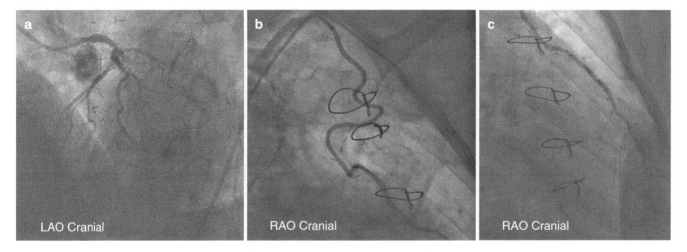

FIG. 35-43

Coronary angiography of a patient with a patent LIMA bypass graft. LAO Cranial (**a**) view of LCA showing a heavily diseased left system. RAO Cranial view early (**b**) and late (**c**) in the injection showing a patent LIMA to LAD bypass graft. Key findings: (**a**) 14. LCx severe stenosis, 13. LAD severe stenosis, (**b**) and (**c**) 50. Bypass graft to LAD

Ventriculograms and Aortograms

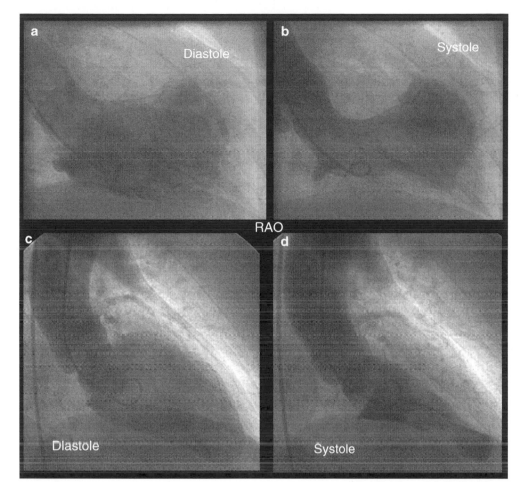

FIG. 35-44

Ventriculography of a patient with an anterior aneurysm seen in RAO view in diastole (**a**) and systole (**b**). The *bottom panels* show an RAO view in diastole (**c**) and systole (**d**) of a patient with apical akinesis or possibly an apical aneurysm

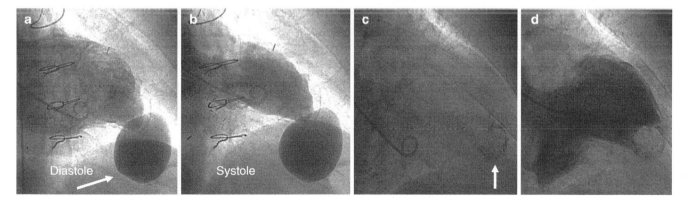

FIG. 35-45

Ventriculography of a patient with an LV pseudoaneurysm in (*arrow*) diastole (**a**) and systole (**b**). The lower panels show a patient with a calcified LV apical thrombus (*arrow*). Notable is the calcified outline of the apex evident in panel (**c**) and subsequently the entire calcified thrombus outline by contrast in panel (**d**)

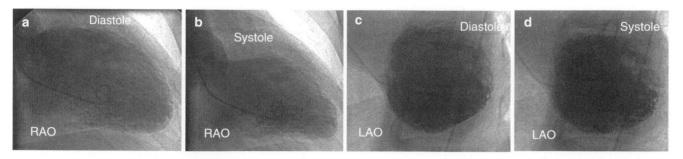

FIG. 35-46

Ventriculography of a patient with dilated cardiomyopathy. The *top panel* shows RAO views in diastole (**a**) and systole (**b**) and the *bottom panels* show LAO views in diastole (**c**) and systole (**d**) of the same patient

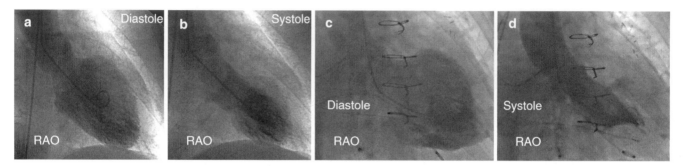

FIG. 35-47

Ventriculography of a patient with Takotsubo (stress) cardiomyopathy in RAO view during diastole (**a**) and systole (**b**). Notable is a hypercontractile base with apical ballooning. The *lower panels* show a patient with apical variant hypertrophic cardiomyopathy in diastole (**c**) and systole (**d**). Notable is the "spade-like" appearance of the apex in systole

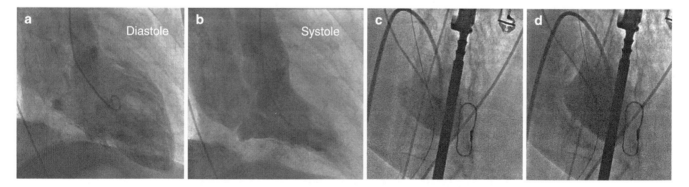

FIG. 35-48

Ventriculography of a patient with severe mitral regurgitation. Notable is the large amount of contrast seen in the left atrium early in systole (**b**) that was not present in diastole (**a**). The *lower panels* show RAO views early in systole (**c**) and later in systole (**d**) of a patient with a VSD. Notable is contrast streaming into the RV

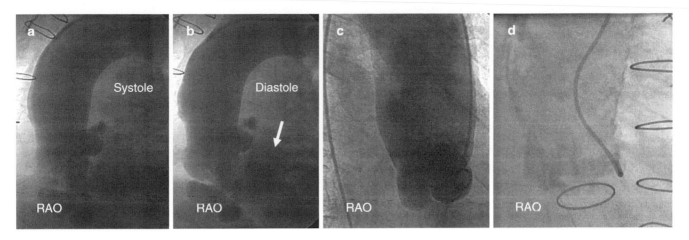

FIG. 35-49

Aortography in LAO view during systole (**a**) and diastole (**b**) of a patient with an aortic root abscess. Notable is the enlarged root with severe AI evidenced by a large amount of contrast streaming into the LV during diastole (*arrow*). Panel (**c**) shows a patient with an enlarged ascending aorta and panel (**d**) is an aortogram of a different patient with a calcified ascending aorta

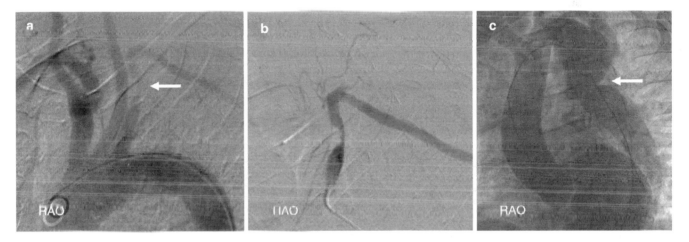

FIG. 35-50

Aortography of a patient with subclavian artery stenosis (*arrow*) (**a**) which is more clearly visualized with a selective angiogram of the subclavian artery (**b**). Panel (**c**) is an LAO view of an aortogram of a patient with a coarctation (*arrow*) of the descending thoracic aorta

CHAPTER 36

Jason Homsy and Philip J. Podrid

Electrocardiography

CHAPTER OUTLINE

ABBREVIATIONS

AIVR	Accelerated idioventricular rhythm
AV	Atrioventricular
AVNRT	Atrioventricular nodal reentrant tachycardia
AVRT	Atrioventricular reentrant tachycardia
CNS	Central nervous system
ECG	Electrocardiogram
IVCD	Intraventricular conduction delay
LA	Left atrial
LAFB	Left anterior fascicular block
LBBB	Left bundle branch block
LGL	Lown-Ganong-Levine
LPFB	Left posterior fascicular block
LV	Left ventricle
LVH	Left ventricular hypertrophy
MI	Myocardial infarction
PVB	Premature ventricular beats
PVC	Premature ventricular complexes
RA	Right atrium
RBBB	Right bundle branch block
RV	Right ventricle
RVH	Right ventricular hypertrophy
VA	Ventriculoatrial
VPB	Ventricular premature beats
VPC	Ventricular premature complexes
VT	Ventricular tachycardia
WPW	Wolff-Parkinson-White

INTRODUCTION

Two most frequent complaints of test takers for the electrocardiography (ECG) section of the board exam were that they did not have enough time and that they did not know the answer options (and therefore they ended up wasting a lot of time looking for the answers that they wanted on the answer options page!). Even if you get everything else on the board exam right, if you fail the ECG section, you still fail the boards. This is the most important part of your board exam. If you don't know the answers, then move on and come back to it. **You must KNOW how to diagnose the answers on the answer options list.** We recommend that you practice coding a set of ECG's in a timed session using the ABIM answer options list (There are typically 37 ECG's in one 2-h session, that's an average of 3.2 min/ECG). Pay special attention to the brief description of the patient. They contain invaluable clues to diagnoses.

You can find the answer option lists on the American Board of Internal Medicine (ABIM) official website, http://www.abim.org/, under the tab, "take the exam *your complete guide*," then under the "Prepare for the Exam: Take the Tutorial" section, near the bottom is a pdf file called "**Sample Cases - Electrocardiograms and Imaging Studies (pdf)**." **Pay extra attention** to the last few pages, which explains the scoring of sample cases.

■ **Key feature descriptions as listed on the answer options list are in italic.**

ECG'S QUICK LIST

1. Normal ECG
2. LAFB and LPFB
3. Low voltage
4. QT interval
5. Juvenile T waves
6. Hyper and hypokalemia
7. Acute subarachnoid bleed
8. ST segment depression
9. Pacemakers: normal atrial and ventricular pacing
10. Pacemakers: normal biventricular pacing
11. Pacemaker malfunction
12. Left atrial abnormality
13. Right atrial abnormality
14. LVH
15. RVH
16. Biventricular hypertrophy
17. Stages of acute MI
18. Inferior and posterior acute MI
19. Chronic MI
20. Acute pericarditis
21. Sinus node exit block and sinus pause
22. First degree AV block
23. Wenckebach block
24. Mobitz type II block
25. 2:1 AV block
26. Complete heart block with escape rhythms
27. IVCD
28. RBBB
29. LBBB
30. WPW and LGL
31. Atrial fibrillation with WPW
32. Sinus bradycardia, tachycardia and arrhythmia
33. Premature atrial complexes
34. Premature junctional complexes and bigenimy
35. Atrial rhythm and atrial tachycardia
36. Wandering atrial pacemaker and multifocal atrial tachycardia
37. Atrial flutter
38. Atrial fibrillation
39. Junctional rhythms
40. AVNRT
41. Orthodromic AVRT
42. Antidromic AVRT
43. Premature ventricular complexes and ventricular parasystole
44. AIVR
45. Nonsustained monomorphic and polymorphic VT
46. Sustained monomorphic VT
47. Torsades de Pointes
48. Ventricular fibrillation
49. Rate-related aberrancy and Ashman's Phenomenon
50. Class I antiarrhythmic drug effect
51. Digoxin effect and toxicity
52. Ostium Primum Atrial Septal Defect
53. Dextrocardia
54. Acute Pulmonary Embolism
55. Pericardial Tamponade
56. Hypertrophic Cardiomyopathy
57. Hypothermia
58. Sick Sinus Syndrome
59. Brugada Syndrome

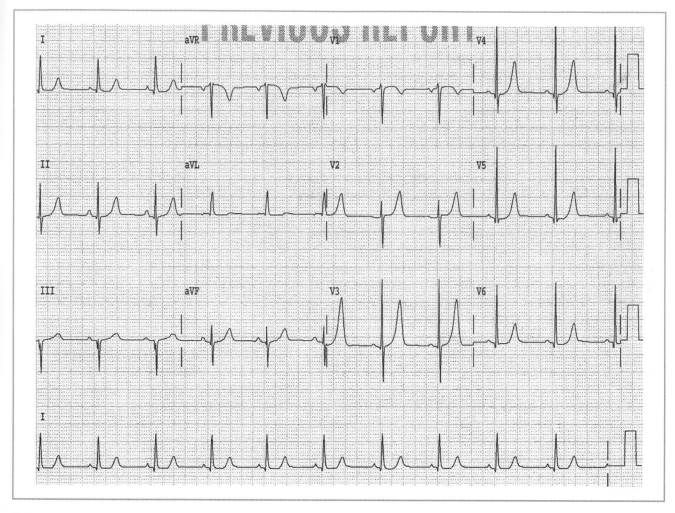

FIGURE 36-1

Normal ECG. Even if you have the correct diagnosis, do not forget to code the underlying rhythm such as *sinus rhythm*

BASICS

A. **Normal electrocardiogram** (ECG) is shown in Fig. 36-1

- **P wave** - Normal duration is ≤0.12 s; Amplitude is ≤0.25 mv (2.5 little boxes); Normal P wave (from sinus node) is upright (positive) in leads 1, 2, aVF, V4–V6; P wave is negative in aVR; P wave is often biphasic (positive–negative) in V1.
- **PR interval** – Interval measured from beginning of P wave to first wave of QRS complex (Q or R wave); Includes P wave (atrial depolarization) and PR segment (conduction through atrioventricular [AV] node and His-Purkinje system); Normal is ≥0.14 s and ≤0.20 s. PR segment changes with rate- shortens with sinus tachycardia, lengthens with sinus bradycardia.
- **QRS complex** – Duration is measured from beginning of QRS complex (Q or R wave) to end of QRS complex (J point); Normal QRS complex duration is between 0.06 and 0.10 s; QRS complex does not change with rate; Normal QRS complex is positive in leads 1, 2, aVF, and V4–V6 and negative in aVR; Small septal Q waves often seen in limb leads and lateral precordial leads.
- **ST segment** – ST segment begins at J point and ends at onset of T wave; ST segment is slightly concave; J point and ST segment are usually isoelectric, which is established by the T-P segment.

- **QT interval** – Interval measured from beginning of QRS complex (Q or R wave) to end of T wave; As QT interval includes QRS complex, need to correct for increased QRS complex duration; QT interval must also be corrected for rate (QTc), using Bazett's formula; Normal QTc < 0.44 s.
- **T wave**– Axis (direction) usually same as QRS complex; T wave is asymmetric (regardless of amplitude), upstroke slower than downstroke; Upstroke and downstroke of T waves are smooth.
- **U wave** – Follows T wave; is not included in the QT interval measurement; U wave is normally seen in right precordial leads (V1-V3).

B. **QRS axis in frontal plane**

- **Normal axis** is 0° to +90° (QRS positive in 1, 2, aVF)
- **Physiologic left axis** is 0° to −30° (QRS positive in 1, 2 and negative in aVF)
- **Pathologic left axis** is −30° to −90° (QRS positive in 1 and negative in 2 and aVF with an rS complex and not Qr which is an inferior wall myocardial infarction [MI]); Called left anterior fascicular block (LAFB) (Fig. 36-2a)
- **Right axis** is ≥+90° (QRS negative in 1 and positive in aVF); is called a left posterior fascicular block (LPFB; Fig. 36-2b) when no other reason for right axis (lateral MI

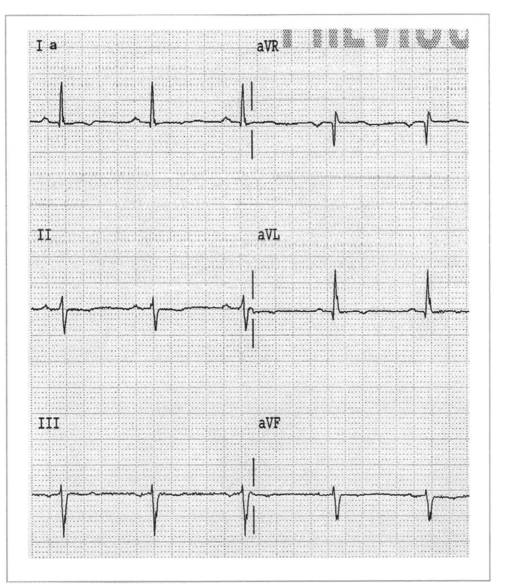

FIGURE 36-2

(**a**) *Left anterior fascicular block,* (**b**) *Left posterior fascicular block*

FIGURE 36-2

(continued)

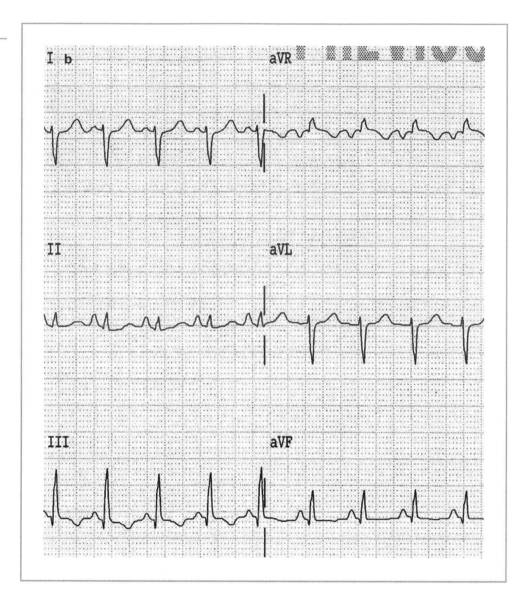

with Qr in leads I and aVL, RVH with tall R wave in V1, **R→L** arm lead switch with negative P wave and T wave in leads I and aVL, dextrocardia which resembles **R →L** arm lead switch and also includes reverse R wave progression V1–V6, Wolff-Parkinson-White with short PR interval and wide QRS complex due to delta wave).

C. QRS complex

- QRS duration does not change with rate.
- QRS ≥ 0.10 s called intraventricular conduction delay (IVCD); if ≥0.12 s may be a bundle branch block (if specific bundle branch block pattern present). Nonspecific QRS complex widening >0.18 and <0.22 s seen with dilated cardiomyopathy. QRS complex width ≥0.24 s is diagnostic of hyperkalemia.
- QRS complex duration may be prolonged if there is rate related aberration or Ashman's phenomenon (see section "Aberration").
- Low QRS voltage or amplitude (recorded at normal standardization, i.e. 1 mV = 10 mm or small boxes in amplitude) is defined as QRS amplitude ≤5 mm in each limb lead and/or <10 mm in each precordial lead. It reflects reduced electrical activity recorded at the surface of the body (Fig. 36-3).

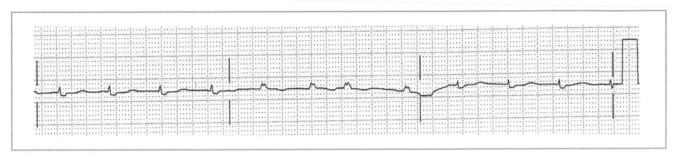

FIGURE 36-3

Low voltage, will need to specify *limb leads or precordial leads.* Note the standardization indicator on the right

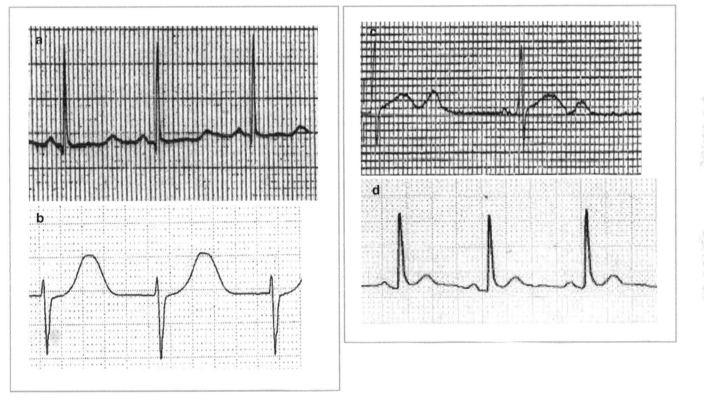

FIGURE 36-4

(**a**) *Prolonged QT interval* with long ST segment (*ST and/or T wave abnormalities suggesting electrolyte disturbances*) seen with *Hypocalcemia,* (**b**) *Prolonged QT interval* from medications, (**c**) *Prolonged QT interval* due to congenital long QT with QTu waves, (**d**) Short QT interval, in *Hypercalcemia,* the short QT interval is mainly due to a shortened ST-segment duration (*ST and/or T wave abnormalities suggesting electrolyte disturbances*)

D. QT interval

- ■ Prolonged QT interval (Fig. 36-4) may be due to:
    - – Delayed repolarization, i.e. the ST segment is long while the T wave duration is normal. Seen with metabolic abnormalities, particularly low calcium (hypocalcemia) or low magnesium.
    - – Prolonged repolarization, i.e. the ST segment is normal in duration but the T wave is broad. This is due to drugs (acquired QT prolongation) or a genetic abnormality

FIGURE 36-5

Normal variant, juvenile T waves.
Two examples of Juvenile T wave
patterns with T wave inversions
in leads V1–V3

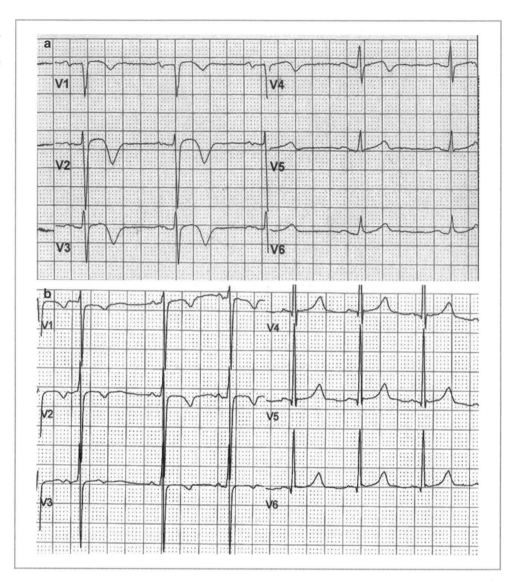

producing a channelopathy (congenital long QT syndrome). Congenital QT prolongation may have a prominent U wave interrupting the T wave (QT-U wave).

- Short QT interval (Fig. 36-4d) is due to metabolic abnormality (hypercalcemia, or
  high magnesium) or a congenital short QT syndrome

E. **T waves**

- Normal T waves are **asymmetric** (upstroke slower than downstroke) and smooth in
  upstroke and downstroke.
- Young patients may have T wave inversions in leads V1–V3, which are normal and
  are termed juvenile T waves (Fig. 36-5).
- Tall, peaked and **symmetric** T waves (hyperacute T waves, see Fig. 36-17a) may be
  seen with acute MI or hyperkalemia. Hyperkalemic changes may also result in prolonged QRS (any QRS duration greater than 0.24 s is pathonomonic for hyperkalemia), atrial asystole (with sino-ventricular rhythm, Fig. 36-6). Hypokalemia
  changes are characterized by prominent U waves (Fig. 36-6c).
- Deeply inverted asymmetric T waves (along with prolonged QT interval) may be
  seen with a central nervous system (CNS) disorder, such as subarachnoid hemorrhage or mass lesion (are termed cerebral T waves) (Fig. 36-7).

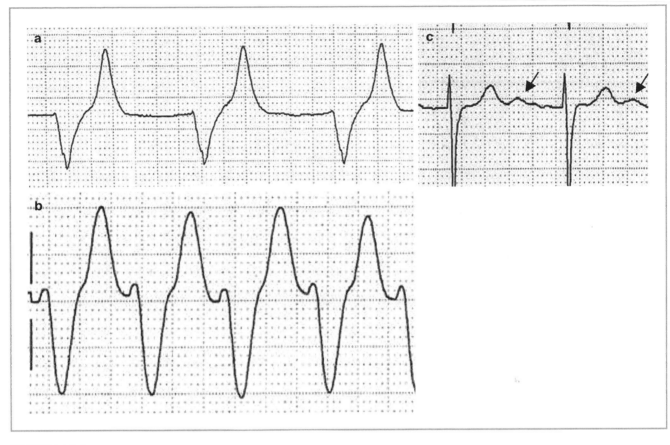

FIGURE 36-6

(a) Tall symmetric peaked T waves (*ST and/or T wave abnormalities suggesting electrolyte disturbances*) with prolonged QRS from *Hyperkalemia*, (b) QRS duration >0.24 s and *ST and/or T wave abnormalities suggesting electrolyte disturbances* (sinusoidal wave forms) diagnostic of *Hyperkalemia*, (c) *Prominent U waves* (arrows) of *Hypokalemia*

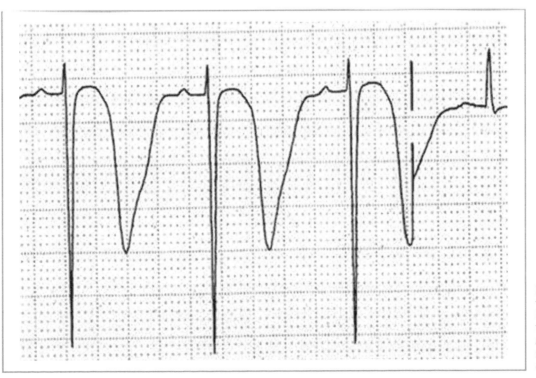

FIGURE 36-7

Deeply inverted T waves from an acute *Central nervous system disorder*, a subarachnoid bleed in this case

FIGURE 36-8

(**a**) Upsloping ST depressions of *Sinus tachycardia* and *Nonspecific ST and/or T wave abnormalities,* (**b**) Downsloping and (**c**) Horizontal ST depressions (*ST and T wave abnormalities suggesting myocardial ischemia*)

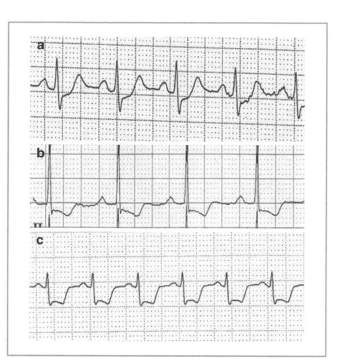

F. **ST segment changes**

■ **J point and ST segment elevation** seen with early repolarization (normal or with left ventricular hypertrophy [LVH]), transmural ischemia, MI, or pericarditis (see section "Myocardial Infarction").

■ **J point and ST depression** upsloping with tachycardia (due to alteration of J point by T wave of P wave, i.e. atrial repolarization, Fig. 36-8a) or horizontal or downsloping seen with subendocardial ischemia (LVH or coronary disease, Fig. 36-8b, c).

PACEMAKERS

■ Single chamber (right atrium [RA] or right ventricle [RV]) or dual chamber pacemaker (RA and RV), see Fig. 36-9.

■ RV paced QRS complex has LBBB morphology (broad R wave in leads 1, V5, V6 and QS in lead V1)

■ Biventricular (RA, RV and left ventricle [LV]). Biventricular paced QRS is RBB-like (QS or initial Q wave in lead 1, V5, V6 and tall R wave V1; Fig. 36-10)

■ Fixed rate (asynchronous) or demand mode

■ Atrial, ventricular, P wave synchronous, or AV sequential pacing

■ Failure of pacemaker sensing generally results in over pacing (atrial and/or ventricular stimuli despite P wave or QRS complex); Failure of myocardial capture is represented by pacemaker spikes with the absence of myocardial depolarization (P wave or QRS complex; Fig. 36-11)

HYPERTROPHY

A. **Left atrial hypertrophy/abnormality** (Fig. 36-12)

■ P wave is broad ≥0.12 s with prominent notching; Left atrial (LA) waveform has an increased amplitude ("P mitrale," >0.25 mv or 2.5 little boxes); P wave in lead V1 (which is normally biphasic) is primarily negative. May also be negative in V2.

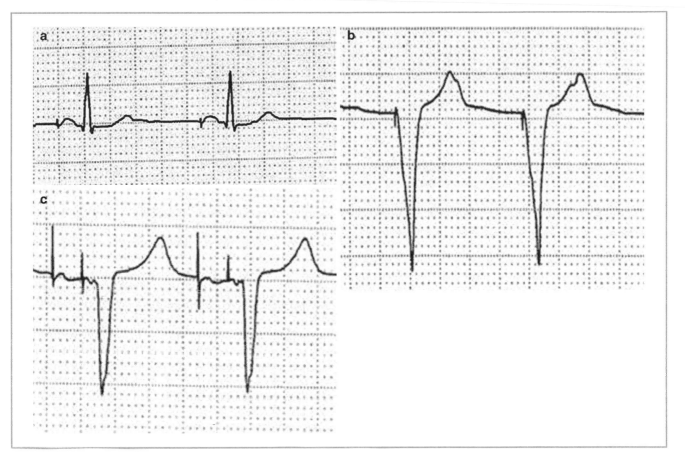

FIGURE 36-9

(a) Atrial pacing (*Atrial or coronary sinus pacing*), (b) Ventricular pacing (*Ventricular demand pacemaker (VVI), normally functioning*). Don't forget to code the underlying rhythm, regardless of pacemaker status. (c) A-V sequential pacing (*Dual-chamber pacemaker (DDD), normally functioning*)

B.   Right atrial hypertrophy/abnormality (Fig. 36-13)

■ The RA waveform has an increased amplitude (>0.25 mv or 2.5 little boxes); P wave is narrow (<0.12 s) and peaked ("P pulmonale," especially in leads I, II, aVF); P wave in V1 (and V2) is very positive, tall and peaked. Normal P wave in this lead is biphasic.

■ Right and left atrial hypertrophy/abnormality may coexist in the same patient-termed biatrial hypertrophy/abnormality.

C.   Left ventricular hypertrophy (Fig. 36-14)
All criteria with ECG recorded at normal standardization (1 mv = 10 mm or small boxes in amplitude)

■ **Sokolow-Lyon.** Depth of S wave V1 (or V2) + amplitude of R wave V5 (or V6) ≥ 35 mm if over age 45, ≥45 mm if under age 45

■ Deepest S wave + tallest R wave in any two precordial leads ≥35 mm (or ≥45 mm if age under 45)

■ S wave depth or R wave amplitude in any one precordial lead ≥25 mm

■ **Sokolow-Lyon.** R wave amplitude in aVL ≥ 11 mm (≥ 18 mm in presence of left axis)

■ R wave amplitude in any one limb lead ≥20 mm

■ **Cornell.** S V3 + R aVL > 28 mm (men); >20 mm (women)

■ **Romhilt-Estes scoring system** (5 points = definite LVH, 4 points = probable LVH)

– Increased voltage = 3 points
– Ischemic ST-T wave changes (repolarization abnormalities) = 3 points

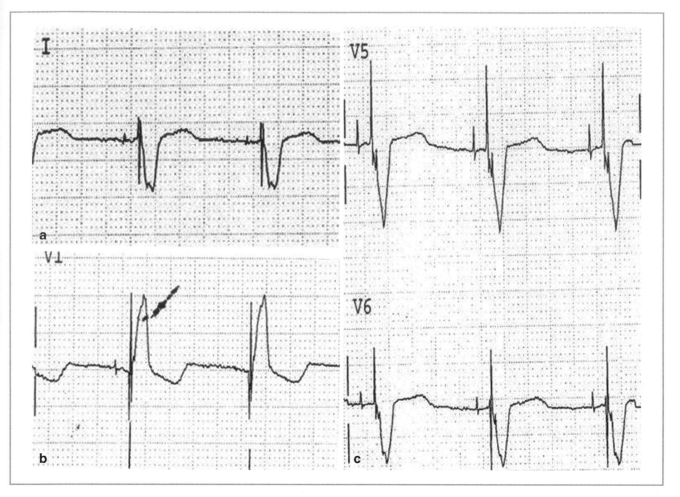

FIGURE 36-10

Paced morphology consistent with biventricular pacing or cardiac resynchronization therapy

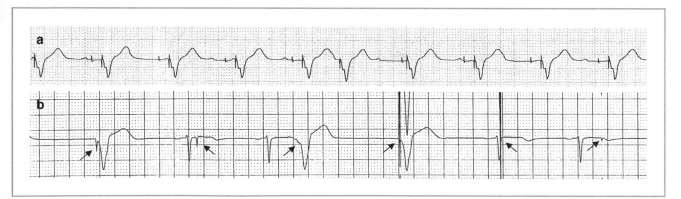

FIGURE 36-11

(**a**) Failure of atrial sensing and intermittent capture (**b**) Failure of ventricular sensing and intermittent capture. *Arrows* in (**b**) denote ventricular pacing spikes. *Pacemaker malfunction, not constantly capturing (atrium or ventricle)* and *Pacemaker malfunction not constantly sensing (atrium or ventricle)*

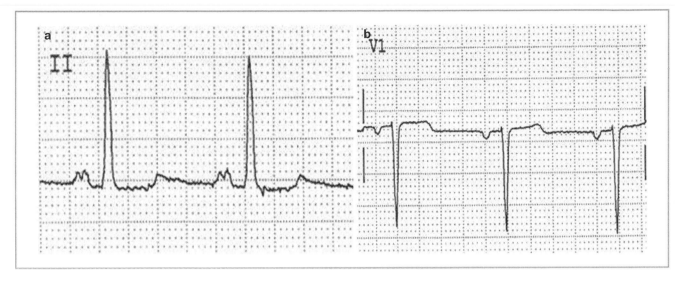

FIGURE 36-12

Left atrial hypertrophy/abnormality a is lead II and b is lead V1

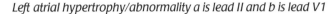

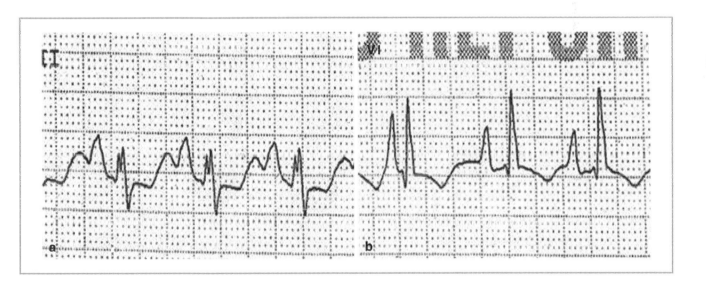

FIGURE 36-13

Right atrial hypertrophy/abnormality a is lead II and b is lead V1

- Left atrial hypertrophy/abnormality = 3 points
- Left axis deviation = 2 points
- Intraventricular conduction delay = 1 point
- Delayed intrinsicoid deflect (upstroke of QRS complex i.e. beginning of QRS complex to peak of R wave >0.05 s) = 1 point

D. Right ventricular hypertrophy (Fig. 36-15)

■ Features characteristic of RVH include the following:

- R in V1 > 7 mm
- R/S ratio in V1 > 1
- S/R ratio in V6 > 1
- Right axis deviation (≥ +90°)

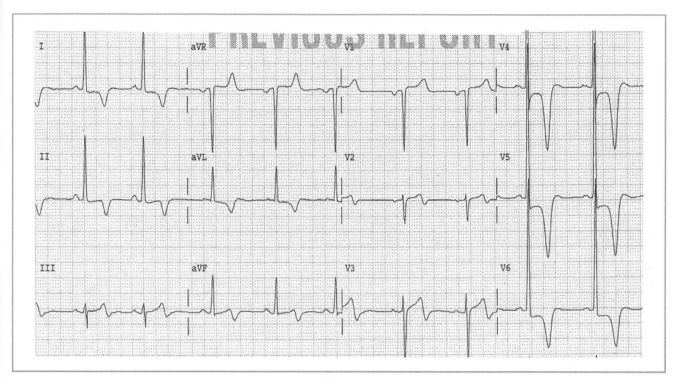

FIGURE 36-14

Left ventricular hypertrophy with *ST and/or T wave abnormalities secondary to hypertrophy* (by all criteria)

- Right atrial hypertrophy (P-pulmonale)
- Associated ST-T wave abnormalities in leads V1–V3

■ Need to exclude other causes for tall wave in V1, including: posterior wall MI, Wolff-Parkinson-White (WPW) pattern, hypertrophic cardiomyopathy, early transition, Duchenne's muscular dystrophy, dextrocardia, lead switch right sided leads

■ LVH and RVH may coexist in the same patient-termed biventricular hypertrophy (Fig. 36-16)

MYOCARDIAL INFARCTION (TABLE 36-1)

A. Acute MI

■ Progression of ECG changes during an acute MI
1. Earliest change of MI is hyperacute T waves (localized hyperkalemia; Fig. 36-17a). They are tall, peaked and **symmetric**
2. ST segments become elevated and are initially concave (Fig. 36-17b).
3. ST segments elevate further and become convex, merging with T wave (looks like monophasic action potential, called a current of injury; Fig. 36-17c).
4. Reciprocal ST segment depression seen in other leads (is the same ST segment shift seen from another direction)
5. R waves lost and Q waves develop (Fig. 36-17d).
6. As ST segment returns to baseline, Q waves become deeper and T waves invert (chronic infarct pattern; Fig. 36-17e).

■ Persistent ST elevation months or longer after the acute event indicates an aneurysm of infarcted wall.

■ Location of acute MI

- Inferior wall MI (Fig. 36-18): ST elevation 2, 3, aVF (ST elevation V1 and on right sided leads rV3–rV4 indicates RV involvement)

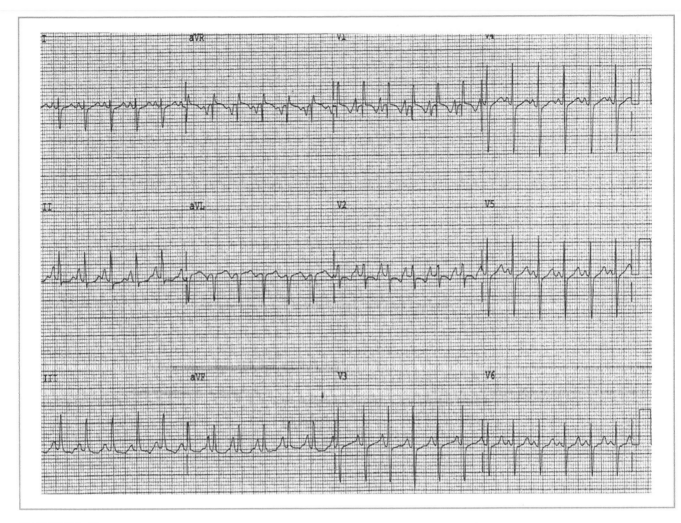

FIGURE 36-15

Right ventricular hypertrophy and *Right atrial hypertrophy/abnormality*

- Anteroseptal MI: ST elevation V1–V2
- Anteroapical MI: ST elevation V3–V4
- Anterolateral MI: ST elevation V5–V6
- Lateral MI: ST elevation 1, aVL
- Posterior MI (Fig. 36-18): suggested by ST depression V1 V2 associated with inferior wall MI; confirm with posterior leads placed under left scapula (V7–V8)

B. Chronic (Old) MI

- ■ Chronic MI is identified by the presence of abnormal Q waves. Any Q wave in leads V1–V3, a Q wave ≥ 0.03 s in leads 1, 2, aVF, or V4–V6 (and in contiguous leads) and ≥1 mm in depth, T wave inversions usually present.

  - Exceptions

    - ■ + Q waves may be normal and are ignored in lead 3 (unless also in lead 2 and aVF)
    - ■ + Q wave in V1–V2 may be normal variant
    - ■ + Q wave in aVL may be normal unless Q is ^{3}50 % R wave height

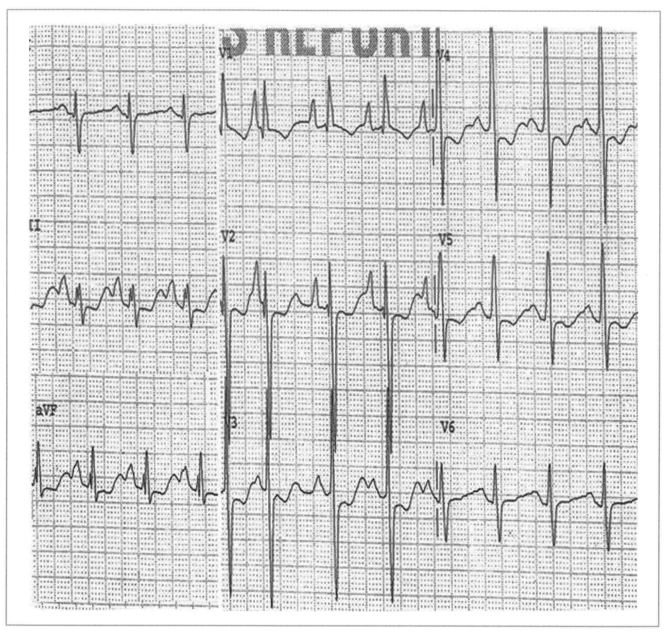

FIGURE 36-16

Left and right ventricular hypertrophy and right atrial hypertrophy/abnormality

- ■ Location of chronic MI

    - Inferior wall MI: Q waves 2, 3, aVF (Fig. 36-19a)
    - Anteroseptal MI: Q waves V1–V2 (Fig. 36-19b)
    - Anteroapical MI: Q waves V3–V4
    - Anterolateral MI: Q waves V5–V6
    - Lateral MI: Q waves 1, aVL
    - Posterior MI: Tall R wave V1 (R/S > 1) with duration ≥0.04 s. Typically seen in association with inferior MI and in the absence of other etiologies for tall R wave in V1 (for example RVH, WPW, lead switch, hypertrophic cardiomyopathy, dextrocardia).

TABLE 36-1

PROGRESSION FROM MYOCARDIAL
ISCHEMIA TO INFARCT

ACUITY	MYOCARDIAL ISCHEMIA	MYOCARDIAL INJURY	MYOCARDIAL INFARCTION
Age recent or probably acute	No Q waves	No Q waves	Q waves
	J point and ST segment depression (upsloping, horizontal, downsloping)	J point and ST segment elevation	ST segment elevation or depression
	Symmetric T wave inversion	Hyperacute- symmetric and peaked T waves	T wave inversion
Age indeterminate or probably old	N/A	N/A	Q waves Isoelectric ST-T segment normal or non-specific ST-T segment abnormalities

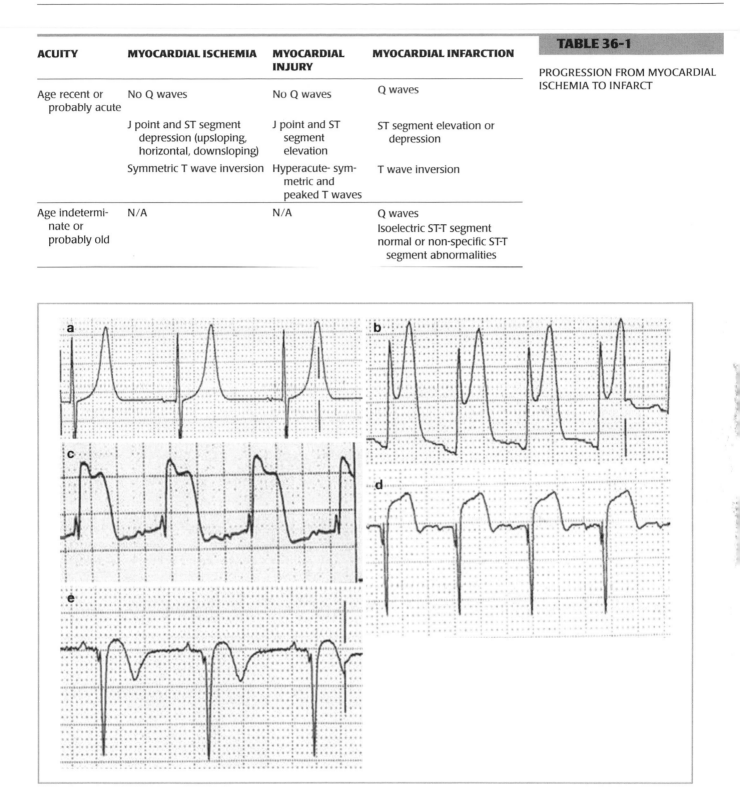

FIGURE 36-17

Stages of acute ST segment elevation myocardial infarction (STEMI). (**a–c**) *ST and/or T wave abnormalities suggesting myocardial injury.* (**d, e**) *Age recent or probably acute Q wave myocardial infarction-though can be old (chronic) myocardial infarction with aneurysm*

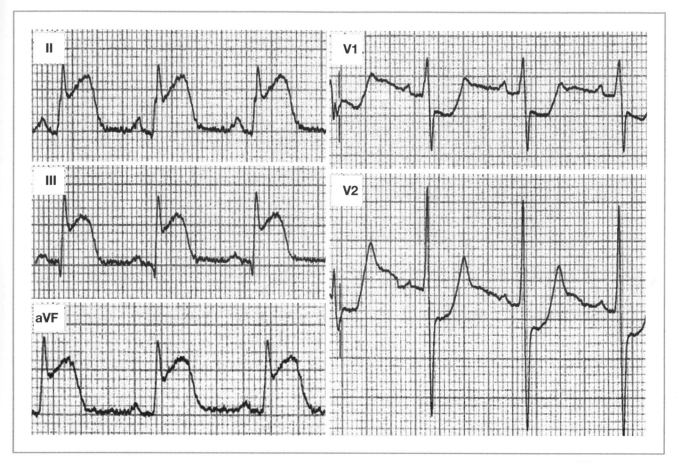

FIGURE 36-18

Probably acute ST segment elevation myocardial infarction (STEMI).

PERICARDITIS

■ Features characteristic of pericarditis (Fig. 36-20)
  - Diffuse ST segment elevation
  - ST segments have normal concave morphology regardless of height of ST elevation
  - No reciprocal ST depression
  - T waves are normal (i.e. asymmetric)
  - PR depression may be seen
  - T wave inversion may occur after ST segments return to isoelectric baseline

CONDUCTION ABNORMALITIES

A. Sinus node pause. A pause in rhythm (long RR interval) with absent P wave during pause

■ **Sinus node exit block**: Duration of pause (PP interval) is twice the underlying sinus rate (equal to 2 sinus pp Intervals; Fig. 36-21a)
■ **Sinus node arrest**: Duration of pause (PP interval) is unrelated to the underlying sinus rate; may be less or greater than two sinus PP intervals (Fig. 36-21b).

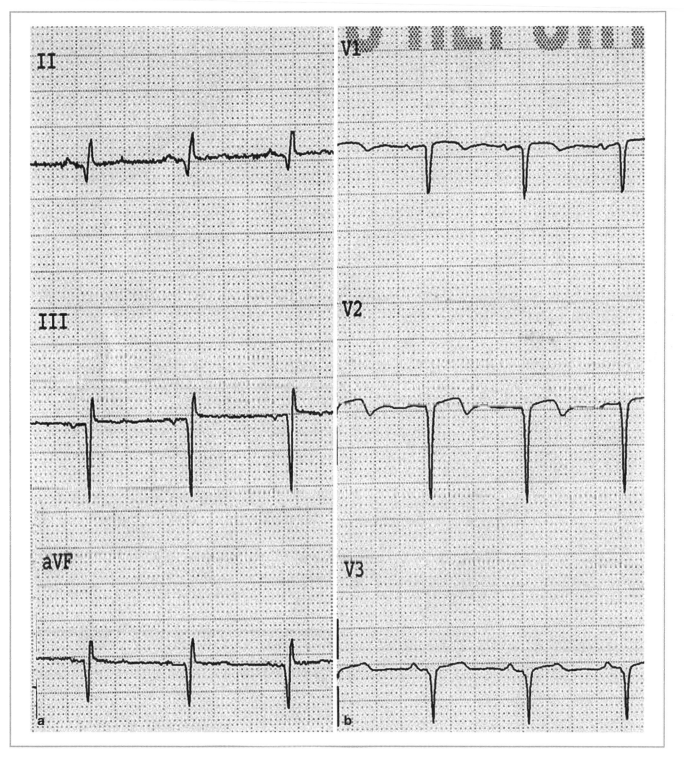

FIGURE 36-19

(**a**) *Inferior Q wave myocardial infarction Age indeterminate or probably old.* (**b**) *Anteroseptal Q wave myocardial infarction Age indeterminate or probably old*

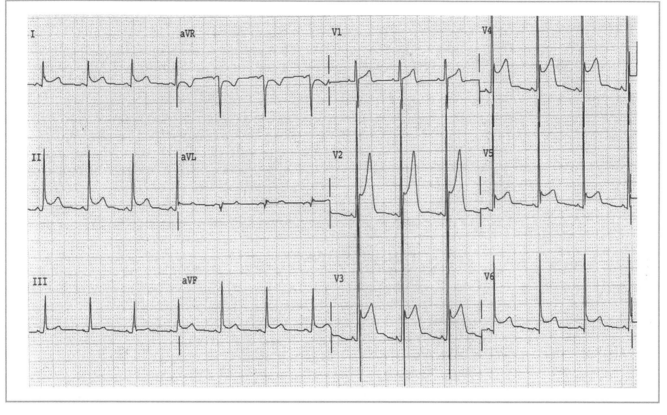

FIGURE 36-20

Acute pericarditis

B. First degree AV block (prolonged AV conduction; Fig. 36-22)

■ Defined by prolonged PR interval i.e. >0.20 s
■ PR interval (PR segment) changes with heart rate.

– It is longer with sinus bradycardia (rate < 60 bpm)
– It is shorter with sinus tachycardia (rate > 100 bpm)

C. Second degree AV block

■ Pause in RR interval due to occasional nonconducted P wave. P wave morphology and PP intervals are constant. First degree AV block may also be present.

– **Mobitz type I (Wenckebach**; Fig. 36-23): Progressive PR interval prolongation before nonconducted P wave and pause; shortening of PR interval (to baseline) after pause. Only one nonconducted P wave, hence one more P wave than QRS complex, Increment of PR lengthening may progressively decrease causing shortening of RR interval. Abnormality is in AV node.
– **Mobitz type II** (Fig. 36-24): Stable PR interval before and after pause. There may be one or more nonconducted P waves. Abnormality is in His-Purkinje system.
– **2:1 AV block** (Fig. 36-25): Every other P wave is nonconducted, PR interval stable; may be Mobitz I or Mobitz II; etiology established if another pattern of AV block seen.

D. Third degree AV block (complete heart block; Fig. 36-26)

■ **AV dissociation** - no association between P waves and QRS complexes, variable PR intervals, atrial rate is faster than ventricular rate, escape rhythm may be junctional or ventricular

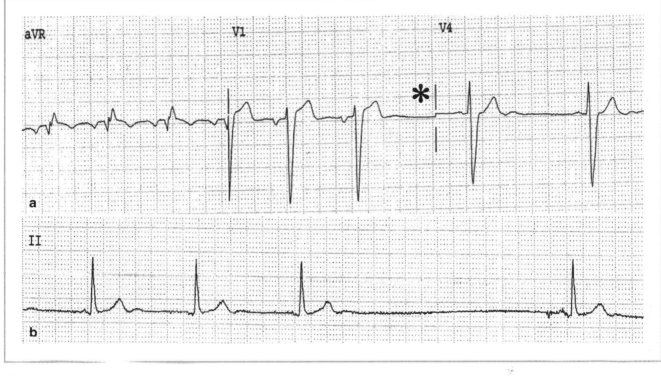

FIGURE 36-21

(**a**) *Sinoatrial exit block*. The pause denoted by * is exactly two P-P intervals. (**b**) *Sinus arrest*

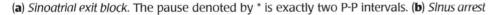

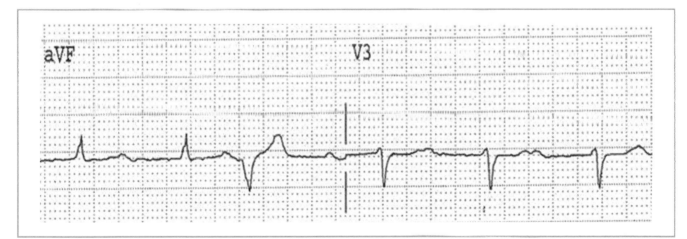

FIGURE 36-22

AV block, 1°

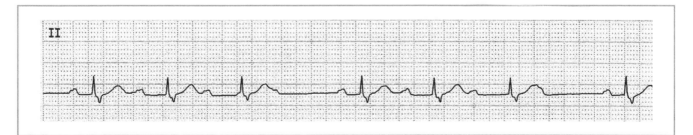

FIGURE 36-23

AV block, 2°-Mobitz type I (Wenckebach block)

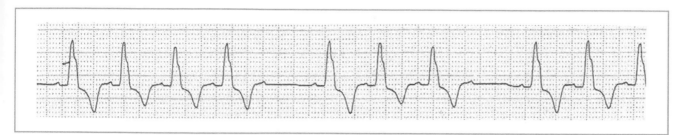

FIGURE 36-24

AV block, 2°-Mobitz type II

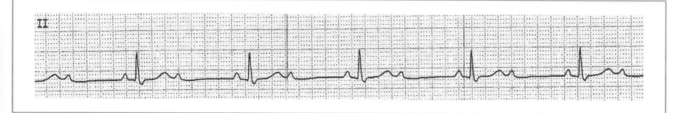

FIGURE 36-25

AV block, 2:1

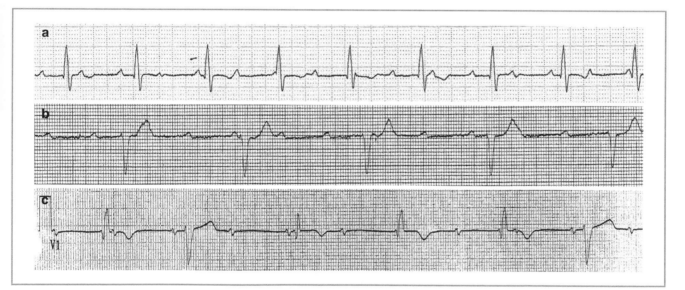

FIGURE 36-26

*AV block, 3°or Complete Heart Block with (**a**) AV junctional rhythm (**b**) Ventricular escape rhythm, and (**c**) Ventricular escape rhythm with intermittent capture/fusion*

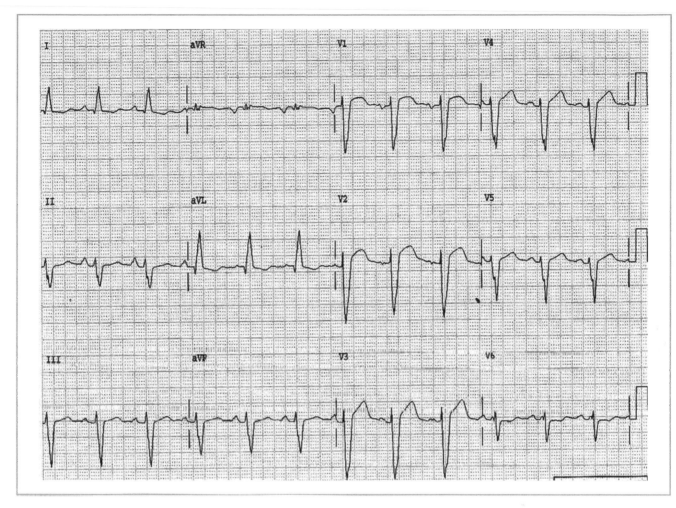

FIGURE 36-27

Intraventricular conduction disturbance, nonspecific type or IVCD consistent with a dilated cardiomyopathy

- ■ Etiology of escape rhythm based on QRS morphology and not rate.
- ■ Intermittent capture may occasionally be present (Fig. 36-26b).

E. **Intraventricular conduction delay (IVCD;** Fig. 36-27)

- ■ Diffuse slowing of conduction through the normal His-Purkinje system
- ■ Nonspecific QRS widening, QRS duration >0.10 s without specific bundle branch block pattern

F. **Right bundle branch block** (Fig. 36-28)

- ■ QRS duration ≥0.12 s due to delayed activation of RV
- ■ RV activation from left bundle and LV directly through myocardium. Terminal forces directed from left to right.
- ■ RSR' complex in lead V1-2 and broad S wave leads I, V5–V6
- ■ RV repolarization abnormal results in secondary ST-T wave changes seen in V1–V3.
- ■ RV activation is abnormal, therefore RVH cannot be recognized.
- ■ LV activation is normal (initial portion of QRS complex normal), therefore LV abnormalities can be recognized (e.g. LVH, infarction, pericarditis); LAFB or LPFB may also be present (bifascicular block)

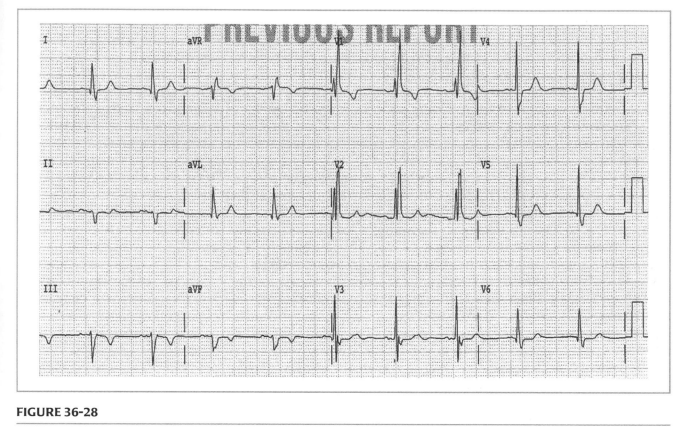

FIGURE 36-28

RBBB, complete

G. **Left bundle branch block** (Fig. 36-29)

- QRS duration ≥0.12 s due to delayed activation of LV.
- LV activation is from right bundle and RV directly through myocardium; all forces directed from right to left (i.e. no terminal S wave in leads I, V6). No septal forces, no Q waves in 1, AVL, V5–V6 or R wave in V1; Broad tall R wave in 1, AVL, V5–V6; deep QS in V1–V2
- Abnormal repolarization. Diffuse ST-T wave abnormalities present.
- Axis may be normal or leftward. Cannot have a right axis.
- LV activation abnormal (not through normal His-Purkinje system). Cannot recognize LV abnormalities

PREEXCITATION PATTERN

A. **Wolff-Parkinson-White** (Fig. 36-30)

- Due to an accessory pathway (bundle of Kent) between atrial and ventricular myocardium.
- The PR interval is short and the QRS is widened as a result of a delta wave that is due to the early, direct and slow myocardial activation via the accessory pathway. QRS complex is a fusion beat representing early, but slow, ventricular activation initiated via the accessory pathway and activation via the normal AV node-His Purkinje system.
- Arrhythmias may occur in patient with WPW (WPW syndrome), including atrioventricular reentrant tachycardia (AVRT), atrial flutter and atrial fibrillation.

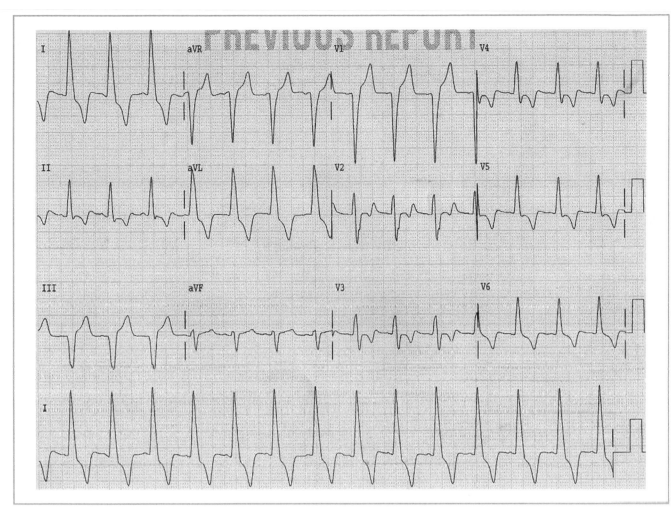

FIGURE 36-20

LBBB, complete

- Atrial fibrillation of particular concern in patient with WPW as rapid ventricular rates may occur and may precipitate ventricular fibrilllation. Needs to be distinguished from rate related aberration before therapy is initiated; in WPW there is no association between QRS width and heart rate-narrow QRS complex with rapid rate and wide QRS complex at slower rate (Fig. 36-31).

B. Lown-Ganong-Levine (LGL) syndrome

- Results from conduction via a bypass tract (bundle of James) that is a connection between atrium and the bundle of His. The PR interval is short but the QRS complex is normal.

SUPRAVENTRICULAR COMPLEXES AND RHYTHMS

A. Sinus rhythm

- P wave upright in leads 1, 2, aVF, V4–V6.Inverted P wave in aVR. One P wave morphology and stable PR interval.

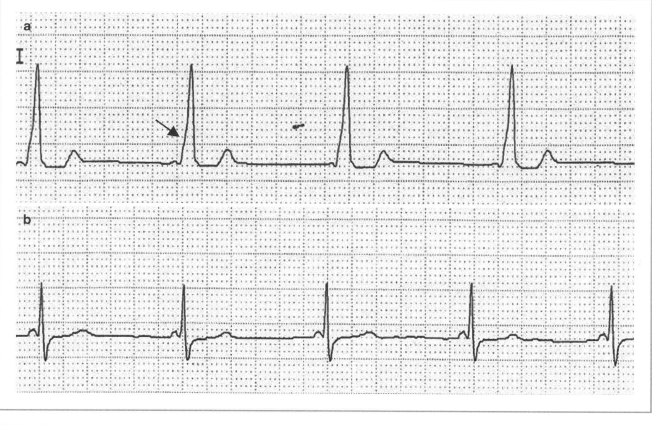

FIGURE 36-30

(**a**) *Wolf-Parkinson-White pattern* in WPW syndrome. *Arrow* denotes the delta wave, (**b**) Lown-Ganong-Levine (LGL)

- **Normal sinus rhythm**: Regular rhythm, rate 60–100 bpm
- **Sinus bradycardia**: Regular rhythm, rate <60 bpm (Fig. 36-32a)
- **Sinus tachycardia**: Regular rhythm, rate >100 bpm; gradual increase and decrease in rate (Fig. 36-32b)
- **Sinus node reentry**: Regular rhythm, rate >100 bpm, similar to sinus tachycardia with abrupt onset and offset
- **Sinus arrhythmia**: Irregularly irregular rhythm – heart rate variable (related to respiration, i.e. respirophasic arrhythmia; Fig. 36-32c)

B. **Premature atrial complex (PAC**, Fig. 36-33)

- ■ Also known as premature atrial beat (PAC); atrial premature complex (APC); atrial premature beat (APB).
- ■ Early (premature) P wave preceding premature QRS complex. P wave morphology and/or PR interval different from that of sinus rhythm.
- ■ Following the PAC there is a pause of variable duration. PP interval surrounding the PAC may be less than, the same as, or greater than 2 PP intervals.
- ■ **Unifocal PACs**:If every PAC has the same P wave morphology
- ■ **Multifocal PACs**: If there are two or more different P wave morphologies associated with PACs
- ■ **Bigeminy PAC**: Every other QRS complex is PAC
- ■ **Trigeminy PAC**: Every third QRS complex is PAC

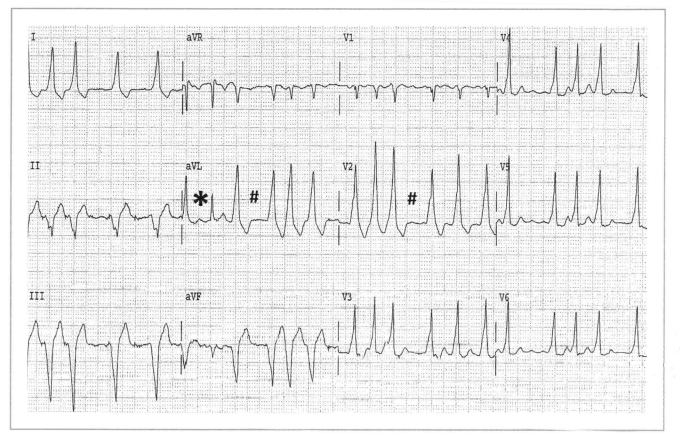

FIGURE 36-31

Atrial fibrillation with *Wolf-Parkinson-White pattern*. Note the width of the QRS complex does not respect a pattern of rate related aberration. Narrow QRS complexes with short RR interval (*) and wide QRS complexes with long RR intervals (#)

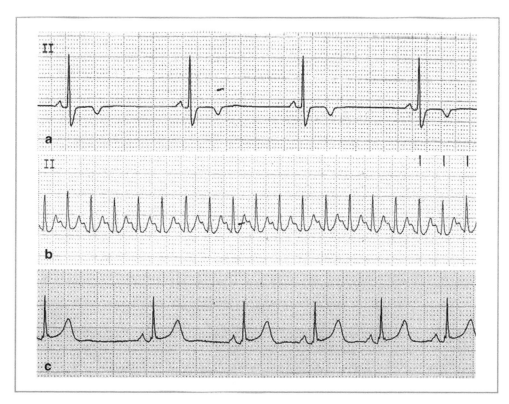

FIGURE 36-32

(a) *Sinus bradycardia*, (b) *Sinus tachycardia*, (c) *Sinus arrhythmia*

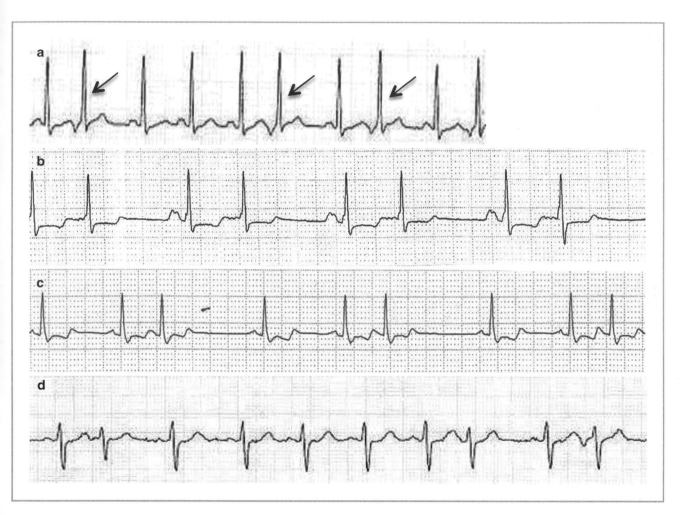

FIGURE 36-33

(**a**) Unifocal PACs (*arrows*), (**b**) PACs in a bigeminy pattern, (**c**) PACs in trigeminy pattern, (**d**) Multifocal PACs

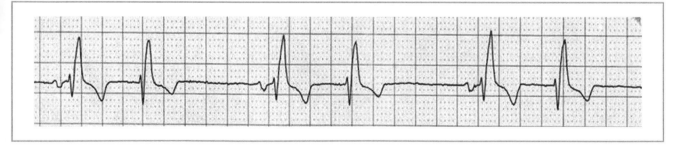

FIGURE 36-34

AV junctional premature complexes in a bigeminy pattern (and RBBB)

C. **Premature junctional complex (PJC,** Fig. 36-34)

■ Also known as premature junctional beat (PJB).

■ Early (premature) QRS complex without a preceding P wave. Morphology of QRS complex is similar to that of sinus rhythm.

■ May be bigeminy, trigeminy, etc. similar as above with PACs.

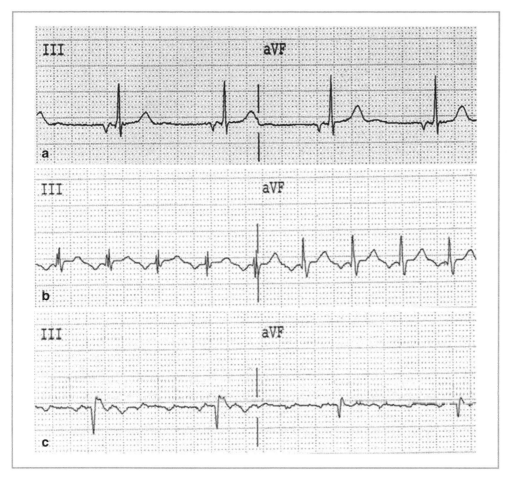

FIGURE 36-35

(a) Atrial Rhythm, (b) *Atrial tachycardia,* (c) *Atrial tachycardia* with block

D. Atrial rhythm (Fig. 36-35a)

- Atrial rate <100 bpm
- Distinct P waves of uniform morphology before each QRS complex
- P wave differs from that of sinus rhythm.
- PR interval constant and may be the same or different from that of sinus rhythm.
- QRS intervals regular.

E. Atrial tachycardia (Fig. 36-35b)

- Stable atrial rate 100–220 bpm
- Distinct P waves of uniform morphology before each QRS complex. Isoelectric baseline between sequential P waves (seen when there is AV block).
- P waves differ from those of sinus rhythm
- QRS intervals regular or regularly irregular (if AV block present). AV block may have constant pattern or may be variable, including Wenckebach (Fig. 36-35c).

F. Wandering atrial pacemaker

- **Multifocal atrial rhythm** (atrial rate <100 bpm; Fig. 36-36a)
- **Multifocal atrial tachycardia** (atrial rate >100 bpm; Fig. 36-36b)
- Irregularly irregular rhythm. PP and QRS intervals irregularly irregular. Distinct P wave before each QRS complex. Presence of ≥3 different P wave morphologies. No dominant P wave seen. PR intervals variable

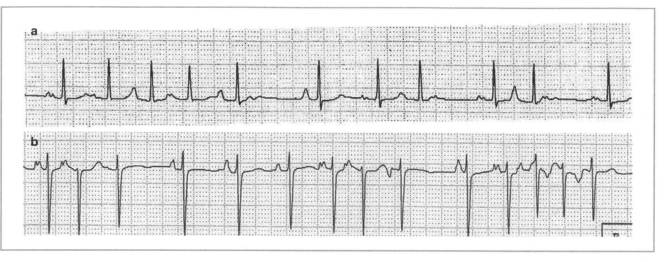

FIGURE 36-36

(**a**) Wandering atrial pacemaker, (**b**) *Atrial tachycardia, multifocal*

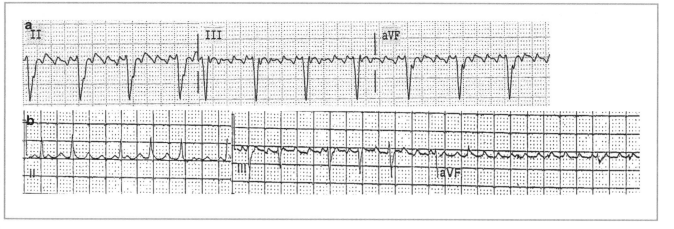

FIGURE 36-37

(**a**) *Atrial flutter*, typical (**b**) *Atrial flutter*, atypical

G. **Atrial flutter** (Fig. 36-37)

■ **Typical atrial flutter** (Fig. 36-37a)

– Regular atrial rate 260–320 bpm
– Flutter waves negative/positive lead 2, 3, AVF
– Flutter waves are uniform in morphology, amplitude and interval.
– No isoelectric baseline between flutter waves (seen when AV block present)-
   Flutter waves are continuously undulating (saw tooth).
– QRS intervals regular or regularly irregular (if variable degree of AV block or
   Wenckebach present).

■ **Atypical atrial flutter** (Fig. 36-37b)

– Atrial rate >320 bpm
– Flutter waves positive in leads 2, 3, aVF

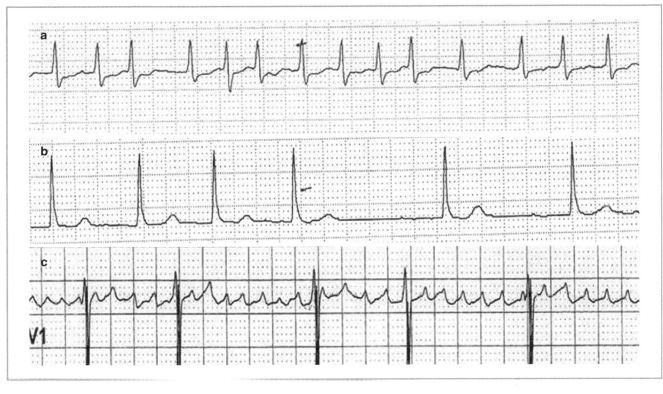

FIGURE 36-38

(a) *ATRIAL FIBRILLATION* **with rapid ventricular rate, (b)** *ATRIAL FIBRILLATION* **with fine fibrillatory waves, (c)** *ATRIAL FIBRILLATION* **with course fibrillatory waves**

H. Atrial fibrillation (Fig. 36-38)

■ Atrial rate >320–450 bpm or even more rapid
■ No organized atrial activity or distinct P wave (fibrillatory waves are present)
■ Fibrillatory waves are irregular in morphology, amplitude, and interval.
■ QRS intervals irregularly irregular (Fig. 36-38c). Ventricular rate depends upon AV nodal conduction

I. Junctional (AV nodal) rhythms (Fig. 36-39)

■ No P wave in front of QRS complex; Inverted (retrograde) P wave may be present following the QRS complex (due to ventriculoatrial [VA] conduction) with stable R-P interval (Fig. 36-38a); QRS intervals regular
■ Junctional rhythm – rate <100 bpm
■ Junctional tachycardia (ectopic) – rate >100 bpm (Fig. 36-39b)

J. Atrioventricular nodal reentrant tachycardia (AVNRT, Fig. 36-40)

■ Reentrant circuit within AV node due to dual AV nodal pathways (fast conducting with long refractory period; slow conducting with short refractory period)
■ Rate 140–220 bpm
■ With typical or common AVNRT (antegrade conduction via slow pathway, retrograde conduction via fast pathway), usually no retrograde P wave seen (no RP tachycardia). P wave may be superimposed on the end of the QRS complex, appearing to be R' or S wave
■ With atypical or uncommon AVNRT (antegrade conduction via fast pathway, retrograde conduction via slow pathway) retrograde P wave seen with long RP interval (long RP tachycardia).

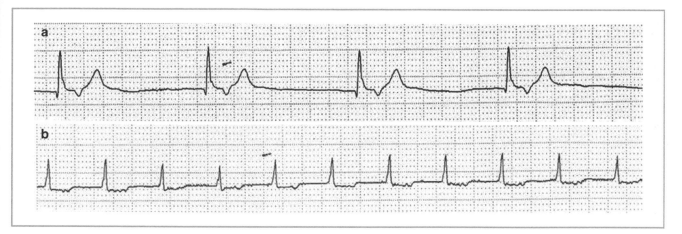

FIGURE 36-39

(**a**) *AV junctional rhythm* with retrograde P waves, (**b**) *AV junctional tachycardia*

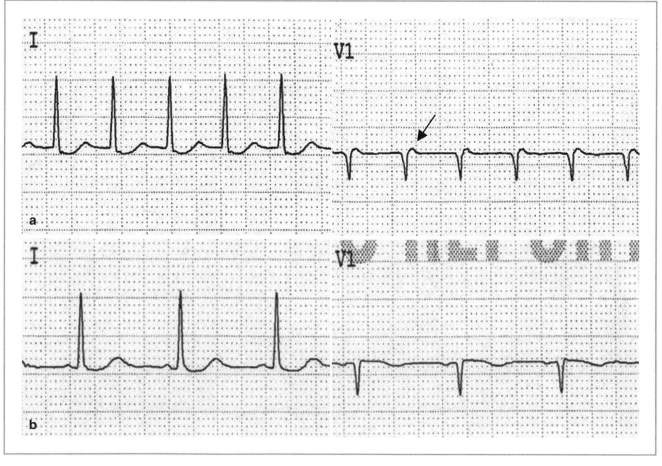

FIGURE 36-40

(**a**) Atrioventricular nodal reentrant tachycardia. Retrograde P wave denoted by the arrow (*Supraventricular tachycardia*). Compare to (**b**) baseline ECG during normal sinus rhythm

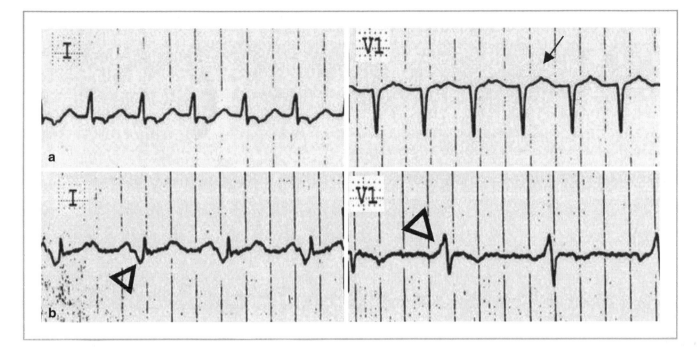

FIGURE 36-41

(a) Orthodromic atrioventricular reentrant tachycardia (*Supraventricular tachycardia*). Retrograde P wave denoted by the *arrow*. Compare to (b) baseline ECG during NSR. Note delta waves on baseline ECG (*arrowheads*) indicating the presence of an accessory pathway

K. **Atrioventricular reentrant tachycardia (AVRT)**

- Reentrant circuit involves accessory pathway as well normal AV node-His Purkinje system (macro reentrant circuit); rate 140–240 bpm; usually a retrograde P wave with short RP interval (short RP tachycardia)
- Orthodromic AVRT- QRS complex is narrow and normal in morphology due to antegrade conduction to ventricles via AV node-His Purkinje pathway; retrograde conduction to the atria is via the accessory pathway (Fig. 36-41).
- Antidromic AVRT- QRS complex is wide and aberrated, resembling QRS (WPW pattern) seen in sinus rhythm although may be wider (i.e. maximally pre-excited complex, not fusion). This results from antegrade conduction to the ventricles via the accessory pathway; retrograde conduction to the atria is via the His-Purkinje AV nodal pathway (Fig. 36-42).

VENTRICULAR COMPLEXES AND RHYTHMS

A. **Premature ventricular complexes (PVC, Fig. 36-43)**

- Also known as premature ventricular beats (PVB), ventricular premature complexes (VPC) or ventricular premature beats (VPB).
- Early wide/abnormal QRS complex without preceding P wave. Does not resemble either a typical LBBB or RBBB.
- P wave after QRS complex may or may not be seen; If P wave is seen it may be retrograde or the on-time sinus P wave, which is unrelated to PVC (dissociated).
- Full compensatory pause (Fig. 36-43a) usually follows PVC, i.e. the PP interval surrounding the PVC is twice the baseline PP interval.
- PVC may be interpolated (Fig. 36-43b), i.e. the PVC does not alter the underlying sinus rhythm and the PP interval surrounding the PVC is the same as the baseline PP interval.

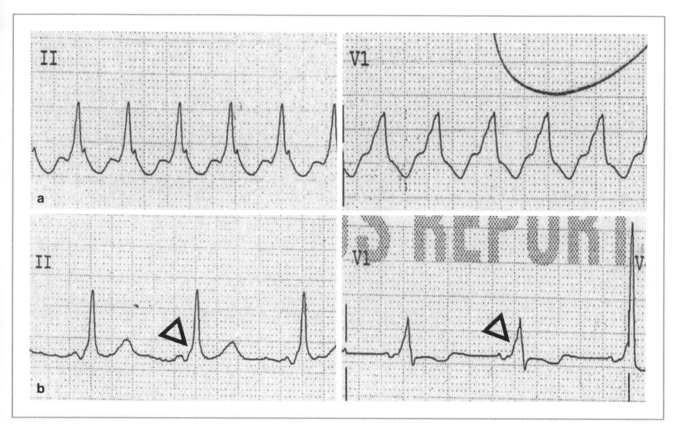

FIGURE 36-42

(**a**) Antidromic atrioventricular reentrant tachycardia (*Supraventricular tachycardia*). The QRS complex is wide, aberrated, and maximally pre-excited. Compare to (**b**) baseline ECG during NSR. Note delta waves on baseline ECG (*arrowheads*) indicating the presence of an accessory pathway

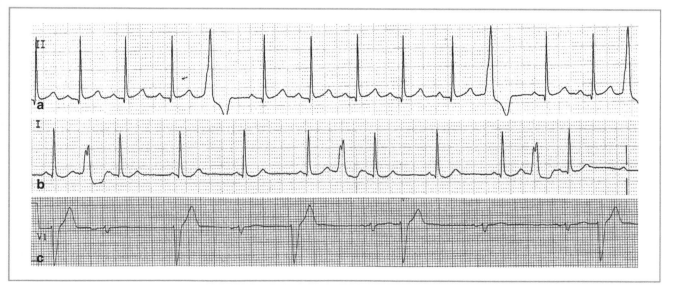

FIGURE 36-43

(**a**) Unifocal Premature Ventricular Complexes (PVCs) with compensatory pause (*Ventricular premature complex[es]*); (**b**) Unifocal interpolated PVCs. (**c**) *Ventricular Parasystole*. Note the unifocal PVCs that occur at varying coupling intervals to the native QRS complexes, as compared to (**a**, **b**) where the coupling intervals are constant

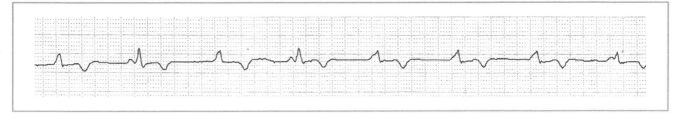

FIGURE 36-44

Accelerated idioventricular rhythm

■ Most common mechanism is reentry; the PVC has a fixed coupling interval with the preceding sinus complex (fixed relationship between the preceding complex and the PVC). Less common mechanism is ectopic focus, known as ventricular parasystole. There is entrance block into this focus (not suppressed) and exit block from the focus (results in activation only when the myocardium is able to respond). Presents with unifocal PVCs with varying coupling intervals (i.e. variability in relationship between the preceding complex and the PVC, Fig. 36-43c).

B. Ventricular rhythms

■ QRS complexes are wide (>0.12 s) and abnormal in morphology (do not resemble RBBB or LBBB. P waves are dissociated from QRS complexes (AV dissociation, i.e. PR interval variable)

■ Ventricular rate > atrial rate. Often P waves not seen; Negative P wave may be seen after QRS complex if VA conduction present (especially if ventricular rate is slow); QRS complexes and ST-T waves may show non-rate related variability in morphology (as ventricular activation not via the normal His-Purkinje system but is by direct myocardial stimulation)

■ Fusion or captured (Dressler) beats may be seen – they are indicative of AV dissociation

■ **Ventricular rhythm**: rate <60 bpm

■ **Accelerated idioventricular rhythm (AIVR or slow VT)**: rate 60–100 bpm (Fig. 36-44)

■ **Ventricular tachycardia (VT)** – rate >100 bpm (rates >260 called **ventricular flutter**)

   – Monomorphic: one QRS morphology
   – Polymorphic: variable QRS morphologies and axis
   – Non-sustained (NSVT): >3 sequential ventricular complexes lasting less than 30 s. NSVT may be monomorphic (Fig. 36-45a) or polymorphic (Fig. 36-45b).
   – Sustained VT: sequential ventricular complexes lasting more than 30 s or terminated within 30 s because of hemodynamic instability (Fig. 36-46).
   – **Torsades des pointes**: polymorphic VT associated with prolongation of QT interval of sinus complex (Fig. 36-47).

■ **Ventricular fibrillation (VF)** – no organized QRS complexes; fibrillatory waves irregular in morphology, interval, and amplitude (Fig. 36-48).

ABERRATION

■ Rate related aberration (functional bundle branch block) is a result of underlying conduction system disease or the reduction in conduction velocity due to a class I antiarrhythmic drug or hyperkalemia. There is a widening of the QRS complex (right bundle or left bundle branch block or a diffuse IVCD) whenever a certain heart rate is achieved (Fig. 36-49a–d).

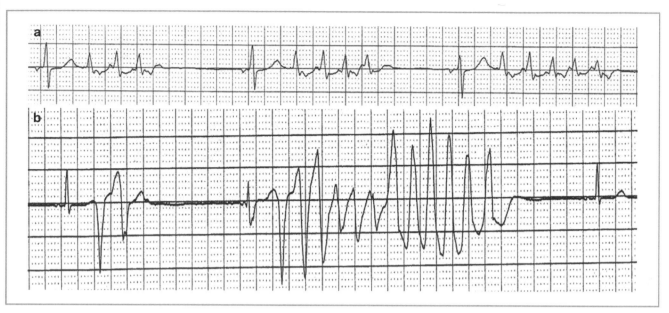

FIGURE 36-45

Nonsustained polymorphic *Ventricular tachycardia* (QTc of sinus complex is normal)

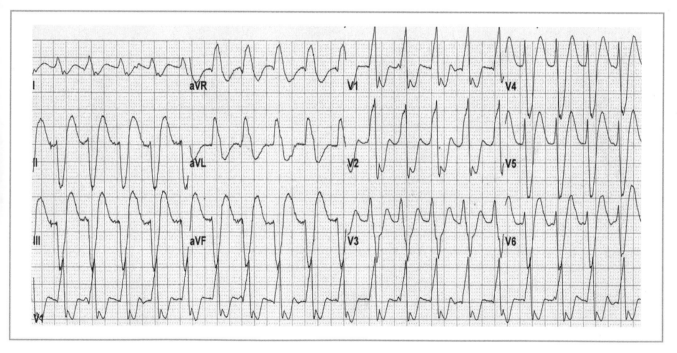

FIGURE 36-46

Sustained monomorphic *Ventricular tachycardia*

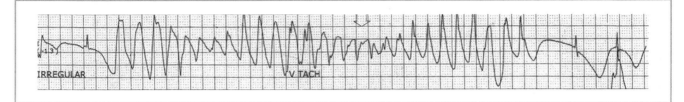

FIGURE 36-47

Torsade des pointes, polymorphic *Ventricular tachycardia* with QTc prolongation of sinus complex

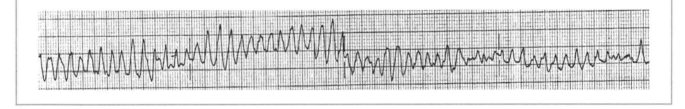

FIGURE 36-48

Ventricular fibrillation

■ Ashman's phenomenon (aberration following a long-short RR cycle, Fig. 36-49e) is a result of normal or physiologic changes in refractoriness of the His-Purkinje system and does not represent underlying pathology. When heart rate is slow His-Purkinje refractoriness prolongs; with fast heart rate His-Purkinje refractoriness decreases. When there is a sudden change in heart rate, i.e. slow (long RR interval) to fast (short RR interval) refractoriness does not adapt immediately and hence one or several QRS complexes are aberrated. Most often there is a right bundle branch block aberration.

CLINICAL DISORDERS

The Brief History Given with Each ECG Provides Clues to the Diagnosis

A. **Digitalis and antiarrhythmic drug effect or toxicity** (Table 36-2).

■ The class I antiarrhythmic drugs slow conduction and therefore prolong the QRS complex duration. This most often seen when the heart rate increases (use dependent effect of these drugs, Fig. 36-50). The class III (and also class IA) antiarrhythmic drugs prolong repolarization and therefore prolong the QT/QTc intervals

■ Digoxin **effect** (Fig. 36-51a) is an ST segment that is depressed, sagging or hammock-like, with a normal J point. A shortened QT interval may be seen.

■ Digoxin **toxicity** is the arrhythmias associated with digoxin excess. These include sinus bradycardia, atrial tachycardia with AV block, accelerated junctional rhythm (Fig. 36-51b), regularization of atrial fibrillation (complete heart block with junctional escape rhythm), bidirectional junctional tachycardia (Fig. 36-51c), ventricular tachycardia

B. **Atrial septal defect (ASD)**

■ ASD with left to right shunting is associated with RVH, rightward axis and P pulmonale.

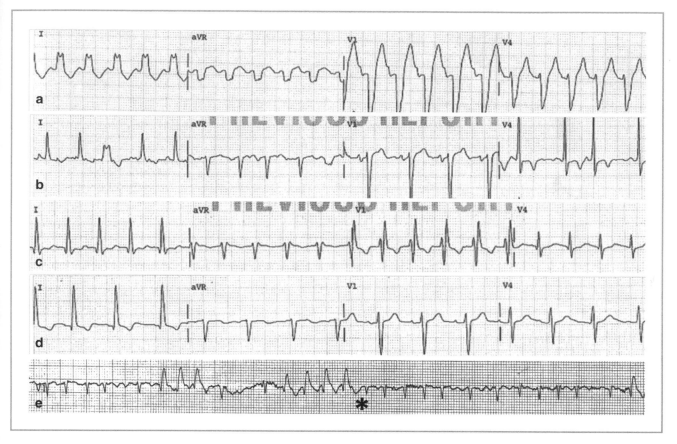

FIGURE 36-49

Aberrant conduction (including rate-related) (**a**, **b**). Rate related LBBB. Aberration occurs consistently above a certain heart rate threshold. Compare the faster heart rate in (**a**) (LBBB) to that of the same patient in (**b**) (normal QRS). (**c**, **d**) Rate related RBBB occurring at a HR threshold in (**c**) (RBBB) above the baseline HR in (**d**) (normal QRS). (**e**) Ashman's phenomenon. When there is a sudden increase in HR, (common in atrial fibrillation shown here), aberrancy occurs for just a few heart beats (usually RBBB pattern) before the His-Purkinje refractoriness adapts to the fast heart rate. Note the complexes following the RBBB beats marked by the * occur at the same interval (heart rate) but are no longer aberrated. This feature distinguishes Ashman's phenomenon from rate related aberration (in which **all** beats above a threshold HR are aberrated)

TABLE 36-2		DRUG EFFECT	DRUG TOXICITY
DIGITALIS AND ANTIARRHYTHMIC DRUG EFFECT OR TOXICITY	Digitalis	ST segment "sagging" with normal J point; shortening of QT interval	Sinus bradycardia, atrial tachycardia with AV block, accelerated junctional rhythm, regularization of atrial fibrillation (complete heart block with junctional escape rhythm), bidirectional junctional tachycardia, ventricular tachycardia
	Antiarrhythmic	Class IA agents- dose related QRS complex widening, dose related QT interval prolongation	Class IA-marked QRS complex widening, proarrhythmia, marked QT prolongation, torsade des pointes
		Class IC-dose related QRS complex widening	Class IC-marked QRS complex widening, complete AV block, proarrhythmia
		Class III-dose related QT interval prolongation	Class III-profound bradycardia, complete AV block, proarrhythmia, marked QT interval prolongation, torsade des pointes

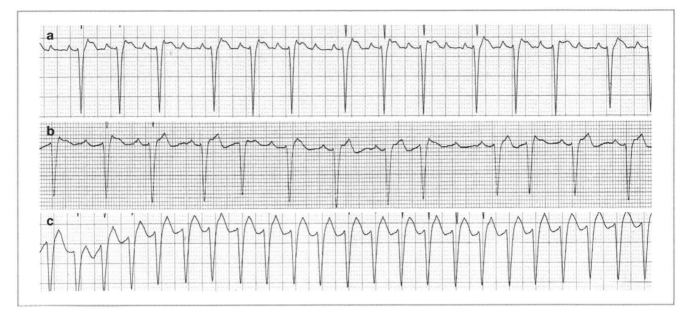

FIGURE 36-50

Use dependent effects of class I antiarrhythmic drugs. (**a**) Baseline rhythm is atrial flutter with variable conduction with an atrial rate of ~220 bpm. (**b**) The atrial rate has slowed to 150 bpm, still with variable AV conduction. (**c**) At the slower atrial rate, there is a risk of conducting at 1:1. As a result there is an acceleration of the ventricular rate and QRS complex widening due to the use dependent effect of the antiarrhythmic drug

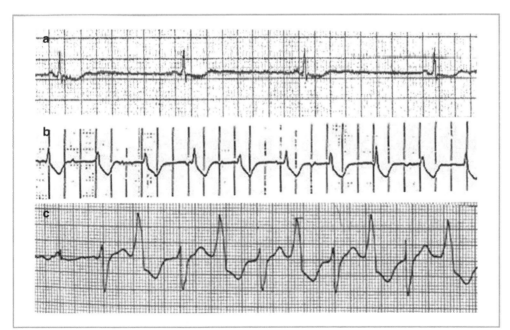

FIGURE 36-51

(**a**) Digoxin effect with "hammock-like" ST segments (**b**) *Digoxin toxicity* manifested by atrial tachycardia with AV block and accelerated junctional rhythm and (**c**) *Digoxin toxicity* manifested by bidirectional tachycardia (alternating RBBB and LBBB)

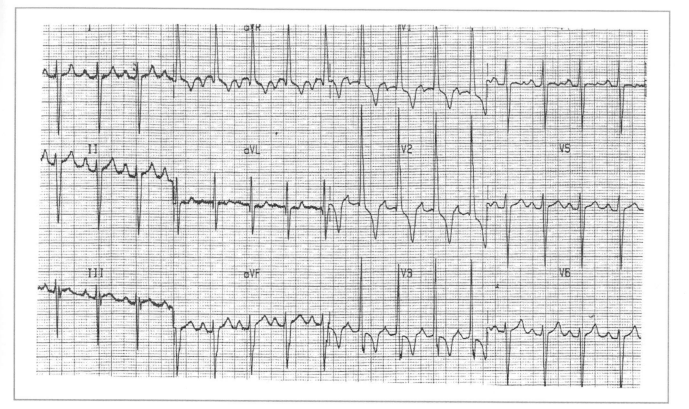

FIGURE 36-52

Ostium primum atrial septal defect

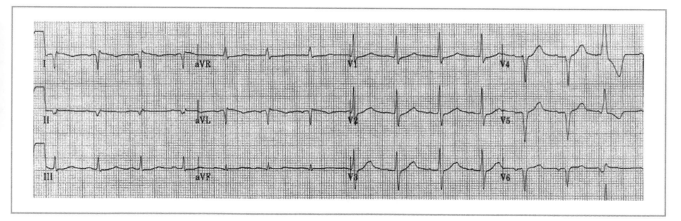

FIGURE 36-53

Dextrocardia

■ Ostium primum ASD (Fig. 36-52) associated with congenital LAFB; axis is therefore indeterminate (negative QRS complex in leads I and aVF) due to left axis from LAFB and right axis from RVH.

C. **Dextrocardia** (Fig. 36-53)

■ With leads in the proper location, dextrocardia looks like R-L arm lead switch with negative P wave and T wave in leads 1 and aVF and right axis (negative QRS complex in lead I and positive QRS complex in lead aVF). The distinguishing feature of dextrocardia is reverse R wave progression in V1–V6.

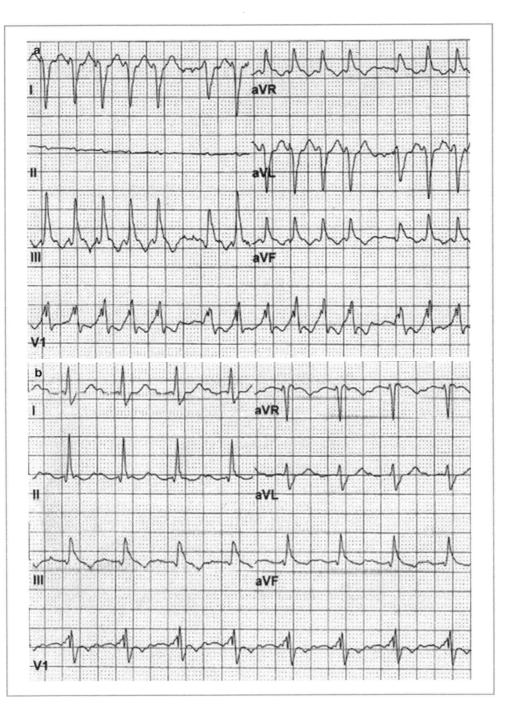

FIGURE 36-54

(a) *Acute cor pulmonale including pulmonary embolus.* Acute pulmonary embolism. Compare to (b) Baseline ECG

D. Chronic lung disease

■ Chronic lung disease pattern is diffuse low voltage and poor R wave progression across precordium (clockwise rotation)

■ When associated with cor pulmonale, produces right ventricular hypertrophy, right axis, P pulmonale.

E. Acute cor pulmonale including pulmonary embolus

■ Acute cor pulmonale or "right heart strain" produces a right axis shift (with S lead 1 and Q in lead III), an intraventricular conduction delay to the right ventricle (RSR' pattern in lead V1) or a right bundle branch block (Fig. 36-54).

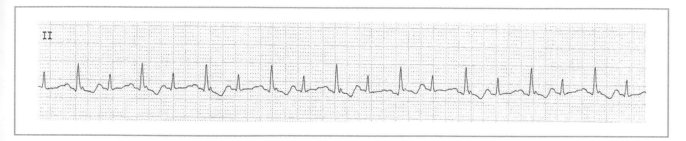

FIGURE 36-55

Pericardial effusion and tamponade. Note QRS, T wave and P wave alternans

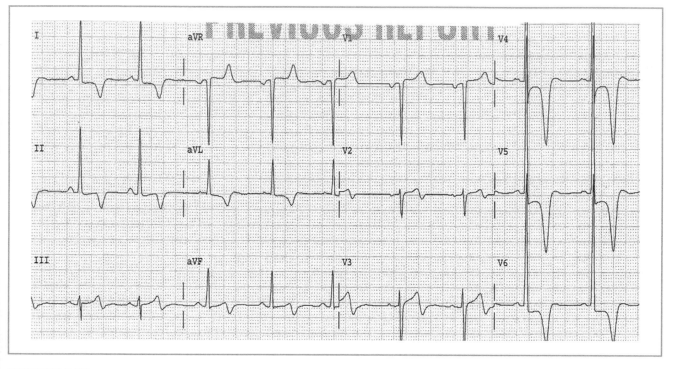

FIGURE 36-56

Hypertrophic cardiomyopathy

F. **Pericardial tamponade**

- Large pericardial effusion and tamponade may result in QRS or **electrical alternans** in which there are beat to beat changes in QRS complex amplitude. T wave alternans (beat to beat changes in T wave morphology and/or amplitude) may also be seen (Fig. 36-55). Rarely seen is P wave alternans.

G. **Hypertrophic cardiomyopathy** (Fig. 36-56)

- Prominent septal Q waves in leads I, V5–V6 and prominent septal R wave in lead V1 may be seen
- Commonly present is significant LVH with associated ST-T wave changes

H. **Myxedema**

- Myxedema results in myxedematous changes of LV myocardium and is associated with diffusely low QRS amplitude (voltage) and diffuse ST-T wave changes.
- Sinus bradycardia and prolonged PR interval also seen

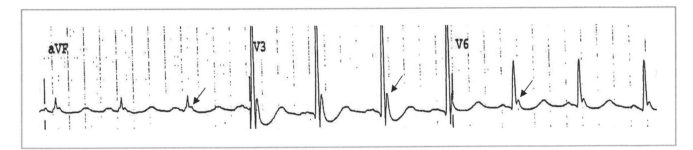

FIGURE 36-57

Osborne waves in *Hypothermia*. The *arrows* denotes the Osborne wave

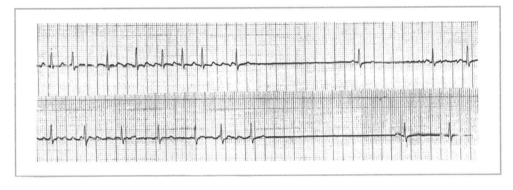

FIGURE 36-58

Offset pauses seen in sick sinus syndrome

I.   Hypothermia

- Hypothermia produces elevated J point (waveform immediately after QRS complex at beginning of ST segment). This is known as Osborne or J wave (Fig. 36-57).

J.   Sick sinus syndrome

Manifestations of sick sinus syndrome (which results from sinus node dysfunction and may involve AV node) include

- Tachycardia-bradycardia, i.e. abrupt termination of an atrial tachyarrhythmia with long offset pause (Fig. 36-58) or if there is intact AV nodal function a junctional rhythm with a prolonged time before there is resumption of sinus node.
- Bradycardia-tachycardia – profound sinus bradycardia with an escape atrial tachyarrhythmia
- Chronotropic incompetence – failure to increase sinus rate with sympathetic stimulation, as with exercise
- Permanent atrial fibrillation with slow ventricular response in the absence of AV nodal blocking agents due to associated AV nodal disease

K.   Brugada pattern

- Results from an abnormality in the early part of repolarization and hence creates an abnormality of the J point.
- There are three patterns seen:
  - Type 1 – there is J point elevation in leads V1 and V2 with a slow descent of the ST segment to a negative T wave (Fig. 36-59a).

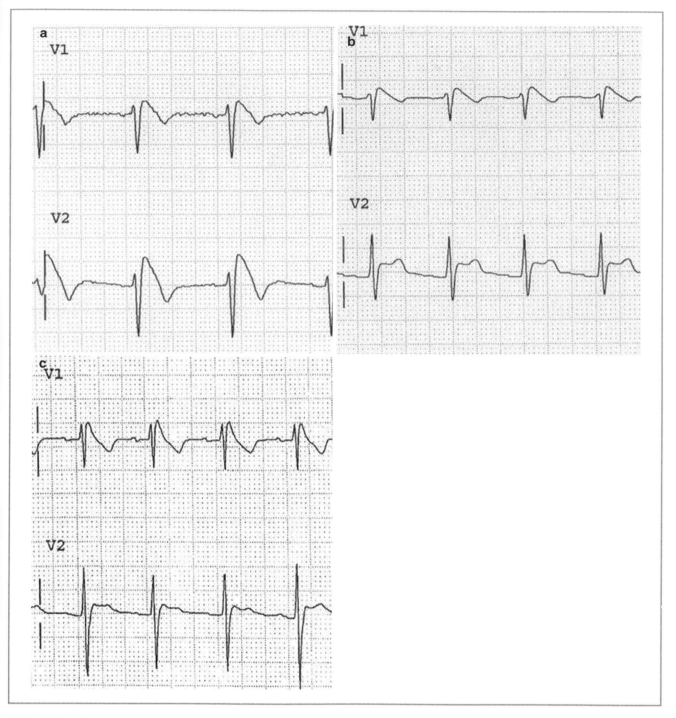

FIGURE 36-59

Brugada Syndrome (**a**) Type 1, (**b**) Type 2, (**c**) Type 3. See text for details

- Type 2 – lead V1 shows J point elevation with a slow descent of the ST segment to a negative T wave. Lead V2 has J point and ST segment elevation; the ST segment is notched, termed "saddle back ," (Fig. 36-59b).
- Type 3 – lead V1 shows J point elevation with a slow descent of the ST segment to a negative T wave. Lead V2 has J point elevation; the ST segment is notched, termed "saddle back" but it is not elevated, rather at baseline (Fig. 36-59c).

Index